ESSENTIALS OF

Electrodiagnostic Medicine

ESSENTIALS OF
Electrodiagnostic Medicine

William W. Campbell, M.D., M.S.H.A.

Professor of Neurology
Chairman, Division of Adult Neurology
Department of Neurology
Virginia Commonwealth University
and
Hunter Holmes McGuire VA Medical Center
Medical College of Virginia
Richmond, Virginia

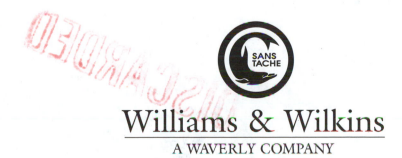

SANS TACHE

Williams & Wilkins
A WAVERLY COMPANY

BALTIMORE • PHILADELPHIA • LONDON • PARIS • BANGKOK
BUENOS AIRES • HONG KONG • MUNICH • SYDNEY • TOKYO • WROCLAW

Editor: Charles W. Mitchell
Managing Editors: Marjorie Kidd Keating and Raymond E. Reter
Marketing Manager: Peter Darcy

Accurate indications, adverse reactions and dosage schedules for drugs are provided in this book, but it is possible that they may change. The reader is urged
to review the package information data of the manufacturers of the medications mentioned.

Printed in the United States of America

Library of Congress Cataloging-in-Publication Data

Campbell, William W. (William Wesley)
    Essentials of electrodiagnostic medicine / William W. Campbell.
       p.   cm.
    Includes bibliographical references and index.
    ISBN 0-683-30239-6
    1. Electrodiagnosis.   I. Title.
    [DNLM: 1. Nervous System Diseases—diagnosis.
    2. Electrodiagnosis—methods.   WL 141 C192e 1999]
    RC77.C327 1999
    616.07'547—dc21
    DNLM/DLC
    for Library of Congress   98-14102
                                                    CIP

*The publishers have made every effort to trace the copyright holders for borrowed
material. If they have inadvertently overlooked any, they will be pleased to make the
necessary arrangements at the first opportunity.*

To purchase additional copies of this book, call our customer service department
at **(800) 638-0672** or fax orders to **(800) 447-8438.** For other book services,
including chapter reprints and large quantity sales, ask for the Special Sales department.

Canadian customers should call **(800) 665-1148,** or fax **(800) 665-0103.** For all
other calls originating outside of the United States, please call **(410) 528-4223**
or fax us at **(410) 528-8550.**

Visit Williams & Wilkins on the Internet: http://www.wwilkins.com **or contact
our customer service department at custserv@wwilkins.com. Williams & Wilkins customer service representatives are available from 8:30 am to 6:00 pm,
EST, Monday through Friday, for telephone access.**

                                      99 00 01 02 03
                                   1 2 3 4 5 6 7 8 9 10

To Rhonda Marie Pridgeon, MD—spouse, companion, colleague, partner and chief tablemaker—without whose patience, support and technical assistance this work could not have been completed.

PREFACE

The impetus to write this book arose from two sources. In training residents and Fellows, both neurologists and physiatrists, in electrodiagnostic medicine we have relied for several years on a hodgepodge, homemade manual because of the lack of a satisfactory intermediate level textbook. Several excellent, comprehensive texts and several short, how-to manuals were available. The how-to manuals are not detailed enough. The comprehensive textbooks are overwhelming to beginning and intermediate electromyographers, and are generally too long to read and assimilate during a standard rotation. Even Fellows are challenged to understand the wealth of information in the excellent full length textbooks. My aim was to write an intermediate work, long enough to adequately discuss major principles and their clinical application, but short enough for the average trainee to read and hopefully understand during a standard rotation. Others obviously noted the same gap, and a couple of intermediate texts have appeared since this project was started.

In preparing for the examination for added qualification in clinical neurophysiology given by the American Board of Psychiatry and Neurology, I had great difficulty finding an adequate but understandable treatment of basic electronics and basic neurophysiology. Too often such sections are written by engineers or PhDs who presume a currency of understanding of these topics that is not realistic for busy clinicians in training or in practice. The material is not as difficult as it first appears, but is usually explained poorly. My second aim in writing this book was to cover the theoretical background of electrodiagnostic medicine, both electronic and biologic, in a concise, clear, comprehensible, and clinically relevant manner. For better or worse, the basic electronics and basic neurophysi-

ology sections of this book were written by an active clinical practitioner.

There can be no serious argument that electromyography, in all the ramifications of that term, is the practice of medicine. Extensive background knowledge is required to perform and accurately interpret electrodiagnostic studies. The necessary preparation spans electronics, biomedical engineering, basic neurophysiology, anatomy, neuromuscular pathology, clinical neuromuscular and musculoskeletal disease, the technical aspects of performing nerve conduction studies and needle electromyography, and, most importantly, the correlations between electrodiagnostic findings and clinical disease. This extensive body of knowledge is reflected by a sizable literature base. Multivolume textbooks are devoted entirely to nerve disease and entirely to muscle disease. Keeping up with the relevant journal literature has become an impossibility.

Clinical practitioners make a diagnosis through a process of making and testing a sequence of hypotheses throughout the clinical encounter to finally find the disease or syndrome that best fits the observed facts. Those who do not have the necessary clinical background to go through a competent differential diagnostic exercise often devolve into rote information gathering, hoping that running one more nerve or sticking one more muscle will somehow magically reveal the answer. Rarely is such an approach rewarded, except financially.

Other authors have made the same point. E.W. Johnson: "only a practicing physician with both theoretical and clinical knowledge of neuromuscular diseases, including their differential diagnosis, is an appropriate electromyographer." J.G. Goodgold: "if meaningful interpretation of the electrodiagnostic observations is to prevail, a solid knowledge of medicine, especially in the neurological realm, must be engrafted on an equally concrete informational base of anatomy, pathology, physiology and fundamental electronics." J. Kimura: "The ample space allocated for clinical discussion. . .reflects my personal conviction that clinical acumen is a prerequisite for meaningful electrophysiologic evaluations." Clinical correlation is always required.

This book is written in a logical sequence, covering first the basic electronics and instrumentation issues and their clinical relevance, and proceeding to discuss the anatomical, physiological, and pathological underpinnings of electrodiagnostic medicine; concluding with the clinical applications and electroclinical correlations of the most common conditions.

I have tried to emphasize the most common and most useful electrodiagnostic procedures and the most common clinical conditions. The esoterica can be found elsewhere, and I have tried to point out sources with further detailed discussions of some conditions. Every book is somewhat idiosyncratic. I must confess to long-standing skepticism about the clinical utility of certain procedures, most notably somatosen-sory evoked responses, less notably F waves. These topics may be given short shrift.

An annotated bibliography is included, with abstracts for many of the cited publications. References have been limited to fairly current or classic articles. The references were carefully selected and no attempt was made at a comprehensive bibliography. Each chapter is preceded by a detailed outline and a summary of the chapter's contents. The summaries are intended for review and overview, the abstracts in the bibliography for detailed reading. The book can then be used on three different levels: overview by reading the outlines and summaries, intermediate level by reading the text, and, when desired, reading in depth is available by perusing the wealth of detailed information available in the bibliography.

I hope this book will provide a useful overview of electrodiagnostic medicine, not too long, not too short, complete but not encyclopedic, practical but not simplistic, current but not inundated with research.

William W. Campbell, MD, MSHA
Richmond, VA

ACKNOWLEDGMENTS

I would like to acknowledge first and foremost the assistance of my wife, Dr. Rhonda Pridgeon. She brought to our marriage not only affection and support, but also a slightly different perspective on neuromuscular disease and electrodiagnostic medicine from her training under Dr. Tulio Bertorini in Memphis. She helped make most of the tables for the book, in addition to proofreading and critiquing large sections. She also gave up many afternoons on the golf course.

Several current and former MCV Neuromuscular Fellows read and critiqued portions of the manuscript. I appreciate the assistance of Drs. Jim Gilchrist, Jobert Vasquez, Steve Otto, Ghazala Riaz, Pat Brancazio, Anthony Quan-Hong, and Jody Vaughan. I also appreciate the assistance of Matt Campbell (neuroscientist and physician-to-be), and Drs. John Cole (former MCV medical student, electrical engineer, and neurologist-in-training), Rich Costanzo and Jim Alexander. Dr. Mike Rivner was kind enough to review the statistics chapter. Dr. Sanjeev Nandedkar of TECA corporation helped clarify and expand important concepts related to electronics and instrumentation.

I must also acknowledge those who kindled my interest in Neurology, Drs. Harold Collings, Don Abbott, and George Mushet, and those who started and finished my training in electrodiagnostic medicine, Drs. Paul Gatens, Don See, Jack Pickett, and Tom Swift. Nearly 20 years of intellectual and professional tête-à-tête with Dr. Bob Leshner has had a uniquely enlivening and enlightening influence.

It was a pleasure to work with Mary Beatty Brooks, medical illustrator at the Hunter Holmes McGuire VA Medical Center, who took my rough sketches and turned them into polished renderings, teaching me a great deal about modern computer drafting in the process. This work would not have been started without the encouragement and assistance of Charley Mitchell, or completed without the aid of Margie Keating or Ray Reter, all of Williams & Wilkins.

Finally, I must acknowledge the contribution of the electropoliticians who created the Certificate of Added Qualification in Clinical Neurophysiology of the American Board of Psychiatry and Neurology. As flawed as I believe that concept to be, it did at least provide the impetus for the review, which ultimately led to writing this book.

CONTENTS

Basic Concepts in Electrodiagnostic Medicine

1

Basic Electronics

Some understanding of basic electronics and biomedical instrumentation is helpful in the clinical arena. It is important to understand such concepts as resistance, impedance, capacitance, circuits, grounding, filtering, and electrical safety. Familiarity with the practical implications of these basic principles helps in making accurate recordings of electrical events, eliminating interference, and avoiding injury to the patient or to the examiner. Several recent reviews of basic electronics concepts relevant to electrodiagnostic medicine are available (1–4).

Electrical Energy

Electricity is a form of energy that can be made from, and converted into, other forms of energy. Electricity and magnetism are intimately related. All matter is composed of atoms, which are in turn composed of subatomic particles: electrically charged protons and electrons, and neutrons. When the positive and negative charges balance, the atom is in a stable configuration. When charges do not balance, the atom is more chemically and electrically active, capable of gaining or losing electrons and interacting with other substances.

The number of electrons in the outer orbital shell of the electron cloud, the valence shell, determines the chemical and electrical characteristics of a substance and governs its behavior. One or two electrons orbiting alone in the valence shell are readily given up, but additional electrons are not readily accepted. Conversely, electrons are easily accepted into a vacancy in an otherwise filled outer orbital, but those already present are not readily released. Substances with only one to three loosely held electrons are good conductors; current flows readily. Those with five or more tightly held electrons in the valence shell are insulators; current flows poorly. Those with exactly four electrons in the outer shell are semiconductors; their ability to conduct current varies. Copper has only one electron in its valence shell and is an excellent conductor. Silver and copper are the best conductors. Glass, quartz, and ceramic are insulators. A material's dielectric constant describes its propensity to conduct. Pure water is a poor conductor, but electrolytic solutions contain charged ions, which do carry charge. Tissue can be viewed as a container of electrolyte solution, the volume conductor, in which ions rather than electrons are the charge carriers. In a good volume conductor, the many ions and free electrons allow electrical events to ramify widely; electrical potentials may be detected at a distance from their site of origin; current may readily spread from one location to another. The human body is an excellent volume conductor, and volume conduction is an important concept in clinical neurophysiology. The practical aspects of volume conduction have a major impact on clinical practice.

The unit of electrical charge (Q) is the coulomb (C), and one electron carries a charge of 1.60×10^{-19} C. One coulomb consists of 6.25×10^{18} electrons. An electric field exists surrounding any charged particle: by arbitrary convention positive fields point radially outward, negative fields radially inward. Like charges repel, unlike charges attract. The law of conservation of charge states that the sum of positive and negative charges in an isolated system cannot change; charge cannot be created or destroyed, but it can move from one location to another. The attractive or repellant electromotive force (emf) between charges is inversely proportional to the square of the distance between the charges. The greater the distance between the charges, the lower the forces between them. This relationship between distance and electrical force is especially relevant to the concept of capacitance and to understanding the correlation between the recorded amplitude of an electrical event and the distance from its source. One volt (V) is the repellant or attractive force between one C of like or unlike charges separated by one meter at a standard temperature. It would require 1 joule of energy to force 1 C of positive charge and 1 C of negative charge 1 meter apart at a specified temperature. Electrical potential is therefore expressed as joules/coulomb, or volts. Electrical potential exists between any charged and uncharged bodies, between two unequal positive or negative charges, or between any positive and any negative charge. Under the influence of an emf, electrons flow creating current (I). When one coulomb of electrons flows past a given point of a circuit in one second, a current of 1 ampere (A) is created: I = Q/t.

Resistivity is the innate capability of a material to conduct current. Resistance is a function of the resistivity, the cross-sectional area available through which to conduct, and the length of the material. Resistivity is defined by the resistance to current flow of a 1-ft long segment of the material 1/100 inch in diameter at 20° C. Resistance is directly proportional to the resistivity and the length of the material and inversely proportional to the cross sectional area. A long, thin wire would have high resistance and a short, fat wire low resistance. Resistance also varies with temperature, usually, but not invariably, increasing with an increase in temperature and decreasing to zero at 0° K. Superconductors are materials that have near zero resistance to conduction at low but achievable temperatures. Resistance is measured in ohms (Ω). The reciprocal of resistance is conductance (G). In an alternating current circuit, the corollary of resistance is impedance (Z), also measured in Ω.

Ohm's law defines the relationship between the emf, the current, and the resistance: V = IR. The emf in volts (V) is equal to the current (I) in amperes (A) $\times$ the resistance (R) in ohms (Ω). At a given resistance, an increase in voltage produces an increase in current. By rearranging the equation, current is directly proportional to voltage and inversely proportional to resistance; and resistance is the voltage divided by the current. The units of measurement help clarify the relationships: amps = coulombs/sec, volts = joules/coulomb, and resistance = coulombs/volt. To work in manageable numbers, these measures are commonly made in mega, milli, and micro units. In clinical EMG, for example, compound muscle action potentials are commonly measured in mV, sensory potentials in μV, leakage current in mA, and impedance in megohms (M Ω).

The driving emf in an electrical circuit is created in a variety of ways, such as by chemical reactions in a battery or by mechanical energy in a generator. The mechanical energy in turn may have been derived from hydraulic energy, combustion, or a nuclear reaction, any of which produce joules of energy. An ordinary 6V battery imparts 6 joules of energy to each coulomb of electrons, which leave the battery terminal. Joules of energy are consumed when electrons travel across resistance and the energy is converted into another form - usually heat or light. The filament of a light bulb is a resistance that converts electrical energy into light energy. A 60-watt light bulb puts out 60 joules of energy/sec as light; the energy originated from the emf source. In conceptual terms, resistance is "good"; it is the mechanism of energy production. A load is an electrical device that performs some useful function, such as the filament in a light bulb. Voltage

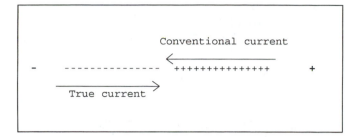

FIGURE 1.1. True current is the flow of negative charges. Conventional or hole current is the flow of positive charges.

drop means the electrical energy crossing the load is being converted into some other form. The voltage drop is the energy per charge going into heat and light. Voltage drop is good and indicates that energy is being consumed to perform some useful function. The concept of voltage drop is important in understanding electrical circuits.

When an electron is displaced from an atom's valence shell, it leaves behind a "hole" of relative positivity. Current flow through a conductor may be viewed as the movement of the negatively charged electrons drawn toward a positive pole, or as the movement of positively charged holes toward a negative pole. Before modern physics clarified the picture, current flow was seen as the movement of the positive charges, and this convention continues in electrical engineering to the present. The movement of positive charges, which in fact do not really exist, is termed conventional current or hole current. The movement of negative charge is true current. For purposes of biology, physiology, and medicine, it makes more sense to think in terms of the movement of electrons, so *current as used in this discussion refers to the flow of electrons* (Fig. 1.1).

Capacitors

A capacitor is a device that can store charge. They are frequently used along with resistors to construct filters for electrophysiology. A capacitor consists of two conductors (plates) separated by an insulating layer (the dielectric). If a capacitor is connected to a battery, the battery pumps charges onto the plates, negative electrons on one plate and positive "holes" on the other. Electrons leave the negative pole of the battery and accumulate on the plate. The electrons on the plate increasingly resist and repel the deposition of more electrons (the capacitor pushes back against the battery) until the resistance to further charge deposition equals the driving emf. The battery will continue

to force charge onto a plate until the repellant force of the accumulated like charges balances the force of the battery and prevents further deposition ($V_B = V_C$) (Fig. 1.2). The amount of charge a capacitor will store depends on the area of the plates, the distance between the plates, the dielectric constant of the insulating material and the voltage of the source. Capacitance describes the amount of charge that can be stored for a given applied voltage and is measured in farads, more often for biologic purposes in microfarads (μF) or picofarads (pF). The higher the capacitance, the more charge can be stored. Capacitors are classified by their dielectrics.

Capacitance can be described as $C = Q/V$, where:

$$\text{Capacitance (C)} = \frac{\text{Charge (Q) stored on one of the plates}}{\text{Potential difference (V) across the plates}}$$

If the charged capacitor is disconnected, the charges will remain stored on the plates for a prolonged period, with only a slow leak to the air. If the capacitor leads are reconnected with the battery out of the circuit, the charges will flow toward the opposite plate until the charges on the two plates are equal and there is zero potential difference (V) across the plates; the capacitor is discharged. Examples of capacitors in everyday use include the flash attachment of a camera, or, better yet for medical personnel, a defibrillator. A finite time is required for a capacitor to charge and to discharge, and the charging and decay curves are exponential. The time constant of a capacitor is the length of time required to charge to 63% of the applied voltage, or to discharge to 37%. The time constant depends on the resistance and capacitance in the circuit ($T = RC$). Time constants are important in understanding filtering in electrophysiology and will be discussed in more detail subsequently.

Tissue has capacitance effects that can influence electrophysiologic recordings. Excitable biologic membranes, such as nerve and muscle cells, are composed of a insulating layer separating positive and negative charges, the same configuration as a capacitor. Tissue has resistive elements as well. These electrical characteristics give tissue filtering properties important to consider in electrodiagnosis.

Electrical Circuits

An electrical circuit requires an emf source, a load, and a ground. Electrons travel around the circuit, receiving joules of energy from the source, delivering the energy to the load, and returning to the source. There are two types of circuits: series and parallel. In

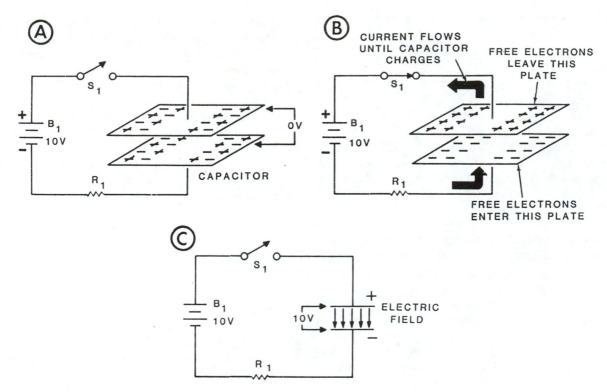

FIGURE 1.2.   A capacitor is two plates separated by an insulator, or dielectric. The emf source deposits negative charge on one plate and positive charge on the other plate until the repellant force from the accumulated charge on the plates balances the driving emf of the source. The capacitor is then fully charged. Electrons cannot flow through the capacitor because of the insulator. In A, the switch is open, no current is flowing, and the capacitor is uncharged with no difference of potential on the two plates. In B, the switch is closed, current flows, and charges are deposited on the plates until the capacitor is fully charged; the time required for this process is the time constant of the capacitor. In C, the capacitor is fully charged and the potential difference between the plates equals the driving emf; the switch is open and the capacitor will remain charged. If the capacitor were allowed to discharge, the time constant would again determine the rate of charge release. Reprinted with permission from Wheeler PE. Electronic Fundamentals. Benton Harbor: Heath Company, 1989.

a series circuit, the loads are sequential; the same current flows through each load and the voltage drops across each load by V = IR. Only one path exists through which current may flow (Fig. 1.3). The total R in a circuit equals the sum of the individual Rs [R_T = R1 + R2 + R3]. The emf source produces a voltage rise—energy imparted to electrons. The loads produce a voltage drop—energy delivered. According to Kirchoff's first law (the voltage law), the sum of the voltage rises must equal the sum of the voltage drops. A series circuit divides the voltage in proportion to the individual resistances and can be used as a "voltage divider"; the voltage varies through each resistor, but the current remains the same ($V_T = IR_1 + IR_2 + IR_3$).

In a parallel circuit, each load is connected directly to the source, and there is more than one path through which current may flow. The same driving emf is supplied to each branch, but the current flowing through a branch varies with the resistance (Fig. 1.4). In a

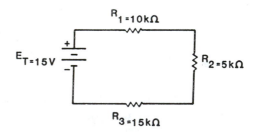

FIGURE 1.3.   A series circuit. The total resistance for this circuit is calculated by:

$$(R_T) = 15k\Omega + 5k\Omega + 10k\Omega = 30k\Omega.$$

The total current (I_T) = 15V/30kΩ = 0.5 mA. The current is the same through each resistor, so the voltage drops across the resistor are given as V = IR, or V = 0.5 mA X R; (R1 = 5V, R2 = 2.5 V, R3 = 7.5 V). The applied voltage equals the sum of the voltage drops (5 + 2.5 + 7.5 = 15). Reprinted with permission from Wheeler PE. Electronic Fundamentals. Benton Harbor: Heath Company, 1989.

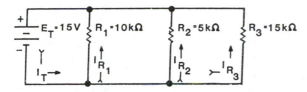

FIGURE 1.4. A parallel circuit. The applied voltage is the same for each branch of the circuit (in this case 15 V), the voltage drop across each R equals the voltage applied to the branch, and the current (I) flowing through the branch varies with the value of R by I = V/R, so that: I_{R1} = 1.5 mA, I_{R2} = 3 mA, I_{R3} = 1 mA). The total current (I_T) is the sum of the branch currents, 5.5 mA. Total resistance is given by the reciprocal method by:

$$R_T = 1/(1/R_1 + 1/R_2 + 1/R_3)$$
$$= 1/(.0001 + .0002 + .00006667) = 2727\Omega$$

Reprinted with permission from Wheeler PE. Electronic Fundamentals. Benton Harbor: Heath Company, 1989.

series circuit, I remains the same and V varies. In a parallel circuit, V remains the same and I varies. The total R in a parallel circuit will be less than any individual R, since more paths exist for current to flow through; in fact, the total R in a parallel circuit will always be less than the smallest R. For a parallel circuit with two resistances:

$$R_T = \frac{(R1 \times R2)}{(R1 + R2)}$$

For a circuit with multiple Rs, the total resistance may be calculated as:

$$R_T = \frac{1}{(1/R1 + 1/R2 + 1/R3)}$$

According to Kirchoff's second law (the node law or current law), the sum of the current flowing into any junction or node must equal the sum of the current flowing out.

Resistance is applicable in situations of direct current (DC) flow. In alternating current circuits, the corollary concept is impedance (Z). The same formulas used to calculate R in a DC circuit are used to calculate Z in an AC circuit. Impedance will be discussed in more detail subsequently.

Some analogies may help illustrate these concepts. The laws of electricity, mechanics, hydraulics, and gravity are all described by similar equations. The electromotive force is comparable to gravity, resistance correlates with friction, and so forth. An electrical circuit can be compared with a hydraulic system. The pump is comparable to the battery, imparting energy to the fluid, which then flows through a pipe (the wire), through a resistance (proportional to the length of the resistance and its material and inversely proportional to its cross sectional area) and back to the pump. The flow of fluid is analogous to the flow of current. A liter of fluid is like a coulomb of charge. One liter passing a point of the circuit in 1 sec corresponds to a current of 1 amp. A capacitor would be analogous to a storage tank on a tower; it requires energy to fill, stores the fluid, and the fluid can then run back into the system when the pump is off.

Magnetism

In 1820, Oerested noted that a compass needle was deflected by an electric current passing nearby. Faraday later found that a magnet moving near a wire could induce current flow in the wire. So, moving charges create magnetic fields and moving magnets create electrical fields. An electric current flowing in a wire induces a magnetic field in the space around the wire. Coiling the wire increases the magnetic field strength; inserting a ferromagnetic core into the coil increases it still further, creating an electromagnet.

Moving a magnet near a wire will induce a current to flow momentarily in the wire, and returning the magnet to its original position will induce current to flow again but in the opposite direction. Current only flows with movement of the magnet. Moving the magnet to and fro induces a reciprocating or alternating current. As long as a relative movement occurs between the wire and the magnet the effect appears; moving the wire and holding the magnet stationary accomplishes the same end. A simple generator can be constructed by rotating a single coil of wire between the poles of a permanent magnet. More current could be induced to flow in the wire by increasing the number of turns of wire, increasing the strength of the magnet, or increasing the rate of movement.

Modern generators are made by moving giant magnets back and forth inside enormous coils of wire, or vice versa. It does not matter whether the magnet moves or the wire moves, as long as they move in relation to one another. The energy to move the magnet or the coil can come from a variety of sources: falling water across a dam, burning coal or oil, or from a nuclear reaction. All convert their energy into electrical energy by using moving magnets to induce current in coils of wire. Because the current reverses direction each time the magnet moves in relation to the coil, the current so created is alternating, or AC. In the US, the frequency of current alternation is 60 Hz.

Inductors

An inductor is a coil of wire carrying current. Moving charges induce magnetic fields, and the flow of current induces a magnetic field around one loop of the coil. This magnetic field in turn induces current in the adjacent loop. The induced current or voltage is that produced by a changing magnetic field acting on a coil. The counter emf (cemf) flows in a direction to oppose the emf that produced it; Lenz's law states that the cemf always acts to oppose the applied voltage. The induced emf is always 180° out of phase with the emf that produced it. Inductance is measured in henrys.

Because the cemf opposes changes in current and AC is always changing, inductors have great resistance to the flow of AC, but DC goes through relatively unaltered. An inductor's resistance to the flow of AC is termed inertia. In a mechanical analogy, an inductor is said to have "mass." As the frequency increases, the impedance, or more precisely the inductive reactance, increases logarithmically. The frequency dependance characteristics of an inductor are the opposite of a capacitor, and this reciprocal relationship can be exploited to construct certain types of filters. More on this subsequently.

Due to the magnetic field created, current flowing in a coil of wire will induce current in an adjacent coil. If two coils are placed side by side and current flows in one coil, current will be induced in the adja-

cent coil in a ratio determined by the number of turns in each coil. Such an arrangement is a simple transformer, which can either step up or step down voltage or current depending on the turns ratio between the two coils. Current flows from the power station at very high voltage to minimize power loss and is stepped down by a transformer to produce useful voltage for everyday consumption.

Alternating Current (AC)

AC power line input cycles as a sine wave at 60 Hz, and the level of voltage and current varies continuously throughout the cycle. The voltage can be expressed as the peak voltage, the peak-to-peak voltage, or the average voltage. The most useful measure is the DC equivalent voltage, termed the effective voltage or the root mean square (rms) voltage. Because half the AC sine wave cycle is negative and half positive, the rms voltage is derived by squaring all values so that all are positive, then taking the square root. So, "110" volts of household current is 110 volts rms and is the work and energy equivalent of 110 volts of DC. In fact, the voltage actually varies from 0 to 154 volts, and the peak-to-peak voltage is up to 308. The rms voltage is equal to the peak voltage $\times$ .707. The average voltage is the peak voltage $\times$ .636. The rms voltage $\times$ 1.4 = peak voltage, and rms $\times$ 2.8 = peak to peak voltage (Fig. 1.5). The concept of rms or effective voltage and the value of .707 $(1/\sqrt{2})$ are important in understanding the cutoff frequencies of filters used in clinical electrophysiology.

The circuits discussed previously were simple DC circuits. With AC circuits, frequency is an added con-

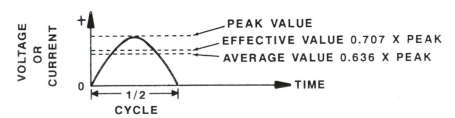

FIGURE 1.5. Alternating current is a sine wave with a frequency of 60 Hz (U.S.). Voltage and current vary continuously so the actual value at any particular point in time is not helpful. Useful concepts include the peak voltage (zero to the positive or negative peak), the peak to peak voltage (positive peak to negative peak) and the root mean square (rms) voltage (peak voltage $\times$ 0.707). The rms voltage or current is also referred as the effective or DC equivalent voltage or current. The rms voltage is the voltage an equivalent DC source would produce. The concept of rms voltage is important in understanding filtering, discussed in Chapter 2. Reprinted with permission from Wheeler PE. Electronic Fundamentals. Benton Harbor: Heath Company, 1989.

sideration. The behavior of some electrical elements depends on frequency. They "react" to the frequency change and are termed reactive elements to distinguish them from resistive elements, which behave the same regardless of frequency. Capacitors and inductors are reactive elements, whereas a resistor is a resistive element. The symbol for reactance is X. X_L is inductive reactance, X_C is capacitive reactance; both are measured in Ω. Impedance (Z) is the total opposition to current flow, including both resistive and reactive elements, in an AC circuit and is also measured in Ω. Impedance is an important concept in clinical neurophysiology. A purely reactive element does not dissipate energy and can only act as a storage device. In reality, all capacitors and inductors also have a resistive element. As a result, a capacitor will slowly lose the charge on its plates over time. Low Z at the recording electrodes and high Z at the amplifier input is necessary for interference free recordings. Most equipment has some method for checking the impedance in different recording channels, and impedance mismatch can greatly increase interference.

Key Points

- Electricity and magnetism are closely related forms of energy. The physics of electricity is analogous in many ways to the physics of hydraulics, mechanics, and gravity; all are described by similar laws and equations.
- The electrical behavior of a substance is determined by the number of electrons in the valence shell. Conductors have 1–3 outer shell electrons, semiconductors have exactly 4 electrons, and insulators have 5 or more.
- The coulomb (C) is the unit of electrical charge (Q).
- An attactant electromotive force (emf) of 1 volt (V) exists between 1 C of positive and 1 C of negative charge separated by 1 meter. The emf decreases as the square of the distance.
- Current is the flow of charges; 1 C of charge flowing past a point in 1 sec creates a current (I) of 1 ampere (A).
- Resistance is related to the resistivity, the length, and cross-sectional diameter of a segment of a material.
- The emf, current, and resistance relationship is given by Ohm's law: V = IR.
- The emf imparts energy to electrons. The electrical energy is converted into other forms of energy when the electrons cross a load such as a resistor. The voltage drop across a load indicates energy is being used to perform some function.
- True current is the flow of electrons; conventional current or hole current is the flow of positive charges.
- Capacitors store charge, the amount proportional to the area and inversely proportional to the distance between the plates, and the intervening material's dielectric constant.
- The charging and discharging of a capacitor is an exponential curve described by the time constant. Capacitors, resistors, and time constants are important in understanding analog filters in electrophysiology.
- Electrical circuits provide for the delivery of energy from the emf source to the load. In a series circuit, V varies and I remains the same across each circuit element; in a parallel circuit, I varies and V remains the same across each circuit element.
- Moving charges create magnetic fields, and moving magnetic fields induce electric current. Relative to and fro movement between a magnet and a coil induces current which changes direction with each movement: alternating current (AC).
- Impedance (Z) is the total resistance to current flow in an AC circuit.
- Inductors are coils of wire carrying current. A transformer is two inductors side by side; the primary coil induces current in the secondary coil even though they are not physically connected.
- The sine wave of 60 Hz (U.S.) power line input can be described in different ways—average, peak, peak-to-peak, or root mean square (rms)—voltage or current.
- The rms voltage is the DC equivalent or "effective" voltage—the amount that would be delivered by an equivalent DC circuit. The rms voltage is an important concept in electrophysiology.
- Inductors have high Z for AC and low Z for DC. Capacitors have high Z for DC and low Z for AC.
- Inductors and capacitors both react to the voltage—they are reactive elements. Their Z is related to frequency. The frequency dependency of capacitors and inductors is an important factor in clinical neurophysiology.

References

1. Misulis KE. Basic electronics for clinical neurophysiology. J Clin Neurophysiol 1989;6:41-74.
   This article reviews the basic electronics that are important to clinical neurophysiology. It is divided into six sections: basic principles of electronics; filters; transistors and amplifiers; displays; electrodes and the electrode-amplifier interface; and electrical safety. In addition, at the end of the review is a brief electronics glossary (Appendix A) and an annotated bibliography (Appendix B) to guide further reading.
2. Barry DT. AAEM minimonograph #36: basic concepts of electricity and electronics in clinical electromyography. Muscle Nerve 1991;14:937-946.
   Fundamental principles of electricity provide a basis for understanding the design and operation of electromyography equipment. An intuitive and quantitative explanation of charge, voltage, current, and impedance provides an introduction to the

concepts of resistance, capacitance, and input impedance. These concepts form the basis for discussion of filters, amplifiers, electrodes, digital electronics, stimulators, and patient safety. The monograph assumes no specialized training in engineering or mathematics. The topics are discussed at an introductory level to provide understanding for readers with no electronics background and intuitive insight for more experienced readers.

3. King JC. Appendix: basic electricity primer. In: Dumitru D. Electrodiagnostic Medicine. Philadelphia: Hanley & Belfus, 1995;93-107.

4. Lagerlund TD. Electricity and electronics in clinical neurophysiology. In: Daube JR, ed. Clinical neurophysiology. Philadelphia: F.A. Davis Co., 1996;3-17.

2

Instrumentation

An electromyograph is a system of interconnected components designed to detect and process a biological signal. Some of the components include filters, differential amplifiers, analog to digital converters, CRT display monitor, stimulation units, stimulus trigger, storage devices, and usually a computer. The signal is detected, amplified, filtered, and displayed. Before going into detail about how these components are configured, we will discuss some of the individual elements.

FILTERS

Biologic signals contain a number of components from multiple sources that have different frequencies, which combine to produce a complex waveform (1). Some of these frequencies are more pertinent than others. In addition, the biologic signal of interest may be contaminated by extraneous noise, contamination, and interference. These considerations make filtering of the signal essential to extract the usable information. But filtering is a trade-off. In cleaning up a signal, important information may be altered or removed. For instance, a 60-Hz notch filter effectively removes AC line interference, but notch filters are usually avoided in electrophysiology because important biologic information can be easily filtered out along with the interference and because they can mask poor patient electrode connections (2). The filtering must be done in such a way as to minimize the inevitable alteration in the desired signal.

In electrodiagnostic medicine, filters are set empirically to optimize the signal to noise ratio. The frequency range of the biologic signal of interest determines filter settings. The low frequency filter (LFF), also referred to as the high pass filter (HPF), removes low frequency components from the signal and allows high frequency components to pass through; conversely with a high frequency (HFF) or low pass filter (LPF). Analog filters use electrical components such as capacitors, inductors, and resistors. Digital filtering is done by computer and is particularly relevant for signals that have already been digitized (3). Current methodology often uses a combination of analog and digital filtering.

Most analog filters are RC circuits, constructed of a resistor (R) and a capacitor (C), arranged to exploit the frequency dependency of the different elements. The resistor is a resistive component, providing about the same amount of opposition to current flow regardless of frequency. The capacitor is a reactive component; its degree of opposition to current flow varies, or reacts to, the frequency of the driving emf. The RC circuit acts as a voltage divider and divides the voltage between R and C. How much of the applied voltage goes to R and how much to C is a function of the frequency of the input signal. It is this frequency-dependent shunting of the input signal voltage between R and C that is the essence of the circuit's ability to filter.

The relationship between X_C, the capacitative reactance (or essentially the impedance, Z) of a capacitor and the frequency is shown in Figure 2.1. As the frequency decreases, Z increases. The relationship between frequency and impedance allows RC circuits to filter. Whether the RC circuit filters out high frequency or low frequency signals depends on where the output is taken in the circuit. If the output is taken across the capacitor, the circuit functions as a LPF, if the output is taken across the resistor, the circuit functions as a HPF (Fig. 2.2). There are several ways to explain this relationship.

The output of an EMG machine is the oscilloscope. Voltage drop will drive the oscilloscope. By Ohm's law (V = IR, or V = IZ), when the impedance is high the voltage drop will be high. Therefore, when Z is high, the signal-induced voltage drop will be most efficiently transferred as a drive to the output oscilloscope. For a capacitor, Z is highest when frequency is lowest, so if the output of an RC filter circuit is taken across the capacitor, then low frequencies will drive the output and will be passed through the circuit; high frequencies will not produce enough voltage drop to effectively drive the output and will be filtered out. This is a LPF/HFF. Low frequencies pass through; high frequencies are filtered out. Voltage drop means that energy is being consumed and used to perform some useful function, and the voltage drop across a capacitor is greatest when the frequency is lowest.

Conversely, if the output of the RC circuit is taken across the resistor, the maximal voltage drop at the output will occur when frequency is high. In this instance, the Z of the capacitor is low at higher frequencies, so little voltage drop appears across the capacitor. The resistor is not frequency dependent, it accepts the "leftovers" depending on whether the capacitor is hungry (low frequencies) or disinterested (high frequencies). At low frequencies, the voltage drop occurs at the capacitor and is shunted off uselessly, i.e., filtered out. At high frequencies, the output will appear across the resistor, creating a high pass or low frequency filter. High frequencies are passed through the resistor, low frequencies are filtered out.

Another way to look at RC circuit filtering is according to the ability of the different components to respond to frequency changes. Again the behavior of

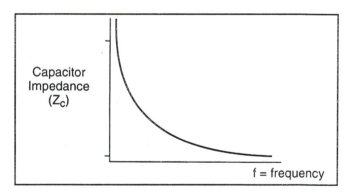

FIGURE 2.1.   The impedance, Z, of a capacitor increases as frequency, f, decreases. At a frequency of zero, Z is infinite. As f approaches infinity, there is insufficient time for any charge movement to occur, so Z approaches zero. The relationship is given as:

$$X_C = \frac{1}{2\pi f C}$$

where X_C is the capacitive reactance, equivalent to the impedance of a capacitor. Reprinted with permission from King JC. Basic electricity and circuit elements: the building blocks of electrodiagnostic instruments. In: 1995 AAEM Course C: Finally, an instrumentation course you can understand, Rochester:AAEM, 1995, p. 7–23.

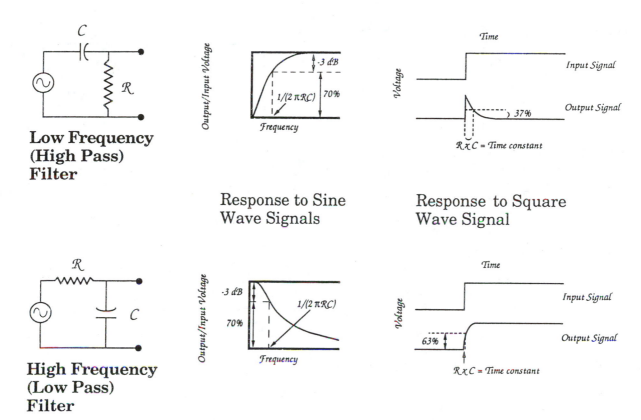

Low Frequency (High Pass) Filter

Response to Sine Wave Signals

Response to Square Wave Signal

High Frequency (Low Pass) Filter

FIGURE 2.2. At the top is an RC circuit with the output taken across the resistor, creating a high pass or low frequency filter. High frequencies pass through to the output; low frequencies are filtered out. At the bottom is an RC circuit with the output taken across the capacitor, creating a low pass filter, or high frequency filter. Low frequencies pass through to the output; high frequencies are filtered out. The center column plots the ratio of output to input voltage for signals of different frequencies. The cutoff frequency is defined as that frequency which is attenuated to 70% (actually .707), or—3 dB. The column on the right demonstrates the filtering effects on a square wave signal. Reprinted with permission from Miller JW, Snyder AZ, Coben LA, et al. Clinical electroencephalography and related techniques. In: Joynt RJ, ed. Clinical Neurology. Philadelphia:Lippincott, 1992, p. 4.

the capacitor determines the filtering behavior, the resistor follows passively. A capacitor is a slow system; it requires time to charge and discharge. The time required is called the time constant and is based on the values of the resistor and capacitor. Because of the time element, the capacitor cannot respond to a high frequency signal, but with a low frequency signal there is adequate time for the capacitor to charge and discharge. Therefore, if the output is taken across the capacitor, high frequencies will be filtered out—the capacitor can't respond quickly enough to follow the frequency changes—but low frequencies will pass through to the output. Exactly which frequencies will pass through is determined by the time constant of the filter.

Recall from Chapter 1 that the charging and discharging of a capacitor can be described by exponential curves. The time constant (TC) is the time required to charge to 63%, or to discharge to 37% of the initial voltage. The TC depends on the resistance and capacitance in the circuit by TC = R × C. In each TC period, the capacitor charges a further 63% of the remaining applied voltage, or discharges a further 37% (Fig. 2.3). So, after one TC, the capacitor is 63% charged or 37% discharged, after the second TC, the capacitor is charged another 63% or discharged another 37%, and so forth until after 5 TCs, the capacitor is fully (99+%) charged or discharged. By lengthening the TC, the capacitor responds more slowly and can react to lower frequencies. Shortening the TC allows a quick filter response and allows higher frequencies to pass through with less attenuation. When the filter setting is changed on an EMG machine, the TC changes so as to more effectively or less effectively filter out certain frequencies.

Filtering does not occur abruptly, but is described best by a "rolloff" curve (4) (Figs. 2.4, 2.5) Recall from Chapter 1 that the effective/rms/DC equivalent (all synonymous) voltage is the peak voltage × .707. The cutoff frequency of a filter is defined as that frequency

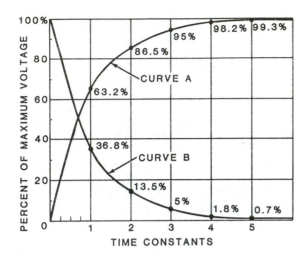

FIGURE 2.3. A DC voltage is applied to a HFF filter circuit (curve A). After the first TC, the capacitor is 63% charged. After the second TC, the capacitor is charged an additional 63%. After 5 TC periods the capacitor is fully (99+%) charged. When the applied voltage is removed, the capacitor has discharged by 37% after the first TC, an additional 37% after the next TC, and fully discharged after 5 TC periods. Changing the TC setting changes the speed at which the capacitor charges and discharges, and thereby changes the frequency response characteristics when used in an RC filter circuit. Reprinted with permission from Wheeler PE. Electronic Fundamentals. Benton Harbor: Heath Company, 1989.

at which the input signal decreases to .707 of its initial value; which is equivalent to a 50% loss of power. Frequencies beyond cutoff produce less than the rms voltage at the output; and below rms the circuit does not have effective voltage to run the output. Consider a HFF. Below the cutoff frequency, the signal is faithfully replicated. As frequencies approach cutoff, the output signal begins to decline. At the cutoff frequency, the output signal = the input signal × .707. Above the cutoff frequency, the output voltage declines at a constant rate, usually described in terms of dB/octave. Frequencies above the cutoff frequency are attenuated and decreased in amplitude, not eliminated entirely (1). The attenuation is 30% at the cutoff frequency, and the attenuation increases steadily as the frequency increases.

The cutoff frequency is sometimes expressed in terms of decibels (dB). Decibels are units that result from taking the logarithm of the ratio of two numbers, as in dB = 20 log (amplitude 1/amplitude 2). The cutoff frequency in dB for an attenuation to the rms value is therefore =

$$20 \log .707 = -3 \text{ dB}$$

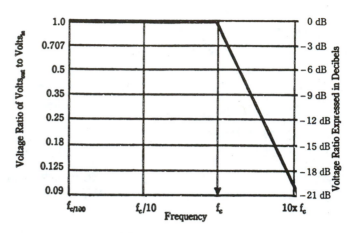

FIGURE 2.4. A simplified diagram of how the volts in/volts out ratio drops rapidly above the cutoff frequency of a HFF. Above this frequency, the capacitive reactance is so low that the circuit starts to become blocking rather than conductive, as an increasing proportion of the input voltage is dropped by the resistor. The cutoff frequency (f_c) is given by:

$$f_c = \frac{1}{2\pi RC}$$

The cutoff frequency is defined as that frequency at which there is a -3 dB loss, or where the volts in/volts out ratio is 0.707. Since the time constant = RC, cutoff frequency can also be described in terms of the time constant. Reprinted with permission from Warring RH. Understanding Electronics. Blue Ridge Summit: Tab Books, 1989; 36–44.

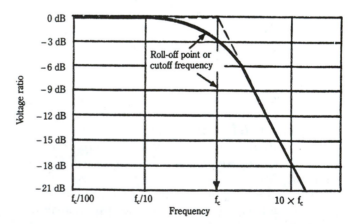

FIGURE 2.5. A close up of the cutoff frequency, showing the change is gradual rather than sharp, termed the rolloff point. At f_c, there is a 50% loss of power. Reprinted with permission from Warring RH. Understanding Electronics. Blue Ridge Summit: Tab Books, 1989;36–44.

the frequency at which the output amplitude is 3 dB less than the input amplitude. Manufacturers may stipulate their filters either in % or in dB. The common mode rejection ratio of a differential amplifier, to be discussed shortly, is also sometimes expressed in dB.

Processing a signal sequentially through a HFF followed by a LFF, or vice versa, attenuates frequencies at each end of the spectrum without affecting frequencies in between, a bandpass filter (Fig. 2.6). The frequency range not attenuated is the bandwidth. The bandpass for a typical EMG machine might extend from 0.1 Hz to 10–20 kHz. Typical filter settings used in clinical EMG are:

Function	LFF	HFF
Motor conduction study	2.0 Hz	20 kHz
Sensory conduction study	20 Hz	2.0 kHz
Needle EMG	10 Hz	20 kHz
Single fiber EMG	500 Hz	20 kHz
Sympathetic skin response	0.1 Hz	100 Hz

Recall from Chapter 1 that inductors have great resistance to the flow of AC because the counter emf (cemf) always opposes the emf that produced it. The constantly changing current in an AC circuit induces constant cemf that opposes the applied voltage, but is 180° out of phase. This opposition is the inductive reactance, X_L, which is essentially the same as the impedance (Z) of an inductor. As frequency increases, X_L increases logarithmically with a curve that is the mirror image of the frequency response of a capacitor (Fig. 2.7). In mechanical terms, the inductor has inertia and mass; the capacitor acts like a spring, its charges pushing back against the driving emf. A ca-

pacitor (c) linked to an inductor (L) in a circuit resembles a mass connected to a spring. The LC circuit will oscillate or resonate. The Z of the capacitor is technically the capacitive reactance (X_C) and the Z of the inductor is the inductive reactance (X_L).

An LC circuit has a resonant frequency, which is the frequency at which $X_L = X_C$, as in Figure 2.7. Parallel and series LC circuits behave differently. In a parallel circuit, impedance is maximal and current is minimal at the resonant frequency; in a series circuit, impedance is minimal and current is maximal at resonant frequency. A series LC circuit could be used as a tuner to maximize current flow at the resonant frequency and "tune in" the desired frequency. Or, a parallel LC circuit could be used to minimize current flow at the resonant frequency and "tune out" a certain frequency. Such circuits are "bandstop" filters as opposed to bandpass filters and the most frequent use in electrophysiology is to construct "notch" filters to remove 60 Hz interference. Be aware that some EMG machines come from the factory with the notch filter on, and some have the notch filter permanently on and not under operator control. A pretty sweep with low interference may not reflect superior equipment, but rather the activation of a notch filter.

Bandpass filters can also be constructed of RL circuits, which exploit the increasing Z of the inductor with increasing frequency. Because of bulk and other technical considerations, RC circuits are generally preferred to RL circuits for analog filtering in electromyography.

Manufacturers are increasingly using digital filtering in EMG machines. The analog signal is converted to numbers by an analog to digital converter (ADC),

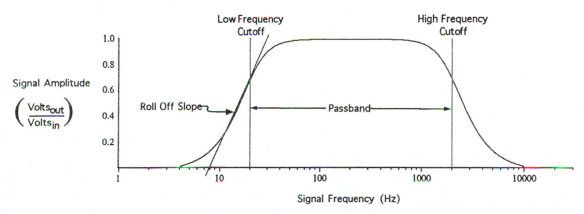

FIGURE 2.6. Frequency response of a 20 Hz LFF in combination with a 2000 Hz HFF. The region between the filters' cutoff points is the bandpass. Because the rolloff is gradual, for the HFF there is some attenuation of frequencies below f_c, and frequencies above f_c continue to appear, although attenuated in amplitude, and similarly for the LFF. Reprinted with permission from Gitter AJ, Stolov WC. AAEM minimonograph #16: instrumentation and measurement in electrodiagnostic medicine—Part I. Muscle Nerve 1995;18: 799–811.

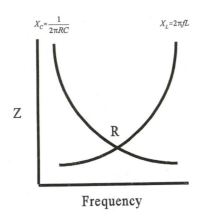

$$X_C = \frac{1}{2\pi RC} \qquad X_L = 2\pi f L$$

Frequency

FIGURE 2.7. The response of a capacitor and an inductor are opposite. The capacitive reactance increases as frequency decreases; the impedance of an inductor decreases. At the crossing point of the 2 curves an LC circuit will resonate. Using either a parallel or a series circuit, the resonant frequency will either tune in or tune out certain frequencies. A notch filter is set to tune out 50 Hz (Europe) or 60 Hz.(U.S. and Canada).

to be discussed shortly. If the sampling rate is high enough (above the Nyquist frequency, see later) and the vertical resolution fine enough, then an accurate replica is created. The digital values are then processed to accomplish the filtering step, after which the revised or modified signal is fed through a digital to analog converter (DAC) and the now filtered analog signal is recovered. The details of the filtering step are beyond the scope of this discussion.

AMPLIFIERS

Biologic signals are of small amplitude and require amplification before processing. In addition, use of a special kind of amplifier, a differential amplifier, is integral in clinical neurophysiology to minimize interference. Amplification is accomplished with transistors constructed of semiconductors. To understand how diodes, transistors, and amplifiers work it is useful to return temporarily to the world of the vacuum tube, or electron tube.

An electron tube is constructed of a filament, the cathode, which emits electrons, and a plate, the anode, which collects the electron stream emitted by the cathode—all enclosed within an airtight shell. A grid, or screen, interposed between the cathode and the anode can be used to control the flow of electrons and to produce amplification (Fig. 2.8). The grid is controlled by a separate circuit. Negatively charging the grid causes the electrons leaving the cathode to be repelled and decreases the flow of electrons between cathode

and anode. Positively charging the grid attracts electrons from the cathode and accelerates them in their flight through the grid and on to the anode. The grid acts as traffic control between the filament and the plate. Relatively small amounts of voltage applied to the grid circuit can control the flux of much larger voltages through the tube.

To amplify a signal, the voltage comprising the signal is used as the input to the grid circuit. A stream of electrons is flowing from filament to plate, the amount depending on the design of the tube. The small and relatively insignificant signal voltage input to the grid circuit causes fluctuations in the charge on the grid, which then controls the flow of electrons by producing varying accelerations and decelerations in the main stream. The signal voltage is then replicated and magnified at the output of the tube. In clinical neurophysiology, tiny biologic signals are the inputs to the grids.

In modern equipment, the vacuum tubes have been largely replaced by solid state devices such as transistors and diodes, and by computers. The first major advance was the invention of the transistor. Although transistors have many advantages over vacuum tubes, their function can be appreciated in the same conceptual terms.

Transistors are constructed of semiconductors. Recall that semiconductors are materials with four electrons in the valence shell and have characteristics that are intermediate between conductors and insulators. A semiconductor can be altered to make it a good

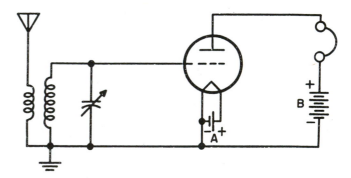

FIGURE 2.8. A vacuum tube with filament (cathode), grid (traffic control) and plate (anode). In this illustration, the input to the grid comes from a resonating LC circuit with an inductor and a variable capacitor which could be set to tune in a given frequency. The small input signal to the grid controls the flow of the much larger current from filament to plate. The output of the tube faithfully replicates on a larger scale the fluctuations of the input signal— amplification. Reprinted with permission from Marcus A, Marcus W. Elements of Radio, 6th Ed. Englewood Cliffs: Prentice-Hall, 1973.

conductor or a poor conductor. Silicon is the most commonly used semiconductor. In its natural state, silicon is not a good conductor but is a fairly good insulator. By adding small controlled amounts of impurities made of other elements to a semiconductor, a process called doping, its conduction characteristics can be manipulated. A silicon chip can be doped with a material such as arsenic, which is pentavalent and provides extra electrons to create an N type ("negativish") semiconductor. Electrons are the "majority carriers" of current. If doped with a trivalent material, such as gallium or indium, there is an excess of holes, the semiconductor is P type ("positivish") and the positive holes are the "majority carriers" of current. The N type is relatively negative in its behavior compared to the P type. Free electrons move about twice as fast as holes, so N type materials have lower resistance and better conductivity than P type materials. A diode is created by joining an N type and a P type semiconductor together. The N type now functions in a manner analogous to the cathode of a vacuum tube and the P type in a manner analogous to the anode. A triode is formed by creating a three-layered semiconductor sandwich—NPN or PNP. This is a transistor. The middle layer of the transistor functions in a manner analogous to the grid of a vacuum tube to control the flow of electrons between the outer layers. One outer layer becomes the emitter (of electrons), the other outer layer becomes the collector and the middle layer, the base, acts as traffic control. Current flow between the layers is controlled by external circuits. A transistor can be envisioned as a miniaturized vacuum tube. A single silicon chip in a modern computer may contain thousands, even millions, of transistors.

DIODES

Complex interactions occur at the interface between N and P type semiconductors. Local attraction between electrons and holes along the NP or PN junction produces some limited, regional transfer of charge back and forth along the border between the N type and P type. Electrons attracted to the holes on the P side leave the N side. This local depletion of electrons leaves the junction zone, immediately adjacent to the interface, of the N type semiconductor with a relatively positive charge in relation to the rest of the chip. Likewise, electrons occupying holes in the borderzone of the P type renders the junction relatively negative in relation to the rest of the chip. This area along the junction of P type and N type materials is referred to as the depletion layer because the majority carriers are depleted and missing.

These local transfers of electrons and holes along the depletion region of the NP junction causes an inversion of polarity along the borderzone that inhibits further transfer of charge and creates a "border potential" or "barrier voltage." The N type semiconductor must force electrons through the relative positivity of its own borderzone before electrons can flow to the P type semiconductor. For a silicon chip, the barrier voltage is 0.6–0.7 V. The barrier voltage can be increased or decreased by an external circuit. Manipulating the barrier voltage is called biasing. Forward biasing results when an external voltage is applied so that the N type is negative with respect to the P type and the voltage across the diode exceeds the barrier voltage. Under these conditions, the diode will conduct. Reverse biasing results when the external voltage is reversed and the P type is relatively negative; conduction through the diode is hampered or blocked. For example, connecting the positive pole of a battery to the P side and the negative pole to the N side is forward biasing and aids the flow of current across the junction.

Semiconductor diodes are all made of N type and P type material and their junction. Changing the construction of the diode and manipulating the doping allows the design of diodes which can serve different functions.

A rectifier converts AC to DC. Most modern electronic equipment requires DC current to function internally, so the AC line input must be rectified. With the advent of solid state physics, semiconductor diodes replaced vacuum tubes as rectifiers. Using a PN junction diode, during AC cycles when the N type material is connected to the negative terminal of the emf (forward biased), electrons flow. When the cycle reverses, electrons cannot flow back. This produces pulsating current, which varies in frequency but does not reverse polarity. Rather than a sine wave of AC, the rectifier yields unipolar half cycles, or pulsating DC. Diodes are also used as voltage regulators, as electronic switches, in tuners, and as detectors in receivers. A forward-biased PN junction generally emits some form of radiation; the frequency of the radiation depends on the design of the diode. Light emitting diodes (LEDs) are commonly used in electronic displays and in remote control devices.

TRANSISTORS

Three individuals working at Bell Laboratories in 1948 were awarded the Nobel prize for developing a device with two PN junctions and devising a method for varying the biasing voltages across these two junctions to create amplification. These breakthroughs led to the transistor, which has become an integral and vital component of modern electronics. The term transistor is an abbreviation for the term *transfer resistor*. Transistors have major advantages over vacuum tubes. They are small, inexpensive, and durable. Their operations consume little energy and they do not produce much heat.

Transistors are either NPN or PNP; the NPN is more commonly used. One outer layer is the emitter, the middle layer is the base, and the other outer layer is the collector. These are analogous to the filament, grid, and plate of a vacuum tube, respectively. The base region is generally thinner and more lightly doped than the emitter and collector. There are two major circuits, the emitter-base circuit and the base-collector circuit. For an NPN transistor, forward biasing the emitter-base circuit (N to P) and reverse biasing the base-collector circuit (P to N) facilitates the flow of electrons from the emitter to the collector. In other words, the base is positive with respect to the emitter and negative with respect to the collector. In a good transistor, less than 5% of the current flow is lost as base current through the emitter-base circuit; the remainder, the "useful current," flows to the collector (Fig. 2.9).

A transistor can amplify when it is connected so as to allow the input signal to control conduction through the transistor. For a simple example of transistor amplification, envision a signal (the input current) applied to the emitter-base circuit, and a separate larger driving emf applied to the emitter-collector circuit (the output current). Fluctuations in the signal input current will induce corresponding fluctuations in the much larger output current, creating amplification. The output of the transistor is a magnified reflection of the input signal to the base, just as the output of a vacuum tube was an amplification of the input to the grid. The term *grid*, commonly used in clinical neurophysiology, is a holdover from the vacuum tube era—input signals are often referred to as "grid 1" and "grid 2" or "G_1" and "G_2". Technically, in the solid state era, we should perhaps refer to "base 1" and "base 2," but the *grid* terminology is firmly entrenched and remains useful.

DIFFERENTIAL AMPLIFICATION

Transistors can be configured with varying connections between the different components. With the common base type, the base is common to both input and output and with the common collector type the collector is common to both input and output; both of these amplify without producing phase reversal. In a common emitter type the emitter is common to

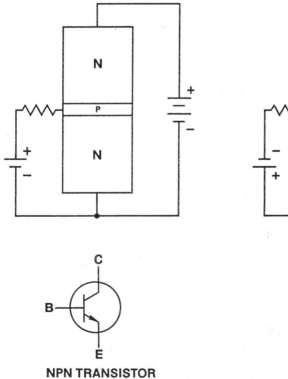

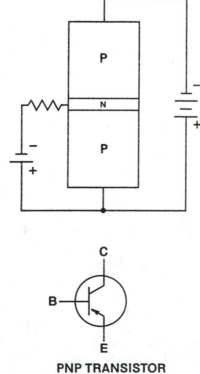

NPN TRANSISTOR   **PNP TRANSISTOR**

FIGURE 2.9. NPN and PNP transistors, and their symbols. The current flows from the emitter (analogous to the vacuum tube filament), through the base (analogous to the grid) and to the collector (analogous to the plate). A small signal input to the emitter-base circuit is amplified by the larger emitter-collector circuit.

both the input and output circuits. This configuration produces high voltage gain but causes a 180° phase reversal of the signal. The phase reversal produced by the common emitter type is exploited to create differential amplification.

The differential amplifier functions by causing a 180° phase reversal of one of the inputs. Any signal that is common to both input leads of the amplifier, the common mode signal, is thus canceled out as equal but opposite and does not appear at the output (Fig. 2.10). The differential amplifier magnifies the difference between the two channels (e.g., an action potential) and cancels or minimizes whatever is common to the two channels (e.g., 60 Hz interference), thereby extracting the biologic signal from the noise. An electromyograph uses multistage differential amplification to achieve high net gain. To achieve further amplification, an additional gain stage is sometimes added to a filter's output.

Signals that are common to both leads into the differential amplifier are referred to as common mode inputs. A true biologic signal, the differential signal, should be different in the two channels, and amplified; noise and external interference, the common mode signal, should be common to the two channels, and suppressed. A perfectly common mode input, equal at the two electrodes, produces complete phase cancellation and a zero differential output from an ideal differential amplifier. It is difficult to create a system with complete cancellation and rejection of the common mode input. The ability to eliminate common mode signals is a function of the quality of the differential amplifier and is expressed as the common mode rejection ratio (CMRR). The gain of an amplifier is the ratio Voltage$_{out}$/Voltage$_{in}$. The CMRR is the ratio of the differential gain to the common mode gain (Fig. 2.10). Modern EMG machines typically have a CMRR of at least 10,000:1. The CMRR of an electromyograph is often given in dB by:

$$CMRR = 20 \log \left(\frac{\text{differential signal gain}}{\text{common mode signal gain}} \right)$$

High quality current EMG machines usually have a CMRR of 90 dB or better (4).

When making clinical recordings, it helps not to sabotage the attempts of the differential amplifier to eliminate interference. Keeping the input electrode impedances equal (<1.5 kΩ difference) ensures any common mode signals will be detected and transmitted to the amplifier equally. Having the active and reference electrode wires twisted or braided together keeps them in proximity and ensures that an extraneous common mode signal will impact on each equally.

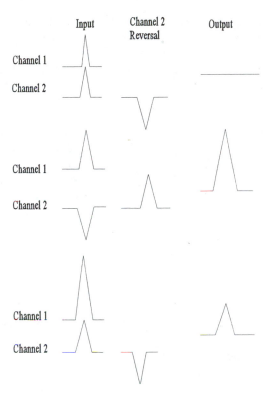

FIGURE 2.10. Differential amplification eliminates a signal that is common to the two input electrodes, and magnifies a signal which is different. In the top set of tracings, the signal is totally common; channel 2 is inverted by the amplifier and the output is the sum of the two, in this case zero. In the middle set, the signal is totally uncommon and the output is twice the size of either input. Channel 2 has been inverted and then added to channel 1. In the bottom set, as in reality, the input is partially common and partially uncommon. The amplifier eliminates the common mode signal and the output consists only of the differential signal. The gain of an amplifier is the ratio V$_{out}$/V$_{in}$. Consider a differential amplifier with a CMRR of 10,000:1. If a 10 mV biologic signal (the differential signal) were input to G$_1$, with a 0 mV input to G$_2$, and the final overall output of the amplifier were then 1,000 mV, then the ratio 1,000/10 = 100 represents the differential signal gain. Now consider an unwanted common mode signal of 50 mV input equally to G$_1$ and G$_2$. If the amplifier's suppression of the common mode signal resulted in an output of only 0.5 mV, then the common mode gain would be 0.5/50 = 0.01. The ratio of the differential gain (100) to the common mode gain (0.01), in this case 100/0.01 = 10,000, is the common mode rejection ratio (CMRR) of the amplifier (10,000:1).

Another desirable characteristic in a differential amplifier is high input impedance (1). Because voltage drop is high when impedance is high (V = IZ) and voltage drop equates to useful work performed, amplification is best when the voltage drop occurs at the amplifier rather than at the patient electrode connections. Maintaining low impedance connections to the patient both minimizes interference and maximizes amplification because less voltage drop is squandered in the periphery. The ideal but unachievable scenario is zero impedance at the patient electrodes and infinite impedance at the amplifier. Practically, the differential amplifier should have a minimum input impedance in the range of 100–200 MΩ and should have an impedance at least 100 times higher than the impedance at the electrodes across all frequencies of the waveform (4). Because concentric electrodes at 10 Hz can have impedance as high as 1.5 MΩ, an amplifier input impedance of 150 MΩ would be required to keep signal attenuation to 1%.(5) An input impedance in the 200–1,000 MΩ range is common in modern electromyography. The patient surface electrode connections should have impedances <5 kΩ.

Unequal impedances of the two recording electrodes produces unequal effects from any common mode signal, impairs the effectiveness of the differential amplifier, decreases the CMRR and increases interference. High amplifier input impedance is especially critical when input electrode Z cannot be equal, as in needle EMG. For both monopolar and concentric needle EMG, the active and reference electrodes are of substantially different size and shape, and therefore have different Z. One can easily record nerve action potentials at a sensitivity of 5 or 10 μV/division with surface electrodes of low and equal Z. A sensitivity setting of 10 μV/division during needle EMG using its electrodes of unavoidably different Z fills the display with artifact and noise.

To minimize interference, the differential amplifier is housed in a remote box, the preamplifier, and connected to the patient by short, preferably braided, wires. The resistive elements of a differential amplifier should be much stronger (megohms) than the reactive (capacitive) elements (picofarads), or the capacitive element's frequency response characteristics may cause the differential amplifier to have filtering effects.

Display

Electrical signals from the patient are detected, amplified, and filtered to put them into usable form. The next step is to present the signals for analysis, both visual and auditory. EMG audio output is generally a filtered and amplified analog signal directed to ordinary speakers. This auditory component is critical. Many things in EMG are recognized as well or better by listening than seeing—from the silence during nerve conduction studies that clues the examiner that the amplifiers are not turned on or the electrodes not connected, to the characteristic, metronomic sound of a distant positive wave otherwise lost in the low grade motor unit action potential (MUAP) output of a poorly relaxed muscle. Various discharges have a characteristic sound—fast firing MUAPs, large and complex MUAPs, "myopathic" recruitment, complex repetitive discharges, fibrillations, positive waves, myotonia, and 60 Hz interference, to name a few. In a teaching environment, a supervisor can often effectively monitor the work of a trainee just from the sounds that emanate from the lab.

The video output is more complex. We are in transition from an era in which the preferred video output is changing from analog to digital. There are advantages and disadvantages for both types.

In older machines, the video display is a cathode ray tube (CRT) oscilloscope. The amplified and filtered signal is fed into a CRT. Electrons stream from the cathode and impact on a photosensitive screen, creating a point of light. The vertical (Y axis) deflections of the electrons are controlled by feeding the signal into deflecting plates arranged above and below the stream. The bioelectric signals control the degree to which the deflecting plates attract or repel the electron stream by causing the charge to vary on the plates. This creates vertical excursions that are an accurate representation of the bioelectric signal. For some displays, the beam deflections are controlled by magnets. The vertical amplification scale is controlled by the examiner as necessary for the circumstances. Properly set, deflections cover most of the available screen but do not "block" at the extremes. Commonly used gain settings are 10–20 μV/div for sensory studies, 2–10 mV/div for motor studies, 100 μV/div for needle EMG spontaneous and insertional activity, and 0.5–2 mV/div for MUAP analysis.

Time (X axis) is controlled by varying the charge on horizontal deflecting plates that cause the electron stream to move across the screen at a constant rate, which can be controlled by the examiner. Gradually increasing positivity on the right plate causes the sweep to progress across the screen at the set rate. At the end of the sweep the polarity of the plates transiently reverses and the electron stream is drawn abruptly back to its far left starting point. The sweep may run freely or be triggered by a stimulus. An accompanying time scale can help ensure accuracy.

Sweep speed is usually measured as either msec per screen division (e.g., a 10 sweep means 10 msec per division) or the time it takes the sweep to cross the entire screen (e.g., a 100 sweep for a 10 msec/division display having 10 divisions across the screen means each sweep consumes 100 msec.) MUAP firing rates can be estimated by their relationship to the sweep (see Chapter 8). For nerve conduction studies

(NCSs), sweep speed is a compromise. It should be set slow enough that the entire potential, either motor or sensory, appears on the screen, but fast enough that it is spread out over all the available display in order to appreciate the details of configuration. Commonly used sweep speeds are 1–2 msec/division for sensory studies; 2, 3, or 5 msec/div for motor studies; and 10 msec/div for needle EMG.

Before discussing digital video output we need to review some of the basics of digital electronics. Analog signals vary continuously and infinitely over time. The electrical events are analogous, more or less, to the physiological or biochemical events. In digital systems, a discrete electronic event is used to represent a physiological or biochemical event. Digital systems are discrete—you may hold up one finger or two, but not 1.346. Modern digital electronics employ a binary number system, based on the number 2, rather than the number 10 as in the decimal system. The digits available are 0 and 1. These digits represent one of 2 states—off/on or inactive/active. A row of numbers, read from right to left represents powers of 2. The first column or place is for ones, the second for twos, the third for fours, the fourth for eights, the fifth for sixteenths, etc. The row of 0's and 1's is a binary digit, or *bit*. An 8-bit processor would use a row of 8 places, a 16-bit processor 16 places, and so on. The binary digit 00001011 represents the decimal number 11. There is one 1, one 2, and one 8 and 1 + 2 + 8 = 11.

An analog to digital convertor (ADC) changes the analog signal into a discrete, digital approximation. How good an approximation depends on the quality of the ADC—its processing speed and sampling frequency. In the early days of digital EMG display, many EMGers developed dizziness, headaches, and a disdain for computerized EMG because the inadequacies of the ADCs and the monitors produced a signal which was only a remote approximation of the analog, real time signal. The situation was further confounded because the digital video display lagged behind the analog audio signal producing a discernible delay between sight and sound. For a considerable period of time, most clinical EMGers continued to prefer real time (analog) display despite some of the other advantages of digital technology.

The accuracy of the digital replication of an analog signal depends on how often the signal is sampled, the sampling frequency, and how many discrete digital steps are available to quantitate the amplitude, the vertical resolution. At each sampling, a discrete digital voltage is assigned which comes closest to the true analog voltage. A high sampling frequency and a large number of steps will produce a more accurate digital replica of the signal than will low sampling frequency and a low number of steps (Fig. 2.11).

The number of available vertical quantitation steps for representing the analog amplitude is the vertical resolution of the system and depends on the number of bits that can be processed. An 8 place binary digit has 256 possible combinations of digits and can represent 256 different decimal system numbers. An 8-bit processor can quantitize a signal into 256 different amplitude levels, a 12-bit resolution can divide a signal into 4,096 discrete steps, a 16-bit into 65,356 discrete

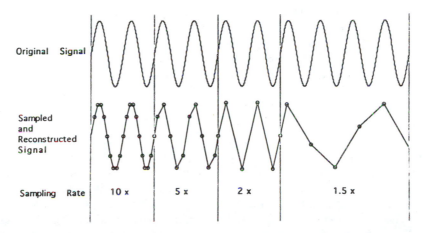

FIGURE 2.11. An illustration of the effect of sampling rate on the fidelity of reproduction of a 2 Hz signal. The Nyquist frequency is twice the fastest frequency in the signal and is the minimal acceptable sampling rate for adequate representation of the frequency content of the signal; in this instance, the Nyquist frequency is 4 Hz. Even at Nyquist frequency there is significant distortion of the waveforms. At lower sampling rates, the distortion is severe and the reconstruction bears little resemblance to the original signal—aliasing. The faster the sampling rate the greater the accuracy of the reconstruction. Reprinted with permission from Gitter AJ, Stolov WC. AAEM minimonograph #16: instrumentation and measurement in electrodiagnostic medicine–Part I. Muscle Nerve 1995; 18:799–811.

steps, and so forth. A high quality modern EMG machine might have a 16-bit vertical resolution, which can digitize an analog signal with a high degree of accuracy.

Sampling must occur sufficiently often to produce a reliable replica of the analog signal (6). The sampling rate must be higher to capture a rapidly changing waveform, such as a MUAP, than a more leisurely waveform, such as a compound muscle action potential. Rapid deflections in a MUAP can occur in 100 μsec or less, which translates into a frequency of 10,000 Hz. For acceptable analog to digital conversion, the sampling rate must be at least twice the fastest frequency (2f) in the sample. This is the Nyquist frequency, the minimal acceptable sampling frequency for accurate reproduction of the frequency content of the sample. Current top end EMG machines may sample at rates up to 350 kHz, and can accurately represent frequency components up to 175 kHz, which corresponds to events transpiring in the 6+ μsec range. Sampling below the Nyquist frequency produces "aliasing," in which the digital representation is so poor than gross inaccuracies occur—the digital version of the signal amounts to a false identity of the real thing (Fig. 2.11). Sampling frequencies below approximately 10–20 kHz are likely to produce aliasing.

After digital processing, the tracing is displayed by using a digital to analog converter (DAC) to change it back into an analog signal. For most monitors, the DAC sends its signals to electron guns at the back of a CRT, which then fires them at a phosphorescent screen. The original analog tracing is then recovered.

Recently manufactured high quality EMG machines have high speed ADCs and high vertical resolution processors, and the digitized tracing is a good replica of the analog tracing. Occasionally the digital limitations are still apparent. The sampling rate quoted (e.g., 200 kHz) may be the rated capacity of the chip, but not necessarily the capability of the system. Similarly for vertical resolution. The resolution of the monitor can impose limitations. A *pixel* (picture element) is the smallest unit that can be used to build an image on a screen. The best and most expensive modern systems have a display 1,600 pixels wide by 1,200 lines high. The information in the tracing must be contained within the limitations of the monitor. With a relatively slow sweep speed such as that used for needle EMG, a rapidly changing waveform such as a small spike fibrillation may not be visible, although clearly audible, because of the limitations of the monitor, despite theoretically adequate sampling frequency and vertical resolution. Because of cost limitations, most EMG machines have less than top of the line monitors. So, under the best of digital circumstances,

clinically significant aliasing can still occur even with the most current equipment.

Averaging

When a small, regularly recurring electrical signal is obscured by random noise, averaging a number of sweeps can often improve the signal to noise ratio and extract the signal. It is sometimes surprising how a nearly invisible sensory potential pops up with averaging. No sensory potential should be interpreted as absent without an attempt to average. There are a variety of ways to accomplish averaging, from simple superimposition of multiple sweeps on a storage scope to sophisticated digital techniques. Modern averagers calculate the algebraic sum of the amplitude of multiple, tiny, discrete segments of the sweep. Randomly fluctuating noise, as often positive as negative, calculated over many sweeps, will have a sum near zero, but the regularly recurring event will summate and grow larger and more conspicuous as the noise grows smaller and less conspicuous (Fig. 2.12). The averaged signal is then = the voltage sum of all sweeps divided by the number of sweeps. The signal to noise ratio (SNR) varies with the square root of the number of sweeps (n), as:

$$SNR \propto \sqrt{n}$$

Therefore, to double the resolution from a 4x extraction to an 8x extraction would require not doubling the number of sweeps, but increasing the samples from 16 to 64.

Triggering

For NCS, the stimulus triggers the sweep. For routine needle EMG, the sweep is retriggered automatically each time it reaches the far right of the screen. A randomly occurring event, such as a MUAP can be captured so as to repeat in the same display position by signal triggering. In this mode, each time a potential exceeds a certain voltage level, the sweep is triggered. Modern signal trigger systems are combined with delay lines. The sweep is retained briefly in memory and then replayed according to the desired trigger criteria. This memorized trace can be frozen for more careful inspection. The trigger and delay are essential for applications such as single fiber and quantitative EMG, and are very useful in obtaining maximum information even during routine needle exams.

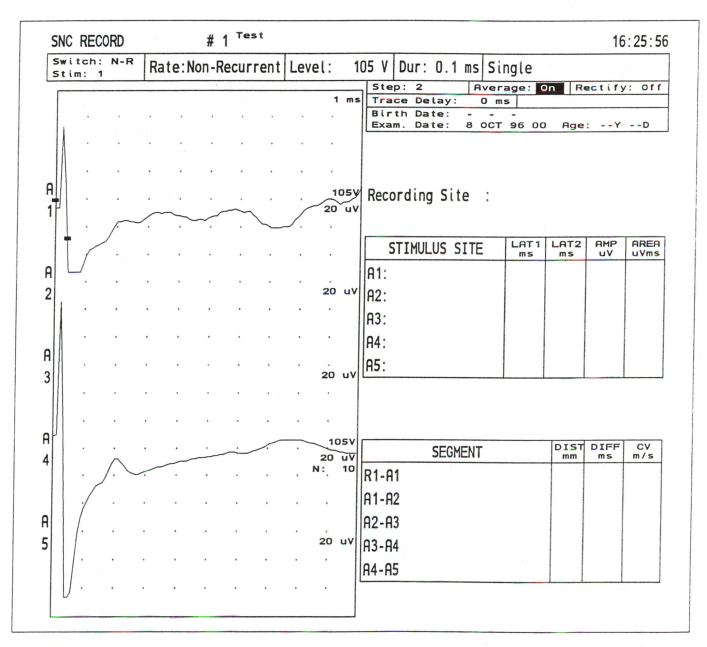

FIGURE 12.12.   In the top tracing, a sensory potential is obscured by overlying muscle contraction artifact. In the bottom tracing, the potential appears unambiguously after averaging only 10 sweeps.

Stimulation

The stimulus for NCSs is usually delivered through a stimulus isolation unit to minimize shock artifact. Isolation is achieved by mating two inductors to create a transformer. The electrical stimulus delivered to the primary coil creates a magnetic field that induces a current to flow in the secondary coil, which is then delivered to the patient. Because the two coils that make up the transformer have no physical connection, the stimulus is isolated and not conducted through the internal electrical system to the recording components of the apparatus, thereby minimizing shock artifact. Some unavoidable shock artifact is still created by surface conduction of stimulus current to the recording electrodes, but this can usually be minimized by good technique. The isolation transformer also affords protection to the patient by guarding against leakage current.

High quality electrical stimulators may be either constant voltage or constant current; some machines permit the operator to switch between these modes. The primary variable in stimulus delivery is the skin impedance. A constant voltage stimulator automatically varies the current to deliver the stipulated voltage to the patient regardless of the skin impedance. A constant current stimulator varies the voltage to deliver the stipulated current. Because nerves are stimulated by current, under most circumstances constant current stimulation is preferable. When trying to localize a nerve, such as identifying facial nerve strands in the bed of an acoustic neuroma, constant voltage stimulation may be more appropriate (7). Stimulus voltages usually range from 0–400 V and stimulus current can range from 0–100 mA. Stimulus intensity can also be controlled by varying the stimulus duration. Most machines permit durations from .05 to 1.0 msec in discrete increments.

The stimulus trigger module fires the stimulator and sends a simultaneous synchronizing signal to the ADC and the computer. It may also generate the machine's calibration signal. Stimulation is usually done with surface electrodes. Under some circumstances a needle cathode offers advantages. A variety of stimulators are available for intraoperative studies. These issues are addressed more fully in Chapter 7.

Other Features

Some machines include ancillary niceties such as temperature probes, devices to quickly check electrode impedance, automated computations, built in report generation, and modules for advanced applications such as single fiber and quantitative EMG. Many of course include evoked potential capability.

FIGURE 2.13. All the components assembled in a idealized EMG machine.

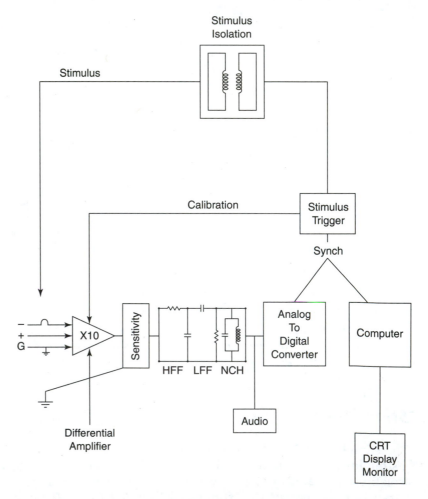

The Electromyograph

An EMG machine consists of an array of all the various components discussed above. The exact arrangements, specifications, and conveniences vary from machine to machine and from manufacturer to manufacturer. Different features are needed for different circumstances. Any EMG machine should be capable of performing basic nerve conduction studies and needle EMG. More advanced machines are used for such things as single fiber EMG and intraoperative monitoring. A basic scheme for an EMG machine is illustrated in Figure 2.13.

An overview of the operation of an EMG machine performing NCS is as follows. The stimulus trigger fires the stimulus isolation transformer, synchronizes the ADC and the computer, and starts the sweep. An electrical stimulus (constant current or constant voltage) is delivered. The evoked signal from the patient is sent first to the differential amplifier, which accentuates the signal from the active electrode and minimizes whatever common mode signal (i.e., interference) might be present, as determined by its CMRR. The amplified signal from the differential amplifier is then processed through a series of filters—HFF, LFF, and perhaps notch—which may be programmed by the operator. Most EMGers engage the notch filter only under the most trying and electrically noisy conditions, such as portable studies, as it may mask electrode problems and filter out important frequencies.

Additional adjustable amplification occurs through a sensitivity adjustment module. The audio signal may come off as an analog signal after sensitivity adjustment or may be processed through the ADC and then reconverted to analog through a DAC for better coordination with the digitized video. The filtered, amplified signal is digitized by the ADC within its limits of sampling frequency and vertical resolution. Further digital filtering may be carried out. The signal is analyzed by the computer's application software. The digitized information is then fed back through a DAC, which converts it back into analog form and sends it to the electron guns of the CRT. The CRT displays the information on a phosphorescent screen within the limits of its pixel and vertical line resolution. The human computer then analyzes and interprets the data and performs clinical correlation.

A possible shopping list of EMG machine specifications is presented in the Table 2.1. For a further discussion of issues related to the selection and purchase of EMG equipment, see reference (8).

Key Points

- Biologic signals contain multiple frequencies, only some of which are of interest. Filtering to extract the frequencies of interest is a trade-off, as important information may be lost.

- Analog filters use electrical components; digital filtering is done by computer. Analog filters are generally resistor-capacitor (RC) circuits which act essentially as frequency dependent voltage dividers and shunt the voltage drop to either the resistor or the capacitor depending on the frequency of the input signal. The filter can be changed by adjusting the capacitor's time constant.

- Filters are high pass/low frequency or vice versa. Filters have rolloff curves. The cutoff frequency is that frequency at which the output falls below the effective (rms, or DC equivalent) voltage. Filtering capability may also be described in decibels.

- Sequential filtering produces a bandpass filter. Different neurophysiologic procedures use different bandpasses. Resonant circuits can be used to create bandstop, or notch, filters to eliminate a given frequency, e.g., 60 Hz.

- Biologic signals require amplification. A vacuum tube analogy is useful in understanding modern electronics. Diodes are made of semiconductors, N type and P type. The barrier voltage must be overcome for a diode to conduct. Biasing manipulates the barrier voltage.

- Rectifiers convert AC to DC.

- Transistors are triodes, either NPN or PNP. The middle layer, or base layer, is analogous to the grid of a vacuum

TABLE 2.1
EMG Machine Shopping List

Desirable features in a basic EMG machine

Differential amplifier
    CMRR $\geq$ 100 dB
    Input impedance $\geq$ 1,000 mΩ
Analog to digital converter
    12 bit vertical resolution
    Sampling frequency $\geq$ 100 kHz
Filters
    Settings from 0 to 20 kHz
    60 Hz notch filter under operator control
Analog audio output
High quality audio speakers
Averager
Signal trigger and delay line
Stimulator
    Constant current/constant voltage option
    Constant current 0–100 mA
    Constant voltage 0–400 V
Current top of the line computer
Current top of the line monitor

tube. A small input signal to the base can control the flow of much larger currents between the emitter and the collector and create amplification.

- A differential amplifier inverts the signal coming into one channel, and since the output is the sum of the two input channels any signal which is equal at the two inputs (a common mode signal) will produce an output of zero. Any signal which is different at the two inputs (a differential signal) will be amplified.

- The common mode rejection ratio defines the ability of a differential amplifier to reject a common mode signal.

- A differential amplifier requires high input impedance in order to direct the voltage drop (the useful work) to the amplifier rather than having it dissipated at the patient electrode connections.

- The function of the differential amplifier can be sabotaged by unequal patient electrode impedances.

- An EMG machine has audio and visual outputs. Current methodology mostly employs digital video displays, while the audio may be analog or a reconverted signal.

- The analog to digital converter (ADC) changes the analog signal into digital form. The accuracy of the digital replica depends on the sampling frequency and the vertical resolution. Sampling below the Nyquist frequency may produce aliasing—where the digital tracing is a grossly inaccurate version of the analog signal, a fabrication.

- The computer monitor poses additional limitations on the display, depending on the number of pixels and vertical lines available. An excellent ADC may be undermined by a low quality CRT display monitor.

- Averaging improves the signal to noise ratio to help extract low amplitude nonrandom events from random background contamination. The averager computes the arithmetic sum of many short discrete segments of the sweep. The recurrent, time-locked event summates as the noise cancels out.

- The signal to noise ratio varies with the square root of the number of sweeps.

- Stimulation for nerve conduction studies is delivered through a stimulus isolation transformer to minimize shock artifact. Stimulation may be constant current or constant voltage. The stimulus trigger unit synchronizes the stimulus, the sweep, the ADC, and the computer.

- A model of an EMG machine demonstrates the relationships between the different components. An EMG machine shopping list is provided for those going to market.

References

1. Barry DT. AAEM minimonograph #36: basic concepts of electricity and electronics in clinical electromyography. Muscle Nerve 1991;14:937–946.
   See Chapter 1 for abstract.

2. Misulis KE. Basic electronics for clinical neurophysiology. J Clin Neurophysiol 1989;6:41–74.
   See Chapter 1 for abstract.

3. Maccabee PJ, Hassan NF. AAEM minimonograph #39: digital filtering: basic concepts and application to evoked potentials. Muscle Nerve 1992;15:865–875.
   Filtering of evoked potentials has been performed in clinical laboratories using both analog and digital methods. Analog methods introduce distortion caused by nonlinear phase shift which may be quite severe. Digital methods, while avoiding distortion caused by phase shift, reveal evoked potential components which may or may not correspond to distinct singular neuroanatomic generators or homogeneous neuroanatomic systems. Thus, components identified with zero phase shift digital filters at restricted bandpass must be compared with components seen in open bandpass recordings. In some specific circumstances, high-pass filtering of short-latency somatosensory-evoked potentials may distinguish slow asynchronous synaptic activity from fast and synchronous synaptic, lemniscal, or axonal activity.

4. Gitter AJ, Stolov WC. AAEM minimonograph #16: instrumentation and measurement in electrodiagnostic medicine—Part I. Muscle Nerve 1995;18:799–811.
   Technical and instrumentation factors play an important role in obtaining reliable information during electrodiagnostic studies. With contemporary electrodiagnostic equipment, neurophysiologic potentials are detected using a variety of electrodes and undergo differential amplification, filtering, conversion to digital form, and finally, analysis and display. Understanding the signal processing principles, limitations, and sources of errors that can occur during this multistep process can improve the technical quality of studies, minimize preventable errors, and improve clinical interpretation. Part I of this minimonograph reviews the basic principles of action potential generation and overviews electrodiagnostic instrumentation. The concept of waveform frequency content is related to the role of filters in suppressing noise while preserving waveform latency, amplitude, and morphology. The electrical characteristics of various surface and needle electrodes influence instrument design and the nature of the potentials recorded. This is especially important in understanding the differences in motor unit characteristics obtained from monopolar and concentric needle electrodes.

5. Dorfman LJ, McGill KC, Cummins KL. Electrical properties of commercial concentric EMG electrodes. Muscle Nerve 1985;8:1–8.
   Five electrical characteristics—impedance, broadband noise generation, line interference sensitivity, signal distortion, and common-mode conversion—were measured in five electromyographic (EMG) concentric needle electrodes (CNEs) from each of six commercial manufacturers. Untreated CNEs showed considerable variation in impedance and broadband noise characteristics, both within and among manufacturers. Electrolytic treatment reduced impedances by a factor between 1.5 and 4.0, and lessened within-manufacturer variability. Average post-treatment impedances at 100 Hz ranged from 31 to 436 kOhms, reflecting in part the range of core surface areas. Treatment also reduced the broadband noise to the level of the instrumentation noise for all but the highest impedance CNEs. Distortion and common-mode conversion were negligible for the lowest impedance CNEs. Line interference from a nearby power cord was completely suppressed only by those CNEs with fully shielded cables, and then only when the electromyographer also was grounded; there was no measurable benefit when the shield was

driven, as opposed to grounded. The authors conclude that there are consistent differences in the properties of CNEs from different manufacturers, reflecting differences in materials, design, and construction.

6. Gitter AJ, Stolov WC. AAEM minimonograph #16: instrumentation and measurement in electrodiagnostic medicine—Part II. Muscle Nerve 1995;18:812–824.
A review of instrumentation and measurement in electrodiagnostic medicine is continued in Part II, which focuses on digital instrumentation principles, gain and sweep effects, noise, nerve stimulation, and conduction measurement limitations. With the adoption of microprocessor-based equipment, the neurophysiologic signal must undergo analog-to-digital conversion (ADC) before analysis and display on a video monitor. ADC resolution and sampling rates affect accuracy and measurement precision. Following waveform display, the visual assessment of latency and duration may be influenced by sweep and gain settings, often overlooked sources of error. Undesired signal or noise typically originates from power-line interference, electronic amplifier noise, background muscle activity, or nerve stimulation artifact. Noise often interferes with clinical studies but techniques exist to reduce noise to acceptable levels in virtually all situations. An awareness and understanding of these technical issues will lead to an appreciation of the limitations of electrodiagnostic testing and improve interpretation and clinical decision-making.

7. Moller AR. Intraoperative recordings that can guide the surgeon in the operation. In: Miller AR, ed. Evoked Potentials in Intraoperative Monitoring. Baltimore: Williams and Wilkins, 1988.104–105.

8. Dorfman LJ. How to buy an EMG machine. In: 1995 AAEM Course C: Finally, an instrumentation course you can understand. Rochester: AAEM, 1995.7–23.

3

Anatomy and Physiology of the Neuromuscular System

The practice of electrodiagnostic medicine requires a detailed appreciation of both the gross and microscopic anatomy, as well as the physiology, of peripheral nerve and muscle. The components of the periph-
eral neuromuscular system particularly relevant to clinical electrodiagnosis are summarized in Table 3.1. A firm anatomical and physiological background is necessary to guide placement of stimulating and recording electrodes during nerve conduction studies (NCS), to ensure accurate placement of needle electrodes for needle electromyography, and to understand the pathophysiology of neuromuscular disease. Atlases are available to assist in the location of muscles for needle examination and for the details of peripheral innervation and anatomy for NCS (1–8). The marvelous monograph *Segmental Neurology* by Wolf contains a wealth of information on peripheral neuroanatomy and the clinical evaluation of the peripheral nervous system (9). This chapter will provide an overview of some of the clinically pertinent anatomy and physiology. Further information is provided in the respective chapters dealing with specific clinical entities. The anatomy of nerves commonly involved in compression syndromes is discussed further in Chapter 17. This chapter is intended to supplement rather than duplicate information which is available from any number of sources.

Motor Unit

The concept of the motor unit is integral to understanding electrodiagnostic medicine and clinical neuromuscular disease. The motor unit consists of an anterior horn motoneuron, its axon and all its subject muscle fibers; it is the final common pathway of the motor system (10). Clinical disorders may affect any portion of the motor unit (cell body, nerve root, plexus,

TABLE 3.1

Components of the Peripheral Nervous System Relevant to Clinical Electrodiagnosis

Motor neurons
Sensory neurons and ganglia
Autonomic neurons and ganglia
Nerve roots
Plexi
Peripheral nerves
    Motor axons
    Sensory axons
    Autonomic fibers
Axon terminals
Neuromuscular junctions
Sensory receptors
Muscle fibers

peripheral nerve, neuromuscular junction or muscle), and disease at different sites has different clinical and electrodiagnostic features.

The anterior horn of the spinal cord and the brainstem motor nuclei contain alpha and gamma motoneurons. The alpha motoneurons innervate common, extrafusal muscle fibers while the gamma motoneurons innervate intrafusal, muscle spindle fibers. The axon arises from the axon hillock and traverses the anterior root and the peripheral nerve enroute to the muscle. The peripheral nerve enters the muscle at the motor point and divides into intramuscular branches. These arborize within a muscle fascicle and terminate as fine twigs, which end as axon boutons. Terminal boutons abut the motor end plates of individual muscle fibers across a synaptic cleft, forming neuromuscular junctions. Each muscle fiber has only a single end plate.

Terminal axonal twigs ramify in the muscle and innervate widely dispersed muscle fibers. Muscle fibers innervated by a given motor unit lie scattered over a large area within a muscle fascicle and are extensively intermingled with muscle fibers innervated by other motor units (Fig. 3.1). A motor unit may have anywhere from a handful of muscle fibers to more than a thousand. The innervation ratio refers to the number of muscle fibers in a motor unit. A low innervation ratio means few muscle fibers are innervated by a single axon and is characteristic of muscles under precise and finely graded voluntary control, such as extraocular or laryngeal muscles. A muscle performing a gross motor movement may have several hundred muscle fibers per motor unit (11). The gastrocnemius has about 2,000. Electrophysiological motor unit counting techniques estimate that an in-

trinsic hand muscle has about 100 motor units (12). Motor units also vary by size within a muscle. Smaller motoneurons have smaller motor unit territories. To produce a smoothly graded muscle contraction, motor units are recruited, more or less, in order of increasing size. Small motoneurons are first recruited, and increasing force of contraction calls forth activity from increasing larger motoneurons: the size principle.

Motor units are classified by histochemical reaction, primarily by the myosin ATPase stain, as type 1 or type 2. The different staining characteristics and the random admixture of type 1 and type 2 units create a microscopic mosaic referred to as the checkerboard pattern (Fig. 3.2). All muscle fibers of a motor unit are of the same type, and there is good correlation between the mechanical properties and other attributes of a motor unit and the histochemical reactions of its muscle fibers (see Table 19.1). Motor unit properties are discussed further in Chapters 8 and 19.

In another functional and physiological scheme, motor units are classified into three different types: FF, FR, and S. Type FF units are fast twitch, fatigue sensitive, type 2B histochemically, rich in glycogen but poor in oxidative enzymes, and designed for brief, phasic activity. Type S units are slow twitch, fatigue resistant, type 1 histochemically, low in glycolytic but high in oxidative enzymes, and designed for sustained, tonic activity. Type FR is intermediate, fast twitch but more fatigue resistant than type FF, type 2A histochemically, high in glycolytic and intermediate in oxidative enzyme activity.

The summated electrical activity of all the muscle fibers of a motor unit, a motor unit action potential (MUAP), can be recorded by a needle electrode inserted into the muscle. The routine needle examination only detects activity from the part of the motor unit near the recording electrode, but special techniques such as macro and scanning EMG can assess the entire motor unit. The needle electrode examina-

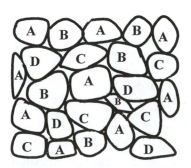

FIGURE 3.1. A representation of muscle cross-section, showing how the fibers innervated by four different units (A, B, C, D) are randomly intermingled.

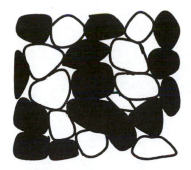

FIGURE 3.2. The muscle fibers of Figure 3.1, have been stained with myosin ATPase at pH 9.4. The type 2 fibers (motor units A and C) stain darkly, while the fibers of the type 1 motor units (B and D) remain light. This alternating staining reaction creates the checkerboard pattern. Different staining reaction with some other histochemical stains can also distinguish between type 1 and type 2 fibers.

tion of normal and abnormal MUAPs, the physiologic determinants of the MUAP, recruitment, the size principle, and motor unit types are discussed further in Chapter 8.

The muscle fibers of one motor unit in concert with fibers of several other motor units form a muscle fascicle, and many fascicles together form a whole muscle. Similarly, the axons of many motor neurons are gathered together into peripheral nerve trunks. Most peripheral nerves also contain sensory and autonomic fibers. Further details of the microscopic anatomy and physiology of peripheral nerve, neuromuscular junction, and muscle are discussed in Chapters 16, 18, and 19.

Gross Anatomy

From a gross anatomical and clinical perspective, the peripheral nervous system begins with the emergence of the anterior and posterior roots from the spinal cord. These join to form the mixed spinal nerve (also referred to as a root), which exits from the intervertebral foramen. The anatomy of the spinal roots and their relationship to the vertebral bodies and discs are discussed in Chapter 14. Immediately after exit, the root divides into anterior and posterior primary rami. The posterior primary ramus turns dorsally to innervate the paravertebral musculature. The anterior primary rami form the cervical, brachial, and lumbosacral plexi, and the intercostal nerves. The peripheral nerves of the limbs then arise from the plexi.

Sensory nerve roots supply cutaneous innervation to specific dermatomes. The generally available dermatomal charts are primarily derived from three

sources: Head and Campbell, Foerster, and Keegan and Garrett, who all used very different approaches (9). Head and Campbell were primarily interested in herpes zoster and mapped dermatomes according to the distribution of herpetic eruptions. Foerster performed posterior rhizotomies in patients with chronic pain. He mapped the distribution of an intact root when one or more of those above and below had been severed, or by electrically stimulating the stump of a severed root and observing the area of cutaneous vasodilation. The observation of dermatomal overlap originated partly from this work, and for a time many believed a lesion of a single root would produce no detectable deficit. Keegan and Garrett examined a large series of patients with clinical involvement of various roots and mapped the sensory deficits; there was surgical correlation in 53% of the patients. The loss of sensation due to isolated involvement of a single root, as occurs clinically, produces a different dermatomal map than the preserved sensation in a zone of anesthesia as found by Foerster. The dermatomal overlap is such that the clinical deficit from an isolated root lesion is typically much more restricted than that expected from the anatomical geography of the dermatome. Deficits to pin prick are smaller than those to light touch. Figures 3.3–3.5 are the dermatome distributions as depicted by Sunderland, which reflect the generally accepted clinical paradigm.

A myotome consists of all the muscles innervated by a specific nerve root. Early anatomists reported myotome innervation from detailed dissections, and some errors have been perpetuated through the years (9). Most skeletal muscles receive innervation from two or more roots, and there is inherent variability in the myotomal patterns between individuals. Many different innervation charts are available, and most vary in some details. Liveson and Ma present charts derived from 7 different sources, separating "new myotomes" derived from electromyographic data (7). Some misinformation remains, such as the inclusion of C6–7 innervation to the thenar muscles, which does not fit apparent clinical reality. The issue has been compounded by observations during intraoperative recordings that indicate contributions from unexpected sources to leg muscles and anomalous innervation so frequent as to be the rule rather than the exception (13,14). More useful for electrodiagnostic medicine is information about which muscles show abnormalities in disease affecting specific roots. Recent electromyographic information is available for both upper and lower extremities and is discussed further in Chapter 14 (15–18). Myotomes of the upper and lower extremities are reviewed in Tables 3.2 and 3.3.

FIGURE 3.3. Dermatomes of the upper extremity.

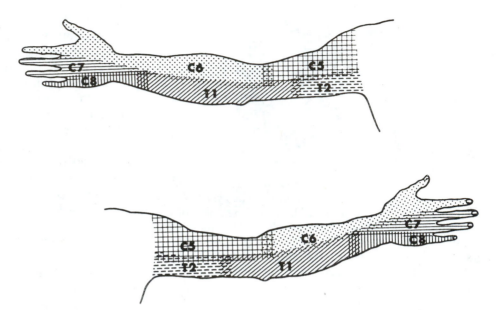

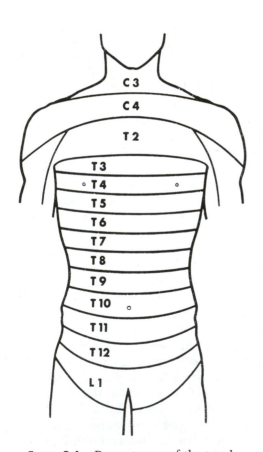

FIGURE 3.4. Dermatomes of the trunk.

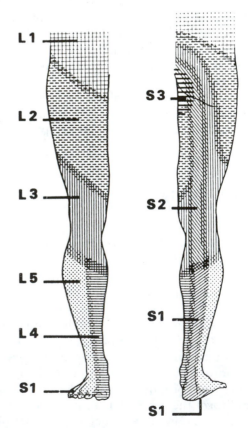

FIGURE 3.5. Dermatomes of the lower extremity.

TABLE 3.2
Upper Extremity Myotomes

Root	Muscles Supplied
C4	Levator scapulae
C5	Levator scapulae, rhomboids, supraspinatus, infraspinatus, teres major and minor, deltoid, biceps, BR, supinator, serratus anterior, pectoralis
C6	Infraspinatus, teres major and minor, deltoid, biceps, BR, supinator, anconeus, serratus anterior, pectoralis, FCR, pronator teres, latissimus dorsi, ECRL, (supraspinatus, triceps)
C7	Serratus anterior, pectoralis, triceps, anconeus, pronator teres, latissimus dorsi, FCR, ECRL, EDC, ECU, (EIP, FCU, FDP, FPL)
C8	Latissimus dorsi, pectoralis, triceps, EDC, ECU, EIP, FCU, FDP, FPL, PQ APB, FDI, ADQ
T1	Pectoralis, FCU, FDP, FPL, EIP, PQ, APB, FDI, ADQ

BR, brachioradialis; ECRL, extensor carpi radialis longus; ECU, extensor carpi ulnaris; EDC, extensor digitorum longus; EIP, extensor indicis proprius; FCR, flexor carpi radialis; APB, abductor pollicis brevis; FPL, flexor pollicis longus; FDP, flexor digitorum profundus; PQ, pronator quadratus; FCU, flexor carpi ulnaris; FDI, first dorsal interosseous; ADQ, abductor digiti quinti.
Parentheses signify minor contribution.

The following sections will briefly review the electrophysiologically pertinent anatomy of selected major peripheral nerves. Tables 3.4 and 3.5 summarize the electrodiagnostically important muscles innervated by different neural structures in the upper and lower extremities, and Table 3.6 reviews the major sensory nerves studied in electrodiagnostic medicine.

Upper Extremity Nerves

The nerves innervating the upper extremity arise from the brachial plexus.(19) The anatomy of the plexus from an electrodiagnostic medicine perspective is discussed in Chapter 15. The upper extremity nerves of major electrodiagnostic importance are diagrammed in Figure 3.6. The cutaneous fields of the head and upper extremity are shown in Figures 3.7 and 3.8.

MEDIAN NERVE

The median nerve has two components: a lateral division and a medial division. The lateral cord of the brachial plexus divides into two terminal branches, one becomes the musculocutaneous nerve, the other

becomes the lateral division of the median nerve. The medial cord of the brachial plexus also divides into two terminal branches, one forms the medial division of the median nerve, and the other continues as the ulnar nerve. The medial and lateral divisions of the median nerve join to form a single trunk, which passes through the upper arm without branching down to the region of the elbow. There the branches begin to separate. Innervating twigs are given off from the lateral head to the pronator teres and flexor carpi radialis muscles. The main trunk passes through the two heads of the pronator teres muscle, and beneath an aponeurosis connecting the two heads of the flexor digitorum superficialis (the sublimis bridge). Just distal to this point, the nerve gives off the anterior interosseus branch, which runs along the interosseus membrane and innervates the median head (lateral portion) of the flexor digitorum profundus, the flexor pollicis longus, and the pronator quadratus. The anterior interosseus branch has no sensory component.

The main trunk of the median nerve continues down the forearm. The palmar cutaneous branch

TABLE 3.3
Lower Extremity Myotomes

Root	Muscles Supplied
L2	Iliopsoas, sartorius, quadriceps, abdominal, (adductors, gracilis)
L3	Iliopsoas, sartorius, adductors, gracilis, quadriceps femoris, abdominal
L4	Gracilis, sartorius, gluteus medius, TFL, quadriceps femoris, adductor magnus, TA, (iliopsoas, adductor longus, internal hamstring, TP, EDL, EDB)
L5	Gluteus maximus, internal hamstring, biceps femoris, gluteus medius, TFL, peronei, FDL, TA, EHL, EDL, EDB, TP, (LG, EDB)
S1	Internal hamstring, biceps femoris, gluteus maximus, FDL, LG, MG, ADQP, AH, FDIP, EDB, (gluteus medius, TFL, peronei, EHL, EDL, TP, TA)
S2	Gluteus maximus, ADQP, AH, soleus, LG, MG, FDIP, (internal hamstring, biceps femoris, EDB, anal sphincter)
S3	Anal sphincter

TFL, tensor fascia lata; TA, tibialis anterior; TP, tibialis posterior; EDL, extensor digitorum longus; EHL, extensor hallucis longus; EDB, extensor digitorum brevis; FDL, flexor digitorum longus; LG, lateral gastrocnemius; MG, medial gastrocnemius; AH, adductor hallucis; ADQP, abductor digiti quinti pedis; FDIP, first dorsal interosseous pedis.
Parentheses signify minor contribution.

TABLE **3.4**

Electrodiagnostically Important Upper Extremity Muscles Innervated by the Various Structures (see Fig.15.1)

Structure	*Muscle*
C3, C4 roots	Diaphragm (via phrenic nerve)
C5 root	Rhomboids and levator scapulae (via dorsal scapular nerve), serratus anterior (via long thoracic nerve)
C6, C7 roots	Serratus anterior (via long thoracic nerve)
Brachial plexus	
Upper trunk	Supra- and infraspinatus (via suprascapular nerve)
Lateral cord	Pectoralis muscles (via lateral pectoral nerve)
Medial cord	Pectoralis muscles (via medial pectoral nerve)
Posterior cord	Latissimus dorsi (via thoracodorsal nerve)
Axillary nerve	Deltoid and teres minor
Musculocutaneous nerve	Biceps, brachialis, and coracobrachialis
Radial nerve	Triceps, brachioradialis, ECRL/B, anconeus
Posterior interosseous branch	Supinator, ECU, EDC, APL, EPL/B, EIP
Median nerve	
Main trunk, lateral head	PRT, FCR
Main trunk, medial head	PL, FDS, APB, OP
Anterior interosseus branch	FPL, $FDP_{1,2}$, PQ
Ulnar nerve	FCU, $FDP_{3,4}$, hypothenar muscles, interossei, $lumbricals_{3,4}$

ECRL/B, extensor carpi radialis longus/brevis; ECU, extensor carpi ulnaris; EDC, extensor digitorum longus; APL, abductor pollicis longus; EPL/B, extensor pollicis longus/brevis; EIP, extensor indicis proprius; PRT, pronator teres; FCR, flexor carpi radialis; PL, palmaris longus; FDS, flexor digitorum sublimis; APB, abductor pollicis brevis; OP, opponens pollicis; FPL, flexor pollicis longus; FDP, flexor digitorum profundus; PQ, pronator quadratus; FCU, flexor carpi ulnaris.

leaves the main trunk 5–8 cm proximal to the wrist crease. The median nerve then enters the hand through the carpal tunnel. The anatomy of this region is discussed further in Chapter 17.

ULNAR NERVE

The ulnar nerve arises as a continuation of the medial cord of the brachial plexus. As it exits from the thorax, it passes through the axilla and into the upper arm lying medial to the brachial artery in a common neurovascular sheath with the median nerve and the medial brachial and antebrachial cutaneous nerves. At about the level of the insertion of the coracobrachialis, the ulnar leaves the common neurovascular bundle and pierces the medial intermuscular septum to gain the posterior compartment of the arm. The nerve then descends toward the elbow in a groove alongside the medial head of the triceps. The point of the ulnar

nerve's penetration of the medial intermuscular septum and the nearby deep fascia binding the nerve in the triceps groove are sometimes referred to as the arcade of Struthers, a potential entrapment site (not to be confused with the ligament of Struthers, a band extending from the medial epicondyle to a supracondylar spur which may compress the median nerve). After piercing the medial intermuscular septum, the nerve proceeds distally on a slanting course toward the ulnar groove. The anatomy of the ulnar nerve in the region of the elbow, the most common area of compression, is discussed further in Chapter 17.

After exiting the flexor carpi ulnaris (FCU) through the deep flexorpronator aponeurosis, the nerve runs in the tissue plane between the FCU and the flexor digitorum profundus. In the distal two-thirds of the forearm, the nerve closely abuts the medial wall of the ulnar artery in a common neurovascular bundle. The palmar cutaneous branch arises in the mid to

TABLE 3.5
Electrodiagnostically Important Lower Extremity Muscles Innervated by Various Structures

Lumbosacral plexus	
Pudendal nerve	Anal sphincter
Superior gluteal nerve	Gluteus medius, TFL
Inferior gluteal nerve	Gluteus maximus
Femoral nerve	Iliopsoas, quadriceps, sartorius
Obturator nerve	Gracilis, adductor longus, adductor magnus
Sciatic nerve	
Peroneal division of sciatic	Short head of the biceps femoris
Superficial peroneal nerve	Peroneus longus and brevis
Deep peroneal nerve	TA, EDL, EHL, peroneus tertius, EDB
Tibial division of sciatic	Long head of biceps femoris, SM, ST, adductor magnus
Posterior tibial nerve	Gastrocnemius, soleus, TP, FDL, FHL
medial plantar nerve	AH, FHB
lateral plantar nerve	ADQP, interossei

TFL, tensor fascia lata; TA, tibialis anterior; EDL, extensor digitorum longus; EHL, extensor hallucis longus; EDB, extensor digitorum brevis; SM, semimembranosus; ST, semitendinosus; TP, tibialis posterior; FDL, flexor digitorum longus; FHL, flexor hallucis longus; AH, adductor hallucis; FHB, flexor hallucis brevis; ADQP, abductor digiti quinti pedis.

distal forearm and pursues a separate course to the hand. It enters the hand superficial to Guyon's canal and supplies sensation to the skin of the hypothenar region. The large dorsal ulnar cutaneous branch leaves the main trunk 5–10 cm proximal to the wrist to wind posteriorly between the tendon of the FCU and the ulna, emerging on the dorsal surface of the wrist to provide sensation to the dorsal, ulnar aspect of the hand and small and ring fingers (20).

The nerve enters the hand through the ulnar tunnel, commonly referred to as Guyon's canal (21). The transverse carpal ligament, which forms the roof of the carpal tunnel, dips downward as it spans medially and forms the floor of Guyon's canal. Just beyond the transverse carpal ligament, the pisohamate ligament, which runs from the pisiform bone to the hook of the hamate, forms the distal part of the floor of the canal. The volar carpal ligament, a thin investment which is basically a continuation of the deep forearm fascia, then arches over and forms the roof of Guyon's canal along with the thin palmaris brevis muscle. The hook of the hamate forms the lateral, and the pisiform bone and FCU tendon the medial, boundaries.

As it emerges from beneath the volar carpal ligament, the ulnar gives a branch to the palmaris brevis, then branches into the superficial terminal sensory division and the deep palmar division. The deep

TABLE 3.6
Electrodiagnostically Important Sensory Nerves

Nerve	Area of Supply
Median, lateral division	Hand, median volar distribution
Ulnar	Hand, ulnar volar distribution
Radial	Thumb; hand, radial dorsal distribution
Dorsal ulnar cutaneous	Hand, ulnar dorsal distribution
Lateral antebrachial cutaneous	Forearm, radial aspect
Medial antebrachial cutaneous	Forearm, ulnar aspect
Sural	Foot, lateral aspect
Superficial peroneal	Foot, dorsal aspect
Medial plantar	Foot, medial sole
Lateral plantar	Foot, lateral sole
Saphenous	Lower leg, medial aspect
Lateral femoral cutaneous	Thigh, lateral aspect

FIGURE **3.6.** The major nerves and branches of electrodiagnostic importance in the upper extremity.

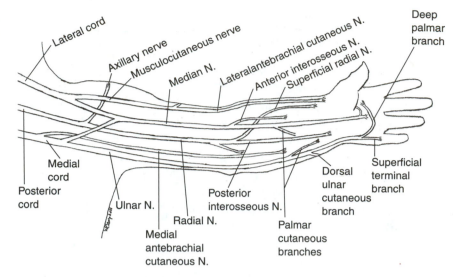

branch exits Guyon's canal, passes through the piso-hamate hiatus, then arches laterally beneath the flexor tendons, innervating the interossei and breaking up into terminal branches on reaching the adductor pollicis and first dorsal interosseous. The deep head of the flexor pollicis brevis is usually supplied by a short twig from the terminal branch to the adductor pollicis.

The Martin Gruber forearm anastomosis is a common anomaly in which ulnar fibers run with the median nerve proximally, then cross over in the forearm to join the ulnar; it is discussed in more detail in Chapter 10 (22). The Riche-Cannieu anastomosis consists of communications between the deep branch of the ulnar nerve and various branches of the median nerve in the palm (23).

RADIAL NERVE

The radial nerve arises as a continuation of the posterior cord of the brachial plexus. It exits through the axilla and then runs down the medial aspect of the upper arm. At about the mid-upper arm it arcs around the mid-humerus in the spiral groove accompanied by the humeral circumflex artery. Branches innervating the long head of the triceps muscle arise before the nerve enters the spiral groove, those to the medial and lateral heads frequently arise in the groove (24). The nerve descends through the lateral upper arm, giving off a branch to the brachioradialis muscle. It then enters the forearm in the groove between the biceps tendon and the brachioradialis. Innervating twigs are given off to the brachioradialis and the extensor carpi radialis longus and brevis, after which the main trunk terminates by dividing into the posterior interosseus branch and the superficial radial branch.

The superficial radial nerve descends along the lateral aspect of the forearm; however, it does not supply the skin in this region, which is instead supplied by the lateral antebrachial cutaneous nerve. The superficial radial branch terminates by arborizing over the skin of the radial aspect of the dorsum of the hand and thumb (25). At its take off, the posterior interosseus nerve sends a branch to the supinator muscle, then passes beneath an aponeurosis in the supinator, the arcade of Frohse (26). The posterior interosseus branch continues along the interosseus membrane supplying the extensor muscles of the fingers: the extensor digitorum communis, extensor indicis, extensor pollicis longus and brevis, as well as the extensor carpi ulnaris (27). It also sends a branch to innervate the abductor pollicis longus. Like its analog, the anterior interosseus nerve, the posterior interosseus has no sensory component.

OTHER UPPER EXTREMITY NERVES

Three nerves arise from the level of the roots: the phrenic, long thoracic, and dorsal scapular. The phrenic arises from C3–5 to innervate the diaphragm; the long thoracic from C4–6 to innervate the serratus anterior; and the dorsal scapular from C5 to innervate the rhomboids. Involvement of these nerves is important in distinguishing between radiculopathy and brachial plexopathy.

The suprascapular nerve arises from the upper trunk of the brachial plexus and passes posteriorly through the suprascapular notch, beneath the suprascapular ligament, to innervate the supraspinatus muscle. It then curves around the glenoid process of the scapula to innervate the infraspinatus. The medial and lateral pectoral nerves arise from the medial and lateral cords of the plexus, respectively, and innervate the pectoral muscles. The thoracodorsal nerve arises from the posterior cord to innervate the latissimus dorsi.

The axillary nerve is a terminal branch of the posterior cord. It travels posteriorly and passes through the quadrilateral space to innervate the deltoid and teres minor. It sends sensory twigs to a small circular area of skin over the deltoid muscle.

The musculocutaneus nerve is a terminal branch of the lateral cord. It passes into the upper arm in the groove between the deltoid and pectoral muscles, traverses a foramen in the coracobrachialis muscle to innervate the biceps and brachialis, after which it continues as the lateral antebrachial cutaneous nerve to innervate the radial aspect of the forearm (28).

LOWER EXTREMITY NERVES

The nerves innervating the lower extremity and hip region arise from the lumbosacral plexus (29). The two major nerves innervating the lower extremity are the femoral and the sciatic. The lower extremity nerves and branches of major electrodiagnostic importance are diagrammed in Figure 3.9. The cutaneous fields of the lower extremity are shown in Figures 3.10 and 3.11.

FEMORAL NERVE

The femoral nerve forms within the belly of the psoas muscle from the L2, L3, and L4 roots. Leaving the cover of the psoas, it runs between the psoas and the

iliacus muscle and exits from the pelvis beneath the inguinal ligament, lateral to the femoral vessels. Its motor branches innervate the psoas, iliacus, sartorius, and quadriceps muscles. Sensory branches innervate the skin of the anterior thigh. Like the musculocutaneous, the femoral nerve terminates as a large sensory branch, the saphenous nerve, which supplies an extensive cutaneous field along the medial aspect of the lower leg and the medial aspect of the foot.

SCIATIC NERVE

The lumbosacral trunk arises from the lower part of the lumbar plexus and fuses with elements of the sacral plexus to form the sciatic nerve. The sciatic, superior gluteal, and inferior gluteal nerves all exit the pelvis through the greater sciatic foramen. The sciatic usually exits beneath the piriformis muscle, but may pierce it or rarely pass above it. The nerve courses in close proximity to the posterior aspect of the hip joint, then enters the thigh. In its course through the thigh it innervates the hamstring muscles and also sends a twig to the adductor magnus.

From its beginnings, the sciatic nerve is made up of two divisions: the peroneal (lateral) and the tibial (medial). The tibial division arises from the anterior divisions of the lumbosacral plexus, and the peroneal from the posterior divisions. The peroneal and tibial divisions run together in a common sheath, forming the sciatic nerve, until the level of the knee where they divide and pursue separate courses. The only portion of the hamstring muscle mass innervated by the peroneal division is the short head of the biceps femoris;

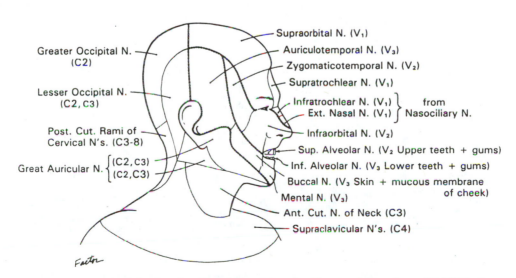

FIGURE 3.7. Cutaneous innervation of the head and neck. Reprinted with permission from Wolf JK. Segmental neurology: a guide to the examination and interpretation of sensory and motor function. Baltimore: University Park Press, 1981.

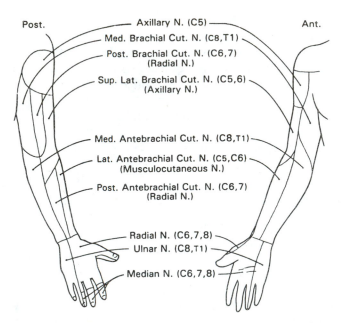

FIGURE 3.8.   Cutaneous innervation of the upper extremity. Reprinted with permission from Wolf JK. Segmental neurology: a guide to the examination and interpretation of sensory and motor function. Baltimore: University Park Press, 1981.

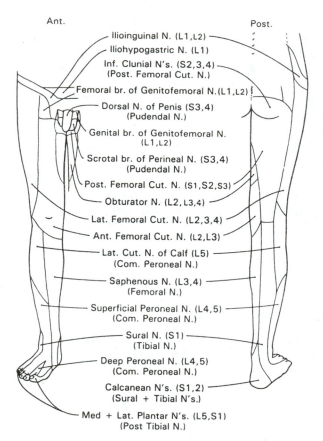

FIGURE 3.10.   Cutaneous innervation of the lower extremity. Reprinted with permission from Wolf JK. Segmental neurology: a guide to the examination and interpretation of sensory and motor function. Baltimore: University Park Press, 1981.

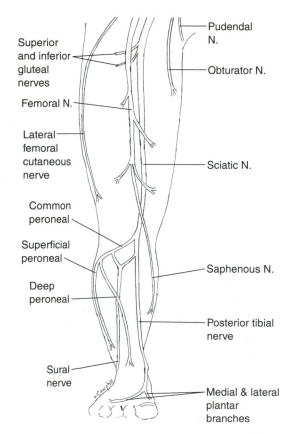

FIGURE 3.9.   The major nerves and branches of electrodiagnostic importance in the lower extremity.

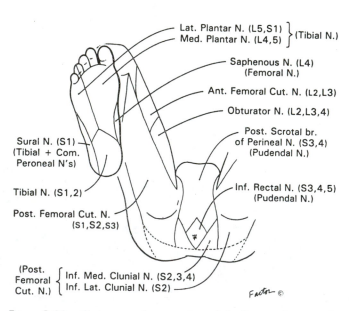

FIGURE 3.11.   Cutaneous innervation of the foot and perineal region. Reprinted with permission from Wolf JK. Segmental neurology: a guide to the examination and interpretation of sensory and motor function. Baltimore: University Park Press, 1981.

all other hamstring muscles are innervated by the tibial division.

After the bifurcation in the popliteal fossa, the peroneal nerve moves laterally and winds around the head of the fibula, then descends toward the foot. The anatomy of the peroneal in the region of the knee is discussed further in Chapter 17.

After the bifurcation of the sciatic, the tibial nerve descends in the midline down the posterior aspect of the leg to innervate the gastrosoleus. In its proximal course it gives off a sural communicating branch, which joins its fellow from the common peroneal nerve to form the sural nerve proper. The sural then moves laterally as it runs distally and pierces the deep fascia to emerge into a superficial position about 15 centimeters proximal to the lateral malleolus, then curves around and beneath the lateral malleolus to supply the skin of the lateral aspect of the foot and toes. Distally the tibial nerve passes beneath the medial malleolus, under the flexor retinaculum, which forms the roof of the tarsal tunnel. The tibial nerve terminates by dividing into the medial and lateral plantar nerves, which innervate the abductors and short flexors of the toes and supply sensation to the skin of the sole.

OTHER LOWER EXTREMITY NERVES

Other important nerves to the lower extremity include the pudendal, the gluteal nerves, and the sensory branches of the lumbosacral plexus. The gluteal nerves exit through the greater sciatic foramen in close proximity to the sciatic; the superior supplies the gluteus medius and tensor fascia lata, the inferior the gluteus maximus (30). The pudendal nerve exits through the sciatic notch to supply the external anal sphincter and other muscles of the perineum, and the skin of the perineal region. There are several sensory branches that arise from the lumbosacral plexus. The most clinically important is the lateral femoral cutaneous, which exits from the pelvis beneath the inguinal ligament just medial to the anterior superior iliac spine to supply the skin of the lateral thigh (31). The posterior femoral cutaneous exits in close proximity to the sciatic and supplies the skin of the posterior thigh and the adjacent buttocks. The genitofemoral and ilioinguinal nerves supply the upper medial thigh and adjacent genitalia.

Key Points

- The motor unit, the final common pathway of the motor system, consists of a motoneuron, its axon, and all its subject muscle fibers.

- The spinal cord and brainstem motor nuclei contain alpha motoneurons that innervate extrafusal muscle fibers. The axon traverses the anterior root and the peripheral nerve enroute to the muscle. At the motor point, the peripheral nerve enters the muscle and divides into intramuscular branches, which end as axon boutons abutting the motor end plates of muscle fibers, forming neuromuscular junctions.

- Muscle fibers innervated by a given motor unit lie scattered over a large area within a muscle fascicle and are extensively intermingled with muscle fibers innervated by other motor units.

- The innervation ratio refers to the number of muscle fibers in a motor unit. A low innervation ratio is characteristic of muscles under precise and finely graded voluntary control. To produce a smoothly graded muscle contraction, small motoneurons are recruited first, followed by activity from larger motoneurons.

- The random admixture of type 1 and type 2 units creates a checkerboard pattern on histochemical stains. There is good correlation between the mechanical properties and other attributes of a motor unit and the histochemical reactions of its muscle fibers. Motor units may also be classified into types FF (fast twitch, fatigue sensitive), FR (intermediate), and S (slow twitch, fatigue resistant).

- The peripheral nervous system begins at the level of the spinal roots. The anterior primary rami form the cervical, brachial, and lumbosacral plexi and the intercostal nerves, and the peripheral nerves of the limbs then arise from the plexi.

- The available dermatomal charts are primarily derived using three different methods. The loss of sensation due to isolated involvement of a single root, as occurs clinically, produces a different dermatomal map than preserved sensation in a zone of anesthesia.

- A myotome consists of all the muscles innervated by a specific nerve root. The many different innervation charts available vary in some details. Recent observations using electrophysiologic techniques indicate contributions from unexpected sources to leg muscles, and that anomalous innervation is common.

- The median nerve has lateral and medial divisions, derived from the lateral and medial cords of the brachial plexus, which join to form a single trunk. At the elbow, branches from the lateral head innervate the pronator teres and flexor carpi radialis muscles. After passing through the pronator teres muscle, the main trunk gives off the anterior interosseus branch, then continues down the forearm. The palmar cutaneous branch arises 5–8 cm proximal to the wrist crease, after which the main trunk enters the hand through the carpal tunnel.

- The ulnar nerve arises as a continuation of the medial cord of the brachial plexus. After piercing the medial intermuscular septum, the nerve proceeds distally on a slanting course toward the ulnar groove. After exiting the FCU distal to the groove, the ulnar traverses the deep flexorpronator aponeurosis. The palmar cutaneous branch arises in the mid to distal forearm, enters the hand superficial to Guyon's canal, and supplies sensation to the skin of the hypothenar region. The dorsal ulnar cutaneous branch exits proximal to the wrist to provide sensation to the dorsal, ulnar aspect of the hand and small and ring fingers. The main trunk enters the hand through Guyon's canal. On emerging from beneath the volar carpal ligament, it branches into the superficial terminal sensory division and the deep palmar division.

- The Martin Gruber forearm anastomosis is a common anomaly in which ulnar fibers run with the median nerve proximally, then cross over in the forearm to join the ulnar.

- The radial nerve arises as a continuation of the posterior cord of the brachial plexus. It curves around the humerus in the spiral groove; branches to the triceps muscle arise before the nerve enters the groove. It enters the forearm in the groove between the biceps tendon and the brachioradialis. Branches are given off to the brachioradialis and the extensor carpi radialis longus and brevis, after which the main trunk terminates by dividing into the posterior interosseus branch and the superficial radial branch. At its take off, the posterior interosseus nerve sends a branch to the supinator muscle, then passes beneath the arcade of Frohse, an aponeurosis in the supinator.

- The femoral nerve forms within the psoas muscle, then exits from the pelvis beneath the inguinal ligament; motor branches innervate the psoas, iliacus, sartorius, and quadriceps muscles, and the nerve terminates as the saphenous nerve.

- The sciatic, superior gluteal, and inferior gluteal nerves all exit the pelvis through the greater sciatic foramen. From its beginning, the sciatic nerve is made up of the peroneal (lateral) and the tibial (medial) divisions, which run together in a common sheath. After the bifurcation in the popliteal fossa, the peroneal nerve moves laterally and winds around the head of the fibula, then descends toward the foot. After the bifurcation, the tibial nerve descends down the posterior aspect of the leg to innervate the gastrosoleus. Sural communicating branches from both the peroneal and tibial nerves join to form the sural nerve proper. Distally the tibial nerve passes beneath the medial malleolus, under the flexor retinaculum of the tarsal tunnel, and terminates by dividing into the medial and lateral plantar nerves, which innervate the abductors and short flexors of the toes and supply sensation to the skin of the sole.

- Other important nerves to the lower extremity include the pudendal and the sensory branches of the lumbosacral plexus.

References

1. Delagi EF, Perotto A, Iazzetti J, et al. Anatomic guide for the electromyographer—The limbs. 2nd ed. Springfield: Charles C. Thomas, 1980.

2. Geiringer SR. Anatomic localization for needle electromyography. Philadelphia: Hanley & Belfus, 1994.

3. Chu-Andrews J, Johnson RJ. Electrodiagnosis: an anatomical and clinical approach. Philadelphia: J.B. Lippincott Co. 1986;232–235.

4. Aids to the examination of the peripheral nervous system. 3rd ed. London: Bailliere Tindall, 1986.

5. Devinsky O. Examination of the cranial and peripheral nerves. New York: Churchill-Livingstone, 1988.

6. Goodgold J. Anatomical correlates of clinical electromyography. 2nd ed. Baltimore: Williams & Wilkins, 1984.

7. Liveson JA, Ma DM. Laboratory reference for clinical neurophysiology. Philadelphia: F.A. Davis Co., 1992; 408–414.

8. DeLisa JA, Mackenzie K, Baran EM. Manual of nerve conduction velocity and clinical neurophysiology. 3rd ed. New York: Raven Press, 1994.

9. Wolf JK. Segmental neurology: a guide to the examination and interpretation of sensory and motor function. Baltimore: University Park Press, 1981.
   A 150 page, profusely illustrated treasure trove monograph on the clinical evaluation of patients with disorders of the peripheral nervous system. Includes unique, sophisticated methods for muscle strength examination, and a historical discussion of the origin of dermatome and myotome charts, useful in providing perspective. Marvelous photographs of the cutaneous distribution of roots and nerves from the writings of Cushing and Foerster. Concludes with signature syndromes of the spinal roots. Unfortunately out of print and probably stolen from your local library.

10. Miles TS. The control of human motor units. Clin Exp Pharmacol Physiol 1994;21:511–520.
    The motor unit, consisting of a single motor neuron and the skeletal muscle fibers that it innervates, is the final output pathway of the motor system. This review briefly summarizes some recent data that has contributed to the understanding of the way that human motor neurons are recruited and controlled during voluntary and reflex movements.

11. Gath I, Stalberg E. In situ measurement of the innervation ratio of motor units in human muscles. Exp Brain Res 1981;43:377–382.
    The attenuation constant K and time constant tau of the muscle tissue transfer function were measured, and the average electrode uptake area calculated for the brachial biceps, tibialis anterior, and deltoid muscles. The average number of muscle fibers in the motor unit, i.e., the innervation ratio, was calculated from the electrode uptake area, data on the motor unit territory, and measurements of fibre density. The innervation ratios for the brachial biceps, tibialis anterior, and deltoid were 209, 329, and 239 fibers, respectively. It was found that the anatomical scatter of fibers belonging to the same motor unit was smaller in brachial biceps than in tibialis anterior, whereas the electrophysiological "fibre density" was higher in tibialis anterior.

12. McComas-AJ. Invited review: motor unit estimation: methods, results, and present status. Muscle Nerve 1991;14:585–597.
    Using motor unit counting techniques in normal subjects, the EDB muscle has approximately 200 motor units while each of the intrinsic muscles of the hand has about 100 units; larger muscles in the limbs contain greater numbers of units. Beyond

the age of 60 years, there is a decline in the number of functioning motor units in both proximal and distal muscles.

13. Phillips LH, Park TS. Electrophysiologic mapping of the segmental anatomy of the muscles of the lower extremity. Muscle Nerve 1991;14:1213–1218.
   Direct electrophysiologic measurements of the root innervation of the lower extremity were done while performing selective posterior rhizotomy for treatment of spasticity. The ventral roots from L2 to S2 were stimulated while recording from all muscles simultaneously, using the size of the evoked CMAP as an indication of the amount of innervation derived from stimulation of a given spinal root. The major root innervation for the 8 muscles studied was: adductor longus, vastus medialis, and vastus lateralis, L3; tibialis anterior; L4; peroneus longus, L5; and medial gastrocnemius, lateral gastrocnemius, and gluteus maximus, S1. In general, each muscle received innervation from 3 or more roots. Prefixed or postfixed innervation patterns were found in 27.9% of legs examined, and there was asymmetry of innervation in 29.8%. The authors conclude that the segmental innervation of lower extremity muscles is broader than previously thought, and anomalous innervation occurs so frequently that caution should be used in attributing any pattern of clinical or EMG findings to a specific spinal level.

14. Liguori R, Krarup C, Trojaborg W. Determination of the segmental sensory and motor innervation of the lumbosacral spinal nerves. An electrophysiological study. Brain 1992;115:915–934.
   Sensory and motor segmental innervation of the lower extremities was examined by electrophysiological methods in 29 subjects by placing needle electrodes close to the spinal nerve at root levels from L3 to S2. Sensory innervation was determined by recording the SNAP evoked by stimulating the saphenous nerve at the medial epicondyle (mainly L3 and L4) and at the medial malleolus (mainly L4 and some L3), the medial plantar nerve at the first plantar interstice (mainly S1, some L5 and S2), the deep peroneal nerve at the first dorsal interstice (mainly L5, some S1), the sural nerve at the dorsolateral aspect of the foot (mainly S1, some L5 and S2) and at the lateral malleolus (mainly S1, some L5 and S2), and the superficial peroneal nerve at the superior extensor retinaculum (mainly L5, S1). The motor innervation was determined by stimulating the spinal nerves supramaximally and recording the evoked responses from the medial and lateral vastus (mainly L3, L4), the anterior tibial (mainly L5), the peroneus longus (L5, S1), the extensor digitorum brevis (mainly S1), the gastrocnemius (mainly S1), the abductor hallucis (mainly S2) and the biceps femoris (mainly L5, S1).

15. Levin KH, Maggiano HJ, Wilbourn AJ. Cervical radiculopathies: comparison of surgical and EMG localization of single root lesions. Neurology 1996;46:1022–1025.
   See Chapter 14 for abstract.

16. Lauder TD, Dillingham TR. The cervical radiculopathy screen: optimizing the number of muscles studied. Muscle Nerve 1996;19:662–665.
   See Chapter 14 for abstract.

17. Lauder TD, Dillingham TR, Huston CW, et al. Lumbosacral radiculopathy screen. Optimizing the number of muscles studies [see comments]. Am J Phys Med Rehabil 1994;73:394–402.
   See Chapter 14 for abstract.

18. Katirji MB, Agrawal R, Kantra TA. The human cervical myotomes: an anatomical correlation between electromyography and CT/myelography. Muscle Nerve 1988; 11:1070–1073.
   The correlation between EMG and metrizamide myelography/computerized tomography was evaluated in 20 patients with cervical radiculopathy. The root involved, using the EMG examination and the myotome chart of the Medical Research Council, was C5 in 3 patients, C6 in 6, C7 in 9 patients, and C8 in 2 patients. The overall correlation with myelography/CT was 65% (33.3, 66.6, 77.7, and 50% for C5, C6, C7, and C8, respectively). EMG done properly has a good correlation of myelography/CT. This correlation is higher (73.3%) for the commonly occurring cervical radiculopathies (C6 and C7).

19. Mukherji SK, Castillo M, Wagle AG. The brachial plexus. Semin Ultrasound CT MR 1996;17:519–538.
   A nice review, profusely illustrated, of the classic, surgical, and radiologic anatomy of the brachial plexus.

20. Botte MJ, Cohen MS, Lavernia CJ, et al. The dorsal branch of the ulnar nerve: an anatomic study. J Hand Surg Am 1990;15:603–607.
   In 24 cadaver dissections, the dorsal ulnar cutaneous nerve arose from the medial aspect of the ulnar nerve at an average distance of 6.4 centimeters from the distal aspect of the head of the ulna and 8.3 centimeters from the proximal border of the pisiform. Its mean diameter at origin was 2.4 millimeters. The nerve passed dorsal to the flexor carpi ulnaris and pierced the deep fascia. It became subcutaneous on the medial aspect of the forearm at a mean distance of 5.0 centimeters from the proximal edge of the pisiform.

21. Lindsey JT, Watumull D. Anatomic study of the ulnar nerve and related vascular anatomy at Guyon's canal: a practical classification system. J Hand Surg Am 1996;21:626–633.
   Thirty-one fresh adult upper extremities were microdissected in order to delineate the regional anatomy of the ulnar nerve and artery at the wrist. Two patterns of division of the ulnar nerve trunk were identified (A and B), and 3 patterns of hypothenar muscle innervation (types 1, 2, and 3) Pattern A occurred in 25 of the specimens where the ulnar nerve bifurcated into a main sensory trunk and a motor branch. Pattern B occurred in 6 of the specimens where the ulnar nerve trifurcated into two common digital sensory branches and a motor branch. The hypothenar innervation patterns were categorized as follows: type 1, 10 cases, single branch; type 2, 14 cases, two branches; and type 3, 7 cases, three or more branches. See also Cobb TK, Carmichael SW, Cooney WP. Guyon's canal revisited: an anatomic study of the carpal ulnar neurovascular space. J Hand Surg Br 1996;21:861–869.

22. Amoiridis G. Median—ulnar nerve communications and anomalous innervation of the intrinsic hand muscles: an electrophysiological study. Muscle Nerve 1992;15:576–579.
   In this study of 100 arms using surface electrodes, a motor median-to-ulnar nerve anastomosis occurred in the forearm in 32% of the cases (Martin-Gruber anastomosis, MGA). No case of motor ulnar-to-median nerve anastomosis could be found. The MGA mainly innervated muscles normally supplied by the ulnar nerve. Stimulus spread must be eliminated. See also: Nakashima T. An anatomic study on the Martin-Gruber anastomosis. Surg Radiol Anat 1993;15:193–195.

23. Ajmani ML. Variations in the motor nerve supply of the thenar and hypothenar muscles of the hand. J Anat 1996;189:145–150.

The distribution pattern of the muscular branch of median and ulnar nerves and motor innervation of the thenar and hypothenar muscles were studied in 68 palmar regions taken from 34 adult cadavers. In 13 of the 68 hands an anastomosis was seen between the ulnar and median nerves.

24. Stanescu S, Post J, Ebraheim NA, et al. Surgical anatomy of the radial nerve in the arm: practical considerations of the branching patterns to the triceps brachii. Orthopedics 1996;19:311–315.

    In 33 cadaveric dissections performed to identify radial nerve branching patterns to the triceps brachii, innervation of the long head of the triceps originated in the axilla in 88% and the brachio-axillary angle in 12%. Innervation of the medial head of the triceps originated in the spiral groove in 52% of the cases, the brachio-axillary angle in 39%, and the axilla in 9%. The lateral head was innervated by branches arising in the spiral groove in 70% of the cases, the brachio-axillary angle in 24%, and the axilla in 6%. On average, the radial nerve crossed the midline in the proximal 45% of the arm, 3 cm superior to the level of the deltoid insertion.

25. Auerbach DM, Collins ED, Kunkle KL, et al. The radial sensory nerve. An anatomic study. Clin Orthop 1994; 241–249.

    In 20 cadaver forearm dissections, the superficial branch of the radial nerve was found to arise between the tendons of the brachioradialis and extensor carpi radialis longus 8.6 cm proximal to the radial styloid, piercing the forearm fascia 6.0 cm from the radial styloid. Innervation to the dorsum of the digits was variable, with 45% of specimens innervating the radial 2½ digits and 30% innervating the radial 3½ digits.

26. Prasartritha T, Liupolvanish P, Rojanakit A. A study of the posterior interosseous nerve (PIN) and the radial tunnel in 30 Thai cadavers. J Hand Surg Am 1993;18: 107–112.

    In 60 cadaver dissections, the radial tunnel began in the furrow between the brachioradialis and brachialis in the distal arm and ended at the distal edge of the supinator muscle in the proximal forearm. The radial nerve pierced the lateral intermuscular septum 13 cm above the elbow joint line. At 1.3 cm above the joint line the nerve divided into its posterior interosseous and superficial radial branches. The extensor carpi radialis brevis muscle received nerve supply from the superficial radial nerve, radial nerve, and posterior interosseous in 43%, 55%, and 2%, respectively. The posterior interosseous passed through the radial tunnel anterior to the radiohumeral joint and then coursed laterally and posteriorly beneath the arcade of Frohse, which is the proximal edge of the superficial layer of the supinator muscle. The arcade was tendinous in 57% of the cadavers and membranous in 43%. The distal edge of the supinator was tendinous in 65% of the specimens and membranous in 35%. No specimens showed evidence of posterior interosseous compression in the radial tunnel. See also: Debouck C, Rooze M. The arcade of Frohse: an anatomic study. Surg Radiol Anat 1995;17:245–248.

27. Abrams RA, Ziets RJ, Lieber RL, et al. Anatomy of the radial nerve motor branches in the forearm. J Hand Surg Am 1997;22:232–237.

    In 20 cadaver dissections of radial nerve motor branch anatomy in the forearm, though variable in individual specimens, innervation order from proximal to distal (based on mean shortest branch lengths) was brachioradialis, extensor carpi radialis longus, supinator, extensor carpi radialis brevis, extensor digitorum communis, extensor carpi ulnaris, extensor digiti quinti, abductor pollicis longus, extensor pollicis longus, extensor pollicis brevis, and extensor indicis proprius. In 10 specimens, branches innervated the brachialis. Mean distances from a point 100 mm proximal to the lateral epicondyle to the muscle measured along the shortest nerve branch ranged from 97.2 mm for the brachioradialis to 299.8 mm for the EIP.

28. Yang ZX, Pho RW, Kour AK, et al. The musculocutaneous nerve and its branches to the biceps and brachialis muscles. J Hand Surg Am 1995;20:671–675.

    In 24 cadavers, the musculocutaneous nerve and its motor branches to the biceps and brachialis were dissected. The motor branch to the biceps exits from the musculocutaneous nerve at 119 mm distal to the coracoid process. Anatomic variations were seen in the innervation of the two heads of the biceps. The motor branch to the brachialis muscle exits from the musculocutaneous nerve 170 mm distal to the coracoid process.

29. Farny J, Drolet P, Girard M. Anatomy of the posterior approach to the lumbar plexus block. Can J Anaesth 1994;41:480–485.

    In 4 cadaver dissections and 22 CT files of the lumbosacral region, the lumbar plexus, at the level of L5, was within the substance of the psoas major muscle. The femoral nerve lies between the lateral femoral cutaneous and obturator nerves. Radiological data provided measurements of the depth of various structures.

30. Akita K, Sakamoto H, Sato T. Arrangement and innervation of the glutei medius and minimus and the piriformis: a morphological analysis. Anat Rec 1994;238:125–130.

    In dissections of 49 pelvic halves of 28 cadavers, the superior gluteal nerve ran on the ventral surface of the piriformis in 89.8% (Type A), and some branches of the nerve perforated the piriformis in 10.2% (Type B). Based on the detailed findings of the innervation of the three muscles, the piriformis is chiefly composed of the caudal element of the gluteus medius (Type A) and in some cases the caudal element of the gluteus minimus as well (Type B).

31. Aszmann OC, Dellon ES, Dellon AL. Anatomical course of the lateral femoral cutaneous nerve and its susceptibility to compression and injury. Plast Reconstr Surg 1997;100:600–604.

    The anatomy of the lateral femoral cutaneous nerve was investigated through dissection of 52 human anatomic specimens. The variability of its course and locations as it exits the pelvis is described and related to soft-tissue and bony landmarks. Five different types are identified: type A, posterior to the anterior superior iliac spine, across the iliac crest (4 percent); type B, anterior to the anterior superior iliac spine and superficial to the origin of the sartorius muscle but within the substance of the inguinal ligament (27 percent); type C, medial to the anterior superior iliac spine, ensheathed in the tendinous origin of the sartorius muscle (23 percent); type D, medial to the origin of the sartorius muscle located in an interval between the tendon of the sartorius muscle and thick fascia of the iliopsoas muscle deep to the inguinal ligament (26 percent); and type E, most medial and embedded in loose connective tissue, deep to the inguinal ligament, overlying the thin fascia of the iliopsoas muscle, and contributing the femoral branch of the genitofemoral nerve (20 percent). The results of this study suggest that the lateral femoral cutaneous nerve is most susceptible to mechanical trauma when the nerve is type A, B, or C.

4

Membrane Physiology and Volume Conduction

This chapter covers concepts of basic membrane physiology and volume conduction pertinent to clinical electrodiagnosis. The origin of the resting membrane potential, mechanisms of depolarization, and genesis and propagation of the action potential are all relevant. Concepts from basic electronics arise frequently, including resistance, capacitance, current and potential difference. For the purposes of this discussion, it is more helpful to think in terms of conventional current (the flow of positive charges, or hole current) rather than true current (the flow of electrons).

Resting Membrane Potential

The cell membrane is a lipid-protein bilayer sparsely studded with specialized pores or channels. The membrane is relatively permeable to lipid soluble substances but impermeable to water and water soluble substances. It separates two electrolytic solutions of different ionic composition and concentrations, the extracellular fluid and the intracellular fluid. An essential feature of excitable membranes is selective ionic permeability, mediated by the action of ion channels that control the passage of ions through the membrane. Under certain circumstances, channels may be open to a particular ion and under other circumstances may be closed.

Ion channels are complex protein macromolecules that are embedded in and span the membrane, connecting the intracellular and extracellular compartments (1,2). The channel has a central pore selective for one or more ions (3). The pore may be open or closed; when open, ions can traverse the channel. Channels may alternate between the open and closed configuration depending on chemical or electrical events in the microenvironment. Some channels are voltage-dependent or voltage-gated; their state varies depending on the transmembrane potential (TMP). For voltage gated channels, changes in membrane potential produce dramatic fluctuations in permeability, from completely closed, to slightly "ajar" (equivalent to having a proportion of the channels open; individual voltage gated channels do not exist in such an intermediate state) to wide open (all channels activated and conducting). Other channels are ligand gated; their configurational changes are induced by neurotransmitters, such as acetylcholine (ACh). The conformational change in the channel can occur rapidly, with the pore snapping open or closed instantaneously, or the channel may remain momentarily in one state before it can revert to the other, becoming transiently refractory to its usual stimuli during the transition.

Abnormalities in the behavior of these channels produces a variety of clinical syndromes, referred to as channelopathies (4). For example, myasthenia gravis attacks the ligand gated ACh receptor on the postsynaptic membrane. The voltage gated Ca++ channels on the presynaptic membrane are involved in Lambert-Eaton myasthenic syndrome (LEMS), K+ channels in Isaac's syndrome, and Na+ channels in paramyotonia congenita. Selected conditions and agents affecting channel function are listed in Table 4.1.

A nerve or muscle cell at rest is in osmotic equilibrium. The osmotically active particles in the extracellular space are primarily ions and other inorganic substances. The intracellular fluid contains vast stores of protein anions, primarily sulfates and phosphates, and some counterbalancing cations. The large protein anions are caged in the cell's interior, unable to cross the membrane because of their size. The smaller, more mobile cations can cross the membrane when their ion channel is open.

Electrolytes on either side of the membrane are distributed in different concentrations related to the electrochemical forces acting on them. Electrical equilibrium requires electrical neutrality intracellularly as well as extracellularly. But the intracellular and extracellular spaces are at different equilibrium levels. Along the boundary between them a charge differential exists, creating an electrical potential across the membrane, which favors the movement of each ion species in a particular direction. There is

TABLE 4.1
Sample of Syndromes and Agents That Affect Channel Function*

Sodium channel
   Hyperkalemic periodic paralysis (dysfunction of inactivation gate)
   Normokalemic periodic paralysis
   Paramyotonia congenita (dysfunction of inactivation gate)
   K+ sensitive myotonia congenita
   Tetrodotoxin (blocks extracellular mouth of ionopore)
   Saxitoxin (blocks channel, similar mechanism to tetrodotoxin)
   Ciguatoxin (opens channel)
   Local anesthetics (block cytoplasmic mouth of ionopore)
   Cardiac antiarrhythmics
   Some anticonvulsants
   Some neuroprotectants
   Cocaine (channel blockade)
Potassium channel
   Episodic ataxia with myokymia
   Continuous muscle fiber activity syndromes
   Tetraethylammonium
   Aminopyridine compounds
   Cocaine (channel blockade)
Chloride channel
   Myotonia congenita (both dominant and recessive forms)
Calcium channel
   Hypokalemic periodic paralysis
   Calcium channel blocking agents

---

* The precise mechanism is known for some (16,17).

also an impetus for ions to diffuse from higher concentration to lower, the chemical potential. These two forces create a net electrochemical potential gradient for each ion. In some cases, both the concentration and electrical gradient favor movement in a given direction; in other instances the forces counterbalance.

The Na+ concentration outside the cell is about 140 mEq/L, K+ about 4 mEq/L, and Cl- about 125 mEq/L, i.e, the levels of normal serum electrolytes. The concentration of different electrolytes inside the cell varies from cell to cell; as an approximation, [K+] is about 30X greater inside than out, and [Na+] is about 12X greater outside than in (Fig. 4.1).

Whether an ion moves across the membrane along its electrochemical gradient depends on the permeability (p), or the conductance (g), of the membrane. The p and g values in turn depend on the TMP. The TMP in turn depends on the electrochemical equilibrium potential of the membrane permeable ions. It is a complex, reciprocal relationship. In the resting state, essentially all the Na+ channels are closed and p is very low, while a small proportion of the K+ channels are open. The membrane at rest is much more permeable to K+ (by a factor of 50–100), and the equilibrium potential for K+ therefore largely determines the level of the resting potential.

The Na/K pump helps maintain the membrane potential. Energy derived from ATP is expended in maintaining the potential by reinforcing the exclusion of Na+. The voltage gated Na+ channels (VGNCs), although mostly closed, permit a slight inward leak. The Na/K pump actively exchanges Na+ and K+, simultaneously moving 3 Na+ ions from inside to outside and 2 K+ ions from outside to inside. The 3:2 ratio causes a continuous net loss of positive charge, and contributes a small additional internal negativity of approximately -4 mV beyond that due to ionic diffusion alone.

When the membrane is permeable to an ion, its electrochemical equilibrium potential (E), at which there is no net flow across the membrane, is described by the Nernst equation. The equation includes the gas constant (R), the Faraday constant (F, relating charge and concentration), the valence of the ion (n), and the temperature, to yield:

$$E_{ion} = \frac{RT}{nF} \ln \frac{[ion]_{outside}}{[ion]_{inside}}$$

At physiologic temperature, the Nernst equation can be reduced to:

$$E_{ion} = 58 \log \frac{[ion]_{outside}}{[ion]_{inside}}$$

The equilibrium potentials vary from cell to cell. The E_K is about -70 to -90 mV, the E_{Na} about $+60$mV, and the E_{Cl} about -70 mV.

The Goldman constant field equation is a refinement of the Nernst equation, which takes into account the conductance of the membrane to each individual ion, as well as its intracellular and extracellular concentration, to yield a value for the membrane potential, E_M. Since the membrane potential depends primarily on Na+ and K+, the Goldman equation can be simplified to:

$$E_M = 58 \log \frac{g_{NaK}[K+]_{outside} + g_{Na}[Na+]_{outside}}{g_{NaK}[K+]_{inside} + g_{NaNa}+]_{inside}}$$

Because the membrane at rest is 50–100 times more permeable to K+ than to Na+, the value of E_M, about -70 for a nerve cell and -90 mV for a muscle cell, is determined primarily by the E_K. (Fig. 4.2).

In summary, the membrane at rest is much more permeable to K+ than to Na+. It is in dynamic equilibrium, a steady state with no net ionic fluxes across it. The concentration of K+ is high on the interior; it tends to move outward down its concentration gradient but is held in check by the strong intracellular negativity. The E_K is at -90 mV and the voltage dependent channels are largely closed. Na+ is at high concentration outside and both the electrical and chemical gradients favor movement inside, but the VGNCs are closed. The few Na+ ions entering the cell are extruded by the Na+/K+ ATPase pump. The Cl- ions tend to follow passively and the membrane permeability to Cl− is fairly constant, so it makes no major contribution. With the membrane more permeable to K+ than Na+, the resting TMP is near the E_K of -90 mV, and far from the E_{Na} of +60 mV. The membrane is poised for action.

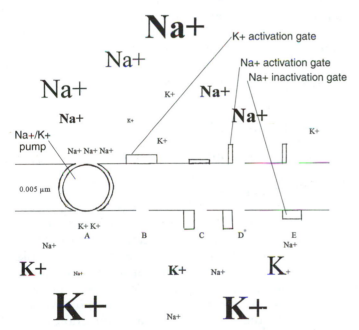

FIGURE 4.1. A representation of the membrane, thickness 0.005 μm, with the relative concentrations of Na+ and K+ on the extracellular (top) and intracellular (bottom) sides. The gaps in the membrane indicate the position of channels. At A is the Na+/K+ pump, which has exchanged 3 Na+ molecules for 2 K+ molecules. At B is the K+ channel in its inactivated (closed) state. At C the Na+ activation gate (top) is closed and the inactivation gate (bottom) is open; the Na+ channel is at rest and ready for activation. At D, the Na+ channel's activation and inactivation gates are both open and the channel is conducting. At E, the inactivation gate has closed, the channel is no longer conducting and cannot again conduct until the channel returns to a resting configuration.

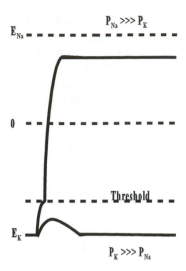

FIGURE 4.2. At rest the membrane's permeability (P) to K+ is much higher than to Na+, and the membrane potential (E_M) is close to the E_K. With subthreshold depolarizations, the P_{Na} increases but Na+ entry remains less than K+ exit and the membrane returns to baseline. With suprathreshold depolarizations, the increase in P_{Na} is overwhelming, Na+ entry greatly exceeds K+ exit and the membrane potential approaches E_{Na}.

Bioelectric Properties of Cells and Membranes

Other biophysical and electrical properties of the membrane are important to consider. The intracellular and extracellular charges separated by the cell membrane constitute a capacitor. Recall from basic electronics that a capacitor is made up of positive and negative charges, separated by an insulating material, or dielectric. In the case of the membrane, the negative charges on the interior are separated from the positive charges on the exterior by the insulating cell membrane. A capacitor can store charge, the amount directly proportional to the size of the "plates," the dielectric constant of the insulator, and the driving voltage of the source; and inversely proportional to the distance between the plates (the thickness of the membrane). The higher the capacitance the more charge can be stored.

$$\text{Capacitance} \propto (\text{dielectric constant}) \times \left(\frac{\text{area of the membrane}}{\text{thickness of the membrane}} \right)$$

The membrane also has resistance to the flow of ionic charges across it. In electronic terms, the membrane can then be viewed as a succession of capacitors and resistors (Fig. 4.3). Capacitors have time constants, which describe the length of time required for the capacitor to charge or discharge. Charging and discharging occur exponentially, and the time constant is the interval necessary to charge to 63% or discharge to 37% of the initial value. The membrane time constant (MTC) is related to the resistance and capacitance of the membrane (TC=R X C); the higher the capacitance the longer the time required for the membrane to charge and discharge. Membrane capacitance is typically about $1\mu F/cm^2$.

Another important bioelectric attribute of the membrane is its ability to filter. Recall from basic electronics that most analog filter circuits are composed of a capacitor and resistor in series (RC circuits). The capacitor is a reactive element, it "reacts to" changes in frequency. Tissue capacitance creates a clinically important filtering effect, tending to remove high frequency components, especially from motor unit action potentials and possibly from fibrillation potential (see Appendix). A motor unit recorded at any substantial distance from the fibers producing it has a blunted main spike, because the high frequency components have been filtered out, with much less change in its duration, because the low frequency components have been passed through.

Cable Properties

Nerve and muscle fibers are long, cylindrical structures, similar to the wires and cables carrying electricity to the EMG machine. All wires have resistance, which is determined by the resistivity of the material, and by the length and diameter of the wire. Cable properties, also referred to as electrotonic properties, are the passive electrical attributes of the excitable cell; they are not related to any permeability changes. An understanding of cable properties aids in appreciating the factors that determine impulse propagation velocity and the changes, such as conduction block and conduction velocity slowing, which occur with demyelination.

The membrane space constant, or length constant (MLC), defines the electrotonic decay of a potential as it spreads down a fiber. As the potential travels along the fiber, there is transverse leakage of current across the membrane, the leakage current. The magnitude of the transverse leakage current is determined by the transmembrane resistance (TMR). In addition, the internal longitudinal resistance (ILR) of the cable acts to oppose the flow of the internal longitudinal current (ILC). As a result of these effects, the peak amplitude of the potential decays exponentially as a function of distance. The MLC is that distance at which the amplitude has declined to 37% of the original value (Fig. 4.3).

Three main effects function to inhibit the spread of an impulse down a nerve or muscle "cable": high ILR, high capacitance, and low transmembrane resistance (TMR). When the ILR is high, the MLC is short, and the potential decrements very rapidly. In small diameter axons, the MLC may be only a few hundred μm. When the TMR is low, the transverse leakage of current is substantial, also serving to shorten the MLC. When capacitance is high, impulse propagation is very slow because of the long MTC; it requires a protracted period of time to discharge the membrane's capacitance at each location before the action potential can move on. So, short space constants and long time constants retard impulse propagation.

In the mammalian nervous system, countermeasures to these impulse propagation impediments are to enlarge and myelinate the fiber. An increase in the diameter of the fiber lowers the ILR and lengthens the space constant. Myelination serves to bolster the TMR, lengthening the space constant, and to decrease the capacitance by increasing the charge separation, thus shortening the time constant.

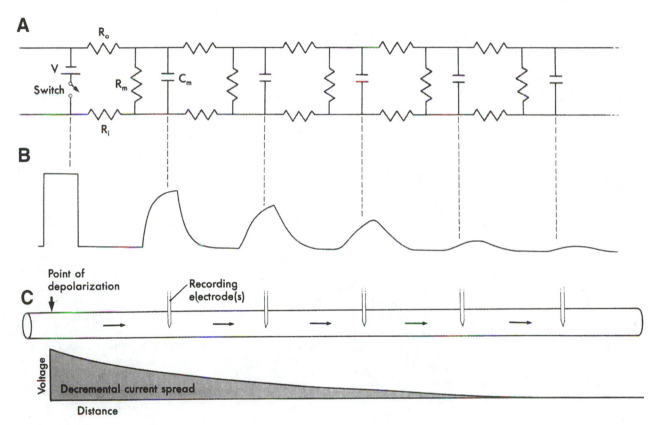

FIGURE 4.3. The membrane acts as an insulator separating internal negative and external positive charges, creating a capacitor. The transmembrane resistance (TMR) opposes the movement of charges across the membrane. The membrane can be viewed as a string of parallel arrayed resistors and capacitors. The thickness of the membrane directly affects the capacitance. A thicker membrane, with a wider separation of charges, as occurs with myelination, has a lower capacitance and a reduced ability to store charge. The internal longitudinal resistance (ILR) opposes the flow of charges down the nerve or muscle fiber. The ILR depends on the resistivity of the fiber and is inversely related to fiber diameter. When a voltage pulse is applied (at the switch), the signals recorded at intervals down the fiber demonstrate decremental conduction, with the pulse amplitude decreasing over distance. The distance over which the amplitude declines to 37% of the initial value is the membrane length, or space, constant. High Cm, high ILR or low Rm shorten the length constant. Cm, membrane capacitance; Rm, transmembrane resistance; Ri, internal longitudinal resistance; Ro, external longitudinal resistance. Reprinted with permission from Brown PB. The electrochemical basis of neuronal integration. In: Haines DE, ed. Fundamental Neuroscience. New York: Churchill Livingstone, 1997;31–49.

The Action Potential

The membrane potential can change in two ways. If it moves toward zero, becoming less negative, it is said to be depolarized. If it moves away from zero, becoming more negative, it is said to be hyperpolarized. There are two basic types of changes in the membrane potential: propagated and non-propagated. Generator potentials and endplate potentials are non-propagated, local or graded responses, whose magnitude depends on the intensity and distribution of the changes in the ion channels. An endplate potential may decay back to normal and never propagate beyond the immediate vicinity. Non-propagated potentials result from changes involving a single type of channel, such as the endplate potential reflecting activation of the ligand gated ACh receptor channel. The action potential is a propagated potential conducted in an all or none fashion down the nerve or muscle membrane, due to the sequential activation and deactivation of the voltage gated Na+ and K+ channels. Whether a propagated potential develops depends on whether a membrane depolarization reaches threshold.

The state of most Na+ and K+ gates depends on the membrane voltage; their conformational state varies as a function of the membrane potential (Fig. 4.1). The voltage gated K+ channel (VGKC) is relatively simple, with a single gate that is either open (activated) or closed (inactivated). With depolarization of the membrane, the gates shift toward the activated state with a time course dependent on the channel's kinetics. The VGNC has both an activation gate and an inactivation gate (5–7). The VGKC channel closes simply by deactivating its single gate; the VGNC closes by mobilizing its deactivation gate. At rest, the VGNC's activation gate is closed and the deactivation gate open. With depolarization, the activation gate opens and the channel transmits freely. The deactivation gate then closes and the channel ceases operations, then returns to its resting state. The closing of the deactivation gates is slow and sluggish in comparison to the opening of the activation gates (Fig. 4.4).

So, in the course of the action potential, three different events, each with its own kinetics, are occurring: activation/deactivation of VGKCs, activation of VGNCs, and deactivation of VGNCs. Of these, the VGNC activation is quickest; VGNC inactivation and VGKC activation/deactivation are both about 10 times slower than VGNC activation. Once triggered, changes in the VGNC cycle according to a fixed time course, but the VGKCs remain open as long as the membrane is depolarized. Each channel alteration produces a corresponding change in membrane permeability.

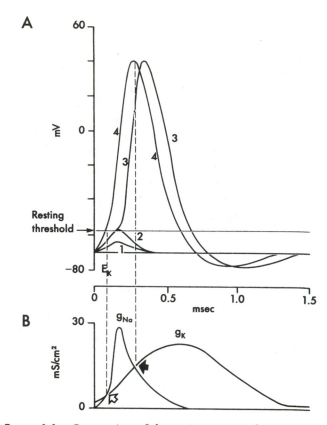

FIGURE 4.4.   Generation of the action potential. Four curves illustrate the response to four different levels of stimulation in A, with membrane conductance changes in B. In curve 1, a subthreshold stimulus produces an increase in g_{Na+}, but the g_{Na+} still remains $< g_{K+}$, and the RMP returns to the resting level without triggering an action potential. In curve 2, a stimulus is just at threshold, teetering on the brink. An action potential will result, by definition, 50% of the time. The rise in g_{Na+} is slow and the action potential, if triggered, requires longer to develop. In curve 4, a suprathreshold stimulus quickly depolarizes the membrane to threshold and triggers an action potential. Once triggered, an action potential has the same amplitude in either case. The conductance changes are shown in B. At the peak of the action potential, g_{Na+} is at its maximum and the E_m approaches E_{Na+}. The decline in g_{Na+} is due to closure of the inactivation gates. The delayed increase in g_{K+} permits the membrane to repolarize much more rapidly than would be the case if only Na+ inactivation and the Na+/K+ pump were available to restore the RMP. The arrows indicate the points at which $g_{Na+} = g_{K+}$, at threshold (open arrow) and at the peak of the action potential (closed arrow).

Threshold

A local, non-propagated potential occurs if the membrane becomes only slightly depolarized. Any depolarization >10 mV produces opening of a few VGNCs and Na+ enters the cell. This neutralizes some of the interior negativity and allows a few K+ ions to flow out of the cell down the concentration gradient. At rest, enough VGKCs are already open for the RMP to approximate E_{K+}, so if only a few VGNCs are activated then K+ permeability is still greater than Na+ permeability. If the depolarization terminates at this point, enough K+ has left the cell to compensate for the Na+ which entered. After about 1 ms, VGNC inactivation and VGKC activation occur, annihilating the paltry results of the VGNC activation, and the membrane is repolarized. This is a subthreshold depolarization. With depolarizations > 15–20 mV, the number of VGNCs opening is great enough to overcome the increased driving force for K+ egress. Increasing depolarization causes the remaining Na+ gates to open *en masse*, and the process becomes overwhelming, generating a self perpetuating, all or none action potential.

Threshold is defined as the level of depolarization that produces an action potential 50% of the time (8). For subthreshold depolarizations Na+ entry is < K+ exit. For threshold depolarizations, Na+ entry is > K+ exit (Fig. 4.4). Just at threshold, the membrane teeters between a potential that fades out and one that produces an action potential.

The action potential can be conceptualized as two separate events: a depolarization cycle and a repolarization cycle (8). Once threshold is exceeded, the opening of VGNCs becomes self perpetuating and the membrane becomes freely permeable to Na+, with a conductance approximately 5,000 fold higher than at baseline. As the most permeable ion, Na+ determines the level of the membrane potential, which very rapidly approaches the E_{Na+} of about +60 mV. This is the main spike of the action potential. The membrane does not reach +60 mV because following close on the heels of VGNC activation is VGNC inactivation, which retards the rise of the action potential spike. If VGNC inactivation were the only process available to restore the RMP, it would slowly return to its resting level of −70 to −90 mV through the loss of K+ via those VGKCs that are always open and the action of the Na+/K+ pump. The activation of VGKCs in response to depolarization allows for the accelerated diffusion of positive charges out of the cell, and speeds repolarization.

There is no separate process of deactivation for the VGKCs as there is for the VGNCs, rather the VGKCs simply close as the membrane is repolarized. This phase requires a certain finite period, so that the VGKCs tend to remain open, and K+ permeability increased, even after the membrane is repolarized (Fig. 4.4). This trailing effect leads to transient membrane hyperpolarization, as K+ continues to flow out of the cell along its concentration gradient, increasing the internal negativity by a further 10–20 mV. As all the ion permeabilities normalize, the membrane potential returns to its baseline, resting level.

The membrane potential depends, in essence, on the ratio of p_{Na+} to p_{K+} (Fig. 4.2). When p_{K+} is much higher, the membrane potential approximates E_{K+}; the normal RMP. When p_{Na+} is much higher, the membrane potential approaches E_{Na+}. Conductances are equal just at threshold and at the peak of the action potential (Fig. 4.4). The resting levels and the ratio of p_{Na+} and p_{K+} vary considerably in different tissues. In skeletal muscle, p_{K+} is higher than in nerve, so muscle fiber action potentials tend to exhibit minimal if any terminal hyperpolarization.

Once initiated, the action potential runs through a fixed cycle of events determined by the inherent kinetics of the different channels. The refractory period (RP) is an interval during the action potential cycle when a second action potential can be produced with difficulty (the relative RP) or not at all (the absolute RP). The absolute RP extends throughout the rising phase and part of the falling phase of the action potential. It reflects the fact that the VGNCs, although inactivated, have not returned to their baseline resting state. Inactivated VGNCs are not excitable, only resting channels are. During the relative RP, many but not all VGNCs have returned to the resting state, and the VGKCs are still activated. During this phase, it is possible to rekindle an action potential, but it requires a higher than normal stimulating current, and the resulting action potential is of lower amplitude and conducts more slowly than normal.

Conduction along Nerve and Muscle Fibers

An action potential tends to crawl along the membrane of an unmyelinated nerve fiber or a muscle cell by continuous conduction (Fig. 4.5). As any finite point is depolarized, the positive charges now on the membrane interior tend to attract and neutralize the negative charges on the immediately contiguous inner membrane. This makes the neighboring segment of membrane less interior negative, depolarizing it to threshold and spawning another action potential. Continuous conduction is a slow process. The depolarization cycle in the active sector must bring the abutting inactive membrane to threshold. The capacitance on the adjoining segment of membrane must be discharged by the flow of depolarizing current.

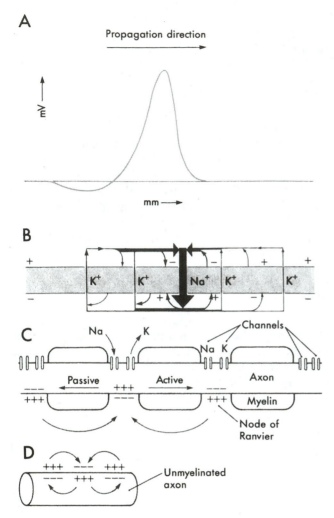

FIGURE 4.5. Current paths during the propagation of the action potential (A) are shown in an electrical circuit of a membrane (B) and in a myelinated (C) and an unmyelinated axon (D).

When capacitance is high, the time constant for discharge of the membrane is long, and the process can be lengthy.

The depolarizing current flowing from the previously depolarized segment must be of sufficient magnitude to bring the newly depolarizing membrane segment to threshold. If the fiber is of small diameter (producing a high ILR) or has low TMR (causing high transverse leakage current), the membrane length constant may be short. With a short length constant, the depolarizing current flow dissipates quickly over a short distance.

The magnitude of the current that is flowing to depolarize the adjacent segment in comparison to that needed for the task is referred to as the safety factor. When safety factor is high, ample current is available to discharge the capacitance of the neighboring membrane and bring it to threshold; perpetuation of the action potential is assured. When current flow is not robust, the safety factor becomes marginal. With a borderline safety factor, depolarization of the adjacent segment is not assured, and, depending on other factors, conduction may fail. When safety factor is too low, the impulse does not propagate. For impulse propagation to proceed, safety factor must be > 1; in large, myelinated fibers it may be up to 7 (8) (Fig. 4.6).

All other things being equal, the impulse conduction velocity (CV) is directly related to fiber size. Resistivity is an innate property of the axoplasm. The resistance is directly related to the resistivity and inversely proportional to the diameter, so a larger fiber has a lower ILR. Current follows the path of least resistance. ILR < TMR favors current flow down the fiber instead of out of the fiber. The lower ILR allows charges to flow more easily down the cable, increasing the ILC and depolarizing the adjacent membrane more rapidly. Because the MTC is the length of time required for the membrane capacitance to discharge to 37% of the applied initial voltage, the stronger ILC flowing down a large fiber discharges the capacitance on the

FIGURE 4.6. Three curves demonstrate a depolarizing current intensity just below safety factor (A) which does not result in propagation of the impulse. The current is above safety factor in both B and C but the greater rate of rise in C results in a shorter time to depolarize the adjacent segment and a more rapid rate of impulse conduction.

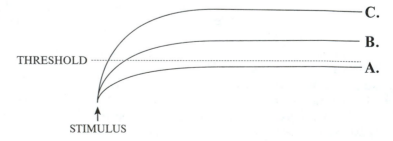

contiguous membrane more quickly, bringing it to threshold more rapidly and speeding impulse propagation (Fig. 4.6).

Increasing fiber size is not a feasible way to increase CV in the mammalian nervous system. To achieve CVs in the range seen with clinical nerve conduction studies, an individual axon might have to be as big around as the median nerve and the nerve as large as the patient's arm! CV can be increased much more efficiently and dramatically by myelination. By insulating the membrane, the myelin sheath increases the TMR, lessens transverse current leakage across the membrane, and thereby increases the space constant. Myelination also decreases capacitance by increasing the separation of the charges. These effects enhance the cable properties of the fiber. More robust current then flows electrotonically for a longer distance down the fiber, enhancing safety factor.

Myelin is laid down in concentric lamellae, with one Schwann cell providing the myelin for a single internodal segment, which is separated by nodes of Ranvier from adjoining segments. The optimal ratio of axon diameter to total diameter is 0.5 to 0.7. The nodal membrane contains predominantly VGNCs. VGKCs are relatively sparse in the nodal region, but more numerous in the paranodal region. A more rapid inactivation cycle of the nodal VGNCs compensates to some degree for the paucity of VGKCs at the node. The long internodal segment is fairly devoid of channels of either type.

Conduction in myelinated fibers is saltatory, jumping from one node of Ranvier to the next (from the Latin *salio*, to leap) (Fig. 4.4). Consider an action potential at node A. The inward flow of Na+ ions creates a flow of positive charges down the fiber. Since the TMR is high due to the insulation of the myelin and the ILR is low because the fiber's diameter is large, the charges readily follow the path of least resistance down the fiber to the next node. On reaching node B, the positive charges neutralize negative charges on the inner membrane. If the ILC is of sufficient magnitude, greater than safety factor, it depolarizes the nodal membrane. The reduced internal negativity on the inner membrane releases positive charges on the outer membrane to flow back to node A, completing the circuit. Node A is in its refractory period so conduction remains unidirectional. An action potential is generated at node B, and the cycle is repeated.

Saltatory conduction is very efficient. A 20 μm myelinated fiber has a CV 10 times faster than an unmyelinated fiber of the same diameter. Larger fibers have longer internodal segments, another factor in the faster CV with increasing fiber size.

TABLE 4.2
Factors That Influence Nerve Conduction Velocity

Fiber diameter
Internal longitudinal resistance
Transverse membrane resistance
Membrane capacitance
Myelination
Clinical effects
   Temperature
   Age
   Height
   Proximal vs. distal
   Upper extremities vs. lower extremities

As an approximation:

CV (m/s) = 6 (the outer diameter of the myelin sheath in μm)

Large myelinated human nerve fibers are in the 6–12 μm diameter range, and conduct at up to approximately 70 m/sec, over 150 miles/hour.

A number of factors have an influence on CV (Table 4.2). Large fibers conduct more rapidly than small ones, and myelinated fibers more rapidly than unmyelinated fibers. Conduction increases with increasing temperature, up to a point at which conduction fails (the blocking temperature, normally about 44– 45° C) (9). Slower CV at lower temperature is likely due to slower opening of the VGNCs. In clinical nerve conduction studies, other factors are important as well, including age and height. These are discussed further in Chapter 10. From a clinical standpoint, the most important variable is temperature.

Nerve fibers are classified according to their size and CV. The largest fibers are spindle afferents and motor fibers arising from alpha motor neurons. The smallest, unmyelinated fibers are slow pain and postganglionic autonomic fibers. The fiber classification systems and their clinical relevance is discussed further in Chapter 16. Muscle fibers conduct more slowly than predicted by their size because the extensive transverse tubular system expands the effective area of cell membrane, vastly increasing membrane capacitance with a consequent slowing of CV.

Volume Conduction

A volume conductor is a container in which electrical events are transmitted over distance (10,11). A poor volume conductor has high resistivity and low conductivity. Charged particles are not present to respond to local current fluxes, and the projection of internal electrical phenomena is consequently limited. A good volume conductor has high conductivity, with an abundance of ambient charged particles that can respond to any electrical event occurring within it. Inside a volume conductor, electricity is conducted at the speed of light. The human body is, in volume conduction terms, a complexly configured container of electrolytic solution. It is an excellent volume conductor. Local current flows are projected widely and can potentially be detected by surface electrodes at a great distance. The body's capability as a volume conductor can cause no end of grief and woe for the unwary electrodiagnostic medicine consultant.

A current "source" is an area of positivity from which charges may migrate toward a negative "sink." No current flows when an excitable membrane is at rest because the system is in a steady state. When an action potential occurs, a negative sink is created. Positive charges from the adjoining membrane flow toward the area of negativity, creating a source (+)/ sink (-) dipole. Since positive charges flow from either side of the actively depolarized segment, in reality two dipoles are created: a sink←source dipole on the leading edge of the propagating wave, and a source→sink dipole on the trailing edge. Viewing the complex in brackets as conducting from left to right along the membrane, from trailing edge to leading edge the configuration is [source→sink:sink←source]. This can also be viewed as a [source→sink←source] tripole (11). In a good volume conductor, charges flow abundantly and their lines of movement form curved paths reminiscent of the field lines of a magnet. Charge density refers to the net charge per unit area. In a good volume conductor, charges move in an infinite number of paths, and the greatest charge density occurs along the straight line between the source and the sink. Current flow and charge density decrease as the square of the distance, so the electrical field exponentially decreases in intensity with movement away from the dipole. Equipotential lines can be drawn perpendicular to the arching lines of current flow. The equipotential lines form concentric rings connecting points at which the electrical potential is the same at two different locations (Fig. 4.7). Increasing separation between flux lines signifies decreasing electrical field intensity. For a dipole, the amplitude of the potential falls off as the square of the distance. Its equipotential lines form a figure 8 (Fig. 4.7B) (10). A quadrupole is a pair of back to back dipoles (Fig. 4.7C). A quadrupole (as in [source→sink:sink← source] above) is the most realistic approximation of

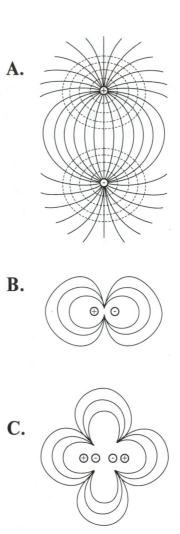

FIGURE 4.7. Current dipoles depicting the lines of current flow (solid) and the equipotential lines (dashed). See text.

an action potential propagating down an axon. The amplitude of a quadrupole decreases inversely with the cube of the distance. Its equipotential lines form a cloverleaf configuration (10).

The action potential recorded with an intracellular electrode is a monophasic, positive event. The waveform recorded with an extracellular electrode depends on the properties of the volume conductor. In a good volume conductor, a triphasic, positive/negative/positive waveform is recorded. The various deflections that produce the waveform can be analyzed by considering the position of the recording electrode in relation to the density and directional flow of charges (11). The classic nerve action potential recorded clinically is a triphasic wave. To understand the configuration of this potential it is helpful to appreciate some of the conventions of clinical neurophysiology.

Electrodes used in neurophysiology are commonly

referred to as grid 1 (G_1) and grid 2 (G_2), as discussed in the chapter on instrumentation. By convention, when G_1 is negative with respect to G_2, the oscilloscope deflection is upwards, and when G_1 is positive with respect to G_2 the deflection is downwards. The negative upwards convention seems foreign to the novice, but quickly becomes familiar.

During membrane depolarization, the negative sink of the intracellular space attracts positive charges. Na+ ions rush toward the sink, toward the area of increased membrane permeability. These positive charges can move great distances in a good volume conductor, and the initial flux for some of the more peripheral ions is away from the sink. This initial movement away from the sink is followed by an arching movement of return towards the sink (Fig. 4.8).

When positive charges move toward G_1, the recording electrode perceives this as positivity. G_1 becomes positive in relation to G_2 and the baseline deflection is downwards. When positive charges move away from G_1, the electrode sees the retreating positivity as negativity; the area has become less positive. Because G_1 then becomes negative in relation to G_2, the baseline deflection is upwards. In summary: when + charges approach G_1 the deflection is $\vee$; when + charges retreat from G_1, the deflection is $\wedge$.

The best analogy for the potentials seen in electrodiagnostic medicine is the traveling tripole of [source→sink←source] or [+++ − +++]. Consider a G_1 electrode positioned to the right of such a tripole as shown in Figure 4.8. The first perturbation it encounters is positive charges moving towards it in their outward arc away from the sink; G_1 then becomes positive in relation to G_2 producing a downward deflection in the baseline (zone A in Fig. 4.8). This is the initial positivity of a traveling wave. As G_1 encounters the main portion of the action potential there is intense movement of positive charges away from it and into the sink; G_1 sees this retreating positivity as negativity and becomes negative in relation to G_2 producing an upward deflection in the baseline (zone B in Fig. 4.8). This is the main negative spike of the traveling wave. As the main portion of the action potential passes, the next thing G_1 encounters is the positive charges from the trailing edge as they arc back toward the sink (zone C in Fig. 4.8). G_1 sees this approaching positivity as positive, producing another positive (downward) deflection. This is the trailing positivity of a traveling wave. The composite of these different deflections is the triphasic positive/negative/positive wave.

Some refinements may be of interest. The current density of the positive charges responsible for the initial and trailing positivity of the triphasic wave is much less than that responsible for the main spike, and the amplitude is correspondingly lower. As the wave propagates, the ionic fluxes on the leading and trailing edges have different densities. Just as the sound waves are packed in front of a moving train, the charges are crowded in a dense swarm in front of the propagating wave. As the wave passes away, the charges are more dispersed and scattered. The effect is much like the doppler shift of sound wave frequency, which abruptly drops as the source passes. This effect is responsible for the typical difference in amplitude and morphology between the initial and terminal positivities. The initial positivity is sharper and deeper,

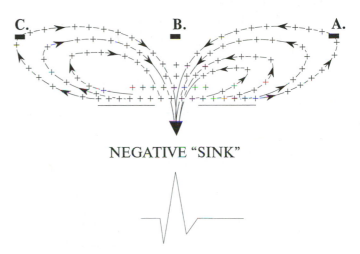

FIGURE 4.8. The origin of the triphasic wave due to a propagating source/sink/source tripole in a good volume conductor. The solid line represents the cell membrane and the gap in the solid line the "defect" in the membrane due to increased Na+ conductance, exposing the negative sink of the intracellular space. In a poor volume conductor, the positive charges immediately outside the "defect," and those on the nearby adjoining membrane would rocket toward the sink, and a recording electrode extracellularly would detect a monophasic event. In a good volume conductor, the charges move in radiating arcs in all directions before heading for the sink. The electrode senses positive charges moving towards it as positivity, and retreating charges moving away from it as less positivity, which is indistinguishable from negativity. Positivity creates a downward deflection and negativity an upward deflection on the oscilloscope. An active electrode at A (G_1), with a distant reference (G_2), sees positivity due to approaching Na+ ions. G_1 becomes positive in relation to G_2, producing a downward deflection. An electrode at B, sees retreating positivity which it interprets as negativity. An electrode at C sees approaching positivity, but more scattered and widespread than the electrode at A. The result is the triphasic action potential shown at the bottom, with a sharp initial positive component, a tall, sharp negative main spike, and a lower amplitude, lower frequency trailing positive component.

while the trailing positivity is of lower amplitude and longer duration (Fig. 4.8).

There are frequent occasions in electrodiagnostic medicine when the expected triphasic wave does not materialize, and a biphasic or even monophasic potential occurs. One of these is when G_1 lies near the terminus of the actively conducting fiber, such as near a tendon or an injured and nonconducting region of the nerve or muscle fiber. The trailing positivity is missing because the potential dies just beyond the electrode and does not retreat into the distance; the so-called killed end effect.

The action potential in reality spreads out along a considerable segment of the fiber; many internodes are active at once. The distance over which activity extends depends on the conduction velocity of the volley and the duration of the action potential. In some instances, G_2 detects activity at a distance through the volume conductor while events are still occurring at G_1. This participation of G_2 as a relatively active electrode can alter the waveform, including eliminating the initial positivity. This occurs especially with antidromic, digital sensory potentials (11).

Interesting events occur at the interfaces where the volume conductor changes shape, as where the finger joins the hand, the hand the arm, and so forth (12–15). As a propagating potential crosses from one area to another, a "standing wave" is created, which is an artifact of the change in shape or conductivity. Also known as boundary or stationary potentials, these waveforms are seen only when the active and reference electrodes are on opposite sides of the boundary and are therefore able to detect the passage from one compartment to another. The stationary wave is projected instantaneously. All electrodes of the proper montage detect the stationary wave at the instant the propagating potential crosses the boundary, and its latency remains fixed since it is not actually related to the conduction velocity of the traveling wave. Changes in the direction of the propagating wave can also generate stationary potentials; merely bending the elbow or abducting the finger can produce these waveforms.

The phenomenon of the stationary wave is most relevant to evoked potentials, especially in trying to sort out the significance of the short latency components of the somatosensory evoked potential. It can occasionally cause spurious and misleading waveforms when performing nerve conduction studies if the active and reference electrodes straddle adjacent body parts.

For the EMGer, volume conduction poses problems primarily in the performance of nerve conduction studies. Current intended to stimulate a particular nerve may also, or instead, stimulate a nearby nerve because the stimulating current has spread through the volume conductor. Recording electrodes may detect activity at a distance. Volume conducted motor responses may be confused with sensory potentials. Impulse traffic in one nerve may be detected by electrodes overlying another nerve. The practical problems of dealing with volume conduction are discussed in Chapters 7, 8, and 10.

Key Points

- The cell membrane is a selectively permeable bilayer separating the extracellular and intracellular fluid. The concentration of Na+ is much higher outside the cell than inside; the reverse is true for K+. The cell's interior has strong negative charge due to impermeable protein anions. Complex macromolecular ion channels embedded in the cell membrane may change permeability depending on chemical or electrical events. The permeability state of voltage-gated channels depends on the transmembrane potential (TMP). Whether an ion moves across the membrane along its electrochemical gradient depends on the permeability of the membrane. In the resting state, essentially all the voltage gated Na+ channels (VGNCs) are closed, while a small proportion of the voltage gated K+ channels (VGKCs) are open. Consequently, the membrane at rest is much more permeable to K+ than to Na+, and the resting TMP, generally −70 to −90 mV (depending on the cell) is near the electrochemical equilibrium potential for K+ (E_K) of −90 mV, and far from the E_{Na} of + 60 mV.

- The membrane can be viewed as a chain of capacitors and resistors. Cable properties are the passive electrical attributes of the cell. The separation of interior negative from positive exterior charges by the insulating cell membrane constitutes a capacitor. The time constant (TC) of a capacitor is an exponential function describing the time required for charging or discharging; the resistance and capacitance of a membrane determine its TC. The membrane length constant describes the distance over which a potential's amplitude decays as it spreads down a fiber. High internal longitudinal resistance, high capacitance, and low transmembrane resistance inhibit impulse spread. In the mammalian nervous system, countermeasures to these impulse propagation impediments are to enlarge and myelinate the fiber. The action potential is conducted down the nerve or muscle membrane due to the sequential activation and deactivation of VGNCs and VGKCs. Whether a propagated or non-propagated potential develops depends on whether a membrane depolarization reaches threshold. When threshold is exceeded, the opening of VGNCs becomes self perpetuating, the membrane becomes freely permeable to Na+ and the TMP approaches E_{Na} (about +60 mV)—the main spike of the action potential. The refractory period (RP) is an interval during the action potential cycle when a second action potential can be produced with difficulty (the relative RP) or not at all (the absolute RP). An action potential conducts along an unmyelinated nerve fiber or a muscle cell by the slow process of continuous conduction. The depolarization cycle in the active region must discharge the capacitance on the adjoining segment of membrane to bring it to threshold. When capacitance is high, the TC is long, prolonging the process. Safety factor is the ratio between the current actually flowing and that necessary to depolarize the adjacent segment. When safety factor is too low, the impulse does not propagate. Conduction velocity is directly related to fiber size and to myelination. Myelin increases the length constant, decreases capacitance, and decreases the TC, enhancing the cable properties of the fiber. Conduction in myelinated fibers is saltatory. The inward flow of Na+ ions at one node of Ranvier creates an electrotonic flow of positive charges down the fiber, which depolarizes the next internode.

- The body's high conductivity makes it an excellent volume conductor. A current source is an area of positivity from which charges migrate toward a negative sink. Positive charges from the adjacent membrane flowing toward the area of negativity created by an action potential constitute a source/sink dipole. In a good volume conductor, charges move in an infinite number of paths; their lines of movement form curved paths. The action potential recorded extracellularly in a good volume conductor is a triphasic, positive/ negative/ positive waveform; its various deflections can be analyzed considering the position of a recording electrode in relation to current density and directional. Charges can move great distances in a good volume conductor; the initial flux for some is away from the sink, followed by an arching return movement towards the sink. The best analogy for the potentials seen in electrodiagnostic medicine is a traveling [source→sink←source] tripole. A G1 electrode along its advancing front first encounters oncoming positive charges in their outward arc away from the sink; G_1 becomes positive, producing a downward baseline deflection. As G_1 encounters the action potential's main portion, it sees a retreating movement of positive charges away from it and into the sink, a relative negativity producing an upward deflection in the baseline: the main negative spike. G_1 last encounters oncoming positive charges from the trailing edge as they arc backwards; registering this as the trailing positive component of a traveling wave. The composite of these different deflections is the classic triphasic wave.

References

1. Catterall WA. Structure and function of voltage-gated ion channels. Ann Rev Biochem 1995;64:493–531.
   Voltage-gated ion channels are responsible for generation of electrical signals in cell membranes. Their principal subunits are members of a gene family and can function as voltage-

   gated ion channels by themselves. Structural elements that are required for voltage-dependent activation, selective ion conductance, and inactivation have been identified, and their mechanisms of action are being explored through mutagenesis, expression in heterologous cells, and functional analysis.

2. Koester J, Siegelbaum S. Ion channels. In: Kandel ER, Schwartz JH, Jessell TM, eds. Essentials of neural science and behavior. Norwalk: Appleton & Lange, 1995; 115–131.
   Channels have three important properties: 1) they conduct ions 2) they are ion specific 3) they open or close in response to specific electrical, mechanical or chemical signals. Up to 1×10^8 ions per second may pass through a channel, comparable to the rate of action of the fastest enzymes. Ion selectivity is achieved through physical-chemical interaction between the ion and various amino acid residues lining the channel wall. The channel's conformation may change in response to voltage changes, a specific chemical ligand, or a mechanical stimulus such as stretch or pressure. Many channels are made up to two or more subunits, which may be identical or distinct. The flux of ions through a channel is passive. Each channel has two or more conformational states, at least one open state and one or two closed states. The transition between different states is called *gating*. There are 3 different physical models for the opening and closing of ion channels: a conformational change in one region of the channel, a generalized conformational change along the length of the channel, or a blocking particle swings into and out of the channel mouth.

3. Favre I, Moczydlowski E, Schild L. On the structural basis for ionic selectivity among Na+, K+, and Ca2+ in the voltage-gated sodium channel. Biophys J 1996;71: 3110–3125.
   Voltage-sensitive sodium channels and calcium channels are homologous proteins with distinctly different selectivity for permeation of inorganic cations. The Lys residue in Domain III of the sodium channel is the critical determinant that specifies both the impermeability of Ca2+ and the selective permeability of Na+ over K+.

4. Ptacek LJ. Channelopathies: ion channel disorders of muscle as a paradigm for paroxysmal disorders of the nervous system. Neuromuscul Disord 1997;7:250–255.
   Hyperkalemic periodic paralysis (hyperKPP) and paramyotonia congenita (PC) result from mutations in a gene encoding a skeletal muscle sodium channel. Hypokalemic periodic paralysis (hypoKPP) is caused by mutations in a gene encoding a voltage-gated calcium channel. The characterization of these diseases as channelopathies has served as a paradigm for other episodic disorders. One example is periodic ataxia, which results from mutations in voltage-gated potassium calcium channels. Long QT syndrome, an episodic cardiac dysrhythmia syndrome, is known to result from mutations in either voltage-gated sodium or potassium channels.

5. Catterall WA. Molecular properties of sodium and calcium channels. J Bioenerg Biomembr 1996;28:219–230.
   Voltage-gated sodium and calcium channels are responsible for inward movement of sodium and calcium during electrical signals in cell membranes. These two channels are built on a common structural theme with variations appropriate for functional specialization of each channel type.

6. Kellenberger S, Scheuer T, Catterall WA. Movement of the Na+ channel inactivation gate during inactivation. J Biol Chem 1996;271:30971–30979.
   Phenylalanine 1489 in the inactivation gate of the rat brain

sodium channel is required for stable inactivation. It is postulated to move into the intracellular mouth of the pore and occlude it during inactivation. This study shows that, upon inactivation, Phe-1489 in the inactivation gate moves from an exposed and modifiable position outside the membrane electric field to a buried and inaccessible position, perhaps in or near the intracellular mouth of the channel pore.

7. Keynes RD. A new look at the mechanism of activation and inactivation of voltage-gated ion channels. Proc R Soc Lond B Biol Sci 1992;249:107–112.
Studies on the kinetics of activation and inactivation of the sodium channels of the squid giant axon, on the sodium gating current, and on the properties of the non-inactivating steady-state current, are briefly reviewed. Taken in conjunction with recent evidence on the structure of voltage-gated ion channels, they have led to the development of a series-parallel model of the sodium channel that can be regarded as a modernized version of the Hodgkin-Huxley model, with some novel features. It is suggested that activation results from conformational changes brought about by voltage sensors operating in parallel. Inactivation is a potential-dependent process which, rather than bringing a ball and chain blocking group into position to close the channels, serves to switch the system so that it passes from an initial activated mode, in which there is a high probability of arriving at an open state with a brief latency, to a second steady-state mode, in which the probability of opening is very much lower.

8. Brown PB. The electrochemical basis of neuronal integration. In: Haines DE, ed. Fundamental neuroscience. New York: Churchill Livingstone, 1997;31–49.

9. Rutkove SB, Kothari MJ, Shefner JM. Nerve, muscle, and neuromuscular junction electrophysiology at high temperature. Muscle Nerve 1997;20:431–436.
An investigation of the effect of elevating limb temperature from 32 degrees C to 42 degrees C on motor conduction studies, antidromic sensory studies, and 3-Hz repetitive stimulation in normal subjects. On average, motor amplitude and duration decreased by 27% and 19%, respectively, whereas sensory amplitude and duration decreased by 50% and 26%, respectively. Neuromuscular transmission remained normal at 42 degrees C. Single motor unit recordings revealed a reduction in amplitude of 26%, similar to the overall reduction in compound motor amplitude. These findings demonstrate that significant reductions in sensory and motor amplitudes can occur in normal nerves at high temperature; these changes may be due to alterations in nerve and muscle ion channel function.

10. Lagerlund TD. Volume conduction. In: Daube JR, ed. Clinical neurophysiology. Philadelphia: F.A. Davis Co., 1996;29–39.
A discussion of volume conduction for the mathematically minded, relying on the principles of solid angle geometry and calculus. Bioelectric potentials generated by sources inside the body may be either active, such as fluxes thru ion channels that cause small currents to flow, or passive, due to cable properties or electrotonic effects. In a purely resistive volume conductor, such as the human body, the conductive properties of the medium are independent of frequency and potentials are always in phase. A single source or sink of current is a monopole; a monopole's potential decreases inversely with distance and its equipotential lines form circles. Many neuronal current generators may be described in terms of a current dipole; a dipole's potential decreases inversely with the square of the distance and its equipotential lines form arcs creating a figure of eight. Two perpendicular dipoles joined together create a quadrupole; a quadrupole's potential falls off inversely as the cube of the distance and its equipotential lines form a cloverleaf. A quadrupole is a fair approximation of an action potential propagating along an axon or a bipolar recording of a dipole along a line parallel to its axis; the potential is triphasic. For a quadrupole, the potential recorded relative to a distant reference at points parallel to its axis is also triphasic, and its sharpness increases with decreasing distance from the source; this most closely approximates the potential expected from an action potential propagating along an axon parallel to the recording electrodes. These calculations all assume a homogeneous medium of uniform conductivity and without any boundaries. The clinical situation is different in that the medium is not homogeneous and boundaries or edges exist where the geometry of the volume conductor changes. When a propagating wave passes through an interface between regions of different sizes or conductivities, a stationary wave (boundary potential) may develop when the first and second electrodes are on opposite sides of the boundary.

11. Dumitru D, DeLisa JA. AAEM Minimonograph #10: volume conduction. Muscle Nerve 1991;14:605–624.
A volume conductor is any medium with the capability of passively conducting a current between regions of potential difference. The monophasic positive intracellular action potential produces a monophasic negative extracellular waveform and a triphasic extracellular waveform in a poor and good volume conductor, respectively. The observed waveform characteristics are dependent upon both the recording electrode montage and the type of volume conductor surrounding the excitable tissue. The extracellular current flow associated with an action potential can be divided into two current sources flanking a central current sink. If a recording electrode is located over the negative current sink, a negative potential is observed. When the two current sources approach a recording electrode, a positive potential is recorded. If a positive deflection of the baseline is observed, one may conclude that the wave of depolarization under investigation did not originate under, but traveled toward, the recording location. Electric currents from external sources are free to propagate extraneurally as the body is a good volume conductor. Care must be taken to not activate nearby nerves and, subsequently, obtain a waveform contaminated with potentials from undesired sources. Additionally, electrical activity from neighboring muscles and nerves can summate in the volume conductor and yield responses capable of masking pathology. An understanding of the principles of volume conduction theory can help the electrodiagnostician avoid artifactual errors and erroneous conclusions.

12. Stegeman DF, Van Oosterom A, Colon EJ. Far-field evoked potential components induced by a propagating generator: computational evidence. Electroencephalogr Clin Neurophysiol 1987;67:176–187.
This study validates current hypotheses for the generation of so-called far-field or stationary somatosensory evoked potential (SEP) components. Changes in the volume conductor configuration and changes in the direction of nerve propagation are capable of generating such components, based on the theory of volume conduction. In an essentially restricted volume conductor, any disturbance of uniform nerve propagation in a homogeneous extracellular medium will lead to the generation of non-moving field components. Realistic changes within the volume conductor can lead to substantial far-field components: 'virtual generators' or 'secondary sources.'

13. Deupree DL, Jewett DL. Far-field potentials due to action potentials traversing curved nerves, reaching cut nerve ends, and crossing boundaries between cylindrical volumes. Electroencephalogr Clin Neurophysiol 1988;70:355–362.

A computer simulation was tested in a biological preparation by recording action potentials from frog sciatic nerves within a volume conductor filled with Ringer's solution. Traveling in a straight line, nerve action potentials traversed a constricted cylinder before crossing into a larger, hemicylindrical volume. Recordings from widely spaced electrodes in the larger volume demonstrated a potential associated with the action potential crossing the boundary between the two volumes. Another potential was associated with the action potential reaching the nerve's cut end. These potentials did not diminish in amplitude with increasing distance from the source. In other recordings, a potential associated with a bend in the nerve was found which was dependent upon the angle of the bend. These results indicate that the simple model of a dipole in a bounded sphere in which potentials decrease as a function of distance from the generator does not explain all potentials that can be observed under conditions that approximate human and animal recordings.

14. Kimura J, Ishida T, Suzuki S, et al. Far-field recording of the junctional potential generated by median nerve volleys at the wrist. Neurology 1986;36:1451–1457.

In 20 arms from 10 healthy subjects, the orthodromic median sensory volleys crossing the wrist gave rise to a stationary, biphasic potential. A pair of electrodes located on each side of the wrist best detected the junctional potential that developed across the partition. Not only positive but also negative peaks of scalp-recorded evoked responses could represent junctional potentials generated along the course of the conduction medium in the absence of fixed neural discharges.

15. Dumitru D, Jewett DL. Far-field potentials. Muscle Nerve 1993;16:237–254.

Far-field potentials are produced by neural generators located at a distance from the recording electrodes. These potentials were initially characterized incorrectly as being of positive polarity, widespread distribution, and constant latency; however, recent advances have clearly demonstrated that far-field potentials may be either positive or negative depending upon the location of the electrodes with respect to the orientation of the dipole generator. Peak latencies in the far-field can vary with alterations in body position; the spatial distribution of far-field potentials, while widespread, is not uniform. Recent studies of far-field potentials suggest how such waveforms are produced when the symmetry of an action potential, as recorded by distant electrodes, is broken by such factors as differing conductivities of volume conductor compartments, direction of action potential propagation, size differentials in adjoining body segments, or the termination of action potential propagation in excitable tissue. Human, animal, and computer experiments support the preceding generalizations. These new explanations are directly applicable to such far-field potentials as the short latency somatosensory-evoked potential. Furthermore, since far-field potentials can also occur in muscle tissue, one should expect that these generalizations will hold with respect to electromyographic potentials.

16. Taylor CP, Narasimhan LS. Sodium channels and therapy of central nervous system diseases. Adv Pharmacol 1997;39:47–98.

Voltage-dependent Na+ channels have long been recognized as targets for anti-arrhythmic and local anesthetic drugs. Since the mid-1980s, Na+ channels have become widely accepted as the primary target of anticonvulsants with pharmacological profiles similar to phenytoin, carbamazepine, and lamotrigine. Results from animal models and a few preliminary clinical trials suggest that this class of drugs may also offer significant potential for reducing the neuronal damage caused by ischemic stroke, head trauma, and perhaps certain neurodegenerative diseases. This review includes an introduction to Na+ channel structure, molecular biology, and physiology as they relate to pharmacology. See also: Meldrum, B.S. Update on the mechanism of action of antiepileptic drugs. Epilepsia 1996;37: Suppl 6:S4–11.

17. Watters MR. Organic neurotoxins in seafoods. Clin Neurol Neurosurg 1995;97:119–124.

Toxins formed by organic micro-organisms may accumulate within certain tissues of predatory fish, which may serve as a source of seafood poisoning for the higher food chain. Distinct clinical syndromes have emerged, and the individual toxins have been identified. Clinical manifestations of each begin with a gastrointestinal prodrome and headache, followed by sensorimotor deficits. Bulbar and cognitive changes are associated with the more lethal tetrodotoxin, saxitoxin, and domoic acid toxin. Tetrodotoxin and saxitoxin block sodium channels, while ciguatoxin opens them. Domoic acid stimulates excitatory amino acids at the NMDA receptors. See also Narahashi T, Roy ML, Ginsburg KS. Recent advances in the study of mechanism of action of marine neurotoxins. Neurotoxicology 1994;15:545–554.

5

Statistics

Interpretation of electrodiagnostic medicine studies is heavily dependent on statistics. The aim is to separate normal individuals from those with disease. Deciding whether a given test result is normal involves comparing the value for the patient with some reference value that defines the limits of normal. Ideally, the test values in normal controls and those with disease would have no overlap, allowing perfect discrimination between the healthy and diseased populations. This is rarely, if ever, the case. Some individuals with mild disease may have test result values that fall into the normal range, and some healthy subjects may have test result values that fall outside the "normal" limit. Although complete and unequivocal separation between the healthy and the diseased is not possible, reference values help to gauge the probability that the patient is normal or has a disease.

The limits of normal, the normative data or the reference values, may be determined in several ways, all of which involve statistics. As with the interpretation of laboratory data in other branches of medicine, it behooves the practitioner to have some familiarity with the statistical methods used to derive the reference values being used. This chapter reviews some basic statistical concepts, their application, and their limitations as used in electrodiagnostic medicine. A glossary is included at the end of the chapter for assistance.

Deriving Reference Values

The methodologies used in clinical electrodiagnosis have inherent variability. When an electrodiagnostic test, such as a median motor nerve conduction velocity determination, is done on different normal subjects, or repeatedly on the same subject, the result obtained varies. The variability occurs for a number of reasons. The same individual might have a slightly different median NCV on 10 successive determinations related to minor differences in the accuracy of measurement of distance or latency, variations in temperature, or even variations in the conduction velocity related to the segment of nerve studied. Different individuals will vary in age, height, and other factors, creating additional intersubject variability. The scatter of results obtained on testing the same individual repeatedly, or on testing different normal individuals creates a range of values. Some of the variability is due to biologic or technical factors, but even after all these have been accounted for, a residual variance remains.

The aim in setting a reference value is to choose a point that best separates diseased from healthy individuals, providing the optimal tradeoff between sensitivity and specificity. Reference values may be established with several different methods, including the range, the percentile, or the mean and standard deviation (SD) (1,2). There are advantages and disadvantages to each of these statistical approaches. The most common procedure is to take the mean ± some arbitrary number of SDs, usually two. The distribution is usually assumed to be Gaussian, the familiar, symmetrical bell-shaped curve of the standard normal distribution; though we have recently recognized that this may not always be the case (1–3) (Figs. 5.1, 5.2). No small consideration is that fewer control subjects are

required to establish reliable reference values with the mean ± SD strategy than with other methods.

Mean and Standard Deviation Method for Establishing Reference Values

Any population has a certain range of values for a particular test. For example, the population of central Virginia has a distribution of values for median NCV. It may range from as low as 3–5 m/s for a patient with Dejerine-Sottas disease, to as high as 65–70 m/s for healthy adolescent. A disease free sample of the population of central Virginia has a much narrower distribution, which will likely be Gaussian. The characteristics of this disease free sample may be used to establish reference values for the study of patients from this population.

The mean ± 2 SDs will include about 95% (actually 95.44%) of the sample. The tails at either end of the curve account for about 2.5% each. Since electrodiagnostic medicine considers only one tail of the distribution as abnormal (conduction velocities cannot be too fast, distal latencies too short or amplitudes too high), only 2.5% of the normal population would fall outside the "normal" range using a two-tailed method (Fig. 5.1). Using a one-tailed method, 2.05 SD beyond the mean includes 97% of the sample. Normal individuals with slightly slow conduction velocity values, in the −2 SD tail, presenting for evaluation might be called abnormal, a type I error or a false-positive (Table 5.1).

The population of patients with diseased median nerves in central Virginia also has a distribution of conduction velocities. The mean conduction velocity in this group will be slower than the mean conduction velocity in the disease free subjects. However, those in the disease group with faster conduction velocities will likely overlap with normal subjects having slightly slower than "normal" conduction velocities. It is this overlap between patients with mild abnormalities (>2 SDs above the mean of the diseased individuals) and outlier normals (<2 SDs below the mean of control subjects) that limits the ability of a test to discriminate between normals and patients with median nerve disease.

Outlier normals with abnormal tests results are false-positives; patients with median nerve disease with normal test results are false-negatives. In establishing normal reference values, there is an inevitable trade-off between false-positives and false-negatives, between sensitivity and specificity (4). Setting the

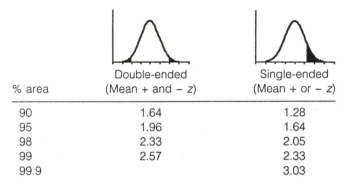

% area	Double-ended (Mean + and − z)	Single-ended (Mean + or − z)
90	1.64	1.28
95	1.96	1.64
98	2.33	2.05
99	2.57	2.33
99.9		3.03

FIGURE 5.1. A Gaussian distribution has two tails. The z score is a measurement of the number of standard deviations a value is away from the mean (see glossary). The mean ± 2SD approach (two-tailed method) to defining normality is appropriate when an abnormal value could be either too high or too low; in which case about 95% of normal values would lie within the span between—2 SD and + 2 SD, and 2.5% would lie in either tail. With a one-tailed method, more appropriate for electrodiagnostic medicine, the mean + 2SD (as for a distal latency) or the mean—2SD (as for conduction velocity or amplitude) would include about 96% of the population. So, using a one- or two-tailed method, the chances of a normal individual having an abnormal test result are about 2.5 – 4.0%. Reprinted with permission from Dorfman LJ, Robinson LR. AAEM minimonograph #47: normative data in electrodiagnostic medicine. Muscle Nerve 1997;20:4–14.

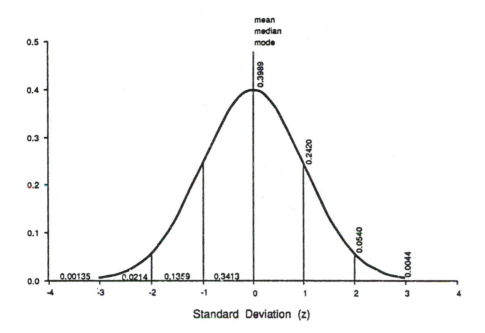

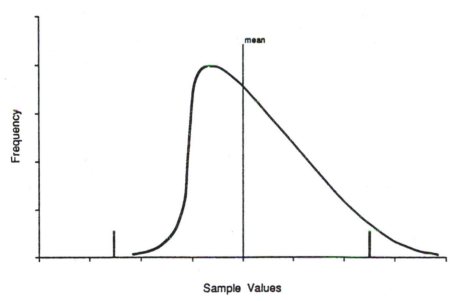

FIGURE 5.2. Frequency distribution curves for a hypothetical Gaussian variable (above) and one with strong positive skew (below). For the Gaussian distribution, the numbers to the right indicate representative frequency values; those to the left indicate the area under the curve for each increment of standard deviation (z score). For the skewed distribution, the vertical bars indicate the values corresponding to ± 2.5SD. Because of the skew, too many cases fall above the upper cutpoint, and the lower cutpoint is nonsensical. Reprinted with permission from Dorfman LJ, Robinson LR. AAEM minimonograph #47: normative data in electrodiagnostic medicine. Muscle Nerve 1997; 20:4–14.

lower normal limit for median nerve conduction velocity to the mean − 3 SD would include 99% of the population, making the risk of a false positive result <1%, virtually eliminating the chance of a type I error and increasing the specificity of the test. However, the cost of this strategy is to increase the likelihood of false negatives in the patient population, the type II error, lowering the test's sensitivity (Fig. 5.3). For most clinical situations a type I error rate, or false positive rate, of 2.5% is an acceptable compromise (5).

These considerations are very important clinically. Never underestimate the ability of the EMG report to

TABLE 5.1

Type I (False-positive) and Type II (False-negative) Errors

		Disease Present	
		Yes	**No**
Test positive	Yes	No error	Type I error, false positive
	No	Type II error, false negative	No error

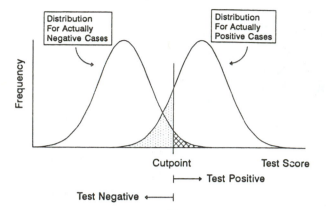

FIGURE 5.3. The distributions of the normal and abnormal populations are rarely free of overlap. False positives are those normal subjects with abnormal test results; false negatives are those patients with disease whose test results fall into the normal range. These Gaussian curves depict the distribution of a test result for normal subjects on the left and individuals with the disease on the right. The test is considered positive when the value exceeds the cutpoint. The stippled area shows the false-negative cases, and the cross-hatched area the false-positive cases. Reprinted with permission from Schulzer M. Diagnostic tests: a statistical review. Muscle Nerve 1994;17:815–819.

bring the knife down upon the patient. One should be as certain as possible that the patient truly has the suspected condition; that the test result is not a false positive. One the other hand, referring physicians are quick to disparage a technology that does not confirm clinically obvious abnormalities; false negatives do not endear the EMG lab to its patients or referral sources. Thus setting the reference value cutoff point becomes pivotal.

The Problem of Multiple Tests

In an attempt to detect an electrodiagnostic abnormality when initial screening results are normal in a patient with a clinically suspected condition, a commonly used tactic is to perform further tests. In carpal tunnel syndrome, numerous techniques have been described to make the diagnosis. If the digital sensory latency is normal, one could then do a palmar sensory latency, compare the "symptomatic" median sensory latencies and amplitudes with the ipsilateral ulnar or contralateral median values, look for a bihumped response recording from the wrist while stimulating the ring finger or the thumb, do short segment studies, do a motor residual latency, or employ other techniques.

The results of one of the ancillary tests may be abnormal, thus "confirming" the diagnosis.

The problem with performing such a battery of tests is that each individual test carries an inherent likelihood of false positivity. If the reference values permit the usual 2.5% type I error rate, the likelihood of a false positive result summates as more test procedures are performed. Table 5.2 summarizes the likelihood of finding an abnormal test result in relation to the number of tests performed. Assuming 10 tests are performed as in the above example, the possibility of finding at least one "abnormality" is 22%. The total type I error rate depends on the independence of the tests. These procedures are not completely independent, but if the tests are correlated by 50%, the false positive rate would be >10%, which is unacceptably high (5). In patients with equivocal symptoms, an isolated abnormality found on a battery of tests must be interpreted cautiously. It is preferable to use a limited number of tests, ideally the one most sensitive test, or to require several positives in a battery of tests before making a diagnosis (5).

Three strategies have been recommended for dealing with the inevitable false positive test result: consideration of the magnitude of the abnormality, clinical correlation, and identification of a pattern of abnormality (2). Trivial abnormalities are less likely to be

TABLE 5.2

Probability of Finding a Positive Test in a Normal Subject Due to Chance Alone (as a Function of the Number of Measurements)

	Number of Positive Tests		
Measurements	*1*	*2*	*3*
1	2.5		
2	4.9	0.1	
3	7.3	0.2	<0.1
4	9.6	0.4	<0.1
5	11.9	0.6	<0.1
6	14.0	0.9	<0.1
7	16.2	1.2	<0.1
8	18.3	1.6	0.1
9	20.4	2.0	0.1
10	22.4	2.5	0.2

* Depending on the statistical measure used, a test always has a certain false-positive rate. Using the mean ± 2SD method, the false positive rate is 2.5%, for each measurement made. The probability of an abnormality summates with the number of tests.
Modified from Dorfman LJ, Robinson LR. AAEM minimonograph #47: normative data in electrodiagnostic medicine. Muscle Nerve 1997;20:4–14.

significant than test results that greatly exceed the normal limit. Abnormalities that have no clinical correlation are less likely to be significant. A pattern of multiple, internally consistent abnormalities that fit the clinical circumstances is most likely to represent a true positive.

Consistency of Technique

Each set of reference values is obtained using some specific electrodiagnostic technique and employing some statistical method. When performing an electrodiagnostic test, the technique used for testing the patient must be the same as that used to obtain the reference values. Although many laboratories establish their own reference values for each common test, this is not always the case. For unusual, less frequently performed procedures, it is common to rely on a technique described in a reference manual or a literature article. All the technical details of distance, temperature, electrode placement, filter settings, and other specifics must be replicated exactly for the stated reference values to have any reliability. The patient should be in the same age range as that of the control subjects. The results of the reference value study should be stated in statistically meaningful terms, including statement of the number of controls. Often, the results will be given as "mean ± SD (range)." View the data with skepticism unless at least 30 subjects (not 30 nerves) were done. The range is not considered a good descriptor of the reference value because of the ability of a single subject (possibly subclinically diseased) to unduly influence the results. If percentiles are given, and the number of subjects is at least 100, taking a given percentile, usually the 2.5th, is usually the most reliable statistical method. Most often, the mean ± 2SD method is the safest.

Because of the shortcomings of the customary statistical approach, other possible methods have been explored. Some electrophysiologic parameters do not have a Gaussian distribution. One method is to use mathematical transformation to convert the distribution to Gaussian, and then to take ± 2 SD of the optimally transformed data (1). The use of Bayes' theorem allows computation of the positive predictive value of a test, taking into account not only its sensitivity and specificity, but the prevalence of the disease in the population (6). Receiver operating characteristic (ROC) curves originated as a method to examine signal to noise discrimination in radar technology. They have been adapted to the evaluation of diagnostic tests, including nerve conduction studies (7).

Glossary

Bayes' theorem- mathematical probability formula that relates the accuracy of a test and the prevalence of a disease in the population to describe the actual performance of the test. Using Bayes' formula, the positive predictive value of a test can be calculated: the probability the disease is present given that the test is positive and considering the true positive rate of the disease in the population (6).

Discriminant analysis- index for a disease is obtained by combining multiple test results using a weighted sum formula of the individual test scores to produce a final discriminant score that separates normal from diseased subjects more efficiently than the original test scores (6,8).

Gaussian distribution- classic bell-shaped curve in which the mean, median, and mode are all close together. The curve is not skewed or kurtotic. As the distribution of values deviates from a Gaussian shape, the mean ± 2 SD loses accuracy in defining normality.

Factor analysis- method for developing subsets from a large number of variables that explain most of the variability present in the larger number (9).

Kurtosis- descriptor for a non-Gaussian distribution in which the curve is tall, narrow, and peaked with long tails (positive kurtosis) or stubby, flat-topped, and broad with short tails (negative kurtosis).

Mean, median, and mode (measures of central tendency)- mean is the arithmetic average of all values. The median is the middle value, halfway between the highest and the lowest. The mode is that value which occurs most often.

Mean related value- description of a particular value in terms of its proximity to the mean, essentially a z score. It succinctly measures how normal or abnormal a value is and implies the likelihood of true pathology as opposed to a normal outlier. A median nerve conduction velocity of −5 MRV is 5 SD below the mean and is highly likely to be abnormal. A conduction velocity of −2.1 SD is only slightly below the normal range and may well represent a normal outlier.

Multivariate analysis- method involving determining multiple, standardized measurements in every patient of a group, then applying discriminant or factor analysis (10).

Normative values- test results derived from a sample of disease free individuals, the reference values.

Percentile- method for describing the frequency distribution of a variable by dividing it into 100 equal parts, then setting some point, e.g., the 2.5th percentile, as the normal reference value. The advantage of the percentile method is that it works equally well for both Gaussian and non-Gaussian distributions, including bimodal or polymodal curves. The major disadvantage is the large sample size required (not < 100). Some argue that percentile analysis should be the gold standard for establishing reference values (2).

Range- highest and lowest values obtained in a group of control subjects. Using the range to establish reference values is problematic in several respects; it requires large sample sizes (at least 120) (1).

Receiver operating characteristic (ROC) curve- graphical representation of the trade-off between the sensitivity and specificity of a test as a function of the reference value used to divide positive from negative tests. The ROC curve depicts the true positive vs. false positive rates at different values for the "cutpoint" reference value (6,7).

Reference values- values used to compare with test results obtained from patients; the "normal" or normative values.

Skewness- descriptor for a discrepancy between a curve and a Gaussian distribution in which the peak of the curve is shifted right or left; one tail is short and the other long; the mean, median and mode are not similar. With positive skew, the peak is shifted to the left with a long tail to the right, conversely for negative skew (Fig. 5.2).

Sensitivity and specificity- sensitivity of a test is its ability to detect a disease; the probability that the test will be positive when the disease is present, or the true positive rate. Specificity is a measure of how definitive the test is, the probability that the disease will be present when the test is positive; or, the probability the test will be negative when the disease is absent. Highly specific tests have a low false positive rate.

Standard deviation- measure of the difference between a value and the mean. SD is calculated by computing the mean, then taking the difference between the mean and each value in the sample, squaring all the differences to produce all positive numbers, dividing by the number of values, then taking the square root. The standard deviation is the square root of the variance.

Transformation- procedure for converting a skewed into a Gaussian distribution by using another mathematical operation, such as taking the square root, cube root, log, or negative inverse (1).

Type I and type II errors- type I error results when the test result is declared abnormal when it is in fact normal; a false positive result. Type I errors are normal subjects incorrectly labeled as abnormal. A type II error is the equivalent of stating that the patient's test result is normal when it is in fact not; a false negative result. Type II errors are abnormal subjects incorrectly labeled as normal.

Variance and variability- variation in the results of a test when given to multiple individuals is due to a number of factors, including the inherent biologic variability, technical factors, age, observer factors, and test-retest variability. Variance is a measure of the scatter of values about the mean, equal to the square of the standard deviation.

Z score- measure of the number of SDs away from the mean. A value with z = 0 is on the mean; z = 1.8 is 1.8 SDs above the mean. Calculated as:

$$z = \frac{(X\text{-}mean)}{SD}$$

Key Points

- By comparing a test result from a patient with some reference value that defines the limits of normal, statistics help to discriminate between normal individuals and those with disease.

- The methodologies employed in clinical electrodiagnosis have inherent variability for a number of reasons. The scatter of results obtained on testing the same individual repeatedly, or on testing different normal individuals creates a range of values. After accounting for all known biologic or technical factors, there remains a residual variance.

- The aim in setting a reference value is to choose a point that best separates diseased from healthy individuals, providing the optimal tradeoff between sensitivity and specificity.

- Reference values may be established in several different ways. The most common procedure is to take the mean ± 2SD, assuming a Gaussian distribution. Any population has a certain range of values for a particular test. A disease free sample may be used to establish reference values for the study of patients from the population. The mean ± 2 SDs will include about 95% of the sample, and the tails at either end of the curve account for about 2.5% each. The overlap between patients with mild abnormalities (>2 SDs above the mean of the diseased individuals) and outlier normals (<2 SDs below the mean of control subjects) limits the ability of a test to discriminate between healthy subjects and patients with disease.

- Outlier normals with abnormal tests results are false-positives; diseased individuals with normal test results are false-negatives. In establishing normal reference values, there is an inevitable trade-off between false-positives and false-negatives, between sensitivity and specificity. Setting the lower normal limit for median nerve conduction velocity to the mean −3 SD would include 99% of the population, making the risk of a false positive result < 1%, virtually eliminating the chance of a type I error and increasing the specificity of the test. However, the cost of this strategy is to increase the likelihood of false negatives in the patient population, the type II error, lowering the test's sensitivity. For most clinical situations, a type I error rate, or false positive rate, of 2.5% is an acceptable compromise.

- To detect an electrodiagnostic abnormality when initial screening results are normal in a patient with a clinically suspected condition, a commonly used tactic is to perform multiple tests. However, each individual test carries an inherent likelihood of false positivity. If the reference values permit the usual 2.5% type I error rate, the likelihood of a false positive result summates as more test procedures are performed. Assuming 10 tests are performed, the possibility of finding at least one "abnormality" is 22%. These procedures are not completely independent, but if the tests are correlated by 50%, the false positive rate would be >10%, which is unacceptably high.

In patients with equivocal symptoms, an isolated abnormality found on a battery of tests must be interpreted cautiously. It is preferable to use a limited number of tests, ideally the *one* most sensitive test, or to require several positives in a battery of tests before making a diagnosis.

- When performing an electrodiagnostic test, the technique used for testing the patient must be the same as that used to obtain the reference values. All the technical details must be replicated exactly for the stated reference values to have any reliability.

- The results of the reference value study should be stated in statistically meaningful terms. View the data with skepticism unless at least 30 subjects (not 30 nerves) were done. The range is not considered a good descriptor of the reference value. If percentiles are given, and the number of subjects is at least 100, taking a given percentile, usually the 2.5th, is usually the most reliable statistical method. Most often, the safest method is to use the mean ± 2SD.

- More advanced and innovative statistical approaches used in electrodiagnostic medicine include Bayesian analysis, receiver operating characteristic curves, and mathematical transformation to correct for non-Gaussian distributions.

References

1. Campbell WW, Robinson LR. Deriving reference values in electrodiagnostic medicine. Muscle Nerve 1993;16:424–428.
   Traditional methods for determining nerve conduction reference values have usually involved studying a group of normal controls, and determining the mean ± 2 standard deviations (SD) for each parameter. Recent studies suggest other factors should be taken into account. Height has a greater effect on conduction velocity than age or temperature. The common assumption that conduction values follow a normal, bell shaped Gaussian distribution appears unwarranted. The curve for some conduction parameters is significantly skewed, making a mean ± 2 SD definition of normality inaccurate to a clinically important degree. In developing and using reference values one should consider height, age, and temperature, and calculate the mean ± 2 SD of the transformed data to remove the effects of skew. Reference values provide only a guide to the probability a given result came from a healthy or diseased individual; one should therefore seek multiple internally consistent abnormalities before diagnosing disease on the basis of electroneurography.

2. Dorfman LJ, Robinson LR. AAEM minimonograph #47: normative data in electrodiagnostic medicine. Muscle Nerve 1997;20:4–14.
   This article reviews, without mathematics, the important principles governing the acquisition and use of normative data in electrodiagnostic medicine. Common flaws in neurophysiological normative data include vague clinical criteria for establishing freedom from disease, samples that are too small and inadequately stratified, and application of Gaussian statistics to non-Gaussian variables. Other problematic issues concern the trade-off between permissible false-positivity and false-negativity in defining the limits of normative from sample data, test-retest variability, and the use of multiple independent test measurements in each electrodiagnostic examination. The following standards for normative data are proposed: (1) standardized objective determination of freedom from disease; (2) appropriately large sample of normal subjects; (3) proportional stratification of normal subjects for known relevant variables; (4) test of Gaussian fit for application of Gaussian statistics; and (5) data presentation by percentiles when Gaussian fit is in doubt. Many existing normative studies in clinical neurophysiology do not meet these standards. High-quality normative data, readily accessible, is essential for the accurate electrodiagnosis of neuromuscular diseases.

3. Robinson LR, Temkin NR, Fujimoto WY, et al. Effect of statistical methodology on normal limits in nerve conduction studies. Muscle Nerve 1991;14:1084–1090.
   This study examined skew in 22 NCS parameters, and compared normal limits derived by several alternative methods in 75 controls. The coefficient of skewness (g1) was significantly positive for 5 of 8 amplitude and 6 of 8 latency measurements. Transformation reduced g1 in 19 of 22 parameters. For each measurement, ideal normal limits were defined as mean ± 2SD of the optimally transformed control data. The percentage of 66 diabetics classified as abnormal by the raw data, but normal by the ideal normal limits, was the positive misclassification rate; while the reverse was the negative misclassification rate. Mean ± 2SD of the raw data produced 11% positive and 12% negative misclassifications. Defining normal limits by the range or 97.5% confidence limits also yielded significant misclassification rates. Conclusion: analyses using the raw data to derive normal limits result in an unacceptable rate of misclassification. Normal limits should be derived from the mean ± 2SD of the optimally transformed data.

4. Redmond MD, Rivner MH. False positive electrodiagnostic tests in carpal tunnel syndrome. Muscle Nerve 1988;11:511–518.
   Of 50 normal subjects, 23 (46%) had at least one false positive electrodiagnostic test for carpal tunnel syndrome (CTS). There were 30% of the subjects who exhibited an abnormal median to ulnar sensory amplitude ratio of less than 1.1. In 7 subjects 8 extremities (14%) revealed prolonged residual latencies, and 4 extremities in 4 subjects (8%) had a difference of 0.4 msec between the median and ulnar palmar sensory latencies. The results of this study indicate that certain reported criteria for CTS are abnormal in a high percentage of normal subjects, thereby making them of limited value in the diagnosis of CTS. Of all the criteria studied, it appears that the comparison of the median to ulnar sensory latency across the carpal tunnel is of greatest potential value. However, even here a more conservative difference of 0.5 msec between median and ulnar nerves must be used to avoid false positive tests for CTS.

5. Rivner MH. Statistical errors and their effect on electrodiagnostic medicine. Muscle Nerve 1994;17:811–814.
   Failure to find abnormalities in patients felt certain to have a disease may lead to performing multiple tests hoping to confirm the clinical suspicion. No diagnostic test perfectly discriminates between normal and abnormal. With common statistical techniques in electrodiagnostic medicine, approximately 2.5% of normals will be mistakenly called abnormal when critical values are set to classify most subjects correctly (type I error).

This error summates when additional independent tests are performed. Even after accounting for interdependency, the total error of combined tests may be unacceptably high. If a single, highly discriminating test is not available and multiple tests are used, abnormalities in more than a single test are needed to distinguish between normals and abnormals.

6. Schulzer M. Diagnostic tests: a statistical review. Muscle Nerve 1994;17:815–819.

Common measures of the accuracy of diagnostic tests are reviewed. The actual performance (predictive value) of these tests depends not only on their sensitivity and specificity, but also on the prevalence of the disease in the population tested (Bayes' theorem). The effect of an inaccurate "gold standard" on the calibration of a new diagnostic test is discussed. Receiver operating characteristic (ROC) curves are introduced as a tool for selecting an optimal cutpoint for a test, and for comparing different tests. Schemes are given for combining tests to improve their accuracy. When multiple continuous measurements are available, methods of discriminant analysis (and logistic regression) are shown to provide measurement combinations with improved accuracy. Examples and key references are provided.

7. Eisen A, Schulzer M, Pant B, et al. Receiver operating characteristic curve analysis in the prediction of carpal tunnel syndrome: a model for reporting electrophysiological data. Muscle Nerve 1993;16:787–796.

Receiver operating characteristic (ROC) curves were used to predict the risk of carpal tunnel syndrome (CTS). Median distal motor latency combined with median-ulnar palmar latency differences had significantly superior discriminant power than other measurements and correlated highly for all groups (r values = 0.71–0.73). These variables were used to construct ROC curves and prediction tables. The approach used allows one to assign a percentage risk of having CTS and can be used in outcome studies.

8. Solders G, Andersson T, Borin Y, et al. Electroneurography index: a standardized neurophysiological method to assess peripheral nerve function in patients with polyneuropathy. Muscle Nerve 1993;16:941–946.

An index based on 12 electrophysiological parameters (conduction velocities, F-latencies, and amplitudes) was constructed to obtain an overall estimation of peripheral nerve conduction. The index was expressed as the mean deviation (in SD) compared to controls standardized for age or height. The stability of the index was tested by repeated examinations during intervals of several months in healthy subjects. The use of a compound index enabled detection of slight impairments of nerve conduction. The relatively low interrecording variability of the index makes it suitable to follow the progression of a polyneuropathy.

9. Robinson LR, Rubner DE, Wahl PW, et al. Factor analysis. A methodology for data reduction in nerve conduction studies. Am J Phys Med Rehabil 1992;71:22–27.

Analyzing multiple nerve conduction study parameters individually is statistically problematic. The goal of this study was to develop a useful factor analysis scheme for assessment of nerve conduction study abnormalities in diabetic neuropathy. 28 NCS parameters were obtained in all subjects and factor analysis extracted five factors from these parameters. These factors were related to conduction velocities (factor 1), distal ulnar function (factor 2), sensory amplitudes (factor 3), distal median function (factor 4) and distal peroneal function (factor 5); together, they explain 57% of the variability in the total data. Diabetic factor scores were significantly ($P < 0.05$) below that of the controls and correlations with fasting blood sugar were significant at the $P \leq 0.001$ level. Use of this technique promises to permit sensible analysis of large amounts of data in clinical studies of diabetic and other types of polyneuropathy.

10. Rondinelli RD, Stolov WC, Fujimoto WY, et al. Electrodiagnosis of diabetic peripheral polyneuropathy. A multivariate analytic approach. Am J Phys Med Rehabil 1988;67:12–23.

Traditional univariate comparisons of nerve conduction data against standard norms may produce conflicting estimates of the presence or absence of a diabetic neuropathy, depending upon the data obtained and the specific nerves sampled. Alternatively, a multivariate analytic approach, using discriminant functions, provides a useful single measure of the degree of neuropathy determined as a weighted combination of the available data. The weights are derived from the linear discriminant function, which maximizes statistical separation of diabetic and nondiabetic subject groups. In this study, 12 electrophysiologic attributes are used to generate a single discriminant function that clearly separates diabetic from nondiabetic subjects and is interpretable as a neuropathic index. For the first time, the degree of diabetic neuropathy can thus be quantified for purposes of comparison and correlation with other quantifiable clinical/somatic measures of diabetes. The index allows for a higher percentage of type II diabetic patients to be classified as neuropathic than previously described and enables determination of degree of neuropathy in affected individuals by an interpolative method.

6

Safety Considerations in Electrodiagnostic Medicine

Electrodiagnostic medicine evaluations are quite safe as long as a few reasonable precautions are followed regarding electrical safety and prevention of bleeding and infection. Although occasional patients are pain intolerant, most tolerate the study well.

Electrical Safety

Patients are at risk for shock any time the body is connected both to a current source and to ground, and the resistance is sufficiently low to allow current to flow from one to the other. If the potential current path includes the heart the risk is much greater. For a 1 sec external contact with 60 Hz AC, currents >100 mA may induce ventricular fibrillation (1). Due to shock-induced involuntary muscular contraction, currents >25 mA may cause inability to let go of the source.

Some amount of current seeps from all electrical equipment. Capacitance may build up between the machine's wiring and any metal components of the chassis. Due to faulty insulation, stray capacitance, stray inductance, liquid spills, electrical faults or other factors, the chassis of the EMG machine and the patient leads harbor an unavoidable amount of leakage current, which can be transmitted along electrode connections to a patient. The leakage current is usually shunted away through the ground connections, but in the event of high leakage current or faulty grounding, unsafe levels of current can flow to the patient. The standard three-prong connector consists of a hot wire and a neutral wire connected to earth ground. The third prong is a safety ground which provides an electrical connection between the instrument chassis and earth ground, separate from the neutral conductor. It provides a low resistance pathway to earth ground for the dissipation of leakage currents (2). Leakage current should not exceed 100 μA (rms) between chassis and ground, or 50 μA from patient input leads to ground (3).

Newer equipment usually uses an isolated power system, in which patient leads are electrically isolated from power lines and earth ground using transformers or other methods. This typically minimizes the leakage current problem, but in some large, isolated power systems it may still be excessive for patient safety (4). In isolated power systems the leakage cur-

TABLE 6.1
Routine Measures to Avoid Electrical Mishaps

Regular preventive maintenance of the equipment by a biomedical engineer to ensure leakage current is within acceptable limits and grounding is intact.

Ensure the ground plug in the outlet to which the machine is connected is intact and functional.

Because of potential power surges, never turn the EMG machine on or off with the patient connected to it.

To avoid current flows between two grounds of unequal impedance, all electrical equipment connected to the patient should share the same outlet, and only one ground should be attached to the patient; disconnect any nonessential equipment during the electrodiagnostic examination.

Do not use ultrasound gel as a substitute for electrode gel; it contains no electrolytes and is a fire hazard.

Newer equipment is fitted with female connectors to avoid having pin connectors on electrode cables. Use female connectors and adapters for older equipment.

Do not ignore apparently trivial unexpected shocks to patient or lab personnel; a machine causing random shocks should be checked and serviced.

Avoid extension cords; they increase the stray capacitive leakage current by about $1\mu A$/foot.

Do not defeat three-pronged, safety grounded connectors with adapters or extension cords.

Keep liquids away from the equipment.

Keep all electrodes, especially the ground, on the same side of the body.

rent from patient leads to ground should not exceed $10\ \mu A$ (5).

When more than one ground is in contact with the patient, current may flow between the grounds if their impedances and connections to earth ground are not identical. As little as 50 mV difference between grounds could lead to significant current flowing in such a "ground loop" and could be hazardous to the patient (4). Leakage current flowing across the body, as from one arm to the other, threatens the cardiac conduction system and is particularly hazardous. All electrode connections should be on one side of the body. When more than one instrument with a ground connection is connected to the patient simultaneously, all grounds should be on one side of the body. Some basic electrical safety measures are summarized in Table 6.1.

Electrically Sensitive Patients

When skin resistance is eliminated, even small currents can pose a significant risk. Macroshock refers to shock through intact skin; microshock refers to shock from very small currents capable of causing arrhythmias if delivered directly to the heart. Patients with central intravenous lines are at particular risk because microshock, delivered directly to the heart through such direct low resistance conduits, can adversely affect cardiac conduction. The threshold for ventricular fibrillation when delivered through a central line is about 180 μA, possibly lower in those with heart disease (1). Patients with implanted cardioverters and defibrillators must be handled with particular care (6,7). Leakage current for electrically sensitive patients in nonisolated systems should not exceed 20 μA. Electrical safety issues are particularly likely to arise when studies are done in the operating room or intensive care unit (8). Isolated power systems effectively protect against macroshock, but do not eliminate the hazard of microshock (9). Some safety measures for the electrically sensitive patient are summarized in Table 6.2.

Bleeding

Patients with bleeding tendencies, usually due to anticoagulants, occasionally present for electrodiagnostic evaluation. At least a limited needle examination can usually be done in patients who are therapeutically anticoagulated, as long as reasonable precautions are

TABLE 6.2
Special Measures to Avoid Electrical Mishaps in a Patient Who Is Electrically Sensitive

Do not perform nerve conduction studies on an extremity with a central line.

Do only those conduction studies absolutely necessary for an adequate electrodiagnostic evaluation, nothing more.

Keep the skin clean, dry, and free of an excessive conductive gel.

Do not stimulate at Erb's point in a patient with a central line.

Get cardiologic clearance before doing conduction studies on a patient with a pacemaker or implanted defibrillator.

Do not perform nerve conduction studies on a patient with an external conductive lead terminating in or near the heart.

TABLE 6.3
Precautionary Measures in Patients with Bleeding Tendencies

Do not perform the study unless it is essential to answering a significant clinical question.

Do a focused, limited exam of the key muscles necessary to settle a clinical issue.

Limit probing of examined muscles to the minimum necessary.

Apply pressure to puncture site after completion of probing.

Do not examine patients with an INR or PTT beyond the therapeutic range, or if platelets are <50,000.

Examine superficial muscles first to ascertain the tendency to bleed, and discontinue the examination if hemostasis is difficult to obtain.

Avoid examining deeply placed or difficult to access muscles.

Don't press your luck.

followed and the study is truly necessary to answer a clinically important question (Table 6.3). When the INR or PTT is extremely prolonged, it is best to forego the study. There have been only rare reports of bleeding complications due to needle electromyography (3,10). Clinically insignificant paraspinal hematomas have been reported even in nonanticoagulated patients (10).

Pain

Most patients tolerate electrodiagnostic medicine evaluations without much difficulty, but occasional individuals find the discomfort unbearable. The patient's level of pain tolerance is in itself sometimes useful clinical information. Usually, women tolerate the study better than men, and older patients better than younger ones, although reports of pain perception may be at odds with these common observations (11). The actual pain experienced during the study is usually less than anticipated (12). When the patient is reluctant to undergo the study, suggest trying a muscle or two with the promise to stop if the pain is unbearable; don't fail to keep the promise. For pain intolerant patients, monopolar needles are preferable. Examine key muscles first and limit the probing to the minimum necessary. NEVER start with the APB. When the examination is incomplete or insufficient, it is often effective to have the patient return at a later

date premedicated with a sedative or analgesic, such as meperidine 50 mg orally. Whether placebo effect or real, patients can frequently withstand a study with this minimal premedication who could not tolerate it previously. Topical anesthetics are rarely worth the trouble (13).

Universal Precautions

Percutaneous or mucocutaneous occupational exposure to blood or body fluids involves a risk of transmission of serious infections, including human immunodeficiency virus (HIV), hepatitis B virus (HBV), hepatitis C, and prion diseases. The spread of HIV and HBV over the past decade has resulted in the development of specific guidelines for the cleaning, disinfection, sterilization, and handling of medical equipment and instruments. The prevalence of these viruses, and the risk of prions with their resistance to conventional sterilization procedures, has fueled the transition to disposable needles. The chances of a health care worker contracting hepatitis B or C is much higher than for contracting HIV infection. In surgeons, the cumulative lifetime risk for hepatitis can be as high as 43% (14).

The Centers for Disease Control established guidelines known as universal precautions (UPs)—a set of work practices designed to minimize exposure to blood and body fluid borne pathogens—to prevent transmission of these infections in hospital settings. UPs consider all bodily fluids an infection risk. Unfortunately, UPs are not universally followed. There is often poor compliance with the established protocols, and body fluid contacts are significantly under-reported (15). Some of the reasons for noncompliance with UPs include old habits, forgetfulness, and the perception that barrier precautions hinder manual dexterity.

Accidental needle sticks and other types of sharps injury represent the greatest hazard. Although the issue has not been specifically assessed for electrodiagnostic medicine, a frequency of needlestick injury in general practice as high as 22 occurences per 100 health care workers per 6 months has been reported (16). The incidence among surgeons, more often faced with risky situations, is significantly higher (15).

The effectiveness of universal precautions training is directly related to compliance, and compliance is directly related to a number of factors. Lack of training in universal precautions and unfamiliarity with its procedures is the greatest impediment to the exercise of reasonable caution. Among health care workers, physicians are least likely to adhere to UPs, older

TABLE 6.4

Measures to Minimize the Risk of Transmissible Disease in the EMG Laboratory

Wash hands and use clean disposable latex gloves for each patient.

Keep lab equipment clean. Disinfect surface electrodes and wires between patients.

Pay attention to your hands; realize the potential for the transfer of body fluids to the EMG keyboard and other ancillary implements.

Protect unavoidably touched lab surfaces, such as countertops and keyboards.

Routinely inspect lab surfaces for evidence of contamination.

Develop the habit of using one hand to manipulate the EMG needle and the other for everything else.

All lab personnel should be vaccinated against hepatitis B and have antibodies assayed.

Avoid using nondisposable needles on demented or ALS patients; if such needles are used they should preferably be sterilized adequately to kill prions. (3) (Some chemical treatments of single fiber needles may damage the needle).

Never attempt to recap a needle; the cleanest and safest place for an EMG needle is in the patient.

Modified from Capazzoli NJ. Aseptic technique in needle EMG: common sense and common practice. Muscle Nerve 1996;19:538.

physicians less likely to comply than younger ones, and men less than women; noncompliance is associated with an increased risk of exposure (17). One of the lowest areas of compliance, particularly relevant for electrodiagnostic medicine, is the recommendation for direct sharps disposal without needle recapping. Training and familiarity clearly help (18). Routine glove wearing can produce a significant reduction in sharps injuries (19).

Capozzolli has recently addressed the issue of aseptic technique in EMG (20). Table 6.4 summarizes some measures to minimize the risk of transmissible disease in the EMG laboratory.

Miscellaneous

Other rare reported complications of EMG include pneumothorax after examination of the supraspinatus or paraspinal muscles; calcinosis cutis; and transmission of mycobacterial infection (21–24).

Key Points

- Some amount of current seeps from all electrical equipment due to faulty insulation, stray capacitance, stray inductance, liquid spills, electrical faults or other factors. The chassis of the EMG machine and the patient leads harbor an unavoidable amount of leakage current, which can be transmitted along electrode connections to a patient. Patients are at risk for shock any time the body is connected both to a current source and to ground, and the resistance is sufficiently low to allow current to flow from one to the other.

- Leakage current flowing across the body, as from one arm to the other, exposes the cardiac conduction system and is particularly hazardous.

- In the event of high leakage current or faulty grounding, unsafe levels of current can flow to the patient. Leakage current should not exceed 100 μA (rms) between chassis and ground, or 50 μA from patient input leads to ground. When more than one ground is in contact with the patient, current may flow between the grounds if their impedances and connections to earth ground are not identical.

- Macroshock refers to shock through intact skin; microshock refers to shock from very small currents capable of causing arrhythmias if delivered directly to the heart. Patients with central lines are at particular risk for microshock. Electrical safety issues are particularly likely to arise when studies are done in the operating room or intensive care unit.

- There have been only rare reports of bleeding complications due to needle electromyography. At least a limited needle examination can usually be done in patients who are therapeutically anticoagulated, as long as reasonable precautions are followed and the study is truly necessary to answer a clinically important question.

- Most patients tolerate electrodiagnostic medicine evaluations without much difficulty, but occasional individuals find the discomfort unbearable. The actual pain experienced during the study is usually less than anticipated. For pain intolerant patients, monopolar needles are preferable. Examine key muscles first and limit the probing to the minimum necessary.

- Occupational exposure to blood or body fluids involves a risk of transmission of serious infectious diseases, especially HIV and hepatitis B virus (HBV). The chances of a health care worker contracting hepatitis B or C is much higher than for contracting HIV.

- Universal precautions (UPs) are a set of work practices designed to minimize exposure to blood and body fluid borne pathogens in hospital settings. Unfortunately, UPs are not universally followed. There is often poor compliance with the established protocols, and body fluid contacts are significantly under-reported. Accidental needle sticks and other types of sharps injury represent the greatest hazard.

- The effectiveness of universal precautions training is directly related to compliance. Lack of training in universal precautions and unfamiliarity with its procedures is the greatest impediment to the exercise of reasonable caution. Among health care workers, physicians are least likely to adhere to UPs. One of the lowest areas of compliance, particularly relevant for electrodiagnostic medicine, is the recommendation for direct sharps disposal without needle recapping. Routine glove wearing can produce a significant reduction in sharps injuries.

- Other rare reported complications of EMG include pneumothorax after examination of the supraspinatus or paraspinal muscles; calcinosis cutis; and transmission of mycobacterial infection.

References

1. Lagerlund TD. Electrical safety in the laboratory and hospital. In: Daube JR, ed. Clinical neurophysiology. Philadelphia: F.A. Davis Co., 1996;18–28.

2. Gitter AJ, Stolov WC. AAEM minimonograph #16: instrumentation and measurement in electrodiagnostic medicine—Part II. Muscle Nerve 1995;18:812–824.
   See Chapter 2 for abstract.

3. Guidelines in electrodiagnostic medicine. American Association of Electrodiagnostic Medicine. Muscle Nerve 1992;15:229–253.

4. Kimura J. Electrodiagnosis in diseases of nerve and muscle: principles and practice. 2nd ed. Philadelphia: F.A. Davis Co., 1989.

5. Barry DT. AAEM minimonograph #36: basic concepts of electricity and electronics in clinical electromyography. Muscle Nerve 1991;14:937–946.
   See Chapter 2 for abstract.

6. Miller RG, Nora LM. Written informed consent for electrodiagnostic testing: pro and con. Muscle Nerve 1997;20:352–356.
   See Chapter 12 for abstract.

7. Nora LM. American Association of Electrodiagnostic Medicine guidelines in electrodiagnostic medicine: implanted cardioverters and defibrillators. Muscle Nerve 1996;19:1359–1360.
   Electrodiagnostic testing should not be carried out without consultation with a cardiologist with expertise in electrophysiology. Roots, plexuses or nerves near the implantation site should not be stimulated. The stimulator must be at least 6 in. from the implanted device. Ground electrodes must be securely in place. Stimulus duration should not be > 0.2 ms., and rate not > 1 per sec.

8. Litt L, Ehrenwerth J. Electrical safety in the operating room: important old wine, disguised new bottles (editorial). Anesth Analg 1994;78:417–419.

9. Day FJ. Electrical safety revisited: a new wrinkle. Anesthesiology 1994;80:220–221.

10. Caress JB, Rutkove SB, Carlin M, et al. Paraspinal muscle hematoma after electromyography. Neurology 1996;47:269–272.
    There have been few reports of complications related to electromyography. Needle examination of certain muscles is sometimes avoided in patients taking anticoagulant agents, although no clear guidelines have been established. This report describes a patient who was not receiving an anticoagulant and developed a large paraspinal muscle hematoma after routine electromyography. Subsequently, a review of all patients who underwent paraspinal muscle EMG and were diagnosed with radiculopathy over a 14-month period disclosed 17 patients who had also underwent MRI of the appropriate spinal levels within 1 week after the needle examination. These images were reviewed for evidence of paraspinal muscle hematomas. Four small hematomas were identified in four different patients. None of these were radiologically significant compared with the large hematoma described in the case report. Radiologically apparent paraspinal hematomas after electromyography are an unusual complication of needle examination and do not appear to have any clinical significance. Nevertheless, the presence of these lesions justifies caution when considering electromyography of paraspinal and other deeper muscles in anticoagulated patients. See also Butler ML, Dewan RW. Subcutaneous hemorrhage in a patient receiving anticoagulant therapy: an unusual EMG complication. Arch Phys Med Rehabil 1984;65:733–734.

11. Richardson JK, Evans JE, Warner JH. Information effect on the perception of pain during electromyography. Arch Phys Med Rehabil 1994;75:671–675.
    The authors hypothesized that anxiety and pain perception associated with EMG would decrease if patients received written material describing the EMG before examination. 42 subjects received written material and 30 did not. Information before the test significantly decreased pain perception for women during the nerve conduction studies (p = .008), but not during the needle examination. A similar effect was not identified for the men. Other results indicate that women perceive the test as more painful than do men, older subjects perceive more pain and experience greater anxiety than do younger subjects, and all subjects perceive greater pain during the performance of needle EMG than during the nerve conduction studies.

12. Kothari MJ, Preston DC, Plotkin GM, et al. Electromyography: do the diagnostic ends justify the means? Arch Phys Med Rehabil 1995;76:947–949.
    Physicians are sometimes reluctant to refer patients for electrodiagnostic studies believing the test is too painful and of little benefit. This study carried out two separate surveys on 126 and 100 consecutive patients referred to a laboratory to determine if EMG/NCS was beneficial to the referring physician and to compare the level of anxiety experienced by patients before the study with the pain actually experienced during the study. The electrodiagnosis was discordant from the referring diagnosis in 39% of the patients. Pretest anxiety levels were low in 59% of the patients, medium in 27%, and high in 14%. After the tests, 82% of the patients said that the test was not as bad as expected, and was generally only mildly painful. Ninety-three responded that they would have the test performed again. The authors conclude that EMG/NCS often suggest alternative diagnoses, and the actual pain experienced during a study is significantly less than expected.

13. Lamarche Y, Lebel M, Martin R. EMLA partially relieves the pain of EMG needling. Can J Anaesth 1992;39:805–808.
    The aim of this study was to evaluate the efficacy of the topical analgesic cream EMLA in alleviating the pains caused by

needling in EMG. The EMLA was spread thickly on the lateral dorsal aspect of the forearm and on the thenar eminence of one arm, and placebo was applied on the homologous sites of the other arm. After at least 45 min of application (range 45–145 min, mean = 72.3 +/− 22.2), the needle was inserted into the skin and into the muscle, after which the patient scored the degree of pain on a visual analogue scale. The pain was less after EMLA than placebo for the forearm site but no different for the thenar site.

14. Pietrabissa A, Merigliano S, Montorsi M, et al. Reducing the occupational risk of infections for the surgeon: multicentric national survey on more than 15,000 surgical procedures. World J Surg 1997;21:573–578.
A probabilistic model was used to predict the cumulative 30-year risk to the surgeon of contracting hepatitis B and C viruses (HBV, HCV) or human immunodeficiency virus (HIV) infection from accidental exposure to blood and body fluids during operations and estimate the effect of preventive strategies in reducing this risk. Accidental exposure to blood or body fluids occurred in 9.2% of 15,375 operations; a needle-stick injury was the commonest accident. The current lifetime risk of acquiring HBV, HCV, and HIV infection was estimated to be as high as 42.7%, 34.8%, and 0.54%, respectively. The adoption of preventive strategies is expected to reduce this risk to 21% for HBV, 16.6% for HCV, and 0.23% for HIV infection.

15. Manian FA. Blood and body fluid exposures among surgeons: a survey of attitudes and perceptions five years following Universal Precautions. Infect Control Hosp Epidemiol 1996;17:172–174.
A survey of surgeons 5 years following adoption of Universal Precautions revealed that 29% estimated having ≥ 1 potentially serious blood or body fluid exposures per month. Failure to report exposures (usually needlesticks) was common.

16. Lum D, Mason Z, Meyer-Rochow G, et al. Needle stick injuries in country general practice. N Z Med J 1997; 110:122–125.
A survey of general practitioners and nurses in of New Zealand revealed an incidence of 22 needle stick injuries in 100 health care workers per 6 month period. Recommended precautionary measures were not being followed by most individuals.

17. Michalsen A, Delclos GL, Felknor SA, et al. Compliance with universal precautions among physicians. J Occup Environ Med 1997;39:130–137.
This study characterized and assessed self-reported levels of compliance with universal precautions (UP) among hospital-based physicians, and determined significant factors associated with both compliance and noncompliance. Compliance with UP was measured through 11 items that examined how often physicians followed specific recommended work practices. Compliance was found to vary among the 11 items: they were high for certain activities (e.g., glove use, 94%; disposal of sharps, 92%) and low for others (e.g., wearing protective clothing, 55%; not recapping needles, 56%). Compliance with all items was low (31% to 38%). Stepwise logistic regression revealed that noncompliant physicians were likely to be age 37 or older, to report high work stress, and to perceive a conflict of interest between providing patient care and protecting themselves. Compliant physicians were more likely to be knowledgeable and to have been trained in universal precautions, to perceive protective measures as being effective, and to perceive an organizational commitment to safety.

18. Diekema DJ, Albanese MA, Schuldt SS, et al. Blood and body fluid exposures during clinical training: relation to knowledge of universal precautions. J Gen Intern Med 1996;11:109–111.
An investigation of the relation between knowledge of universal precautions and rates of exposure to blood and body fluid during clinical training in a cohort of 155 students. Knowledge of universal precautions was inversely associated with the frequency of mucous membrane exposures (p < .001).

19. Ben-David B, Gaitini L. The routine wearing of gloves: impact on the frequency of needlestick and percutaneous injury and on surface contamination in the operating room. Anesth Analg 1996;83:623–628.
The impact of wearing gloves on surface contamination and on the incidence of percutaneous injury were prospectively compared for two 4-mo periods in a single anesthesia department. Period I was immediately prior to the institution of mandatory glove wearing, and Period II followed a 1-mo adjustment period of mandatory glove use. Recording of all needlestick and other percutaneous injuries was performed on an ongoing basis, and incident reporting was actively and regularly solicited. The implementation of a mandatory glove use policy was associated with nonsignificant trends toward reduction in the incidence of needlestick and other percutaneous injury and in the level of surface contamination in the anesthesia workplace. Compliance with glove use resulted in a significant reduction in needlestick injury and overall percutaneous injuries.

20. Capazzoli NJ. Aseptic technique in needle EMG: common sense and common practice. Muscle Nerve 1996; 19:538.

21. Reinstein L, Twardzik FG, Mech KF, Jr. Pneumothorax: a complication of needle electromyography of the supraspinatus muscle. Arch Phys Med Rehabil 1987; 68:561–562.
A patient developed a 10% pneumothorax during needle EMG of the right supraspinatus muscle. The patient was treated conservatively with complete resolution. A review of the pertinent anatomy indicates that the supraspinatus muscle overlies the pleural cavity. Indications for needle EMG of the supraspinatus muscle are reviewed, and a new technique described that minimizes the risk of pneumothorax when performing needle EMG of the supraspinatus muscle.

22. Honet JE, Honet JC, Cascade P. Pneumothorax after electromyographic electrode insertion in the paracervical muscles: case report and radiographic analysis. Arch Phys Med Rehabil 1986;67:601–603.
A patient developed pneumothorax after needle electrode examination of the paracervical muscles. Cadavers and cervical spine radiographs were studied to assess the vulnerability of lung tissue to paracervical muscle needle insertion. In five of 23 patient radiographs studied, lung tissue extended above the clavicle with a distance from skin surface to lung tissue of approximately 3.3 cm. The electromyographer examining the paracervical musculature should be aware that needle electrode penetration of lung tissue is possible. Examination must be conducted with care, especially in thin patients with long necks. Needle insertion close to the midline is the safest technique. See also Miller J. Pneumothorax: complication of needle EMG of thoracic wall. N J Med 1990;87:653; and Honet JC. Pneumothorax and EMG. Arch Phys Med Rehab 1988;69:149.

23. Johnson RC, Fitzpatrick JE, Hahn DE. Calcinosis cutis

following electromyographic examination. Cutis 1993; 52:161–164.

24. Nolan CM, Hashisaki PA, Dundas DF. An outbreak of soft-tissue infections due to Mycobacterium fortuitum associated with electromyography. J Infect Dis 1991; 163:1150–1153.

During a 6-week period, six patients who received EMG in one laboratory by one physician and assistant developed soft-tissue Mycobacterium fortuitum infections, manifested by slowly ex-panding suppurative nodules at sites of needle electrode inser-tion. Standard procedures included use of reusable needle elec-trodes disinfected with 2% glutaraldehyde and then rinsed with tap water. On recognition of the outbreak, the procedure was changed to include autoclaving of needle electrodes. Active surveillance for 1 year revealed no further cases. M. fortuitum could not be isolated from the laboratory, EMG equipment and reagents, or skin of the medical personnel. The outbreak demonstrates that nontuberculous mycobacterial infection may be associated with EMG.

7

Nerve Conduction Studies

Standard procedures used in electrodiagnostic medicine include: motor and sensory conduction studies, late responses, repetitive nerve stimulation, blink reflexes, and the needle electromyographic exam. Other procedures are available for assessment of certain clinical situations, such as the mini-exercise test for suspected periodic paralysis, root stimulation, and intraoperative electrodiagnosis. This section will discuss basic nerve conduction studies. Subsequent chapters will cover special studies such as blink reflexes, repetitive nerve stimulation studies, and the needle examination.

Motor Conduction Studies

Motor conduction studies are performed by stimulating a motor nerve at one or more points while recording the compound muscle action potential (CMAP) or, preferably, the M wave, from a muscle innervated by that nerve. The active recording electrode (G_1) is placed over the motor point on the belly of the muscle to be studied, and the reference electrode (G_2) is placed over the tendon of the muscle distally. The motor point is that site where the intramuscular nerve enters the muscle belly. The muscle action potential originates at the motor point and spreads throughout the muscle. The tendon is used for G_2 since it is presumably electrically inactive. After nerve stimulation, the potential difference between the active and reference electrodes is displayed and the time between delivery of the stimulus and the onset of the M wave determined. This technique is referred to as the belly-tendon method. Parameters evaluated include the motor nerve conduction velocity, the distal motor latency, the proximal motor latency, and the characteristics of the M wave.

By convention in clinical electrophysiology, when G_1 is negative in relation to G_2, the deflection of the baseline is upward. Relative positivity at G_2 also causes an upward deflection, and relative positivity at G_1 or relative negativity at G_2 cause downward deflections. Electrical events occurring at a distance in the volume conductor are detected by both G_1 and G_2 and may influence the direction of deflection (1).

The M wave is the summated, "compounded" response of all the muscle fibers that lie within the recording area of the electrode and have responded to the electrical stimulation of the nerve. The M wave is usually recorded via a 10 mm surface disc electrode, which "sees" the electrical activity in the whole muscle, or at least over a large area. The configuration of the M wave is significantly affected by the size and shape of both the recording and reference electrodes

(2–4). A subcutaneous electrode, such as a 1 cm EEG needle electrode, also sees nearly the entire muscle and has advantages under some circumstances, such as for intraoperative recordings. An intramuscular needle recording can rarely be useful, such as for recording from a deeply placed muscle, but only detects the activity from a limited number of muscle fibers within the circumscribed recording area of the needle tip. The intramuscular recording, while accurately recording the latency of the response, is highly unreliable for evaluating response amplitude or configuration. Because M wave amplitude and configuration are very important attributes, intramuscular needle recording has only limited applicability.

Figure 7.1 depicts a typical M wave. Characteristics usually measured include the onset latency, amplitude, and configuration. Under some circumstances,

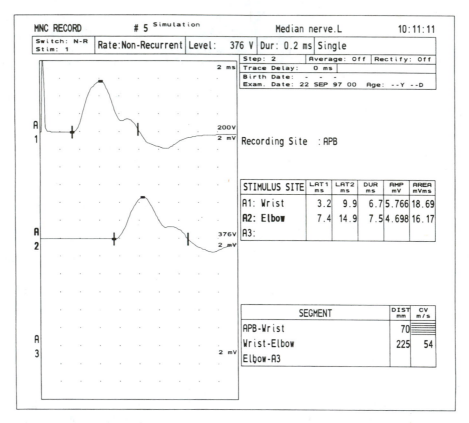

FIGURE 7.1. An M wave, or compound muscle action potential (CMAP). Tracing A1 was obtained by stimulating the median nerve at the wrist, recording with G_1, the active electrode, over the belly of the abductor pollicis brevis and G_2, the reference electrode, over the tendon. Tracing A2 was obtained by stimulating the median nerve at the elbow. Parameters measured include the latency at the onset, the latency at the termination of the negative spike, the duration, the negative spike amplitude, and the negative spike area. The distal distance, from the wrist stimulation site to the active electrode was 70 mm, the distance from the elbow stimulation site to the wrist stimulation site was 225 mm, and the conduction velocity from elbow to wrist was 54 m/s. Note the higher stimulus intensity required to obtain a supramaximal response at the elbow. The M wave amplitude is lower on proximal stimulation, but the duration is increased and the area under the curve is decreased proportionately much less than the amplitude. These changes are a reflection of temporal dispersion over distance.

measurement of the duration and area may provide useful additional information.

The M wave onset latency marks its initial deflection, the point at which the waveform leaves the baseline. The negativity at G_1, the active electrode, produces an upward deflection of the sweep. When the surface disc electrode is properly placed over the motor point of the muscle, the onset is a clean, initially negative deflection from the baseline. When the recording electrode is off the motor point, this initial deflection is positive (downward) as the electrode detects the motor point negativity at a distance through the volume conductor. The negative deflection follows as the wave of depolarization passes beneath the electrode. This sequence produces a "dip" of initial positivity followed by the main negative deflection. When such a dip occurs, the electrode should be repositioned so as to obtain a clean, initially negative deflection. Rarely, usually when recording from an atrophic muscle, the dip cannot be eliminated. In this case, the latency is always taken from the onset of the M wave, even if this is a positive deflection.

The configuration or shape of the M wave is constant for any given positioning of the recording electrodes. The M wave amplitude may be measured from the baseline to the height of the negative peak (negative peak amplitude), or from the height of the negative peak to the depth of the positive peak (peak to peak amplitude). Either method is acceptable so long as the clinical study follows the same conventions and procedures as that used to obtain the normal reference values. The M wave negative spike duration extends from the initial deflection to the return to the baseline. Modern computerized electromyographs can calculate the total area under the M wave curve, which can be particularly useful for distinguishing between true conduction block and loss of amplitude due to temporal dispersion.

A peripheral nerve consists of a population of axons of different sizes and different degrees of myelination, and therefore different conduction velocities. Stimulation at increasing distances from the recording electrodes produces an increasing dispersion of the M wave as the volley of impulses arriving at the recording electrode becomes progressively less synchronized due to the differing conduction velocities. This is the phenomenon of physiologic temporal dispersion and produces a lower amplitude, longer duration M wave on proximal as compared with distal stimulation (Fig. 7.1). There is less change in total area under the curve because the same number of muscle fibers is eventually activated. With a significant disparity in the conduction velocity of individual axons, the positivity of the repolarization phase of muscle fibers activated by the first arriving impulses begins to balance and ne-

gate the negativity created by later arriving impulses: the phenomenon of phase cancellation.

Because of temporal dispersion and phase cancellation, M wave amplitude normally decreases on proximal stimulation vs. distal stimulation. With the usual proximal stimulation sites at the knee and elbow, there is no more than a 20% decrease in M wave negative peak amplitude, and no significant change in M wave configuration. A decrease in amplitude > 20%, an increase in amplitude, or a significant change in waveform on proximal as compared with distal stimulation suggests either: submaximal proximal stimulation, inadvertent spread of the stimulus to adjacent nerves (either proximally or distally), a demyelinating lesion in the nerve between the two sites or anomalous innervation.

The normal range of fiber sizes and CVs is different in motor and sensory nerves. Sensory fibers vary from very small, unmyelinated slow pain axons to large, myelinated spindle afferents. The spectrum of size for motor fibers is much less. The range from slowest to fastest sensory fiber CV is about 25 m/s, while the range for motor fibers is only about half that. Phase cancellation is not a significant factor in normal motor conduction studies, but can become a major influence on M wave amplitude in the face of severe conduction velocity slowing, or when studies are done over very long distances. Phase cancellation is a major factor in determining the amplitude of sensory potentials on proximal stimulation (5).

Nerve conduction studies are done by delivering an electrical stimulus to depolarize the nerve and generate an action potential. The cathode delivers the stimulus. Its negativity draws positive charges away from the surface of the axolemma, decreases the transmembrane potential and depolarizes the nerve to threshold, which causes an action potential to fire. Stimulation is usually done percutaneously with surface electrodes, but occasionally a needle cathode is advantageous. With surface stimulation, the anode and cathode are usually separated by about 2 cm. Measurements are made from the center of the stimulating cathode to the center of the recording electrode. Small stimulating electrodes, as often used for pediatric studies, are actually more painful because the smaller surface concentrates the stimulation and delivers a higher local current density, which is more painful. The unnecessary sharpness of the stimulating electrodes made by most manufacturers is another often unrecognized source of pain. The rounded sides of the electrodes deliver the stimulus just as effectively.

Two types of stimulators are possible. A constant voltage stimulator delivers the same voltage at any given voltage setting. A constant current stimulator delivers the same current at any given stimulator setting, varying the voltage as necessary, depending on the tissue resistance, to deliver the same current (recall V = IR). Since it is current flow, not voltage, that depolarizes the nerve, a constant current stimulator is usually preferable. For locating nerve strands in the bed of a tumor or a scar during intraoperative studies, constant voltage stimulation may be better (6). One point of potential minor confusion is that when the EMG machine stimulator is set to deliver constant voltage stimulation, the stimulation intensity readout is in volts, and the setting changes with rotating the stimulus intensity knob; vice versa with constant current. The point is that, although the mA readout may change with rotating the knob, the current delivered at any given setting is constant.

Motor nerve conduction velocity (MNCV) is determined by stimulating a nerve at two sites separated by a known distance. By convention, the maximal MNCV is assessed for clinical studies. Determining maximal MNCV requires supramaximal stimulation at both sites; this ensures that all fibers have been activated, including the fastest fibers in the nerve. Supramaximal stimulation is assured by progressively increasing the stimulus intensity (in volts or mA) until there is no further increase in M wave amplitude, then increasing the intensity by a further 20–50% for the final stimulation. Taking the onset latency of the M wave further ensures that maximal MNCV is determined since the initial deflection reflects the activity in the first fibers to arrive at the motor point.

Theoretically, MNCV could be assessed for any subpopulation of axons by measuring the latency to an identical point on the two M wave waveforms. The average (really the modal) MNCV could be measured by taking the peak latencies. The slowest fibers could be assessed by taking the latencies to the tail of the M wave. These other conduction velocities are sometimes determined experimentally (7). In clinical studies, for all practical purposes, the maximal NCV is always determined, and the term NCV inherently connotes maximal NCV.

The distal motor latency (DML) is the onset latency of the M wave elicited by supramaximal stimulation at the distalmost site, usually the wrist or ankle. Most laboratories determine the DML at a fixed, premeasured distance proximal to the recording electrode, the same distance used for determining reference values. Some labs determine the DML from a fixed anatomical point, such as the distal wrist crease, and allow the distance to vary within a set range. The proximal motor latency (PML) is the onset latency after supramaximal stimulation at some proximal point, usually the elbow or knee. The distance between the two sites is measured over the skin surface, usually

with a tape measure, occasionally with calipers. The maximal MNCV is then calculated by

$$MNCV = \frac{Distance}{PML\text{-}DML}$$

For example, for a median nerve where wrist stimulation produces an onset latency of 3.0 msec, elbow stimulation a latency of 8.0 msec and the distance from wrist to elbow is 250 mm, then:

$$MNCV = 250 \text{ mm} / (8.0 \text{ ms}-3.0 \text{ ms})$$
$$= 50 \text{ mm/ms, or } 50 \text{ m/s}$$

By convention, conduction velocity (CV) is expressed in m/s. For motor studies, the CV cannot be determined by stimulating at a single site and measuring the distance to the active electrode, because the timing of distal events is uncertain. More is involved than simply the CV of the nerve. The length of time required for conduction in terminal axons, for neuromuscular transmission and for generation of the muscle action potential is indeterminable: the events constitute a "black box." The time required for the main trunk of the nerve to conduct from the proximal to the distal site is therefore reflected by the value of PML-DML. The distance is always measured between the proximal and distal stimulation points, *NEVER* from the stimulation point to the recording electrode. In contrast, for sensory studies the nerve action potential is measured directly and the maximal sensory NCV can be determined by taking the onset latency from a single stimulation site and measuring the distance from the stimulation site to the center of the recording electrode. See the following discussion on sensory conduction studies for further discussion of this method.

The recording setups and normal values for commonly done motor conduction studies are summarized in Table 7.1. The topic of motor conduction studies has recently been reviewed in detail (8).

Sensory Conduction Studies

Sensory conduction studies are done differently. A nerve is stimulated and the evoked nerve action potential (NAP) is recorded directly by electrodes placed over the nerve. Orthodromic sensory studies are done by stimulating distally and recording proximally, in the direction of normal impulse flow. Antidromic studies are done by stimulating proximally, e.g., at the wrist, and recording the retrogradely transmitted potential distally, e.g., at the finger. Latency is the same with either technique as long as the recording interelectrode separation is the same, but amplitude

TABLE 7.1
Techniques for Commonly Studied Motor Nerves (with the Normal Reference Values Used at the Medical College of Virginia)

Nerve	Active Electrode Site (G1)	Reference Electrode Site (G2)	Distal Stimulation Site	Distal Distance (cm)	Proximal Stimulation Site 1	Proximal Stimulation Site 2	Distal M Amp (mV)	Distal Motor Lat	CV	Minimal F Latency	Traps and Frequent Problems
Median	APB	tendon	wrist	7	elbow		>3	<4.5	>48	<32	1) spread to the ulnar n. at the wrist. 2) submaximal stimulation at elbow 3) anomalous innervation
Ulnar	ADQ	tendon	wrist	7	BE	AE	>5	<3.6	>48	<32	1) spread to the median n. at the wrist 2) CV from AE varies with elbow position 3) anomalous innervation
Peroneal	EDB	tendon	ankle	8	BFH	AFH	>2	<6.6	>42	<55	1) spread to tibial n. at AFH site 2) pseudodip on proximal stimulation 3) anomalous innervation
Tibial	AH	tendon	ankle	8–14	PF		>2	<6.6	>42	<55	1) spread to peroneal n. at PF 2) submaximal proximal stimulation

APB, abductor pollicis brevis; ADQ, abductor digiti quinti; EDB, extensor digitorum brevis; AH, abductor hallucis; AE, above elbow; BE, below elbow; BFH, below fibular head; AFH, above fibular head; PF, popliteal fossa; CV, conduction velocity is lower with the orthodromic method. Most electrodiagnostic medicine consultants prefer antidromic techniques for all but palmar and plantar studies.

Technically, a sensory nerve action potential (SNAP) study can only be done by either simulating and recording from a purely sensory nerve (e.g., the sural), stimulating a mixed sensorimotor peripheral nerve and recording from a purely sensory branch (e.g., median antidromic digital) or stimulating a sensory nerve while recording from a mixed nerve (e.g., median orthodromic digital potential). In fact, the compound nerve action potential (CNAP) recorded from a mixed nerve (e.g., the median at the wrist) after stimulation of a mixed nerve (e.g., the median in the palm) is still commonly referred to as a SNAP. In customary usage, SNAP refers to any nerve action potential, whether truly sensory or in fact compound.

Assessment of a SNAP (Fig. 7.2) is analogous to that of an M wave but with important differences. Recording of a SNAP over the midportion of a nerve produces the classic triphasic potential. The initial and terminal positivities are a normal phenomenon; their genesis is discussed in detail in Chapter 4. The onset of the negative wave (equivalent to the initial positive peak) indicates the time of arrival of the depolarization wave beneath G_1, and is the time of onset of the NAP. The peak latency represents arrival of the main volley at G_1. For complicated reasons related to physiology and volume conduction, the initial positivity is frequently not present. If G_2 overlies an electrically inactive end of the nerve, such as a tendon, the terminal positivity does not occur (killed end effect).

Because of the relatively slow CV of muscle fibers, the M wave is a slowly evolving, long duration event. The NAP, in contrast, is a short duration, compact wave in which the minimal separation between the fastest and slowest fibers causes phase cancellation to occur to a much greater degree than with motor studies. SNAPs recorded over long distances can normally lose significant amplitude because of this effect (5,9). Amplitude can also decrease by up to 70%, and the initial positivity become less apparent, if the active electrode is not precisely over the nerve (10).

In contrast to the belly-tendon bipolar method employed for recording the M wave, sensory potentials are recorded with a bipolar method in which G_2 is placed distally along the nerve. For NAP recordings, the separation between G_1 and G_2, the interelectrode distance, becomes critical because the summated NAP amplitude is the algebraic total of the electrical activity recorded at the two electrodes. If G_1 and G_2 are too close together, both become active, distorting the

FIGURE 7.2. Sensory potential studies. Tracing A1 is an orthodromic median palmar potential stimulating the palm and recording from the wrist; peak latency and peak to peak amplitude are marked. Tracing A2 is an orthodromic median digital potential, stimulating the index finger and recording over the same wrist site used for tracing A1. A3 is a digital potential obtained antidromically, reversing the stimulation and recording points used in A2. Again the peak latency and peak to peak amplitude are indicated. Tracing A4 is the same potential, marked at the onset for performing a single site CV (55 m/s over the distance of 13 cm). Tracing A5 is the antidromic digital potential on elbow stimulation. The sensory CV over 230 mm from elbow to write is 61 m/s.

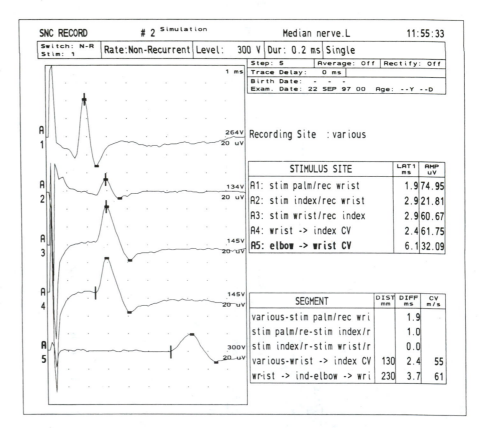

waveform and lowering its amplitude (11). Ideally, the wave of depolarization should clear G_1 before activity begins at G_2. The duration of an action potential is typically about 1 msec. The usual *average* CV of a NAP is about 30 mm/msec so that action potentials in various stages extend along about 30 mm of nerve at any given instant. An interelectrode separation of about 3 cm usually suffices to allow the potential to clear G_1 before activity begins at G_2. Greater separation, while desirable from a theoretical standpoint, has a potentially deleterious countereffect. Large G_1-G_2 distances magnify interference because increasing separation increases the potential difference between the electrodes, magnifying the NAP but also magnifying the noise. A compromise separation of 3–4 cm is usually employed for clinical recordings. NAPs can also be recorded using a monopolar montage with G_1 over the nerve and G_2 at a distant site lateral to G_1. This is the standard technique for near nerve needle recording, but is seldom used otherwise.

The distal sensory latency (DSL) is often done over a relatively short distance, which may allow the shock artifact to contaminate the initial portion of the SNAP, making it difficult to accurately determine the onset latency. As a result, the DSL is usually taken to the peak of the potential, which is a more stable and reproducible point. Sensory CV must still be determined as a maximal CV using onset latencies (Fig. 7.2). Rather than using a peak latency over a fixed, predetermined distance, some labs compare the SNCV from a single stimulus using the onset latency; the distance is thus not a critical factor. This can be done because sensory studies analyze the NAP directly; motor conduction studies must take into consideration the unmeasurable events in the "black box" beyond the nerve, and direct determination of MNCV from a single stimulus is invalid. When doing SNCV from a single point, care must be taken to use the onset of the negative deflection as the latency; initial positivity is a normal physiological event and is not analogous to being off the motor point in motor conduction studies (Fig. 7.3). The SNCV thus determined is compared to normal reference values. SNAPs can also be recorded using near nerve needle electrodes. Amplitude can be determined either as baseline to negative peak, or peak-to-peak depending upon how normal reference values were obtained. The majority of labs in North America assess peak latency over a fixed distance; using surface recording and stimulation; bipolar, antidromic techniques (except for palmar and plantar studies); and a fixed distance of 3–4 cm between G_1 and G_2.

Sensory responses are even more sensitive to temperature effects than are motor responses (12). A de-

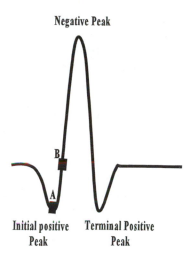

FIGURE 7.3. A sensory potential depicting the different peaks. The initial positive peak is equivalent to the onset of the negative wave and is the true onset of the potential. The initial positivity is frequently absent. The point where the negative spike crosses the baseline (B) may be as much as 0.4 ms after the onset (A) of the negative potential (see Oh SJ. Clinical Electromyography: Nerve Conduction Studies, Baltimore: Williams and Willkins, 1993;289). When performing single point sensory conduction velocities, account should be taken of the latency of activation (approximately 0.15 ms) required to depolarize the nerve and initiate the action potential (see Krarup C, Horowitz SH, Dahl K. The influence of the stimulus on normal sural nerve conduction velocity: a study of the latency of activation. Muscle Nerve 1992;15:813–821).

layed DSL will more often prove to be due to low temperature than to nerve pathology. An important clue to slow sensory conduction due to temperature is that the response amplitude will be normal or even unusually high. Decreased temperature slows down the channel fluxes and ionic shifts; currents flow for a longer period and the apparatus detects this as a delayed latency, high amplitude, long duration NAP. In contrast, a prolonged DSL due to nerve pathology is usually accompanied by a reduction in amplitude. Correction factors to compensate for cold extremities, such as subtracting 1 ms for each 1° C below the reference level, may not be valid for diseased nerve and should be used with caution (13). A better procedure is to warm the part to the temperature at which the reference values were obtained. The clinical importance of this temperature effect cannot be overemphasized. Patients without median nerve pathology have undergone carpal tunnel release because they had cold hands on the day of their EMG. Many "peripheral neuropathies" are "cured" with simple warming.

Sensory potential studies are very sensitive to nerve pathology. Sensory conduction changes tend to occur earlier than motor conduction changes in both focal and generalized neuropathies. SNAP amplitude is the most sensitive indicator of nerve pathology. The exact reasons why SNAP amplitude is a more sensitive indicator for axon loss than M wave amplitude is not entirely clear (11). Despite their sensitivity, however, distal sensory potential abnormalities are nonspecific and nonlocalizing. Axon loss due to a lesion at any point along the nerve will decrease the number of functioning fibers, decreasing the amplitude and prolonging the latency to the mild degree consistent with axon loss. Distally depressed SNAP amplitude could result from a focal lesion anywhere along a nerve trunk, or from a generalized polyneuropathy. Detecting conduction block or temporal dispersion is more problematic with sensory nerves because of the pronounced dependence of NAP amplitude on the distance from the generator source and the buried position of most proximal nerve trunks, and because of the effects of phase cancellation.

It is important to understand that lesions involving nerve roots do not change the sensory potentials. The pathology in radiculopathy involves the nerve root proximal to the dorsal root ganglion; between the ganglion, which lies in or just distal to the neural foramen, and the spinal cord. A lesion in this location does not involve the dorsal root ganglion neurons, which remain healthy and are able to maintain their peripheral processes in a robust state despite the root lesion. Normality of the SNAP is an important differential electrodiagnostic point favoring radiculopathy over plexopathy or neuropathy (14). See Chapters 14 and 15 for further details.

Sensory studies are technically demanding. Accuracy is improved and aggravation lessened by a few simple measures. The skin should be clean to minimize electrode impedance. Gentle abrasion with a pumice preparation (such as OmniPrep, used frequently for EEG recordings), followed by cleaning the skin with alcohol and reapplication of electrodes will sometimes turn a vexatious study into a simple one. Shock artifact can usually be controlled by rotation of the anode. When this fails, cleaning and prepping, maximally separating the stimulator cable from the recording wires, wadding up the electrode lead wires and placing them under the extremity under study while bringing the headbox in as closely as possible, and dousing the fluorescent lights usually help.

The recording setups and normal values for commonly done sensory conduction studies are summarized in Table 7.2. The topic of sensory conduction studies has recently been reviewed in detail (11).

Late Responses

Late responses, F waves and H reflexes, are special techniques used to assess the proximal portions of the peripheral nervous system which are largely inaccessible to routine conduction studies (15). Stimulation of a peripheral nerve always evokes an action potential that travels both directions, both orthodromically and antidromically, from the site of the stimulus. Routine conduction studies assess only the result of the distally traveling potential. The cathode of the simulator is the origin of the nerve stimulus, and it is placed distal to the anode for all routine conduction studies. Anodal block is a theoretical, but equivocally significant, problem that could delay or obliterate the stimulus arising from the cathode and traveling proximally. For late responses, the usual procedure is to reverse the simulator so that the cathode is placed proximally. This generates an action potential that travels centripetally. The sweep is changed to 5 or 10 ms/division, as late responses do not appear on the sweep at the usual settings employed for routine motor conduction studies. The gain is increased for F wave determinations; 500 μV/division usually suffices. H reflex amplitude may match or exceed M wave amplitude, so no change in sensitivity is usually required.

The F wave results from the antidromic activation of motor fibers. The nerve action potential travels proximally, traverses the brachial or lumbosacral plexus, and enters the spinal cord ventral horn through the anterior root. The impulse invades the anterior horn cell retrogradely, causing it to depolarize. In response to this unexpected incursion through its normal egress portal, the anterior horn cell in effect "backfires" and generates an action potential that then travels orthodromically over motor fibers back to the muscle of origin, where it is recorded with surface electrodes.

Each individual F response involves a discharge of about 2–3% of the motor neuron pool. The F wave can be elicited from any muscle, although it is usually not done with proximal recording sites as the F wave becomes lost in the trailing components of the M wave. This limits its applicability for studying proximal muscles, and the F is usually done only in small hand and foot muscles. It is best elicited by supramaximal stimulation and its amplitude is small in relationship to the amplitude of its associated M wave; the normal F amplitude does not exceed 10% of the associated M wave amplitude. At any given stimulus intensity the F wave varies in both latency and amplitude, and the response is usually absent with some stimuli. The F wave persistence is the percentage of stimuli that produce an F wave and is generally in the range of 60–

TABLE 7.2
Techniques for Commonly Studied Sensory Nerves (with the Reference Values Used at the Medical College of Virginia)

Nerve	Active Electrode Site (G1)	Reference Electrode Site (G2)	Stimulation Site	Distal Distance (cm)	SNAP Amplitude (µV)	Distal Sensory Latency (ms)	Traps and Common Problems
Median, antidromic digital	index or middle finger	3–4 cm distal to G1	wrist	13	>15	<3.7	1) low temperature 2) M wave contamination
Median, orthodromic digital	wrist crease	3–4 cm proximal to G1	index or middle finger	13	>5	<3.7	1) low temperature 2) painful
Median orthodromic palmar	wrist crease	3–4 cm proximal to G1	palm	8	>40	<2.3	1) low temperature 2) shock artifact
Ulnar, antidromic digital	small finger	3–4 cm distal to G1	wrist	11	>5	<3.1	1) low temperature 2) M wave contamination
Ulnar orthodromic digital	wrist crease	3–4 cm proximal to G1	small finger	11	>5	<3.1	1) low temperature 2) painful
Ulnar, orthodromic palmar	wrist crease	3–4 cm proximal to G1	palm	8	>11	<2.2	1) low temperature 2) shock artifact
Sural, antidromic	lateral malleolus	3–4 cm distal to G1	posterolateral leg proximal to G1	14	>5	<4.2 under age 30 <4.8 over age 30	1) low temperature 2) submaximal stimulation 3) stimulation too medial or lateral 4) motor artifact
Superficial peroneal, antidromic	anterior aspect of ankle*	3–4 cm distal to G1	anterolateral leg proximal to G1	12	>10	<3.5	1) low temperature 2) stimulation too medial or lateral 3) G1 too medial or lateral

* Midway between peroneal motor stimulation site and lateral malleolus.

FIGURE 7.4. A series of F waves obtained with supramaximal stimulation of the median nerve at the wrist, recording from the APB. Sixteen consecutive stimuli were delivered, of which 14 elicited an F response (persistence 88%). The minimum latency of all the F waves was 28.2 ms, the maximum 33.6 ms, the mean 31.3 ms, and the chronodispersion 5.4 ms.

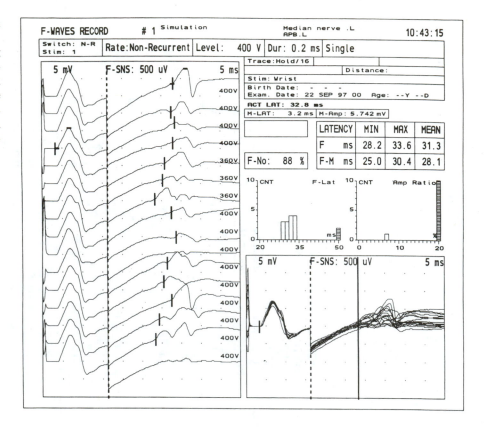

80%. Elicitation of the F wave with every stimulus is unusual and may signal hyperexcitability in the motoneuron pool, such as occurs with upper motoneuron lesions. The F is best elicited by slow irregular stimuli, e.g., once every 2–3 s. It can be fatigued by rapid regular stimuli. Some stimuli will elicit the same F response, a so-called repeater F wave, of the same amplitude, latency and configuration as a previous response.

The variability in F wave latency with a series of stimuli is its chronodispersion or scatter, a measure of temporal dispersion. Most frequently, the minimal F wave latency out of series of 10–20 stimuli is determined. In addition, maximal latency, mean latency, chronodispersion, and persistence may be analyzed, but their use is not routine and normal reference values are scanty (Fig. 7.4). For most applications in most electrodiagnostic medicine laboratories, the minimal latency out of a series of at least 10–20 stimuli is determined, and this value is usually in the range of 28–32 ms in hand muscles and 50–55 ms in foot muscles. The side-to-side difference between upper extremity F waves of homologous nerves or between ipsilateral median and ulnar F waves should not exceed 2 ms. Side-to-side or nerve-to-nerve differences in the lower extremities should not exceed 4 ms. With

borderline values, a more precise calculation taking into account the patient's height and NCV should be carried out.

Recommendations are not consistent regarding how to elicit the F. Some authorities recommend analysis of the F from 10–20 stimuli, others recommend analysis of 10–20 F waves, eliminating repeater waves, which involves a considerably different number of stimuli. Others have recommended eliciting at least eight different F waves before attempting analysis and interpretation and refusing to attempt judgment from a lesser number of responses. This approach leaves many F determinations in limbo—not absent but not adequate for analysis.

Some have advocated calculation of the F wave conduction velocity by deducting the distal motor latency from the minimal F latency, deducting an additional 1 ms for central delay, dividing the remainder by 2 and dividing that figure into the distance from wrist to sternal notch or C7 spinous process, or from ankle to xiphoid or T12 spinous process. This approach introduces a potential measurement error and a somewhat arbitrary central delay into an already marginal determination and has not been widely adopted.

Several types of potentials can be confused with the F response. The A wave, or axon reflex, is a small amplitude potential, usually of short latency and near 100% persistence, that is elicited by submaximal stimuli and usually abolished by supramaximal stimuli (16). It is due to normal or pathologic axon branching and is essentially a "ricochet" of the nerve action potential off a proximal axonal branch point. It is seen most often in neuropathies, presumably the result of collateral sprouting. A submaximal stimulus distal to the sprout generates a centripetal impulse that glances off some reflection of the axolemma at the branch point, activating the subpopulation of the motor units innervated by the collateral. The wave bounces immediately back to the recording electrodes and is recorded as a short latency wave of fixed latency and amplitude, which occurs with every sweep. The A wave amplitude is similar to that of the F. It does not vary in latency or amplitude as the F does, and the latency may be as short as 10–20 ms. Occasionally an A wave may follow the F response. Elicitation of A waves is not uncommon, and they may be readily confused with F responses by the unwary examiner. Low amplitude, surface-recorded MUAPs due to poor relaxation may produce undulations in the baseline simulating F waves. Turning the audio volume up helps monitor relaxation and ensure a flat baseline before delivering the stimulus. Occasionally, the trailing late components associated with a complex, fragmented M wave can be mistaken for F waves.

The H reflex is elicited by activation of large myelinated, type Ia, muscle spindle afferent fibers, generating an impulse that travels centripetally through the brachial or lumbosacral plexus, enters the spinal cord via the posterior root and monosynaptically or oligosynaptically activates an anterior horn cell pool. The anterior horn cell pool then generates a motor action potential that travels centrifugally over motor fibers back to the muscle of origin. The H reflex is approximately the electrodiagnostic equivalent of ankle jerk, and there is a close correlation between the characteristics of the H reflex and the clinical status of the ankle jerk.

An H reflex can be elicited from any muscle in neonates and very young children. In adults, it can normally be elicited only from the gastrosoleus after stimulation of the tibial nerve in the popliteal fossa and from the flexor carpi radialis (FCR) after stimulation of the median nerve at the elbow. It can sometimes be elicited from other muscles with special activation techniques, but its occurrence in any relaxed muscle other than the soleus or FCR usually signifies motor neuron hyperexcitability and suggests the presence of an upper motor neuron lesion. The H reflex was originally recorded from the gastrosoleus and described by Hoffman, hence the designation. It is best elicited by submaximal, long duration stimuli. The long duration stimulus most efficiently activates the large myelinated fibers, which subserve the reflex (17). The H reflex habituates and decreases in amplitude with stimuli delivered more rapidly than 0.5 Hz.

The classic H reflex is large in relation to the M wave elicited from the same muscle and in fact the H may have maximal amplitude when the M is not even visible. The H/M ratio is the ratio of the maximal H amplitude to the maximal M amplitude in a given muscle and normally does not exceed 0.7. At a given stimulus intensity, the H is fairly constant in amplitude and latency and is present with each stimulus. As the stimulus intensity is increased, the H reflex becomes smaller and eventually disappears with high intensity supramaximal stimuli, then reappears as the intensity is decreased (Fig. 7.5). With supramaximal stimulation, an F wave of approximately the same latency may appear instead of the H reflex. In electrodiagnostic medicine, the natural inclination is to increase the stimulus intensity when the examiner is having difficulty eliciting some particular potential. This is a major trap with H reflex determinations because the supramaximally elicited F wave may be readily confused with the H reflex. The greatest potential for error occurs when the H reflex is in fact absent, the stimulus intensity is progressively increased to elicit it, and a normal F wave of approximately the same latency is mistaken for the absent H reflex.

In summary, the F wave is antidromic motor/orthodromic motor; the H is orthodromic sensory/orthodromic motor. The F can be elicited from any muscle; the H has a restricted distribution in normal adults. The F wave is elicited with supramaximal motor nerve stimulation; the H is best elicited with a long duration, submaximal stimulus. The F wave has variable latency and amplitude at a given stimulus intensity and may not appear at all from some stimuli; its amplitude is small in relation to the amplitude of the M wave recorded from the same muscle. The H reflex has a constant latency and amplitude at a given stimulus intensity and can be nearly as large in amplitude as the M wave recorded from the same muscle. The F wave is most often confused with an A wave or with surface-recorded MUAPs; the H is most often confused with an F wave. Normal reference values for late responses depend on the length of the arm and leg studied and on the body height of the individual patient, as well as on the CV of the nerves under study.

FIGURE 7.5. An H reflex elicited by stimulation of the tibial nerve in the popliteal fossa, cathode proximal, recording from the soleus muscle. The active electrode was placed anteriorly, about 1 cm medial to the medial border of the tibia, at the level where the curve of the calf muscles flattens out, approximately halfway between the popliteal fossa and the medial malleolus, with the reference electrode on the medial malleolus. A 1.0 ms, low intensity stimulus best elicits the response. With increasing intensity the H reflex decreases in amplitude as the M wave increases; the H reflex is of highest amplitude when the M wave is merely a nubbin.

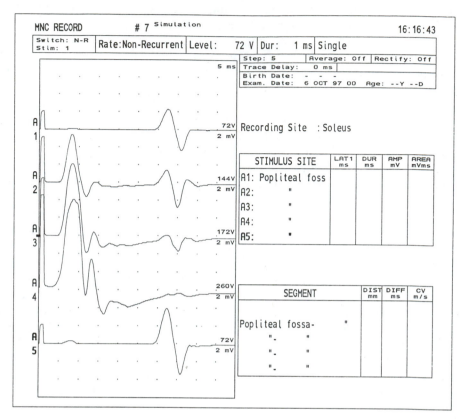

Nomograms and formulas taking these factors into account are useful. Table 7.3 summarizes the attributes of H and F responses.

Utility of the F Wave

The F wave has potential usefulness in several clinical situations: evaluation of a focal demyelinating lesion affecting an otherwise untestable proximal portion of a nerve, evaluation of an axonopathy, and evaluation of a demyelinating peripheral neuropathy. Other applications are primarily experimental. Even in these clinical situations, the F has distinct limitations. When a purely demyelinating focus involves a proximal nerve segment, e.g., the median nerve in the axilla, all the peripheral conduction studies may be normal, including the SNAP, since there is no axon loss. In this situation, absence or prolongation of the F response may provide the only confirmation of an abnormality. However, the F has low sensitivity and is not uncommonly normal or not helpful, in part for the following reasons: 1) since the abnormal segment is relatively short, it may not affect overall conduction through the very long loop that comprises the F pathway. 2) only one axon must survive through the lesion to yield a single F wave of normal latency to produce a normal value by the criterion of the shortest latency of a group of 10–20 stimuli 3) even if abnormal, the F change is non-localizing.

Mild or early axonopathies may produce only equivocal amplitude loss and CV slowing. In this situation, the F wave may theoretically provide additional useful information since the abnormality may summate over the long up and back course of the response (18). The F might thus be abnormal when peripheral conduction studies are normal or equivocal. However, when peripheral conduction studies already clearly indicate an axonopathy, such as with moderate slowing and amplitude loss, the F adds no additional information. In the demyelinating peripheral neuropathies in which peripheral conduction studies are equivocal, the F may add additional evidence of demyelination

TABLE 7.3
Attributes of F and H Responses

	F-wave	*H-reflex*
Ideal stimulus intensity	Supramaximal	Long duration, submaximal
Distribution	Widespread	Restricted
Afferent limb	Antidromic motor	Orthodromic sensory
Efferent limb	Orthodromic motor	Orthodromic motor
Latency at a given stimulus intensity	Variable	Constant
Amplitude/ configuration at a given stimulus intensity	Variable	Constant
Persistence at a given stimulus intensity	Variable	Constant
Amplitude	Small	Large
Confused with	A-wave, surface recorded MUAPs	F-wave

by showing disproportionate prolongation indicative of involvement of proximal structures, primarily nerve roots. But when the peripheral conduction studies have already shown clear evidence of demyelination, such as with severe slowing or conduction block, F wave determinations add little or no additional useful information.

The F wave has theoretical but little practical value in the evaluation of radiculopathies. In the upper extremity, only the C_8 root can realistically be tested; recording from other muscles is limited because the F is lost in the trailing component of the M wave. C_8 radiculopathies are rare, and the F has no practical role to play in evaluation of the much more common C_6 and C_7 radiculopathies. The F wave may be more useful in the relatively common L_5 radiculopathy. Its abnormality in the face of normal peripheral conduction studies and a consistent needle examination could be construed as soft electrical confirmation of a root lesion. In S_1 radiculopathy, the H reflex has more demonstrated utility than the F. The utility of the F wave is limited in all radiculopathies because 1) the limitations for any proximal lesion related to the length of the abnormal segment as discussed; 2) its lack of sensitivity to pathology involving the posterior root; 3) most muscles have redundant innervation by at least 2 roots and the F may remain normal by conducting through the unaffected root.

Electrodiagnostic medicine consultants tend to have one of three philosophies regarding the F wave. Some never do it at all and consider the F response essentially worthless. Some do an F wave as part of the study of every nerve, essentially as a cross check on the accuracy of the nerve conduction velocity. Most perform F wave studies selectively when searching for specific information in certain clinical circumstances, as summarized in Table 7.4. To do F waves mainly to increase reimbursement is despicable.

Utility of the H Reflex

The primary clinical application of H reflex studies is in the evaluation of suspected S_1 radiculopathy. Normal H reflex latency is typically 25–35 ms. Most laboratories use the side-to-side latency comparison as the criterion of abnormality. There is no firm agreement on how much asymmetry is permissible.

TABLE 7.4
Primary Usefulness of F-Wave Determinations

1. Evaluation of a suspected axonopathy when peripheral conduction studies are normal or equivocal.
2. Evaluation of a suspected demyelinating peripheral neuropathy when peripheral conduction studies do not show clear evidence of demyelination.
3. Suspected proximal focal mononeuropathy.
4. Suspected plexopathy.
5. Suspected early Guillain-Barre syndrome.

Some authors contend that a difference as little as 1.2 ms between the two sides is significant. Many EMGers prefer to see a difference of about 3 ms between the two sides before suggesting the presence of S_1 radiculopathy. Amplitude asymmetry is not considered important, but some labs attach significance to this parameter and may use it in addition to, or in lieu of, latency determinations. A side-to-side amplitude asymmetry of up to fourfold can occur in normal controls (15). In most situations, H reflex findings closely correlate with the clinical status of the ankle jerk. Bilateral absence of H reflexes is not necessarily abnormal, especially in elderly patients or those who have undergone lumbar spine surgery.

The wisdom of diagnosing radiculopathy solely on H reflex abnormalities is dubious. When unequivocal and clearly localizing abnormalities are present on needle examination, the H become superfluous. Its greatest utility is in providing another indicator of disease when needle examination is equivocal or nonlocalizing, as when fibrillations are limited to the lumbosacral paraspinal muscles. H reflexes may be useful in evaluating peripheral neuropathy following the same principles as the F wave, but its restricted distribution limits applicability. The H reflex has also been used to investigate motor neuron excitability in upper motor neuron lesions and in dystonia.

Key Points

- Motor conduction studies are performed by stimulating a motor nerve at one or more points while recording the M wave from a muscle innervated by that nerve, using the belly-tendon method with the recording electrode over the motor point on the belly of the muscle and the reference electrode over the tendon.
- Parameters evaluated include the motor nerve conduction velocity (MNCV), the distal motor latency (DML), the proximal motor latency (PML), and the characteristics of the M wave. The configuration of the M wave is significantly affected by the location, size, and shape of both the recording and reference electrodes.
- The M wave onset latency is the point at which the waveform leaves the baseline, its initial deflection. When the surface disc electrode is properly placed over the motor point of the muscle, the onset is a clean, initially negative deflection from the baseline. Because of temporal dispersion and phase cancellation, there is normally a decrease in M wave amplitude on proximal stimulation, which should not exceed 20%.
- For routine nerve conduction studies, the cathode delivers a percutaneous stimulus to depolarize the nerve and generate an action potential. Measurements are made from the center of the cathode to the center of the recording electrode. A constant voltage stimulator delivers the same voltage at any given stimulator setting. A constant current stimulator delivers the same current at any given setting, automatically varying the voltage to adjust for tissue resistance.
- The DML is the onset latency of the M wave at the most distal site. Maximal motor nerve conduction velocity is determined by performing supramaximal stimulation at two nerve sites separated by a known distance, subtracting the distal from the proximal latency and dividing the latency difference into the distance.
- For sensory conduction studies, the evoked nerve action potential (NAP) is recorded directly by electrodes placed over the nerve. Orthodromic sensory studies are done in the direction of normal impulse flow, conversely with antidromic studies. In customary usage, SNAP refers to any nerve action potential, whether truly sensory or in fact compound.
- Phase cancellation occurs to a much greater degree with sensory than motor studies.
- For NAP recordings, an interelectrode distance of 3–4 cm is optimal.
- Because of the frequent shock artifact interference with the NAP onset, the distal sensory latency is usually taken to the peak. The majority of labs assess peak latency over a fixed distance using surface recording and stimulation, bipolar, antidromic techniques (except for palmar and plantar studies), and a fixed distance of 3–4 cm between G_1 and G_2.
- Sensory responses are more sensitive to temperature effects than are motor responses. A normal or high amplitude is an important clue to slow sensory conduction due to low temperature. Mathematical correction factors to compensate for cold extremities may not be valid for diseased nerve. A better procedure is to warm the part to the temperature at which the reference values were obtained.
- Sensory conduction changes tend to occur earlier than motor conduction changes in both neuropathies, and SNAP amplitude is the most sensitive indicator of nerve pathology. Despite their sensitivity, however, distal sensory potential abnormalities are nonspecific and nonlocalizing.
- Lesions involving nerve roots do not change the sensory potentials. Normality of the SNAP is an important differential electrodiagnostic point favoring radiculopathy over plexopathy or neuropathy.
- Late responses, F waves and H reflexes, are special techniques used to assess the proximal portions of the peripheral nervous system which are largely inaccessible to routine conduction studies. The usual procedure is to reverse the simulator so that the cathode is placed proximally, generating an action potential traveling centripetally. The F wave is antidromic motor/orthodromic motor; can be elicited from any muscle; has variable latency, amplitude, and persistence at a given stimulus intensity; is of

relatively small amplitude; and is most often confused with an A wave or with surface recorded MUAPs.

- The H reflex is an orthodromic sensory/orthodromic motor; has a restricted distribution; is best elicited with a long duration submaximal stimulus; has a constant latency and amplitude at a given stimulus intensity; is relatively large; and is most often confused with an F wave.

- The F wave is especially useful for evaluation of a focal demyelinating lesion affecting an otherwise untestable proximal portion of a nerve, and evaluation of some generalized polyneuropathies; but the F has distinct limitations. It has theoretical but little practical value in the evaluation of radiculopathies.

- The primary clinical application of H reflex studies is in the evaluation of suspected S_1 radiculopathy. Its greatest utility is in providing another indicator of disease when needle examination is equivocal or non-localizing.

References

1. Dumitru D, DeLisa JA. AAEM Minimonograph #10: volume conduction. Muscle Nerve 1991;14:605–624.
   See chapter 4 for abstract.

2. Lateva ZC, McGill KC, Burgar CG. Anatomical and electrophysiological determinants of the human thenar compound muscle action potential. Muscle Nerve 1996;19:1457–1468.
   Clinical interpretation of the compound muscle action potential (CMAP) requires a precise understanding of its underlying mechanisms. The authors recorded normal thenar CMAPs and MUAPs using different electrode configurations and different thumb positions. Computer simulations showed that the CMAP has four parts: rising edge, negative phase, positive phase, and tail which correspond to four distinct stages of electrical activity in the muscle: initiation at the end-plate, propagation, termination at the muscle/tendon junctions, and slow repolarization. The shapes of volume-conducted signals recorded beyond the muscle are also explained by these four stages. Changes in CMAP shape associated with thumb abduction are due to changes in termination times resulting from changes in muscle-fiber lengths. These findings demonstrate that the negative and positive phases of the CMAP are due to different mechanisms, and that anatomical factors, particularly muscle-fiber lengths, play an important role in determining CMAP shape. See also Wee AS, Ashley RA. Relationship between the size of the recording electrodes and morphology of the compound muscle action potentials. Electromyogr Clin Neurophysiol 1990;30:165–168 (size of the M wave decreases with increasing electrode size).

3. Kincaid JC, Brashear A, Markand ON. The influence of the reference electrode on CMAP configuration. Muscle Nerve 1993;16:392–396.
   The ulnar, hypothenar CMAP often shows a double-peaked configuration in the negative phase component while the median, thenar potential has a simple dome shape. To investigate the origin of these differences the authors evaluated the activity at the belly and tendon electrode locations by referencing those sites to an electrode on the contralateral hand. The tendon sites are not electrically inactive. The ulnar tendon electrode contributes a large amplitude potential which corresponds to the second peak of the ulnar belly-tendon potential. The median tendon electrode contributes only a minimal component to the negative phase of the belly-tendon potential. The distribution of such potentials throughout the hand is evaluated and possible mechanisms for the presence of a tendon potential as well as the differences between ulnar and median sites are discussed.

4. Brashear A, Kincaid JC. The influence of the reference electrode on CMAP configuration: leg nerve observations and an alternative reference site. Muscle Nerve 1996;19:63–67.
   Peroneal and tibial compound motor action potentials (CMAP) recorded using the standard belly-tendon montage have different configurations. The peroneal CMAP is a smooth dome shape, while the tibial CMAP has a slow-rising initial component followed by a higher amplitude negative peak. To evaluate possible causes of these differences we investigated the individual activity recordable at the belly and tendon electrodes by using a referential montage with the opposite foot as the reference. This type recording shows that the peroneal belly site produces most of the nerve CMAP, whereas the tendon site generates most of the high tibial CMAP. Some features and technical problems of referential CMAP recording using an opposite limb reference are shown. An alternative method using an ipsilateral distal leg reference site is described. A montage which separately records the activity at the belly or tendon electrodes may provide new insight into mechanisms of commonly observed nerve conduction phenomena.

5. Kimura J, Machida M, Ishida T, et al. Relation between size of compound sensory or muscle action potentials, and length of nerve segment. Neurology 1986;36:647–652.
   In 24 median nerves from 12 healthy subjects, antidromic digital sensory potentials progressively diminished in size, averaging 40.4, 37.0, 30.7, and 23.9 uV with stimulation at the palm, wrist, elbow, and axilla, respectively. In contrast, compound muscle action potentials changed minimally, measuring 19.4, 19.8, 19.0 and 18.2 mV, respectively. Similar studies of the ulnar and radial nerves showed identical trends. Physiologic temporal dispersion can mimic conduction block of sensory nerves by summating the peaks of opposite polarity generated by fast- and slow-conducting axons. This type of cancellation affects muscle responses much less because motor unit potentials of longer duration superimpose nearly in phase, given the same latency shift as the sensory potentials. See also Felsenthal, G. and Teng, C.S. Changes in duration and amplitude of the evoked muscle action potential (EMAP) over distance in peroneal, median, and ulnar nerves. Am J Phys Med 1983;62:123–134; and van Dijk JG, van der Kamp W, van Hilten BJ, et al. Influence of recording site on CMAP amplitude and on its variation over a length of nerve. Muscle Nerve 1994;17:1286–1292.

6. Moller AR. Intraopertive recordings that can guide the surgeon in the operation. In: Miller AR, ed. Evoked potentials in Intraoperative Monitoring. Baltimore: Williams and Wilkins, 1988;104–105.
   For a discussion of the physics and physiology of constant current vs. constant voltage stimulation see: Rose RD. Selective

posterior rhizotomy and constant voltage stimulation. Muscle Nerve 1997;20:1044–1045.

7. Dorfman LJ. The distribution of conduction velocities (DCV) in peripheral nerves: a review. Muscle Nerve 1984;7:2–11.
    Advances in digital signal processing have permitted the development of clinically relevant, noninvasive, computer-based methods for estimating the distribution of conduction velocities (DCV) in motor, sensory, and mixed populations of large myelinated nerve fibers. Preliminary investigations using DCV methods have clarified some issues concerning conduction of impulses in the different fiber subpopulations of normal and diseased human nerves. In the presence of severe nerve disease, DCV analysis is usually either impractical or superfluous; additional studies are needed to define its range of clinical applicability. Extension of this technology to clinical analysis of small myelinated and unmyelinated fiber populations will require improvements in the techniques of nerve stimulation and recording.

8. Falck B, Stalberg E. Motor nerve conduction studies: measurement principles and interpretation of findings. J Clin Neurophysiol 1995;12:254–279.
    An exhaustive review of the subject of motor conduction studies. Principles of electrode placement, stimulus intensity, algorithms for measurement of parameters, causes of variability, reference values, and reporting are discussed. Pathophysiological interpretation of findings is also presented.

9. Kimura J. Principles and pitfalls of nerve conduction studies. Ann Neurol 1984;16:415–429.
    Reviews fundamental principles and changing concepts of nerve stimulation techniques and discusses their proper application in the differential diagnosis of peripheral nerve disorders. NCS help delineate the extent and distribution of the neural lesion and distinguish two major categories of peripheral nerve disease: demyelination and axonal degeneration. Although the method is based on simple principles, pitfalls abound in practice. Variability in nerve conduction measurement may result from temperature change, variations among nerve segments, and the effects of age. Other sources of error include excessive spread of stimulation current, anomalous innervation, temporal dispersion, and inaccuracy of surface measurements. Unlike a bipolar derivation, which selectively records near-field potentials, a referential recording may give rise to stationary far-field peaks from a moving source. Overlooking this possibility can lead to an incorrect interpretation of findings. Conventional NCS deal primarily with measurements of the distal nerve segments in an extremity. More recent techniques are applicable to less accessible anatomical regions, as illustrated by the elicitation of the blink reflex, F wave and H reflex, and the use of the inching technique. Other methods used to assess special aspects of nerve conduction include the ischemic test and studies of slow-conducting fibers.

10. Raynor EM, Preston DC, Logigian EL. Influence of surface recording electrode placement on nerve action potentials. Muscle Nerve 1997;20:361–363.
    Computer modeling predicts that displacement of the active recording electrode laterally off the ideal recording site produces an action potential that is of lower amplitude, less clearly triphasic, with an earlier onset, longer duration, and displacement of the negative peak to the right. This study of sural and median sensory potentials recorded 1–3 cm laterally from the ideal site, found that active electrode misplacement produces a change from a triphasic, initially positive, wave to a biphasic,

initially negative, wave; a reduction in amplitude of up to 70% with a lateral displacement distance of 2–3 cm; a decrease in SNAP onset latency with little change in peak latency; and an increase in the maximal NCV. These changes in the SNAP result from differences in current density at each of the recording sites. Accurate G1 placement is thus especially important when assessing amplitude in side-to-side comparison studies.

11. Wilbourn AJ. Sensory nerve conduction studies. J Clin Neurophysiol 1994;11:584–601.
    Sensory NCSs are an indispensable component of the electrodiagnostic examination. Variables regarding them include: (a) bipolar vs. monopolar recording; (b) antidromic vs. orthodromic technique; needle vs. surface stimulating electrode(s); (d) needle vs. surface recording electrodes; (e) fixed vs. variable distances between cathode and active recording electrode; (f) measuring latencies to onset vs. to peak; and (g) measuring amplitudes baseline to peak vs. peak to peak. "Tier 1" studies are performed routinely in most labs (median and ulnar digital, sural); "tier 2" studies are performed frequently in many labs (radial, median and ulnar palmar, superficial peroneal); "tier 3" studies are performed infrequently in most labs (median and lateral antebrachial cutaneous, medial and lateral plantar); "tier 4" studies are performed rarely, if at all, in most labs (posterior antebrachial cutaneous, saphenous, lateral femoral cutaneous). Benefits of sensory NCS include a) they may be the only part of the electrodiagostic assessment that is abnormal b) they generally are more sensitive than motor NCS to pathophysiologic processes occurring along mixed nerves, regardless of the particular type of pathophysiology c) sensory NCS frequently prove to be extremely helpful in the localization of proximal axon loss lesions of moderate or greater severity d) because sensory NCS do not assess any aspect of the "motor unit," they aid in distinguishing generalized disorders affecting the PNS from those involving the neuromuscular junctions or muscles e) sensory NCS are highly sensitive to sensory axon dysfunction and can be grossly abnormal at a time when large fiber sensory deficits cannot be demonstrated clinically f) with longstanding axon loss lesions, the sensory responses are sometimes the only component of the electrodiagnostic exam that remain abnormal. Limitations of sensory NCS include a) they are technically far more difficult to perform than motor NCS b) sensory responses are often difficult to record for technical reasons, e.g., limb edema c) SNAPs may be of low amplitude or unelicitable because of coincidental nerve fiber injury d) SNAPs are more sensitive to physical/physiological variables, e.g., temperature, age e) because of these limitations, interpreting changes found on sensory NCS is a more difficult task than interpreting those found on motor NCS f) sensory NCS do not evaluate the most distal segments of the sensory nerves, where pathology often begins g) in comparison to motor NCS, sensory techniques are much less standardized from lab to lab h) physiologic temporal dispersion has a marked effect on the SNAP, in contrast to the effect on the CMAP. The value of sensory NCS with various peripheral nerve fiber lesions, including plexopathies, mononeuropathies, and polyneuropathies, is discussed. See also Walker FO, Gitter AJ, Stolov WC. Optimal interelectrode recording distances. Muscle Nerve 1996;19: 536–538.

12. Denys EH. AAEM minimonograph #14: The influence of temperature in clinical neurophysiology. Muscle Nerve 1991;14:795–811.
    Temperature affects biologic and neurophysiologic processes and is, therefore, always well controlled in vitro experiments.

Its role is equally important in the clinical laboratory but has often been neglected. Lower temperatures cause slower nerve conduction velocities (NCVs), and increased amplitudes of muscle and nerve potentials. Fibrillations may disappear, and muscle contraction will be slower and weaker. Neuromuscular transmission improves. Somatosensory evoked potentials (SEPs) are similarly vulnerable in the peripheral segments, or with changes in central temperature. As a result, abnormalities are artificially created or existing defects are not detected, resulting in false or missed diagnoses. Control of temperature, albeit somewhat time consuming, will result in greater diagnostic accuracy.

13. Ashworth NL, Marshall SC, Satkunam LE. The effect of temperature on nerve conduction parameters in carpal tunnel syndrome. Muscle Nerve, in press.

    A study of the effects of temperature on motor and sensory conduction parameters in CTS using the normal ipsilateral ulnar nerve as a control. Both median and ulnar nerves showed the expected changes with increasing temperature: a decrease in distal latency, duration, area and amplitude. However, statistically significant differences were present in the rate of change. In CTS, the focally demyelinated nerve reacts differently to temperature changes compared with normal control ulnar nerves. The use of correction factors based on the responses of normal nerves may not be valid in this setting.

14. Benecke R, Conrad B. The distal sensory nerve action potential as a diagnostic tool for the differentiation of lesions in dorsal roots and peripheral nerves. J Neurol 1980;223:231–239.

    Median and ulnar amplitude and sensory CV were measured in 194 patients and 20 controls. In dorsal root lesions attributable to degenerative changes of the cervical spine and/or discs, SNAP amplitude and sensory CV were normal. In peripheral nerve lesions, located in the brachial plexus, or at the elbow or wrist, diminished SNAP amplitudes and/or slowing of SCV were found. Conclusion: in patients with sensory deficits in the hands, recordings of SNAPs can differentiate between lesions of dorsal roots and peripheral nerves.

15. Fisher MA. AAEM Minimonograph #13: H reflexes and F waves: physiology and clinical indications. Muscle Nerve 1992;15:1223–1233.

    Motoneurons can be activated both reflexly and antidromically following electrical stimulation of peripheral nerves. These H reflexes and F waves are clinically useful responses which interface at the level of the peripheral nerves and the spinal cord. Because these responses are commonly employed in the electrodiagnostic evaluation of patients, an understanding of their physiology and clinical applications is important. Reasoning from the physiology, both the value and limitations of H-reflex and F-wave studies are considered for disorders of peripheral nerves, roots, and the central nervous system. Theoretical concepts about the physiology and pathophysiology of the nervous system based on H-reflex and F- wave data are also discussed. See also Nishida T, Kompoliti A, Janssen I, et

al. H reflex in S-1 radiculopathy: latency versus amplitude controversy revisited. Muscle Nerve 1996;19:915–917.

16. Bischoff C, Stalberg E, Falck B, Puksa L. Significance of A-waves recorded in routine motor nerve conduction studies. Electroencephalogr Clin Neurophysiol 1996; 101:528–533.

    The occurrence of A-waves during routine F-wave studies was investigated in 2367 nerves in the upper and lower extremities in 556 consecutive patients with various neuromuscular disorders. An A-wave, with a nearly constant latency and a uniform shape on consecutive stimulations, could be recorded in 184 nerves (7.8%) out of 124 patients (22.3%). More than 50% of patients with A-waves had various types of polyneuropathies. Of all patients with polyneuropathy, 65% had at least one nerve with A-waves. A-waves occurred somewhat less frequently in patients with radiculopathies. In other proximal local nerve lesions they were found less often and only exceptionally in patients with distal nerve lesions. A-waves were present in 6 out of 10 patients with motor neuron diseases. There was no correlation between the number of A-waves found in one nerve or the number of nerves in a given patient with A-waves and the etiology or severity of the underlying disease. A-waves were found in 11 patients referred for various neurological symptoms in whom other neurophysiological findings were normal. This might be interpreted as an early sign of underlying disease because in 100 healthy controls no A-waves could be elicited, with the exception of 3 subjects who had A-waves in the abductor hallucis muscle when the tibial nerve was stimulated. The authors conclude that the appearance of A-waves should be considered a sign of either a local nerve lesion or a generalized neuropathy in all other nerves except for the tibial nerve.

17. Panizza M, Nilsson J, Hallett M. Optimal stimulus duration for the H reflex. Muscle Nerve 1989;12:576–579.

    In order to find the optimal stimulus duration for recording H reflexes, the recruitment curves for H reflexes and M responses were studied in 10 healthy subjects. The H reflex was recorded in the upper and lower extremities, and the durations of the electrical stimulus used ranged from 0.1 to 3 msec. The amplitude of the H reflex and the relation between the H reflex and M response changed with stimulus duration. H reflexes are brought out to advantage using a stimulus duration between 0.5 and 1 msec.

18. Andersen H, Stalberg E, Falck B. F-wave latency, the most sensitive nerve conduction parameter in patients with diabetes mellitus. Muscle Nerve 1997;20:1296–1302.

    A study of the diagnostic sensitivity of minimal F-wave latency, F-wave persistence, motor NCV, CMAP amplitude, and sural sensory NCV and SNAP amplitude in patients with diabetes. The Z scores of the minimal F-wave latency were significantly larger than for the other measurements. F-wave persistence did not differ from reference values. The investigators concluded that minimal F-wave latency was the most sensitive measure for detection of nerve pathology in diabetics. See also Fraser JL, Olney RK. The relative diagnostic sensitivity of different F-wave parameters in various polyneuropathies. Muscle Nerve 1992;15:912–918.

8

Needle Electrode Examination

The needle electrode examination (NEE) is performed by inserting a needle electrode into a muscle and assessing its activity at rest, its response to small movements of the needle, and the activity on volitional contraction. Different patterns of abnormality, albeit with some overlap, permit the differentiation of diseases which affect nerve from those which affect muscle. In addition to the pattern of abnormality in an individual muscle, the distribution of abnormalities and the temporal evolution of changes helps in differential diagnosis. The NEE is a complex undertaking, and sophistication in its performance and interpretation comes only with experience. Many pitfalls exist which may lead to overinterpretation or underinterpretation. Abnormalities may be subtle, such as in a mild metabolic myopathy, or widespread and flagrant, such as in an advanced motor neuron disease.

Before the examination, inquiry should be made regarding possible transmissible illnesses or coagulopathy. The patient should be briefed regarding the nature of the examination, but not in such detail as to frighten them out of undergoing the study. Most patients tolerate NEE reasonably well, but some do not. The examination should be terminated promptly should the patient so request.

Needle Electrodes

Two types of needle electrodes are used for most NEEs: the concentric needle electrode (CNE) or the monopolar needle electrode (MNE). Single-fiber, macro, and scanning electrodes are generally used only in specialized centers. Table 8.1 compares the attributes of the CNE vs. the MNE. Whether to use one or the other is generally a trade-off depending upon circumstances. Monopolar needles are often better tolerated by the patient and are perfectly adequate for routine NEE in patients with suspected radiculopathies or neuropathies. Traditional CNEs were considerably more painful than comparable MNEs of the same era. Patient tolerance of the newer disposable CNE is generally much better (although recent "improvements" in some disposable concentrics have resulted in an electrode that is again painful for the patient and difficult to slide freely through tissue).

CNEs have generally better recording characteristics with a more stable baseline, less noise, and more reliable and consistent motor unit action potential (MUAP) amplitude and duration. Essentially all available data regarding quantitative EMG is based on concentric electrodes. A CNE is clearly preferable when motor unit quantitation is particularly important, as in suspected myopathy. It is not widely appreciated that the manufacturers' recommended low frequency filter setting is different for the two types of electrodes (Table 8.1).

An important difference between CNE and MNE is in the size of the MUAP recorded. Numerous investigators have found that MNEs tend to record MUAPs of higher amplitude than do CNEs. A recent study used the two needle types to record the same MUAP simultaneously (1). These investigators found that the MUAP amplitude when recorded by a MNE was, on average, twice as high as the amplitude recorded by a CNE. The duration recorded with a MNE was about 50% longer. There was no difference in the number of phases or turns recorded. Presumably some of the variability in the reported amplitudes and durations of other wave forms, such as fasciculation potentials, fibrillation potentials and positive sharp waves, also reflects differences in the needles used to record them.

Each type of electrode has its advocates. The CNE school tends to view the MNE school as lax and indulgent; the MNE school tends to view the CNE school as sadists. A skilled electrodiagnostic medicine consultant can use either of these needle electrodes with equal facility depending on the circumstances.

Another issues is expense, particularly in the era of disposable needles. A MNE is considerably less expensive than a CNE. A disposable monopolar electrode runs about $3.00, as compared with about $10.00 for a disposable concentric. The trade-off between expense, tolerance, and recording characteristics led one prominent Scandinavian electromyographer to say, "In America, they are very rich. They throw away monopolar needles after they use them. But in my country, we throw them away before we use them."

A MNE consists of a 22 to 30 gauge stainless steel needle covered with Teflon except at the very tip (Fig. 8.1). The active recording surface at the needle tip

TABLE 8.1

Comparison of Concentric (CNE) and Monopolar (MNE) Needle Electrodes for Needle Electromyography

	CNE	*MNE*
Recording area	0.08 mm² hemisphere (?, see reference 2)	0.17 mm² sphere
Recording surface	125 × 580 μm	500 μm diameter, tapering to point
Active electrode (G_1)	Core	Solid shaft
Reference electrode (G_2)	Hollow cannula	Surface
Patient tolerance	Lower (disposables much better than reusables)	Higher
MUAP amplitudes	Lower	Higher
MUAP durations	Shorter	Longer
MUAP complexity	Same	Same
LFF setting	2 Hz	20 Hz
Expense	Higher	Lower

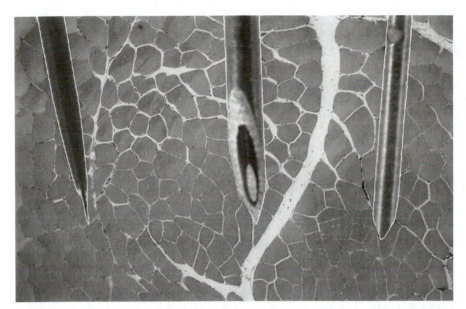

FIGURE 8.1. From left to right, monopolar, concentric, and single fiber needle electrodes superimposed on a section of muscle. Muscle fibers are, on average, about 40–50 μm in diameter. All these needle electrodes are huge in comparison.

(G_1) is referenced to a remote electrode (G_2), usually a disc electrode on the skin surface. A CNE is a 24 to 26 gauge hollow cannula, which serves as G_2, with an inner core of fine wire which serves as the active electrode. Less impedance mismatch and a shorter G_1-G_2 interelectrode distance likely account for most of the superiority in recording characteristics of the CNE. With the MNE, variations in the degree of Teflon covering produce changes in the dimension of the recording surface area, particularly with repeated use, and consequent variability in recording characteristics. This problem is minimal with disposable electrodes. The recording area of a MNE is a 0.17 mm² sphere. The recording area of a CNE is a 0.08 mm² hemisphere. The beveled edge of the CNE acts as a shield between the recording surface and those muscle fibers located on the side away from the bevel. The hemispherical shape of the CNE's recording area has been questioned (2). These differences in the size, shape, and orientation of the recording area, as well as the differences in G_1-G_2 interelectrode distance, likely account for most of the tendency for MNEs to record MUAPs at larger amplitude as compared to CNEs.

The single-fiber EMG (SFEMG) needle is similar to the concentric needle, except that the active recording surface is located on the shaft of the electrode proximal to and on the side opposite the bevel. The recording surface is comparatively tiny, about 25 μm in diameter. The cannula of the needle serves as the reference electrode. The small recording surface creates a circumscribed hemispheric recording area that generally will pick up no more than 1 or 2 active muscle fibers. SFEMG studies are used primarily in

the assessment of neuromuscular transmission (NMT) disorders, but have other applications as well.

General Principles

The routine NEE assesses three types of electrical activity in the muscle: spontaneous, insertional, and voluntary. Spontaneous activity is that which occurs with the muscle at complete rest. A normal muscle contains no spontaneous activity other than in the region of the end plate. Insertional activity is that created by small movements of the electrode, and normally consists of a brief burst of potentials. Voluntary activity is that created by the patient's volitional contraction of the muscle. With low grade, mild to moderate contraction only a handful of motor units become active. With forceful maximal contraction many units become active, and the chaos of many simultaneously active but unrelated MUAPs produces constant turmoil on the screen, an effect termed the interference pattern (IP). The MUAPs "interfere" with each other and with the baseline. Provided there is full effort, a "decreased" IP at maximum contraction implies that segments of flat baseline are discernible, indicating that recruitment is decreased and that there is a reduction in the number of active motor unit potentials. A decreased IP is usually a sign of a neuropathic process. An increased IP means that a complete IP is seen at mild to moderate contraction, rather than at maximal contraction. This reflects an excess of active motor units for the force of contraction and usually indicates a myopathic process.

Waveforms seen in both normal and abnormal muscle can be categorized into three groups: potentials that arise from single muscle fibers, potentials that arise from motor units, and potentials that arise from electrically linked muscle fibers firing synchronously. The amplitudes and durations of these potentials as reported in various publications and textbooks show considerable variability. Hopefully, the following scheme will provide some clarity. As recorded with a CNE, the action potential of a single muscle fiber has a duration of 1–5 ms and an amplitude of 50–200 μV. A normal MUAP at mild to moderate contraction is in the range of 5–15 milliseconds in duration and 2–3 millivolts in amplitude. Potentials recorded with an MNE are, on average, about twice the amplitude and 1.5x the duration of potentials recorded with a CNE.

Potentials that arise from single muscle fibers include: endplate spikes (EPS), fibrillation potentials, and positive sharp waves (PSWs). Potentials that arise from MUAPs include: normal motor units, fasciculations, myokymia, neuromyotonia, cramp discharges, and tetany. The discharge that arises from linked muscle fibers firing synchronously is the complex repetitive discharge (CRD). Miniature endplate potentials (MEPPs) are very small amplitude potentials that occur in the region of the end plate.

Repetitive discharges, or grouped discharges, are action potentials with identical or similar form which fire recurrently. Repetitive discharges under voluntary or quasivoluntary control include iterative firings of a motor unit taking the form of doublets, triplets, or multiplets. Repetitive discharges not under voluntary control include those that arise from muscle fibers (CRDs) or those that arise from motor units (myokymia).

Needle Electrode Examination in Normal Muscle

The following sections will discuss the findings on NEE of normal muscle. Thorough familiarity with normal findings is necessary, not to mistake normal phenomena for evidence of disease. The variety of waveforms seen in needle electromyography in both normal and abnormal muscle are summarized in Table 8.2.

INSERTIONAL ACTIVITY

Insertional activity is induced by small movements of the exploring needle electrode and evaluated at a gain of 50–100 μV/division. It is seen as a burst of activity due to injury or mechanical stimulation of muscle fibers, causing them to generate action potentials. Normal insertional activity consists of a burst of amorphous spike discharges, the duration of which does not exceed 300–400 ms. The duration depends to some degree on the velocity of needle movement, in addition to the size and sharpness of the electrode. Adequate evaluation of insertional activity requires a brief pause between needle insertions to ascertain whether the insertional activity will be prolonged. This pause should be at least 0.5–1.0 seconds in duration. Hurried, "type A" NEEs with frequent insertional movements and brief pauses can easily miss mildly increased insertional activity and low grade spontaneous activity, especially in myopathies. A good technique is to rest the heel of the hand on the surface, grasp the needle like a pencil and make high velocity, small amplitude thrusting movements. The motion pattern should be thrust and hold, not jab and withdraw or "jiggle." About 50 discrete needle movements made in the course of several random passes in different directions through the muscle should suffice for an adequate sampling. Any hint of increased insertional activity should prompt another 50 discrete insertional movements. Any electrical activity persisting for more than 300–400 milliseconds after needle movement is referred to as increased insertional activity. This most commonly takes the form of a train of PSWs. Unsustained positive waves will die out over the next 1 to 2 seconds. Activity persisting beyond that time crosses the boundary into becoming spontaneous activity.

Increased insertional activity and unsustained runs of positive waves may constitute an early manifestation of pathologic muscle membrane instability. However, there are two types of increased insertional activity that occur in otherwise normal individuals: "EMG disease" and "snap, crackle, pop." The picture of "EMG disease" consists of runs of PSWs following needle movement which occur in a widespread distribution and are not accompanied by spike fibrillations or abnormal motor units indicative of a denervating process (3). This widespread increased insertional activity appears to be inherited in a dominant pattern and may represent a *forme fruste* of myotonia. In contrast to the short runs of unsustained regular positive waves of EMG disease, the picture of snap, crackle, pop consists of trains of potentials made up of individual components which fire at irregular intervals, varying in form and amplitude from one component to the next. It is a benign form of increased insertional activity most often seen in the medial gastrocnemius muscles of young muscular males. It can be mistaken for pathologic increased insertional activity, and there is

TABLE 8.2

Characteristics of Various Waveforms Seen on Needle Electromyography (as Recorded with a Concentric Needle Electrode)

	Amplitude (μV)	Duration (msec)	Frequency	Firing Pattern
Potentials arising from single muscle fibers				
MEPPs (end plate noise)	10–20	0.5–1.0	Very high	Irregular, hissing
End plate spikes	100–300	1–5	50–100 Hz	Irregular, sputtering
Spike fibrillation potential	20–200	1–5	0.5–15 Hz typically and sometimes faster	Regular
Positive sharp wave	20–200	10–30 typically, sometimes up to 100	Same as spike fibrillation	Regular
Myotonic discharge	20–200	1–5 (spikes) and/or 5–20 (PSWs)	20–80 Hz	Waxing and waning, vary in amplitude and frequency
Potentials arising from motor units				
Motor unit action potential	300–3000*	5–15 ms	5–50 Hz*	Slightly irregular
Fasciculation potential	Very variable	Very variable	0.1–10 Hz	Extremely irregular; sporadic
Myokymic discharge	Variable	Variable	2–60 Hz intraburst 1–5 Hz interburst	Semiregular bursts
Neuromyotonic discharge	Variable	Variable	150–300 Hz	Waning
Cramp discharge	Variable	Variable	Up to 150 Hz	Resembles interference pattern
Potentials arising from linked muscle fibers				
CRD	100–1,000	Variable	5–100 Hz	Very regular; start and stop abruptly

* Dependent on the level of contraction.

a particular danger of misdiagnosis of S1 radiculopathy (4).

SPONTANEOUS ACTIVITY

There are two types of spontaneous activity that occur normally, and do not signify any pathology; both are seen in the region of the endplate. Endplate noise is due to MEPPs, which are non-propagated, subthreshold depolarizations due to the spontaneous release of acetylcholine quanta (Fig. 8.2). MEPPs consist of very brief monophasic negative spikes, which are so tiny and so numerous they fill the baseline and produce a hissing, buzzing, or roaring sound. Endplate noise has been classically likened to that of a sea shell held to the ear, but also resembles the white noise and static

of a radio off station. When endplate noise is seen on the screen, the patient commonly feels increased discomfort; moving the electrode through the area of endplate noise lessens the pain and causes the potentials to disappear.

Endplate spikes (EPS) or "nerve potentials" are high amplitude, spiky potentials with an initially negative deflection which are also encountered in the region of the endplate, often accompanied by the static hissing of the MEPPs (Fig. 8.2). EPS arise from single muscle fibers. They fire irregularly, making a sputtering sound or a high pitched buzz, which has been likened to the sound of fat frying in a pan. Although referred to as nerve potentials in the past, EPS are the action potentials of single muscle fibers, probably the result of mechanical activation of intramuscular

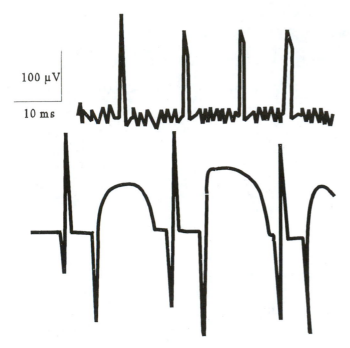

FIGURE 8.2. In the upper tracing, low amplitude, high frequency, monophasic negative end plate noise (MEPPs) are mixed with high amplitude, irregular, initially negative endplate spikes ("nerve potentials"). The lower tracing demonstrates initially positive spike fibrillations and positive sharp waves.

nerve terminals. The initial positive component is missing because the recording electrode is at the point of origin of the potential and does not see an approaching wave of depolarization through the volume conductor. Recorded in the endplate region, fibrillation potentials can also have an initial negative deflection, but they fire regularly. EPS can thus be mistaken for fibrillation potentials, but the irregular firing pattern and close analysis of the initial component should help avoid error. A potential should never be called a fibrillation unless the initial deflection is positive. EPS are always multiple. Although spike fibrillations can fire in isolation, when many spike fibrillations are present there are always PSWs also, which should further help to distinguish these two waveforms.

VOLUNTARY ACTIVITY

Volitional activity is assessed by having the patient contract the muscle with a needle in place. The initial assessment should take place at mild to moderate contraction. Many examiners include an analysis of the inference pattern at maximal contraction as part of the routine exam, but it is debatable whether this provides much additional useful information. The re-

ward for assessing activity at maximal contraction is more likely to be pain and bent needles than further knowledge.

Voluntary contraction causes motor unit action potentials (MUAPs) to appear on the screen. At minimal levels of contraction only 1–3 MUAPs will be firing. As the force of contraction is increased the MUAPs present increase their firing rate, and additional MUAPs are recruited. Recruitment of MUAPs is done, more or less, in order of increasing size. The Henneman size principle describes the relationship between the size of an alpha motor neuron and its function. Recall that the muscle is composed of a mosaic of type 1 and type 2 motor units. The first MUAPs recruited with volitional contraction are type 1. These units have the smallest motor neurons, the lowest threshold for activation, and fire in a slow, slightly irregular fashion. These smaller motor neurons give rise to smaller motor axons. The muscle fibers that they innervate tend to be of smaller diameter, are high in oxidative enzymes, are resistant to fatigue, and generate low twitch tension. In summary, minimal voluntary contraction tends to recruit small amplitude MUAPs which generate low levels of force, and are capable of sustained firing over a long period of time (5).

With an increase in the force of contraction, more and more type 2 units begin to fire. Type 2 units arise from larger motor neurons, which have larger axons and which innervate larger diameter muscle fibers. They have a high threshold for activation and tend to fire in high frequency bursts. Their muscle fibers are rich in glycogen and phosphorylase, and sparse in oxidative enzymes; they are designed for short duration, high twitch tension contraction. Type 2 units are highly susceptible to fatigue and cannot sustain their high firing rate and contraction for very long. These motor unit attributes are summarized in Table 8.3.

Imagine the muscle at minimal contraction. A single, low threshold, type 1 MUAP begins to discharge. The usual firing rate at the beginning of contraction is 3–5 Hz, which is termed the onset frequency (the frequency at the onset of firing). The discharge tends to be slightly irregular, a consistent attribute of all MUAPs. The motor unit activates all its subject muscle fibers, some of which lie within the recording area of the exploring needle electrode. In response to the neuronal input, each muscle fiber belonging to the motor unit generates an action potential. Although all muscle fibers are responding to the same neural input, their action potentials are not precisely synchronous. The muscle fibers are scattered over a wide spatial area; preterminal axonal twigs which innervate individual muscle fibers are of different lengths; the neuro-

TABLE 8.3
Henneman Size Principle and the Attributes of Motor Units and Motor Unit Action Potentials

	Type I	*Type II*
Motor neuron		
Size	Small	Large
Threshold for activation	Low	High
Firing characteristics	Slow, steady	High frequency bursts
Axon diameter	Small	Large
Muscle fibers		
Diameter	Small	Large
Oxidative enzymes	High	Low
Glycogen	Low	High
Tension	Low	High
Fatigue resistance	High	Low
MUAP attributes		
Size	Small	Large
Recruitment sequence	Early	Late
Level of contraction	Minimal	Maximal
Firing rate	Lower	Higher

Modified from Brown WF. The Physiological and Technical Basis of Electromyography. Boston: Butterworths, 1984;235.

the filtering effects of the tissue, high frequency components are rapidly filtered out. The amplitude of a potential falls off as the square of the distance. The high frequency spike components of those muscle fibers which are lying at the periphery of the electrode's recording area are thus filtered out, and only the low frequency components are detected by the electrode. Only a handful of muscle fibers lying very close to the electrode tip contribute the high frequency components that comprise the main spike.

The proximity of the electrode to the generator source is reflected by the rise time of the MUAP (Fig. 8.3). The rise time is that interval between the onset of the negative deflection and the peak of the negative deflection. It is a high frequency component. Moving the electrode only a slight distance away from the active generator source blunts the rise time. The electrode's proximity to the generator source, as indicated by its rise time, is also reflected by the sound created. Fibers active at a distance from the electrode create a dull, thumping sound (low frequency components), while those close to the recording electrode create a sharp, clicking sound (high frequency components). Rise time should be < 0.5 ms to indicate that the electrode is close enough to the MUAP for analysis. This criterion may be too restrictive, and crisp sounding MUAPs may sometimes have a rise time > 0.5 ms (6). Acoustically, duration and rise time determine the pitch of a MUAP; amplitude determines loudness.

muscular junctions are, while generally along the midportion of the fiber, slightly variable in location; and the events of NMT require a slightly variable length of time. Conduction of the action potential down the muscle fiber is relatively slow, 3–5 meters per second, and is dependent on the fiber diameter; it is not identical for all the muscle fibers of the motor unit. As a result of these factors, all the fibers in the motor unit fire together, but not perfectly together.

The needle electrode can only detect the electrical activity of the fibers which lie within its recording area. Those fibers which lie closest make the largest contribution, and generate the main spike of the potential. Fibers lying at a distance contribute low frequency components to the onset and determination of the MUAP. Recall that tissue has capacitance. The positive and negative charges lined up on either side of a dielectric (the biologic membrane) in effect create myriad tiny capacitors. When the output of an RC filter circuit is taken across the capacitor, the filter acts as a low pass, or high frequency, filter—filtering out high frequency components and allowing low frequency components to pass through. As a result of

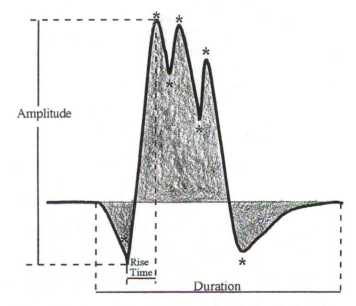

FIGURE 8.3. A motor unit action potential. The shaded areas represent phases. Asterisks indicate turns, or changes in baseline direction. There are three phases, two baseline crossings and seven turns.

Because of the filtering effects of tissue, the amplitude of the spike component of the MUAP decreases by over ninety percent with movement only 200–500 μm away from the generator source. The width of most motor unit territories is in the range of 5–10 mm, so the majority of muscle fibers belonging to a motor unit make little or no contribution to the recorded potential. Using a CNE, the main spike of the MUAP is probably generated by no more than 5–15 muscle fibers, which represent less than ten percent of the total number of muscle fibers in the unit. Those fibers which are in an intermediate zone—close enough to be detected but too far away to contribute to the main spike—produce the low frequency components at the onset and termination of the MUAP. Computer simulations suggest that the MUAP duration primarily correlates with the number of fibers within 2.5 mm of the electrode (2).

Asynchrony of firing of those muscle fibers within the striking area to contribute a spike potential creates "complexity" in the MUAP. Just as the spike potential from one fiber is declining, the spike from another fiber(s) arrives at the recording electrode to regenerate a negative deflection. If the second fiber lies near the first and its timing is only slightly off, there is simply a change in direction of the potential, a "turn." If the second fiber is further away, the spike from the first fiber(s) may have already returned to baseline and crossed it in the positive direction, signaling the beginning of repolarization. A second spike arriving at this time creates another negative spike, a whole new "phase" of the MUAP. A turn is defined as a change in direction of the wave form, a reversal of polarity, of 100 μV or more. A turn does not necessarily produce a voltage change large enough to cross the baseline. A phase is defined as that portion of the wave between the departure from and the return to the baseline (7). The number of phases in a MUAP can also be defined as the number of baseline crossings plus one. A normal MUAP may have up to four phases. A MUAP with five or more phases is termed polyphasic. A MUAP that contains an increased number of turns without actual phase changes is termed "serrated." Both serrated units and polyphasic units have the same implication: a loss of synchrony of motor unit firing. Sometimes polyphasic and serrated potentials are lumped together under the term "complex" MUAPs. A given complex MUAP may be both polyphasic and serrated. Normal muscles may contain a proportion of complex MUAPs, the number varying with the age of the patient and the muscle studied. A conservative figure is 10–15% of the MUAPs in an otherwise normal muscle may be polyphasic. The incidence is especially high in the deltoid and tibialis anterior.

NORMAL MUAP

It is very difficult to find information on the acceptable limits of normal MUAP amplitude. When asked if he knew of a reference on the topic, one well known EMGer replied that it was like "finding a reference on how to palpate the spleen." Amplitude is the most variable and least precisely defined of the MUAP parameters that are commonly measured. Ironically, it is critically important because it is the parameter that most EMGers pay most attention to most of the time when doing a screening examination on most patients. MUAP duration is a more constant and reliable indicator of motor unit size, but its determination requires quantitative, or at least semi-quantitative, EMG with trigger and delay line analysis of a representative sample of MUAPs. Buchthal and colleagues laboriously established the range of normal mean MUAP durations in various commonly studied muscles for every decade from infancy to age 79 (8). They did not, however, assess amplitude. Most references rely heavily on Buchthal's data and are precise in discussing normal MUAP duration, but very vague in discussing amplitude. Even Dumitru's heroic compendium skirts adroitly around the issue (9). The problem is that relying primarily on duration to assess motor unit size is too time consuming and impractical for routine needle electromyography. The examiner wants to perform a semi-quantitative analysis and place the patient into one of three broad categories: clearly normal, clearly abnormal, or borderline. Peak to peak MUAP amplitude can be quickly and simply assessed on most modern electromyographs with several motor units simultaneously active, or even during a maximal IP assessment. Duration measurement, in contrast, requires the isolation and measurement of single MUAPs. In addition, marking the onset and termination of the MUAP is often somewhat arbitrary, as the slow frequency components leave and return to the baseline gradually, and at times merge almost imperceptibly. MUAP amplitude and duration generally parallel each other. Long duration units are generally high amplitude units as well, provided the MUAP is analyzed only after ensuring a rise time less than 0.5 ms to ensure proximity to the active muscle fibers. With experience, electrodiagnostic medicine consultants learn to subjectively judge normal, long duration, and short duration units. When the study is clearly normal or clearly abnormal, there is little to be gained by efforts at precise quantitation. If the clinical situation or equivocal electrodiagnostic findings dictate, then careful quantitative analysis is useful (10). It is best to assess the duration of simple units only, avoiding complex or polyphasic potentials.

Another consideration is that a MUAP of abnormal size will almost always be associated with other evidence of abnormality. Size is not the only consideration. A pathologically large, neurogenic unit will be accompanied by other evidence of neurogenic disease. Thus, it is the internal consistency between MUAP amplitude, duration, configuration, and recruitment pattern that is most useful in diagnosis, rather than one parameter alone.

In addition to the critical dependence of amplitude on proximity to the active muscle fibers, numerous other physiological variables influence MUAP amplitude. First recruited, low threshold, type 1 units are lower in amplitude than later recruited, high threshold, type 2 units. "Large" MUAPs firing on strong volitional contraction may well be normal. The same size unit firing at minimal to moderate contraction may be clearly abnormal, again emphasizing that most of the useful information is gathered with low grade contractions. MUAP amplitudes tend to be larger in older individuals and larger in peripheral muscles than in central muscles.

With some trepidation, the following is offered as a general guideline. Using a CNE, the first recruited, low threshold units tend to have an amplitude in the range of 300–700 μV. With moderate contraction, peak-to-peak MUAP amplitudes tend to run 1–3 mV. Amplitudes larger than three millivolts should be regarded with suspicion. It is hazardous to assess amplitude during maximal contraction when high threshold, large units may be firing. Peak-to-peak MUAP amplitudes < 1 mV during moderate contraction are suspiciously low amplitude. Higher amplitude units are to be expected in the distal muscles of older patients, and lower amplitude units in the proximal muscles of younger patients. According to Chan and Hsu, who simultaneously recorded the same potentials with both MNE and CNE, the expected amplitudes with an MNE are about 2x, and the expected durations about 1.5x, those seen with a CNE (vida supra) (1).

The widely referenced data of Buchthal and colleagues contains detailed information about normal MUAP duration in different muscles at different ages. For general purposes, most MUAPs in most patients will have a duration of 5–15 ms. When more precise enumeration is necessary, consult a reference source (8).

Satellite potentials are small waveforms which are part of, but trail behind, the main body of the MUAP, separated by a variable isoelectric interval (7,11). They occur because of very slow conduction through some component of the motor unit, such as a regenerating axon or a small, slowly conducting muscle fiber. Also referred to as parasites, late components, or linked potentials, they occur most often in chronic neurogenic disease with reinnervation, but can be seen in long-standing myopathies as well.

The component muscle fibers of mature, healthy motor units fire in near synchrony. Each discharge of the MUAP reveals the same components in the same locations. The MUAP is then said to be stable. Minor variations in conduction along axonal twigs, across neuromuscular junctions and along muscle fibers introduces slight variation in the arrival times of different muscle fiber action potentials at the recording electrode. This mild, inherent instability is termed the jitter. When disease is present in the motor unit, especially in neuromuscular transmission disorders, jitter may increase. Slight jitter is detectable only with the special techniques of SFEMG. Blocking occurs when some component of the MUAP intermittently suffers complete transmission failure and fails to fire altogether. When jitter is very high, especially when accompanied by blocking, gross instability of the MUAP may be detectable with ordinary monopolar or concentric electrodes. The technique of modified SFEMG employs a MNE or CNE and a low frequency filter of 500 Hz to better appreciate MUAP instability without resorting to formal SFEMG studies. With neuromuscular transmission disorders, blocking is reflected by a beat to beat variability in MUAP amplitude. Complex, polyphasic potentials due to either nerve or muscle disease may also display instability, with beat to beat variability in amplitude or configuration. Main spike components may come and go, or satellite potentials may overtly jitter and block. MUAP instability implies an ongoing, dynamic process with changes in motor unit architecture which are still evolving. A stable MUAP implies a static process. Stalberg recently introduced the concept of the "jiggle," an attempt to quantify the MUAP shape variability using conventional electrodes and a modified SF technique (12).

RECRUITMENT

MUAPs are recruited in an orderly manner, as previously discussed. At the most minimal level of voluntary contraction, a single MUAP will begin to fire at about 3–5 Hz. To increase the force of contraction slightly, that unit will increase its firing rate to about 10 Hz. To increase the force of contraction still more, another unit will be recruited, and will fire initially at 3–5 Hz. To increase the force of contraction still further, the motor units already present discharge at an increasingly rapid rate, and more and more units are recruited. The orderly recruitment of MUAPs by increasing numbers, firing rates, and sizes results in a smoothly graded voluntary muscle contraction. At maximal contraction, the MUAPs of 6–10 motor units will be firing, some of them very rapidly (at rates greater than 50 Hz). Maximum contraction thus produces a chaotic pattern with multiple overlapping MUAPs: the interference pattern. At full contraction, the characteristics of individual MUAPs cannot be discerned in normal muscle.

Electrodiagnostic parameters have been devised to describe this orderly pattern of recruitment. The *onset frequency* is the frequency of a motor unit when it first begins to discharge. The *recruitment frequency* is the firing rate of a MUAP when the next unit is recruited. The *onset interval* and *recruitment interval* are the interpotential time intervals at these respective recruitment levels, which allow onset frequency and recruitment frequency to be determined mathematically. A recruitment interval of 100 milliseconds reflects a MUAP firing rate of 10 Hz (1000 milliseconds divided by 100 milliseconds equals 10 iterations of the MUAP in one second). One problem is that MUAPs tend to fire slightly irregularly—one of their defining characteristics. This makes assessment of firing rate at best an approximation.

Recruitment can be further defined by the *rule of 5's*, which describes the relationship between the firing rate of the fastest firing unit and the number of units which are active, as illustrated by the following. The onset frequency of unit 1 is 5 Hz (onset interval 200 ms); it's recruitment frequency is 10 Hz, at which time unit 2 is recruited and begins to discharge at 5 Hz. With further contraction, unit 1 increases its firing rate to 15 Hz, unit 2 to 10 Hz, and unit 3 begins to fire at 5 Hz. With further contraction, unit 1 increases its firing rate to 20 Hz, unit 2 to 15 Hz, unit 3 to 10 Hz, and unit 4 begins to fire at 5 Hz. The recruitment ratio is defined as the firing rate of the fastest firing unit divided by the number of units active on the screen. In the aforementioned example, the recruitment ratio is 5 (20 Hz/4 units). A recruitment ratio > 10 implies decreased recruitment with high firing rates and low numbers of units. A recruitment ratio of < 5 implies increased recruitment with a high number of units firing at normal rates (9,13). One thing many novices have trouble understanding is that an increased firing rate means decreased recruitment.

Only top of the line EMG machines have the capability to display MUAP firing frequency. Although recruitment intervals and frequencies can be useful, many EMGers eschew these techniques for routine examinations. Instead, they judge recruitment by the timing pattern of MUAP firing in relationship to the sweep, and by the sounds the units create. At a sweep of 10, there are 10 ms/division and usually 10 divisions/screen, so that one sweep lasts for 100 ms and 10 sweeps occur in 1 second (see Chapter 2). In effect, the sweep is running at 10 Hz. Thus, a MUAP firing at 10 Hz will appear once during each sweep, and at the same point on the screen, even without a delay line. A unit firing faster than 10 Hz recurs slightly early in the cycle of the sweep, and will be displayed slightly to the left of its position on the previous sweep. As the sweep recurs, the unit will seem to dance to the left across the screen. This is easiest to appreciate in raster mode (Fig. 8.4). When the MUAP is firing slower than 10 Hz it will recur later and later with each sweep and will seem to dance across the screen to the right. At a firing rate of 15 Hz, the unit will move to the left, and on every other sweep it will appear twice. At a firing rate of 20 Hz, the unit appears twice each sweep, at 30 Hz, three times each sweep. Thus, the examiner can estimate firing rate from the appearance and timing of the unit in relationship to the sweep.

Even more useful is the sound a unit makes. One can quickly learn to estimate firing rate by ear. Try the following exercise. Set up the EMG machine for repetitive stimulation. Place the stimulator about an inch from the activated preamp and trigger the run.

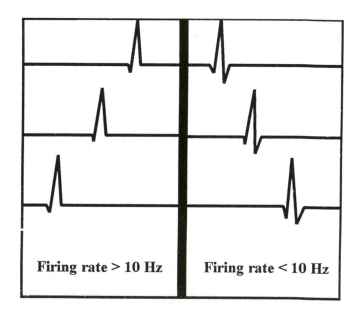

FIGURE 8.4. A depiction of an EMG running on a 10 sweep, with 10 ms per division and 10 divisions across the display. In the screen on the left, a MUAP firing at > 10 Hz reappears early in the sweep with each successive discharge and moves across the display to the left, firing "ahead of the sweep." On the right, a MUAP firing at < 10 Hz shows up slightly later with each successive discharge and moves to the right; it is firing "behind the sweep."

The sound of the stimulator firing should be audible. Some minor adjustment of volume and stimulus duration and intensity may be necessary. Set the repetitive nerve stimulation (RNS) program to deliver a long train of stimuli at 5 Hz. This simulates the sound of a MUAP at onset frequency. Although the RNS stimulation will be regular and MUAPs are by nature slightly irregular, the simulation is otherwise fairly accurate. Increase the RNS delivery rate to 10 Hz. When a MUAP makes this sound, a second unit should be appearing on the screen. Increase the rate to 20 Hz. When an individual MUAP's sound can be discerned from the background at this rate, there should be at least four units on the screen. If there are only one or two, then recruitment is decreased and the firing rates of individual units are disproportionately fast for the number of units present.

The sound of 20 Hz is particularly important. A maximal IP is present at about 30% of maximum isometric contraction. At this level the "acoustic signature" of individual units, determined by the size and rate of firing, cannot be discriminated. Individually discernible MUAPs firing at 20 Hz or greater are pathologically fast at this level of contraction ($\geq$ 3 SD above the mean rate), and certainly at lower levels of contraction (14). Conversely, early recruitment, common in myopathies, produces a full IP at moderate or low levels of contraction. The activation of three or more MUAPs with slight effort or a barely perceptible muscle contraction suggests early recruitment, the firing of an inappropriately high number of units to generate only minimal force (14).

In myopathic disorders, the IP consists of more high-frequency components; spikes are of shorter duration and lower amplitude than normal, and the peak to peak voltage of the IP is lower than normal (14). Unfortunately, this change in recruitment is a late feature in myopathies, and other abnormalities are generally apparent much earlier (15). In contrast, an increased frequency of low frequency components typifies the IP in neuropathic processes. In central disorders, such as spasticity, MUAPs display "erratic" recruitment with greater irregularity of firing, inability to sustain firing, and greater variability of discharge rates. In ALS, firing rates and variability are both increased; in neuropathy, firing rate is increased but variability is not (14,16). Erratic, irregular, variable recruitment due to unsustained central activation also occurs with pain, hysteria or simply poor cooperation. It is often difficult to achieve complete activation in some very strong muscles, such as the gastrocnemius. Abnormalities found on NEE are discussed in more detail in the following sections.

Needle Electrode Examination in Abnormal Muscle

A host of abnormalities can occur in the needle examination in the face of neuromuscular disease. Changes may be seen in motor unit size, shape, stability and recruitment. Insertional activity may be increased or decreased. If increased, a variety of forms can occur. Spontaneous activity may be present or absent. It is the pattern of changes in these different parameters on needle examination that allows an etiologic diagnosis. Table 8.4 summarizes some of the patterns that may be seen.

Either nerve disease or muscle disease may produce membrane instability of the surviving fibers. The electrodiagnostic marker for membrane instability is increased insertional and spontaneous activity. The pathophysiologic basis for this membrane instability will be discussed subsequently.

ABNORMAL INSERTIONAL AND SPONTANEOUS ACTIVITY

The mildest form of abnormally increased insertional activity is trains of PSWs, which persist for more than about 300 ms. Mildly increased insertional activity without definite spontaneous activity is sometimes referred to as "irritability." Other forms of insertional activity include myotonia, complex repetitive discharges, myokymia and neuromyotonia. These abnormal discharges are frequently provoked by needle movement, and are therefore a form of insertional activity, but often persist well past the end of needle movement, thus evolving into a form of spontaneous activity. The dividing lines between what is insertional activity and what is true spontaneous activity are obviously somewhat arbitrary.

Under some circumstances, insertional activity may be abnormally decreased. This most often happens in chronic myopathies when there has been replacement of muscle by fat and fibrous tissue. Other circumstances of decreased insertional activity include: periodic paralysis during an attack, phosphorylase deficiency during an electrically silent contracture, and ischemic muscle. In obese patients, an insufficiently long electrode may fail to sample muscle tissue.

FIBRILLATION POTENTIALS

The normal resting membrane potential of a muscle fiber is approximately -70 to -80 mV, and the normal threshold for depolarization approximately -55 to

TABLE 8.4
Changes in Needle Electrode Examination in Different Conditions

	MUAP				Insertional Activity	Spontaneous Activity
	Size	*Configuration*	*Recruitment*	*Stability*		
Normal	N	N	N	N	N	None
Neuropathic process						
-acute, active, progressive	N, I, rarely D	N, variable polyphasics and complexity	D	D	I	Yes
-chronic, nonprogressive	I	Polyphasics common	D	N	±I, CRDs common	±, may have tiny fibs
Myopathic process, acute						
-without myonecrosis	D	Small polyphasics common	N or I	N	N	None
-with myonecrosis	D	Small polyphasics common	N or I	D	I	Yes—small fibs that may initially fire slowly
Myopathic process, chronic						
-without myonecrosis	D	Small polyphasics	I	N	Maybe D	None
-with myonecrosis	D	occ. LDPP, satellites	I	N or D	Maybe D, CRDs	Variable
Neuromuscular transmission disorders						
-post synaptic	N or D	N	N	D	N	Rarely?
-pre-synaptic	N or D	N	N	D	Maybe I	Sometimes

N, normal; I, increased; D; decreased, LDPP, long duration polyphasic potential.

−65 mV. A number of physiological changes occur in a muscle fiber deprived of its innervation. One of these is a change in the resting membrane potential to a level much closer to threshold, −65 to −75 mV, and the beginning of oscillations that spontaneously depolarize the fiber and cause it to discharge. After depolarization, the action potential cycle leads to repolarization and a brief period of hyperpolarization, after which the membrane begins to oscillate toward its new, near threshold resting level, spontaneously spawning another discharge. The fiber falls into a rhythmic cycle of depolarization and repolarization. This is the fibrillation potential: the spontaneous, periodic depolarizations of a single, unstable muscle fiber.

Another consequence of denervation is spread of acetylcholine receptor, normally confined to the region of the neuromuscular junction, along the surface of the fiber. Denervation supersensitivity due to extrajunctional receptor responding to ambient acetylcholine also may play a role in the genesis of fibrillations.

When recorded outside the endplate region, fibrillation potentials may have one of two configurations: the spike fibrillation or the PSW (sometimes referred to as a positive sharp fibrillation) (Fig. 8.2). Both have an initial positive component followed by a negative phase, and both usually fire with monotonous, metronomic regularity, although a small proportion may fire irregularly (7). Spike fibrillations have the dimensions of a single muscle fiber action potential as discussed above: 1–5 ms in duration, with a peak to peak amplitude of <1 mV. PSWs may be much longer in duration due to the leisurely trailing negativity; the duration is usually 10–30 ms, occasionally up to 100 ms.

Abnormal insertional and spontaneous activity does not appear immediately after denervation, but usually takes several days to several weeks to appear. PSWs are frequently seen in isolation as the only abnormal waveform when denervation is early; they may trail out of the insertional activity and fire briefly before subsiding. This is the earliest manifestation of pathologic membrane instability. The usual sequence of changes is: increased insertional activity with trains of unsustained PSWs induced by needle movement, evolving into sustained PSWs which persist for several seconds before dying out, evolving into a mixture of sustained PSWs and spike fibrillations. Spike fibrillations seldom occur in isolation; they are most often accompanied by PSWs. Fibrillations (both forms) typically discharge at a rate of 1–10 Hz. Faster rates, up to about 30 Hz, occur when spontaneous activity is abundant. The usual fibrillation firing in isolation discharges at a rate of 0.5–2.0 Hz.

PSWs are low frequency potentials that produce a dull "pop" on the speaker. Spike fibrillations are high frequency potentials that produce a sharp ticking sound. The sound of spike fibrillations has been likened to crinkling cellophane, or "rain on a tin roof"; however, few modern EMGers have ever heard rain on a tin roof. There are a few clinical situations in which positive waves occur without fibrillations, but most often the two waveforms are seen together (17). When present in abundance, they create a symphony of ticks and pops. See the Appendix on waveform modeling for a further discussion of the frequency components of fibrillation potentials and PSWs.

The amplitude of fibrillation potentials and PSWs roughly correlates with the duration of disease. An atrophic muscle fiber may elaborate a small, sometimes tiny, fibrillation. Larger, nonatrophic fibers in recently denervated muscle may generate a very high amplitude fibrillation. Kraft assessed fibrillation potential amplitude at various intervals after peripheral nerve injury and found it useful in estimating the time since injury. Amplitudes >100 μV were not seen after the first year (18). Fibrillations in myopathy are particularly likely to be small and to recruit slowly (15).

MUAPs may sometimes have the configuration of PSWs, but these can usually be distinguished by their irregularity of firing and volitional control. Myotonic discharges commonly have a PSW configuration. Very brief myotonic discharges may be difficult to distinguish from trains of PSWs. The electrical myotonia reported in some unlikely clinical situations, such as hypothyroid myopathy, may reflect this sometimes difficult distinction.

PSWs and fibrillation potentials are intimately related. Sometimes a spike fibrillation will transmogrify into a PSW over the course of a few discharges with no movement of the needle or other interference. The nature of the relationship has been a long-standing matter of conjecture, and was recently debated by two authorities (17,19). The primary difference is in the configuration. A spike fibrillation has a brief initial positive component followed by a tall, sharp negative spike. The PSW has a deep and prolonged initial positive component, followed by a low amplitude, blunted component of trailing negativity. Both arise from the discharges of single muscle fibers, both fire regularly, and both generally have the same clinical significance.

There are two primary theories that seek to explain the difference in configuration. The first theory holds that positive waves are intracellularly recorded potentials, which detect an inrush of cations during depolarization to produce the positive phase, and the slow return to internal negativity and overshoot that marks the repolarization phase. One problem with this formulation is that both the MNE and the CNE are gigantic in relation to the size of the muscle fiber (Fig. 8.1). It is difficult to see how such a large and relatively blunt instrument could pierce a muscle fiber and leave intact membrane around it still able to carry out membrane events.

The other theory is that a PSW represents a "blocked fibrillation." In this situation, the electrode is in contact with the muscle cell surface. During depolarization a wave of approaching negativity is seen through the volume conductor, producing the positive component of the wave. However, the mechanical presence of the needle prevents the membrane in the immediate vicinity of the needle from depolarizing normally, so that when the wave arrives beneath the electrode, instead of a sharp negative spike potential there is a long, slow, blunted negativity representing a thwarted attempt by the local membrane to generate an action potential. The negative spike is "stifled" (17).

Mechanical distortion of an unstable fiber may explain why PSWs are frequently seen before spike fibrillation potentials in the time course of denervation. As the resting membrane potential decreases after nerve injury, there may be a level before spontaneous discharges begin, but at which the fiber is sensitive to mechanical stimuli. Deformation by the needle electrode might then initiate a train of provoked PSWs at a time too early for frank spontaneous activity to appear (17).

Another factor in the two different faces of the fibrillation potential may be the effects of tissue filtering and the distance of the electrode from the generator source. Using waveform modeling with the electromyograph, the shock artifact of the stimulator can be made to simulate either waveform simply by changing the filters. See Appendix on waveform modeling for further discussion.

Whatever the mechanism for their dissimilarity, PSWs and sharp fibrillations are much more alike than different; in most instances they have the same clinical significance. Although originally recognized as a consequence of denervation, it soon became clear that fibrillation potentials could occur in primary muscle disease and in other circumstances as well (Table 8.5). After initial reports describing their occurrence in dermatomyositis, investigators reported fibrillation potentials in muscular dystrophies and other myopathies. The primary attribute in common of muscle diseases which are associated with fibrillation potentials is muscle fiber necrosis. Currently, the

TABLE 8.5
Conditions Associated with Fibrillation Potentials

Denervation
  Anterior horn cell disease
  Radiculopathy
  Plexopathy
  Neuropathy
Myonecrotic myopathies
  Inflammatory myopathy
  Muscular dystrophy
  Rhabdomyolysis
Congenital myopathies (some)
Metabolic myopathies (some)
Hyperkalemic periodic paralysis
Neuromuscular transmission disorders
  Myasthenia gravis (rare, debatable)
  Botulinum toxin effect, including therapeutic injections (common)
Upper motor neuron lesions with transsynaptic anterior horn cell degeneration (very controversial)

---

occurrence of fibrillation potentials is used to separate myopathies into the broad groups of bland myopathies, those without fibrillation potentials, and necrotizing or myonecrotic myopathies, those with fibrillation potentials (Table 8.6). See Chapter 19 for further discussion. There is some evidence that fibrillation potentials may be related to muscle fiber regeneration, rather than denervation and degeneration, which might explain their occurrence in so many disparate conditions (20).

When present, fibrillation potentials vary greatly in abundance, from a few, scattered potentials to profuse activity everywhere. Their amplitude may vary greatly depending on the chronicity of the process. Sparse, low amplitude fibrillation potentials may be difficult to discern, especially with modern, digital EMG machines where the fibrillation potential is sometimes better heard than seen. Clinicians commonly grade fibrillation potentials on a poorly standardized scale of 1+ to 4+ intensity (Table 8.7). They should be called as definitely present only if unequivocal fibrillation potentials are seen in at least two different areas of the muscle remote from the endplate.

COMPLEX REPETITIVE DISCHARGES (CRDs)

Complex repetitive discharges (CRDs) were formerly called bizarre high frequency or bizarre repetitive discharges, but that term was dropped in favor of CRD (7). The concomitant loss of the adjective bizarre was unfortunate; it was an apt term, as the quintessential attribute of these discharges is that they sound very strange, remarkably odd and often outlandish. Sometimes it is difficult to believe such noise could emanate from human muscle, and the wild sound of a CRD coming from a lab often brings curiosity seekers. Despite the spectacle, one CRD should be considered as of approximately the same significance as one fibrillation potential (15). CRDs have also been referred to as pseudomyotonia, a term best avoided.

CRDs are felt to be due to a group of adjacent muscle fibers discharging together, due to ephaptic spread from fiber to fiber. They occur in situations wherein muscle fibers with unstable membranes lie adjacent to one another, as in neurogenic group atrophy or myopathic disorders with fiber necrosis and splitting. CRDs imply chronicity of the disease process. A circus movement, similar to that causing cardiac atrial tachyarrhythmias has been postulated. The discharge may begin with the spontaneous depolarization of a pacemaker fiber, then spread to a fixed sequence of adjacent unstable fibers, then return to the starting point. If the discharge returns to the generator fiber during its refractory period the cycle may stop. CRDs characteristically have very low jitter on SF analysis, which is typical of split fibers. This supports the concept that transmission is from muscle fiber to muscle fiber, with no intervening neuromuscular junction.

CRDs are complex, having two or more components, and they reverberate repetitively, rumbling and rasping. They typically begin and end abruptly, as if someone had thrown a switch. Their sound has been likened to machinery running, or a roughly idling outboard motorboat engine. CRDs typically discharge at 5–100 Hz. The entire complex may change amplitude or frequency because of the acquisition or loss of a subcomponent, but the frequency of subcomponents does not change. The changes are abrupt, discrete, quantal jumps. This is in contrast to myotonia, where the frequency and amplitude are ever changing, waxing and waning, and the shifts are gradual (see above). CRDs may occur normally in the iliopsoas muscle, and have no significance when found there. Refer to the Appendix on waveform modeling for a method to simulate a CRD on the electromyograph.

FASCICULATION POTENTIALS

Fasciculation potentials are due to the spontaneous discharge of all or part of a motor unit. A group of muscle fibers contracts and a potential suddenly and unpredictably pops out of an otherwise silent background. Fasciculations resemble MUAPs in amplitude, duration and configuration. However they do not fire in trains as MUAPs do. Rather they fire once, then disappear—a single, isolated twitch. The same or a different fasciculation potential may fire one to several seconds later. The normal initial firing rate of a MUAP at minimal contraction is 3–5 Hz; a fasciculation can hardly muster two successive contractions, much less fire at anything approaching the rate of even a minimal, spasmodic, voluntarily controlled MUAP.

A simple and convenient method to grade fasciculations is as follows. The rare or occasional fasciculation is described as rare or occasional. If fasciculations are occurring frequently enough to grade, wait for one to fire, then begin slowly counting to 10 at 1 count/sec. If one fasciculation fires over the next 10 s, the grade is 1+, if 2 fire the grade is 2+, and so on up to 4+.

Fasciculations occur in a number of clinical circumstances. They are typically prominent in ALS, but can occur as well in any condition causing chronic denervation, including radiculopathies and neuropa-

---

TABLE 8.6
Possible Patterns of Abnormality on Needle Electrode Examination in Myopathies

Normal examination
  Steroid myopathy (most)
  CPT deficiency (between attacks of rhabdomyolysis)
  Myoadenylate deaminase deficiency
  Congenital myopathies (some)
  Periodic paralysis (between attacks)
Bland myopathies (MUAP abnormalities only)
  Steroid myopathy (some)
  Inflammatory myopathy in remission
  Mitochondrial myopathy (most)
  Critical illness myopathy (most)
  Hypothyroidism (most)
  Hyperthyroidism (may have fasciculations and myokymia)
  Carnitine deficiency (most)
  FSH dystrophy
  Oculopharyngeal dystrophy
  Scapuloperoneal syndrome
  Congenital myopathies (most)
  Periodic paralysis with fixed weakness
Myonecrotic myopathies (MUAP changes plus fibrillation potentials)
  Dystrophinopathy (Duchenne and Becker dystrophy and related conditions)
  Limb girdle dystrophy
  Congenital muscular dystrophy
  Distal dystrophy
  Inflammatory myopathy (polymyositis, dermatomyositis, inclusion body myositis)
  Rhabdomyolysis
  Trichinosis
    Sarcoidosis
  Glycogen storage diseases (most)
  Carnitine deficiency (some)
  CPT deficiency (during attack of rhabdomyolysis)
  Nemaline myopathy
  Myotubular myopathy
  Toxic myopathies (some)
Myopathies with myotonic discharges
  As a relatively isolated abnormality
    Myotonia congenita (dominant and recessive forms)

Paramyotonia congenita
Myotonic subtype of K⁺ sensitive periodic paralysis
Adult acid maltase deficiency
Toxins (rare)
With major accompanying evidence of myopathy
  Myotonic dystrophy
  Myotubular myopathy
  Infantile acid maltase deficiency
  Proximal myotonic myopathy (most)
Myopathies with fibrillation potentials only
  Inflammatory myopathy (early)
Myopathies with occasional long duration, polyphasic potentials
  Inflammatory myopathy (very chronic)
  Muscular dystrophy
  Nemaline myopathy
Myopathies with an abnormal response to repetitive stimulation or brief isometric exercise
  Myotonic dystrophy
  Myotonia congenita
  Phosphorylase deficiency
  Inflammatory myopathy
  Periodic paralysis
Myopathies that may have both myopathic and neuropathic features
  Inclusion body myositis
  Alcoholic myopathy
  Emery-Dreifuss dystrophy
  Far advanced, severe chronic myopathy with long duration polyphasic potentials
  Oculopharyngeal dystrophy
  Mitochondrial myopathy (with accompanying neuropathy)
  Chronic spinal muscular atrophy masquerading as limb girdle dystrophy
Myopathies with frequent bizarre potentials (myotonic discharges or CRDs): the raucous myopathies
  Myotonic disorders
  Acid maltase deficiency
  Debrancher deficiency
  Continuous muscle fiber activity syndromes

CPT, carnitine palmityl transferase; FSH, facioscapulohumeral; MUAP, motor unit action potential.

TABLE 8.7
Grading of Fibrillation Potentials

Grade	Intensity
0	No definite fibrillation potentials
+/−	Equivocal; a single sustained fibrillation potential or examiner thinks fibrillation potentials were present but is not certain
1+	Unequivocal fibrillation potentials in at least two areas, but sparse and difficult to demonstrate, requires many needle movements, elicitation is tedious
2+	Fibrillation potentials demonstrated with ease in many areas of the muscle, demonstration is not laborious
3+	Fibrillation potentials almost everywhere, demonstration is very easy, difficult to find areas that are not fibrillating
4+	Fibrillation potentials constantly fill the screen in all locations, high amplitude, may resemble an interference pattern

thies. Benign fasciculations occur in the absence of any other clinical or electrical evidence of neuromuscular disease (see Chapter 13). A contention that malignant fasciculations, i.e, those due to ALS, have a lower firing rate and that this permits differentiation from benign fasciculations has not been widely accepted. Current evidence suggests that fasciculations arise distally in the axon (21)

MYOTONIA

Myotonic discharges are wonderfully peculiar. They are usually elicited by needle movement, but may be brought out by muscle contraction or percussion, all of which mechanically excite muscle fibers. After the triggering stimulus, the discharges erupt from the muscle in a high frequency, high amplitude cacophony which then gradually but spasmodically wanes in frequency and amplitude to die down toward silence, only to burst out again with a minimal mechanical excitation. Myotonia is pandemonium in the muscle. The discharges are due to the independent, repetitive discharges of single muscle fibers at rates of 20–80 Hz, and are typically composed of a mixture of spike fibrillations and PSWs. Both the amplitude and the frequency must wax and wane to qualify as true myotonia. The sound of myotonic discharges is classically likened to a dive bomber. However, the modern EMGer is no more likely to have ever heard a real dive bomber than to have heard rain on a tin roof. One of the few EMGers to know the sound of a real dive bomber denies the similarity (22). A better auditory analogy is to the sound of a chainsaw or a two-cycle motorcycle engine revving and dying (the Kawasaki discharge; the muscle as motocross event).

The essential difference between myotonia and CRDs is that myotonic discharges spontaneously and continuously vary in amplitude and frequency, have a gradual offset, and are retriggered by needle movement. CRDs have an abrupt onset and offset, vary only by gaining or losing subcomponents, and slight needle movement may cause the discharge to disappear.

Myotonic discharges occur in myotonic dystrophy, myotonia congenita, paramyotonia congenita, hyperkalemic periodic paralysis, acid maltase deficiency and myotubular myopathy. Whether true myotonia occurs in inflammatory myopathies, hypothyroid myopathy or chronic denervation is disputed.

MYOKYMIA

Myokymia is a type of grouped or repetitive discharge that consists of a burst of motor unit potentials recurring regularly or semiregularly. The sound has been likened to that made by marching soldiers—the near but not perfect synchrony of multiple footfalls, recurring as a group—brrrruup, brrrruup. Picture a platoon of goose-stepping, jack-booted storm troopers, maybe slightly ragged recruits, and imagine the sound they would make. The myokymic discharge appears as a flurry of spikes—at least two, usually a dozen or so and rarely many dozen—grouped together, separated by an interval of silence. As with CRDs, the group may gain or lose subcomponents and thus abruptly change in duration or amplitude. The interdischarge interval may vary slightly or markedly; the discharge is typically slightly irregular. The frequency of the bursts is usually 2–10 Hz, while the frequency of the spikes comprising the bursts may range from 5–60 Hz (23).

Myokymic discharges, the electrical phenomenon, are seen only rarely, and may or may not be accompanied by clinical myokymia, the visible, vermicular undulations on the skin surface. Myokymia is thought to arise because of biochemical perturbations in the nerve microenvironment due to demyelination, a toxin (such as rattlesnake venom or gold salts), edema or other factors (23). It may be generalized or focal/segmental. Generalized myokymia is most often a part of a continuous muscle fiber activity syndrome (24,25). Focal limb myokymia is particularly characteristic of radiation damage to a nerve or plexus. Myokymia is only very rarely associated with nerve compression syndromes. It sometimes occurs in the facial muscles in patients with MS or other lesions of the brainstem or cranial nerves, such as pontine glioma, syrinx or Guillain-Barre syndrome. The pacemaker site varies with the condition. The response pattern of myokymic discharges to sleep, anesthesia, nerve blocks and curare suggests a distal origin in many instances.

CRAMP DISCHARGES

Cramps are involuntary muscle contractions that occur in a variety of clinical circumstances. A needle electrode in a muscle during a cramp records a cramp discharge: multiple MUAPs indistinguishable from the IP of a maximal voluntary contraction, except that it originates from a tetanic involuntary contraction. With a minimal cramp only a few units may fire together at a high rate, 20–150 Hz. In contrast, the muscle "contraction" which occurs in some metabolic myopathies, classically in McArdle's disease, while clinically a painful muscle shortening resembling a cramp, is electrically silent—a muscle contracture and not a true cramp. Cramps appear to result from high frequency nerve discharges and do not arise primarily from the muscle. In some patients, cramps, fasciculations, and myokymia all occur in various combinations (25–27).

NEUROMYOTONIA

Neuromyotonic, or neurotonic, discharges are bursts of multiple spikes firing at a very high frequency, up to 100–300 Hz, in a decrescendo pattern. The frequency does not change but the amplitude gradually wanes, perhaps due to the muscle membrane's inability to sustain such high firing rates. They create a unique musical piiiiinnnngggggggg'ing sound. Neurotonic discharges are very rare. They are due to the discharging of a single motor unit and are seen primarily in continuous motor unit activity syndromes, but in some very chronic denervating syndromes as well (28). Neurotonic discharges are also induced by mechanical stimulation of the nerve, and are useful for monitoring the status of a nerve during intraoperative recordings, especially the facial nerve during acoustic neuroma surgery. When the surgeon stretches or otherwise mechanically stimulates the nerve, the muscle responds with an alerting chorus of neurotonic discharges.

ABNORMAL VOLUNTARY ACTIVITY

Diseases of nerve and diseases of muscle both produce changes in the architecture of the motor unit. The primary change seen in muscle disease is atrophy of individual muscle fibers. Fibers may become necrotic, undergo splitting, or exhibit a variety of other pathological changes. With more severe myopathies, the muscle fibers may be replaced by electrically inactive fat and fibrous tissue. Atrophic muscle fibers may ultimately lie scattered in a matrix of electrically inactive tissue.

With neurogenic disease, the motor unit's territory is altered in a different way. Denervation is accompanied by reinnervation. After reinnervation, the total number of functional motor units is decreased due to a dropout of neurons or axons, depending on the specific process, but each unit has an enlarged territory with an increase in its total number of muscle fibers. The electrodiagnostic picture depends on when in the course of denervation and reinnervation the study is done. Satellite cells become mobile and proliferate after muscle injury, and play a part in regeneration. Their role in primary muscle diseases is more clear cut than their role in recovery from denervation.

The range of normal MUAP amplitude and duration is fairly restricted, at least for the low threshold, first recruited units that appear with minimal to moderate voluntary contraction. A normal, generic MUAP as recorded with a CNE at mild to moderate contraction can be summarized as having a duration of 5–15 ms, up to four phases, and a variable amplitude depending on needle position, but generally in the range of 2–3 mV. MUAPs may be of abnormal size because they are either too large or too small. Most often they are large or small in both dimensions, amplitude and duration; and, as a broad generalization, large units are typical of neuropathic disease and small units of myopathic disease. This is only a generalization, and there are important exceptions. Although small amplitude, short duration units are typical of muscle diseases, there are other conditions in which bantam units can occur, such as early reinnervation or neuromuscular transmission disorders. Large amplitude, long duration units are typical of neurogenic diseases, but can be seen in some long-standing, severe myopathies. MUAPs may be of long duration but low amplitude, as in the "nascent" units of early reinnervation, or of short duration but normal amplitude as is not uncommon in myopathies (29). A brief overview of neuromuscular pathophysiology will help to understand the nuances.

Any disease process affecting the motor unit initially results in dysfunction of individual muscle fibers. In myopathies, the fibers are affected at random; in neuropathic disease, whole motor units may be involved, but their fibers lie randomly within the muscle fascicle. Early muscle fiber dysfunction may result only in the inability to generate a normal action potential. This could be the result of a myopathic process involving individual, random muscle fibers; defective neuromuscular transmission with failure of some fibers to achieve activation; a neuropathy selectively affecting terminal axonal twigs, as may occur with early Guillain-Barre syndrome producing terminal conduction block or with the distal twig neuropathy of hyperparathyroid neuromuscular disease; or the very early stages of axon loss due to neuropathy or neuronopathy. At this stage, regardless of etiology, the picture on NEE may be similar. Functional loss of random muscle fibers at the periphery of the electrode's recording area removes the low frequency early and late components from the MUAP, shortening its duration. Dysfunction of those relatively few fibers at the heart of the recording zone that make up the main spike may result in a lowered MUAP amplitude. Any of these mechanisms may result in short duration, low amplitude MUAPs. Although classic for myopathy, such potentials may also be a feature of NMT disorders, periodic paralysis, or very early denervation (Table 8.4). The term pseudomyopathic is sometimes applied in such circumstances.

(A feel of the sight and sound of short duration, small amplitude units can be easily obtained by simply increasing the low frequency filter to 500 Hz (the setting for SFEMG studies) during the course of a routine, normal needle examination. This effectively removes the low frequency components at the onset and termination of the MUAPs, and simulates the short duration and early recruitment of a myopathic process. Conversely, to simulate neuropathic units filters should be wide open to increase the amplitude and duration [See the Appendix on waveform modeling for further discussion.]

With continued progression of the disease process, the pathophysiologies of nerve and muscle disease begin to diverge, only to converge again in the very late stages. To increase power in myopathy, additional motor units are recruited, producing the picture of early or increased recruitment. To increase power in neuropathy, the surviving units discharge more rapidly, producing the picture of decreased recruitment and fast firing units. After several days to several weeks deprived of nerve supply, the muscle fiber membranes become unstable and fibrillations emerge. The loss of trophic influences on muscle fibers incites nerve fiber sprouting and attempts at regeneration and rescue.

With continued evolution, reinnervation restores function to some muscle fibers. When denervation has been severe, this early return of function may produce small, short units for the same reasons discussed; thus, small amplitude, short duration units may be a feature of early reinnervation. As reinnervation proceeds, more and more muscle fibers are brought under neural control. These fibers are in various stages of atrophy, have various sizes, disparately mature neuromuscular junctions, and collateral sprouts of different lengths; all of which combine to produce asynchrony of discharge, jitter and blocking. The result is low amplitude, long duration, complex, polyphasic, unstable MUAPs which may have satellite potentials: the so-called "nascent" units of early reinnervation. Because of low amplitude and polyphasia, these have also been dubbed pseudomyopathic.

With further evolution of a necrotizing myopathy, a variety of pathologic changes may occur in individual muscle fibers, such as necrosis, degeneration, and splitting. Variably effective regeneration may occur concomitantly. The result is the marked random variation of fiber size typical of many myopathies, with atrophic, normal sized and occasionally even hypertrophic fibers haphazardly admixed. These changes cause marked desynchronization of the MUAP due to varying conduction velocity along different size muscle fibers. Many fibers may die, to be replaced by fat and fibrous tissue. Fibers undergoing segmental necrosis or splitting may develop "myogenic" denervation as part of the fiber is functionally or anatomically separated from its neuromuscular junction. These fibers certainly, and other necrotic fibers probably, develop membrane instability and fibrillate. The electrophysiologic result is predictable: early recruitment; small amplitude, short duration units; complex, polyphasic, fragmented, often unstable units; and fibrillations. Desynchronization may be so severe as to result in the formation of long duration, polyphasic units that may resemble those of neurogenic disease—the "pseudoneurogenic unit" (30).

In end stage disease, myopathic and neuropathic processes again share similarities. In neurogenic disease, reinnervation results in an enlarged motor unit territory with many more muscle fibers per motor unit than normal. With maturation of reinnervating sprouts and neuromuscular junctions, the asynchrony of firing decreases, the amplitude increases and stability improves. More fibers belonging to the same motor unit may lie at the tip of the electrode, resulting in high amplitude, and more fibers may be active at the periphery of the recording zone, resulting in long duration. Synchrony seldom improves to normal, so increased complexity is common. The end result: the long duration, high amplitude, stable, complex, polyphasic MUAP of chronic denervation with reinnervation. If reinnervation is incomplete, or the reinnervated unit itself later dies (as in ALS) the muscle may undergo atrophy with fibrous replacement and leave scattered, small atrophic fibers, resulting in the small, short MUAP of late neurogenic atrophy.

In end stage myopathy, replacement of the muscle by fat and fibrosis is the rule, sometimes leaving islands of muscle tissue imbedded in a sea of scar. Whole motor units may have disappeared, and "myogenic denervation" and other processes may have resulted in significant remodeling of the surviving motor units. Split or regenerated fibers may lie in clusters. Thus, a decreased number of fast firing, long duration, sometimes high amplitude, polyphasic, "chronic neurogenic" MUAPs may be prominent in far advanced, severe myopathy (30).

Thus, comparable pathophysiology may underlie the electrodiagnostic similarities in very early and very late myopathic and neuropathic processes. Various mechanisms may result in either large or small MUAPs in either nerve or muscle disease. As Wilbourn stated, "The MUAP changes seen with early Guillain-Barre syndrome and myasthenic syndrome may not merely "resemble" those seen with recent onset polymyositis, they may be *identical* to them" (15); and similarly the chronic neurogenic features of endstage myopathy. Fortunately, most patients are seen in the intermediate stages of disease when the electrodiagnostic changes are sufficiently different to allow the distinction between neuropathic and myopathic disorders.

Key Points

- The routine needle electrode examination (NEE) assesses three types of electrical activity in the muscle: spontaneous, insertional and voluntary. A normal muscle contains no spontaneous activity other than in the region of the end plate. Insertional activity is created by small movements of the electrode, and normally consists of a burst of amorphous spike discharges, the duration of which does not exceed 300–400 ms. Voluntary activity is created by the patient's volitional contraction of the muscle.

- Waveforms seen in both normal and abnormal muscle can be categorized into three groups. Potentials arising from single muscle fibers include endplate spikes, fibrillation potentials, and positive sharp waves (PSWs). Potentials arising from motor units include normal motor unit action potentials (MUAPs), fasciculations, myokymia, neuromyotonia, cramp discharges, and tetany. Complex repetitive discharges (CRDs) arise from electrically linked muscle fibers firing synchronously.

- As recorded with a concentric needle electrode (CNE), single muscle fiber action potentials have a duration of 1–5 ms and an amplitude of 50–200 μV. A normal, generic MUAP as recorded with a CNE at mild to moderate contraction has a duration of 5–15 ms, up to four phases,

and a variable amplitude depending on needle position, but usually in the range of 2–3 mV.

- Distinctive types of increased insertional activity may occur in otherwise normal individuals. Two types of normal spontaneous activity occur in the region of the endplate: endplate noise and endplate spikes.

- Volitional activity is assessed by having the patient contract the muscle with a needle in place. The orderly recruitment of MUAPs by increasing numbers, firing rates, and sizes results in a smoothly graded voluntary muscle contraction. First recruited, low threshold, type 1 units are lower in amplitude than later recruited, high threshold, type 2 units.

- Using a CNE, the first recruited, low threshold units tend to have an amplitude in the range of 300–700 microvolts. With moderate contraction, peak to peak MUAP amplitudes tend to run 1–3 mV. The expected amplitudes with a monopolar needle electrode (MNE) are about 2x, and the expected durations about 1.5x, those seen with a CNE.

- The main spike of the MUAP is probably generated by no more than 5–15 muscle fibers. Amplitude is the most variable and least precisely defined of the MUAP parameters that are commonly measured. MUAP duration is a more constant and reliable indicator of motor unit size.

- Maximum contraction produces a pattern of multiple overlapping MUAPs: the interference pattern. At full contraction, the characteristics of individual MUAPs cannot be discerned in normal muscle.

- Onset frequency is the frequency of a motor unit when it first begins to discharge; recruitment frequency is the firing rate of a MUAP when the next unit is recruited. Recruitment is most often judged by the timing pattern of MUAP firing in relationship to the sweep and by the sounds the units create.

- The mildest form of abnormally increased insertional activity is trains of PSWs that persist for more than about 300 ms. Other forms of insertional activity include myotonia, complex repetitive discharges, myokymia and neuromyotonia.

- Fibrillation potentials are spontaneous, periodic depolarizations of a single, unstable muscle fiber. Recorded outside the endplate region, fibrillation potentials may have one of two configurations: the spike fibrillation or the PSW. PSWs and fibrillation potentials are intimately related. The nature of the relationship has been a long-standing matter of conjecture. Whatever the mechanism for their dissimilarity, PSWs and sharp fibrillations are much more alike than different; in most instances they have the same clinical significance.

- Fibrillations can occur in many disparate conditions.

- Myopathies can be broadly grouped into bland (without fibrillations) and necrotizing or myonecrotic myopathies (with fibrillations).

- CRDs occur in situations wherein muscle fibers with unstable membranes lie adjacent to one another, permitting ephaptic spread from fiber to fiber. They imply chronicity of the disease process.

- Fasciculation potentials are due to an isolated spontaneous discharge of a motor unit and resemble MUAPs in amplitude, duration, and configuration. They occur in any condition causing chronic denervation.

- Myotonic discharges result from the independent, repetitive discharges of single muscle fibers at rates of 20–80 Hz, with waxing and waning of both frequency and amplitude.

- Myokymia is a type of grouped or repetitive discharge consisting of a burst of MUAPs recurring regularly or semiregularly, thought to arise because of biochemical perturbations in the nerve microenvironment.

- Neuromyotonic discharges are bursts of multiple spikes firing at a very high frequency, up to 100–300 Hz, in a decrescendo pattern.

- Diseases of nerve and diseases of muscle both produce changes in the architecture of the motor unit. MUAPs may be either too large or too small. As a broad generalization, large units are typical of neuropathic disease and small units of myopathic disease, but there are significant exceptions.

- Various mechanisms may result in either large or small MUAPs in either nerve or muscle disease at certain stages in their evolution. Comparable pathophysiology may underlie the electrodiagnostic similarities in very early and very late myopathic and neuropathic processes. Fortunately, most patients are seen in the intermediate stages of disease when the electrodiagnostic changes are sufficiently different to allow the distinction between neuropathic and myopathic disorders.

References

1. Chan RC, Hsu TC. Quantitative comparison of motor unit potential parameters between monopolar and concentric needles. Muscle Nerve 1991;14:1028–1032.
   This study quantitatively compared the simultaneous recording of the "same" motor unit potentials recorded by closely positioned concentric and monopolar needles. The motor unit potentials from the anterior tibialis of 12 young subjects were analyzed independently by both needles being connected to 2 sets of EMG-computer combinations. Recordings of the same motor unit potentials were confirmed by triggering and averaging of the 2 sets of motor unit potentials with identical firing patterns on both EMG screens. Automatic analysis disclosed the monopolar recordings had a significantly higher mean amplitude (2.05 times), larger surface area (2.64 times), and longer duration (1.86 times) than the concentric recordings, while the mean number of phases (1.58 times) and turns (1.35 times) revealed no statistical differences. Both active recording and reference electrodes contributed to these differences. See also: Pease WS, Bowyer BL. Motor unit analysis. Comparison between concentric and monopolar electrodes. Am J Phys Med Rehabil 1988;67:2. These investigators found no statistically

or clinically significant difference in MUAP measurement parameters between monopolar and concentric electrodes, a minority opinion.

2. Nandedkar SD, Dumitru D, King JC. Concentric needle electrode duration measurement and uptake area. Muscle Nerve 1997;20:1225–1228.
   Computer simulations of CNE MUAP recordings assume the cannula shields muscle fibers on the side away from the bevel from detection by the active electrode, producing a hemispheric recording area radiating outwardly from the bevel. This model predicts that the MUAP amplitude depends on 1) fibers within 0.5 mm of the CNE core 2) size of the muscle fibers 3) distance of the closest fibers. The MUAP spike is defined by those fibers within 1 mm of the core, the duration depends on the number of fibers within 2.5 mm of the core, and the area depends on fibers within 2 mm of the core and on the amplitude. In this study, MUAPs were recorded with different orientations of the bevel to the muscle fibers. Contrary to computer simulation predictions, the MUAP duration remained constant during needle rotation, although amplitude and configuration changed. The authors question the shielding effects of the cannula, hypothesize the recording area may be spherical rather than hemispherical, and re-emphasize that duration is a "robust" MUAP feature. See also: Nandedkar SD, Sanders DB, Stalberg EV, Andreassen S. Simulation of concentric needle EMG motor unit action potentials. Musc & Nerve 1988;11:151–159.

3. Wright KC, Ramsey-Goldman R, Nielsen VK, et al. Syndrome of diffuse abnormal insertional activity: case report and family study. Arch Phys Med Rehab 1988;69:534–536.
   In 1979 Wiechers and Johnson described ten patients with diffuse abnormal insertional activity on EMG examination in the absence of neuromuscular disease. This report presents a family group with identical findings. The propositus is a 53-year-old woman who presented with back pain. EMG studies revealed trains of positive sharp waves with needle movement in all muscles studied. Nerve conduction studies, radiographs, and laboratory studies were all unremarkable. Eight additional family members were recruited who underwent a screening EMG of five muscles. Four patients had trains of positive sharp waves present in all five muscles. This report confirms the findings of Wiechers and Johnson. The abnormality appears to be genetically transmitted in an autosomal dominant pattern. Although without clinical significance, it is important for electromyographers to be aware of this entity so as not to mistakenly ascribe serious neuromuscular disease to these patients.

4. Wilbourn AJ. An unreported, distinctive type of increased insertional activity. Muscle Nerve 1982;5:S101-S105.
   Movement of a recording needle electrode in normal muscle provokes a brief burst of action potentials due to the mechanical excitation of muscle fibers, which usually lasts < 1/3 of a second. One type of increased insertional activity, referred to as "Snap, Crackle, Pop" (SCP) follows the normal brief burst of insertional activity and consists of trains of potentials in which the individual components fire at irregular intervals and vary in both configuration and amplitude with sequential firings. The potentials may be mono-, bi-, tri-, or multi-phasic and often have a positive wave form. The total number of potentials in each train ranges from 2 to > 10; rarely does the same potential recur. The interpotential interval and length of train are variable; most commonly they last approximately

1 s, but can persist for up to 3 s. Rarely, SCP is accompanied by 1 or 2 fibrillation potentials, having either the biphasic spike or positive wave form. SCP has a distinctive sound because each successive potential tends to vary in wave form and sound from those preceding it. The overall prevalence is 5%, but SCP is 4X more common in males, and is seen with the highest frequency in the medial gastroc muscles of young, muscular males. SCP has no clinical significance itself, but may be mistaken for more significant types of increased insertional activity.

5. Ertas M, Stalberg E, Falck B. Can the size principle be detected in conventional EMG recordings? Muscle Nerve 1995;18:435–439.

According to Henneman's size principle, small motor units are recruited before large ones. It is commonly believed that this can be detected in routine conventional EMG recordings even among the earliest recruited motor units. That is, the motor unit potential (MUP) amplitude, area, and thickness should increase with recruitment order. This study examined the first four MUPs recruited within the pickup area of the electrodes. Data were obtained from 179 different sites in monopolar recordings and in 153 concentric recordings from 5 healthy subjects. In the pooled material, amplitude, area, and thickness increased slightly between consecutively recruited MUPs. However, at individual recording sites the size of consecutively recruited MUPs varied considerably. At some recording sites the first recruited MUP had the largest amplitude and the later MUPs had successively smaller amplitudes. The authors conclude that, at individual recording sites, the size principle cannot be detected in low threshold motor units with monopolar or concentric EMG electrodes. The reason for this is the small uptake area of these electrodes in relation to the motor unit territory.

6. Barkhaus PE, Nandedkar SD. On the selection of concentric needle electromyogram motor unit action potentials: is the rise time criterion too restrictive? Muscle Nerve 1996;19:1554–1560.

Concentric needle electromyogram motor unit action potentials (MUAPs) were recorded from the biceps brachii muscle of normal subjects and in patients with neuromuscular diseases. Although the MUAPs had a crisp sound and appeared sharp, their rise time (RT), measured from the maximum negative peak to the preceding maximum positive peak before it, was often > 500 microseconds. All MUAPs with an RT < or = 500 microseconds were recorded from within the motor unit (MU) territory. MUAP recordings from outside the MU territory had a long RT but also low amplitude (< 50 μV) and/or a characteristic initial negative deflection. In the remaining recordings from within the MU territory, MUAP duration remained relatively constant while MUAP amplitude and RT varied inversely with each other. These MUAPs may be useful in electrodiagnosis but discarded due to their longer RT. The authors feel that while the current RT criterion for MUAP selection ensures that the electrode tip is within the MU territory, it is also too restrictive.

7. Jablecki CK, et al. AAEE glossary of terms in clinical electromyography. Muscle Nerve 1987;10:G1-G60.

8. Liveson JA, Ma DM. Laboratory reference for clinical neurophysiology. Philadelphia: F.A. Davis Co., 1992; 408–414.

Summarizes data on CNE mean durations from: Buchthal, F. and Rosenfalck, P. Action potential parameters in different human muscles. Acta Psychiatr Neurol Scand 1955;30:125; Rosenfalck, P. Electromyography in normal subjects of different age. Methods Clin Neurophysiol 1991;2:47; and Sacco, G., Buchthal, F., and Rosenfalck, P. Motor unit potentials at different ages. Arch Neurol 1962;4:366. Data on MNE parameters from: Chu-Andrews J, Johnson RJ. Electrodiagnosis: an Anatomical and Clinical Approach. Philadelphia:J.B. Lippincott Co., 1986;232.

9. Dumitru D. Electrodiagnostic medicine. Philadelphia: Hanley & Belfus, 1995.

10. Dorfman LJ, McGill KC. AAEE minimonograph #29: automatic quantitative electromyography. Muscle Nerve 1988;11:804–818.

A review of different computerized methods of automatic quantitative electromyography. Interference pattern methods-turns analysis, spectral analysis- are efficient, but the results usually cannot be directly related to the physiological properties of the motor units. Integration analysis does not currently have a major role in diagnostic electromyography. Traditional measurement of single motor unit action potentials during weak contraction can be facilitated and made more objective with computer assistance, but only the lowest-threshold motor units in the muscle are amenable to study. A new class of methodologies under development permit the decomposition of interference patterns into their constituent motor unit action potentials for measurement of configurational and behavioral properties. Patient data from these various methods can be statistically compared with normative data bases available online in computerized electromyographs. See also: Stalberg E, et al. Quantitative motor unit potential analysis. J Clin Neurophysiol 1996;13:401; and Engstrom JW, Olney RK. Quantitative motor unit analysis: the effect of sample size. Muscle Nerve 1992;15:277.

11. Finsterer J, Mamoli B. Satellite potentials as a measure of neuromuscular disorders. Muscle Nerve 1997;20: 585–592.

The study was carried out to investigate the characteristics of satellite potentials and their validity in clinical electromyography. Conventional needle electromyography was applied to the right biceps brachii and tibialis anterior muscles of 41 controls, 22 neuropathies, and 17 myopathies. Satellites were defined as small extrapotentials, preceding/following the main motor unit action potential (MUAP) component and separated from it by an isoelectric interval of > 1 ms. The normal mean satellite rate was 1.6% (biceps brachii) and 1.2% (tibialis anterior). In the biceps brachii (tibialis anterior) muscle it was 5 (5) times higher for neuropathies (P = 0.005, P = 0.006) and 5 (6) times higher for myopathies (P = 0.006, P = 0.003). MUAP parameters were not significantly different, whether satellites were considered or ignored. Evaluation of the satellite rate increased detection rates of neuromuscular disorders by up to 13%. The satellite rate proved a valuable and easily available, supplemental electromyographic parameter for the discrimination and detection of neuromuscular disorders.

12. Stalberg EV, Sonoo M. Assessment of variability in the shape of the motor unit action potential, the "jiggle," at consecutive discharges. Muscle Nerve 1994;17:1135–1144.

A method for quantifying shape variability, the jiggle, or motor unit potentials (MUPs) recorded with conventional EMG electrodes is presented. Amplitude variability at each point of time of the MUP was analyzed. Two new parameters are proposed: the normalized value of the consecutive amplitude differences (CAD), and the cross-correlational coefficient of the consecutive discharges (CCC). Simulations showed that increased jitter of the constituent single fiber potentials increases the jiggle as expressed by an increase in CAD and decrease in CCC values. Even when the jitter value of each component was fixed, increased temporal dispersion increased the jiggle whereas an increased number of fibers decreased the jiggle. This new method has been applied in normal subjects, patients with chronic neurogenic diseases and patients with ALS. Jiggle was significantly increased in the ALS group, in agreement with visual observations. This method for quantifying jiggle will increase the information obtainable from routine EMG investigations.

13. Daube JR. AAEM minimonograph #11: Needle examination in clinical electromyography. Muscle Nerve 1991;14:685–700.

The physiologic and histologic principles underlying clinical electromyographic studies are briefly reviewed as an introduction to the normal and abnormal findings in human subjects. Technical aspects of recordings as well as the specific types of discharges and their significance are discussed.

14. Petajan JH. AAEM minimonograph #3: motor unit recruitment. Muscle Nerve 1991;14:489–502.

Motor unit recruitment is the process by which different motor units are activated to produce a given level and type of muscle contraction. At minimal levels of muscle contraction (innervation), muscle force is graded by changes in firing rate (rate coding) of individual motoneurons (MNs). At higher levels of innervation, recruitment is accomplished by the addition of different motor units firing at or above physiologic tremor rate. During slowly graded and ballistic increases in force, motor units are recruited in rank order of their size. In addition to MN soma diameter, other factors contribute to the selectivity of MN activation. The central drive for motor unit activation is distributed to all the MNs of the pool serving a given muscle. Size-structure organization of the MN pool determines the order of recruitment and how MNs interact with each other. A method for the clinical EMG assessment of recruitment is suggested. Assessment is made at three levels of innervation: minimal contraction for onset and recruitment firing rates; moderate contraction required to maintain the limb against gravity for the maximum number of motor units, their firing rates, and motor unit spikes; maximal voluntary contraction (MVC) for detection of high threshold enlarged motor units characteristic of reinnervation and completeness of the interference pattern (IP). Loss of muscle fibers results in early and excessive recruitment at minimal and moderate levels of innervation. Loss of motor units can result in both an increased rate and range of single motor unit firing at all levels of innervation. With reinnervation and enlargement of motor units, firing rates increase significantly and the interference pattern during MVC is incomplete.

15. Wilbourn AJ. The electrodiagnostic examination with myopathies. J Clin Neurophysiol 1993;10:132–148. See Chapter 19 for abstract.

16. Dorfman LJ, Howard JE, McGill KC. Motor unit firing rates and firing rate variability in the detection of neuromuscular disorders. Electroencephalogr Clin Neurophysiol 1989;73:215–224.

This investigation used automatic decomposition electromyography (ADEMG) to study 41 muscles in 29 patients with well-defined peripheral and central motor disorders. In motor neuron diseases motor unit action potentials (MUAPs) showed increased amplitudes, firing rates and firing variability. In myopathies the MUAPs showed reduced amplitudes, durations and turns, and sometimes dramatic increases in firing rates. Also, the mean number of MUAPs per recording site was often increased, indicating excessive recruitment. In polymyositis, the nature and magnitude of the MUAP shape and firing abnormalities were usually similar at different levels of contractile force, suggesting that motor units are affected without regard to recruitment order. In upper motor neuron paresis (multiple sclerosis), the shape properties of the MUAPs were normal, but mean firing rates were reduced, and firing variability increased. These findings confirm many of the traditional criteria for distinguishing neurogenic from myopathic disease electrophysiologically at the level of the individual MUAP. In addition, they demonstrate the potential diagnostic sensitivity of MUAP firing rate measurements for detecting neuromuscular dysfunction, and for differentiating between some cases of central and peripheral paresis, but not for distinguishing peripheral neurogenic from myopathic weakness, since firing rates tend to increase in both. Increased firing rate variability may be a marker of central or peripheral neurogenic weakness.

17. Kraft GH. Are fibrillation potentials and positive sharp waves the same? No. Muscle Nerve 1996;19:216–220.

Electrodiagnostic medicine consultants report electrical activity in muscle recorded at rest and during voluntary movement by means of waveform and firing rate characteristics. This principle allows us to distinguish fibrillation potentials from positive sharp waves. Although in most cases these two potentials have the same clinical significance, there are at least five different situations in which they do not have an identical meaning: (1) positive sharp waves can be recorded earlier after a peripheral nerve injury than can fibrillation potentials; (2) occasionally, nonclinically significant diffuse positive sharp wave activity may be seen in the absence of fibrillation activity (i.e., "EMG disease"); (3) positive sharp waves may be seen in distal muscles of "normal" subjects without the presence of fibrillation activity or clinical significance; (4) positive sharp waves without fibrillation potentials may be seen following local muscle trauma; and (5) positive sharp waves may be seen alone in some demyelinating polyneuropathies. By accurately describing the observed potentials, the electrodiagnostic medicine consultant may be able to obtain more clinically useful information from an electrodiagnostic study. See also: Kraft GH. Fibrillation potentials and positive sharp waves: are they the same? Electroencephalogr Clin Neurophysiol 1991; 81:163–166.

18. Kraft GH. Fibrillation potential amplitude and muscle atrophy following peripheral nerve injury. Muscle Nerve 1990;13:814–821.

Maximum peak-to-peak fibrillation potential amplitude was measured in 69 subjects between 7 days and $10\frac{1}{2}$ years post complete or partial peripheral nerve injury. Mean amplitude during the first 2 months was 612 μV; third and fourth months 512 μV, fifth and sixth months 320 μV. After the first year, no population of fibrillation potentials greater than 100 μV was recorded. The sciatic nerve was sectioned in 13 guinea pigs and animals studied up to 17 weeks. Fibrillation potential amplitude in gastrocnemius muscles declined paralleling that in humans. By the end of the study, type I fibers had lost almost half of their initial diameter and type II fibers had atrophied more than twice this amount. Fibrillation potential amplitude may be useful in estimating the time post nerve injury and appears to correlate with the surface area and fiber diameter of a type I muscle fiber.

19. Dumitru D. Single muscle fiber discharges (insertional activity, end-plate potentials, positive sharp waves, and

fibrillation potentials): a unifying proposal. Muscle Nerve 1996;19:221–226.

The exact origin and precise morphologic explanation of positive sharp waves (PSWs) are presently lacking. Observing normal needle electromyographic insertional activity reveals two types of waveforms: (1) biphasic negative/positive spikes, and (2) positive spikes followed by a small negative phase. In the end-plate region, it is possible to occasionally observe a biphasic end-plate spike transform into a monophasic positive end-plate waveform. It is postulated that this waveform is simply a form of intracellular recording for the biphasic end-plate spike or a form of extracellularly recorded but blocked single muscle fiber discharge. Similarly, the observed monophasic positive insertional activity may be an intracellularly recorded single muscle fiber discharge or a blocked extracellular discharge originating about the needle electrode. Applying this reasoning to PSWs suggests that they may also be an intracellular recording of a fibrillation potential, or needle-induced extracellular blocked local single muscle fiber discharge. This unifying concept is applied to various clinical situations purported to demonstrate "different" types of PSWs.

20. Heuss D, Claus D, Neundorfer B. Fibrillations in regenerating muscle in dystrophic myopathies. Clin Neuropathol 1996;15:200–208.

This study attempted to demonstrate a correlation between muscle regeneration and fibrillations in electromyography in dystrophic myopathies. Especially in Emery-Dreifuss muscular dystrophy there is much abnormal spontaneous activity, and NCAM (neural cell adhesion molecule) and cytoskeletal protein vimentin expressing myocytes are predominantly seen. Therefore, definitely regenerating fibers are identified apart from only a few remnants of previous necrosis. Moreover, in the other biopsies of dystrophic myopathies there are also scattered and clustered NCAM and vimentin expressing regenerating myofibers. Here, regressive fiber changes, like necrosis, are more prominent. Furthermore, most regenerating fibers show pseudo-cholinesterase activity indicating innervation. Interestingly, motor end-plate changes in regeneration and in disuse atrophy are very similar. They predominantly consist of terminal sprouting and pseudo-cholinesterase spread. However, in disuse atrophy there is no abnormal spontaneous activity on EMG. Therefore, in regenerating muscle not innervation, but regeneration itself is likely to be the cause of fibrillations. In conclusion, a correlation is evident between regenerating muscle and fibrillations in electromyography.

21. Layzer RB. The origin of muscle fasciculations and cramps. Muscle & Nerve 1994;17:1243–1249.

The anatomic site of origin of muscle fasciculations and cramps has been debated for many years. Many authors have argued for a central origin of the abnormal discharges in the anterior horn cells. However, most of the evidence favors a very distal origin in the intramuscular motor nerve terminals. The factors giving rise to these discharges are not well understood. Fasciculations may be related to chemical excitation of motor nerve terminals, whereas cramps may result from mechanical excitation of motor nerve terminals during muscle shortening.

22. Kimura J. Electrodiagnosis in diseases of nerve and muscle: principles and practice. 2nd ed. Philadelphia: F.A. Davis, 1989:254.

"Despite common belief, a myotonic discharge does not closely simulate the sound of a dive-bomber, judged from my extensive personal experience (with dive-bombers)."

23. Gutmann L. AAEM minimonograph #37: facial and limb myokymia. Muscle Nerve 1991;14:1043–1049.

Myokymia is a clinical phenomenon associated with characteristic electromyographic activity referred to as myokymic discharges. These are spontaneously generated bursts of individual motor unit potentials with each burst recurring rhythmically or semirhythmically, usually several times per second. It involves facial muscles more commonly than those of the extremities, and is most often seen in association with Guillain-Barre syndrome, multiple sclerosis, radiation plexopathy, pontine tumors, and timber rattlesnake envenomation. An alteration in the biochemical microenvironment of axon membranes at one of the various sites along the motor axon is the likely basis for the altered membrane excitability that underlies the myokymic discharges in most cases. The similarity of these discharges to those seen with hypocalcemic tetany, and the ability to manipulate myokymic discharges by altering serum-ionized Ca^{++}, suggests that decrease in the ionized Ca^{++} in the microenvironment of the axon may play an important role.

24. Auger RG. AAEM minimonograph #44: diseases associated with excess motor unit activity. Muscle Nerve 1994;17:1250–1263.

See Chapter 19 for abstract.

25. Jamieson PW, Katirji MB. Idiopathic generalized myokymia. Muscle Nerve 1994;17:42–51.

Idiopathic generalized myokymia (IGM) is a rare, heterogeneous, and poorly understood syndrome. This study analyzed 75 reported cases in the world literature. IGM affects men and women equally, with a mean age of onset 29 +/− 19 years. Patients' common presenting complaints are stiffness (60%), cramps (12%), weakness (12%), and muscle twitching (4%). Family history is positive in 30%. In addition to generalized clinical myokymia (92%), abnormal neurologic findings include: hyporeflexia (70%), weakness (45%), grip myotonia (39%), and calf hypertrophy (16%). Electrical activity consisting of spontaneous continuous motor unit activity and/or electrical myokymia was documented in all patients. When electrical myokymia was observed (66%), the grouped discharges were irregular and had an interburst frequency of 2–300 Hz. Both phenytoin and carbamazepine are effective treatments. IGM has a wide spectrum of symptoms and severity and should be considered in all patients that present with stiffness, cramps, or muscle twitching. EMG greatly aids in diagnosis.

26. Tahmoush AJ, Alonso RJ, Tahmoush GP, et al. Cramp-fasciculation syndrome: a treatable hyperexcitable peripheral nerve disorder. Neurology 1991;41:1021–1024.

See Chapter 19 for abstract.

27. Smith KK, Claussen G, Fesenmeier JT, et al. Myokymia-cramp syndrome: evidence of hyperexcitable peripheral nerve. Muscle Nerve 1994;17:1065–1067.

A report of 2 patients with myokymia, cramps, myokymic discharges and repetitive discharges following the CMAP on nerve stimulation. The authors hypothesize that the myokymia-cramp syndrome is an intermediate form of hyperexcitable peripheral nerve disorder between cramp-fasciculation syndrome (mild) and Issac's syndrome (severe).

28. Torbergsen T, Stalberg E, Brautaset NJ. Generator sites for spontaneous activity in neuromyotonia. An EMG study. Electroencephalogr Clin Neurophysiol 1996;101:69–78.

A 16-year-old female patient with symptoms and signs compatible with neuromyotonia was studied with various neurophysiological tests and muscle biopsy. NCSs revealed signs of axonal motor neuropathy. EMG showed denervation in distal muscles, and moderate neurogenic changes in other muscles. Abundant spontaneous motor unit activity was recorded in all muscles. This activity did not disappear upon proximal nerve blockade with local anaesthetics. Based on the shape of spontaneous discharges and their behavior on nerve stimulation and during voluntary effort, the site of generation was suggested. This varied for different discharges, from proximally in the nerve, to various sites along the intramuscular nerve tree. In some axons there were signs of conduction block proximal to the generation site for the spontaneous discharges. Different axons showed various degrees of abnormality; local hyperexcitability triggering new impulses only after the passage of a preceding impulse, increased hyperexcitability generating spontaneous activity, total impulse blocking, and finally axonal degeneration. Treatment with dihydantoin reduced the spontaneous activity with concomitant clinical improvement.

29. Trojaborg W. Quantitative electromyography in polymyositis: a reappraisal. Muscle Nerve 1990;13:964–971.
Manual analysis of motor unit action potentials (MUAPs) was performed in 33 patients with polymyositis of whom 16 were studied in the acute stage and 17 in the chronic stage. Contrary to common description of "myopathic potentials" as being of low amplitude, short duration, and polyphasic shape, the quantitated study revealed no difference as to amplitude of short duration MUAPs in patients and normal subjects though short-duration MUAP and short duration polyphasic potentials were 4 and 3 times, respectively, more common in patients than in controls. Although the mean duration of MUAPs usually was significantly shorter in polymyositis than in controls, the average scatter of MUAPs' duration was the same in the 2 groups. The average incidence of polyphasic MUAPs was 4 times higher in patients than in controls, as was the incidence of those of long duration. To avoid misinterpretation of EMG findings due to an excess of polyphasic MUAPs, a greater number of individual potentials than usually recommended should be collected allowing a valid estimate of the mean duration of MUAPs of simple configuration.

30. Uncini A, Lange DJ, Lovelace RE, et al. Long-duration polyphasic motor unit potentials in myopathies: a quantitative study with pathological correlation. Muscle Nerve 1990;13:263–267.
See Chapter 19 for abstract.

9

Special Electrodiagnostic Medicine Techniques and Procedures

Techniques other than routine conduction studies and needle electromyography are frequently useful. This chapter briefly reviews some commonly and not so commonly performed procedures that are applicable under specific circumstances. This discussion is intended as an overview. Details regarding specific aspects are covered under individual clinical syndromes in Part II.

Blink Reflexes

The blink reflex (BR) is a complex response elicited by electrical or mechanical stimulation of the trigeminal nerve while recording from a muscle innervated by the facial nerve (1). It is most often done by stimulation of V_1, but can sometimes be recorded after stimulation of other trigeminal divisions. The BR is usually recorded from the orbicularis oculi or nasalis muscle after stim-

ulation of the supraorbital nerve; the recording site is modified for stimulation of other trigeminal divisions.

Elicitation of the BR should usually be preceded by conduction studies of the facial nerve to ensure normality of the peripheral motor pathways. Facial nerve conduction studies are done by stimulating VII either at the stylomastoid foramen or just anterior to the tragus, recording from the orbicularis oculi or the nasalis. It is frequently difficult to obtain a clean initial negative M wave deflection because of uncertainty about the motor points of facial muscles. Volume conducted potentials from inadvertent stimulation of the masseter muscle can be mistaken for a facial muscle response. Close inspection and palpation of the face and jaw during stimulation helps avoid this trap. Normal facial nerve onset latency with stimulation anterior to the tragus is <4.2 ms. Side-to-side amplitude difference should not exceed 20%.

Once facial nerve conduction studies establish the normality of the peripheral VII component, the BR is elicited using the same recording site while stimulating the supraorbital nerve both ipsilaterally and contralaterally. The gain is usually increased to 200–500 μV per division and the sweep slowed to 5 or 10 ms/division. The normal BR consists of an early ipsilateral response, the R_1, with a latency of 10–13 ms and a late bilateral response, the R_2, with a latency of 30–41 ms ipsilaterally and 30–44 ms contralaterally (Fig. 9.1). The side-to-side difference should be <1.2 ms for R_1 and <8.0 ms for R_2 (1). It is helpful in interpretation to have a specially designed worksheet to keep track of the results of BR studies (Fig. 9.2).

The impulses that elicit R_1 travel into the brain stem via V_1 and make oligosynaptic connections in the pons

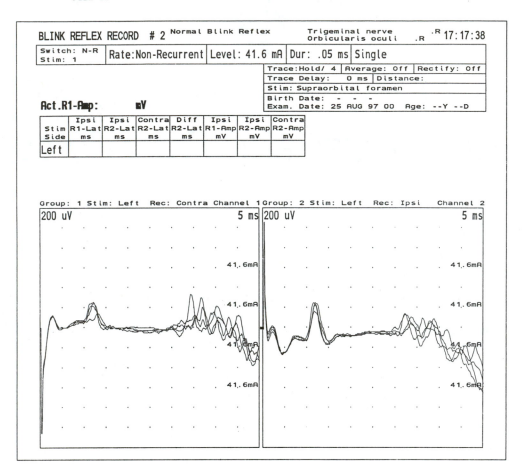

FIGURE 9.1. Blink reflexes, with superimposition of four sweeps. The sweeps on the right were recorded from stimulation of the left supraorbital nerve and recording from the left nasalis. The R_1 response has a latency of 10 ms and the R_2 a latency of 28 ms. The sweeps on the left demonstrate an R_2 recorded from the right nasalis on stimulation of the left supraorbital nerve with a latency of 30 ms. The initial peak shown in the sweeps on the left is a "contralateral R_1" deliberately produced by rotating the anode medially; the initial portion of the sweep with contralateral recording is ordinarily flat.

with VII, generating reflex activation of facial muscles. R_1 is orthodromic sensory and orthodromic motor, with oligosynaptic central connections, analogous to the H reflex. The impulses that elicit R_2 travel into the brain stem via V_1, then ramify along complex polysynaptic pathways to make eventual connections with VII bilaterally. Impulse traffic mediating R_2 may descend far caudally into the brain stem along the spinal tract of V. R_2 is associated with the visible contraction of the orbicularis oculi and corresponds to the clinically observed blink. The latency of R_2 varies, and the response shows habituation. The R_1 latency is minimally variable and it shows less habituation. As with late responses, irregular stimulation at a slow rate mini-mizes habituation and variability; rates >0.2 Hz should be avoided. In about 10% of normals, an R_1 may appear on contralateral stimulation (Fig. 9.1). In some such instances, rotation of the anode too far medially has inadvertently elicited an R_1 response on the opposite side, in effect eliciting bilateral simultaneous BRs. However, there is an increased incidence of a true contralateral R_1 in some conditions.

The BR is potentially useful in a number of clinical situations: unilateral disease of V or VII, intrinsic brain stem disease, cerebellopontine angle lesions, multiple sclerosis, and evaluation of the patient in coma. BRs may be markedly delayed in patients with either hereditary or acquired demyelinating neuropathies, but are usually normal in patients with axonopathies. BRs may also be useful in the evaluation of aberrant regeneration following Bell's palsy and in hemifacial spasm (2).

The pattern of BR abnormality may permit a localizing diagnosis. Absence of R_1 and ipsilateral R_2 with an intact contralateral R_2 suggests an ipsilateral VII lesion. Absence of both R_1 and R_2 on the same side with an intact R_2 on that side after contralateral stimulation suggests a lesion of V on the side of BR absence. Delay of R_2 bilaterally with normal R_1 responses suggests intrinsic brain stem pathology below the level of the pons.

Repetitive Nerve Stimulation (RNS) Studies

RNS consists of delivering a train of stimuli at a given frequency to a nerve, while recording the M wave from a muscle innervated by that nerve (Fig. 9.3). The stimulus train may be of various lengths and various frequencies. The responses of the M wave provide information about the integrity of the peripheral nerve, neuromuscular junction (NMJ), and muscle fiber (3,4).

RNS studies are used primarily to investigate disordered neuromuscular transmission (NMT). The physi-

BLINK REFLEX WORKSHEET

Date _____ Name _____ SS# _____

Age ____ dx. _____ EMG# _____ Ward _____

Ht. ____ Wt. _____ Code _____

FIGURE 9.2. A worksheet that tracks the results and aids in the interpretation of blink reflexes.

FACIAL NERVE STUDY

Stimulate	Record	Lat. (nl < 4.0)	Amplitude
Right Facial n	Nasalis		
Left Facial n	Nasalis		

BLINK STUDIES

Supraorbital nerve	Record right	Record left
Stimulate right	R1(ipsi) =	
	R2(ipsi) =	R2(contra) =
Stimulate left		R1(ipsi) =
	R2(contra) =	R2(ipsi) =

SUMMARY:

IMPRESSION:

CODE:

Electromyographer

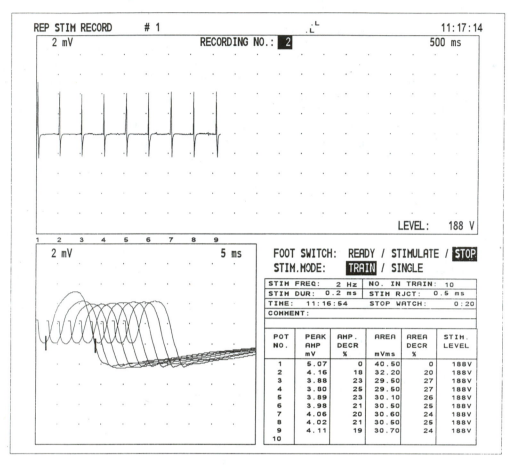

```
Nicolet Viking IV                    Nicolet Biomedical
FILE ID: 6483010        4.1.0       25 SEP 97  11:17
```

REP STIM RECORD   # 1   11:17:14
2 mV   RECORDING NO.: 2   500 ms

LEVEL: 188 V

2 mV   5 ms

FOOT SWITCH: READY / STIMULATE / STOP
STIM.MODE: TRAIN / SINGLE

STIM FREQ:	2 Hz	NO. IN TRAIN: 10
STIM DUR:	0.2 ms	STIM RJCT:	0.5 ms
TIME:	11:16:54	STOP WATCH:	0:20
COMMENT:		

POT NO.	PEAK AMP mV	AMP. DECR %	AREA mVms	AREA DECR %	STIM. LEVEL
1	5.07	0	40.50	0	188V
2	4.16	18	32.20	20	188V
3	3.88	23	29.50	27	188V
4	3.80	25	29.50	27	188V
5	3.89	23	30.10	26	188V
6	3.98	21	30.50	25	188V
7	4.06	20	30.60	24	188V
8	4.02	21	30.50	25	188V
9	4.11	19	30.70	24	188V
10					

FIGURE 9.3. Repetitive nerve stimulation of the left spinal accessory nerve recording from the trapezius muscle in a patient with myasthenia gravis. A train of 10 stimuli was delivered at a frequency of 2 Hz. There is a marked decre-ment of both amplitude and area which reaches a maximum at the fourth stimulus, after which it remains relatively stable.

ological, technical, and clinical details of NMT studies are discussed in detail in Chapter 18. In brief, pre-synaptic and post-synaptic NMT disorders produce different patterns of abnormality on RNS. The primary pre-synaptic disorders of concern are Lambert-Eaton myasthenic syndrome (LEMS), hypermagnese-mia, and botulism. The only post-synaptic disorder of any significance is myasthenia gravis (MG). Pre-synaptic disorders tend to have a low baseline M wave amplitude to single shock, as opposed to MG where it is normal. Both pre-synaptic and post-synaptic disorders produce a decrement on repetitive stimulation at 2–3 Hz. This is the stimulation frequency at which NMT is physiologically most tenuous, and where the safety factor for NMT is lowest. Artifact and technical pitfalls abound in RNS studies, and careful attention

must be paid to procedural detail. A reproducible decrement in excess of 10% is considered abnormal. In MG, a demonstrable decrement is most likely to be present in warm, proximal, and clinically involved muscles. In pre-synaptic disorders, the transmission disturbance is more widespread and may be demonstrable in distal muscles.

In MG, brief isometric exercise repairs the decrement and is followed 2–5 minutes later by an increase in the decrement due to post-activation exhaustion. In pre-synaptic disorders, brief isometric exercise not only repairs the decrement but produces marked facilitation with an increase in the low amplitude baseline M wave amplitude by a factor of 2–10.

Abnormal responses to RNS have been found in a number of conditions other than NMT disorders. In

TABLE 9.1
Causes of an Abnormal Response to Repetitive Nerve Stimulation

Primary disorders of neuromuscular transmission
  Myasthenia gravis
  Lambert-Eaton myasthenic syndrome
  Botulism
  Hypermagnesemia
  Drugs
  Toxins
Probable secondary disorders of neuromuscular transmission
  Amyotrophic lateral sclerosis
  Inflammatory myopathy
  Peripheral neuropathy
Primary disorders of muscle or the muscle membrane; channelopathies
  McArdle's disease and variants
  Myotonia congenita

some of these, the abnormal response to RNS is likely due to secondary changes in the neuromuscular junction due to axonal damage. In other instances, the abnormal response is due to pathology involving the muscle membrane or muscle fiber. The conditions causing abnormal responses to RNS are summarized in Table 9.1. Details regarding the patterns of abnormal response are provided in Part II.

Proximal Nerve Stimulation Techniques

Some proximal and relatively inaccessible nerves can be studied after a fashion using proximal stimulation. This includes stimulation of nerve roots, the brachial plexus and the lumbosacral plexus. Components of the brachial plexus can be stimulated in the supraclavicular fossa at Erb's point, located at about the junction of the clavicle and the posterior border of the clavicular head of the sternocleidomastoid muscle. Nerves are stimulated at Erb's point and the M wave recorded from the target muscle, comparing the M wave latency, amplitude and configuration with reference values (5,6). Because only a single site of stimulation is used, no CV data is obtainable. Similarly, the lumbosacral plexus may be stimulated directly with a monopolar needle electrode 3 cm lateral to the caudal margin of L_5. Nerves that arise directly from the plexus are evaluated in this manner. Proximal stimulation can also be done to evaluate the phrenic, femoral,

lateral femoral cutaneous and others, as summarized in Table 9.2. Rarely, stimulation at Erb's point provides additional useful information in the evaluation of the median, ulnar or radial nerves. Techniques have been described for stimulation of cervical and lumbosacral nerve roots by the placement of a deep stimulating needle electrode (7,8). The utility of many proximal stimulation techniques is not universally accepted.

Short Segment Studies

The experimental error inherent in NCV determinations primarily results from variability in measuring latency and distance. Maynard and Stolov examined the experimental error in NCV determinations using sophisticated mathematics (9). They were attempting to construct error curves, which related the experimental error to the CV and the distance, to better define the limits of reliability of NCV determinations. From this paper evolved the traditional teaching that distances less than 10 cm not be employed for NCV determinations because of an excessive amount of experimental error—the "10 cm rule." Electrodiagnostic medicine practice commonly requires the detection of focal nerve pathology, and in some instances precise localization of the pathology. Unfortunately, as increasing conduction distance lowers experimental error and avoids inadvertent overdiagnosis, it also decreases the likelihood of detecting a focal lesion. The abnormality present is masked by the adjacent normally conducting segments which raise the average NCV through the studied segment. Experimental error and sensitivity for lesion detection are reciprocally

TABLE 9.2
Nerves Evaluated with Proximal Stimulation Techniques

Stimulate	Record
Long thoracic	Serratus anterior
Phrenic	Diaphragm
Spinal accessory	Trapezius
Dorsal scapular	Rhomboids
Suprascapular	Supraspinatus or infraspinatus
Axillary	Deltoid
Thoracodorsal	Latissimus dorsi
Musculocutaneous	Biceps
Femoral	Quadriceps
Sciatic	Foot muscle

related. So, *pari passu* with low experimental error comes underdiagnosis.

Very short nerve segments have been studied reliably and successfully, both percutaneously and intraoperatively (10–12). Kimura advocated short segment studies to localize conduction abnormalities in carpal tunnel syndrome, commenting that "a large per-unit increase in latency more than compensates for the inherent measurement error associated with multiple stimulation in short increments" (13).

There are two types of short segment studies. Inching, strictly defined, refers to the technique of moving the stimulator along the nerve in sequential steps in search of points of abrupt change in M wave amplitude or configuration indicative of conduction block or differential slowing due to underlying focal demyelination. It does not necessarily include measurement of latency changes over consecutive segments, or precise measurement of segment lengths. The other type of short segment study includes measuring both latency and amplitude changes over precisely measured segments of 5 to 20 mm. This latter, more quantitative type of inching study is sometimes referred to as a short segment incremental study (SSIS). Inching technique that evaluates only amplitude and configuration changes is useful only when conduction block or differential slowing is present, and conduction block occurs in a minority of chronically compressed or entrapped nerves. If the predominant pathophysiology is focal slowing, conventional inching may fail to detect the lesion. Remyelination with short internodes may adequately eliminate significant degrees of conduction block, leaving only a "footprint" of focal slowing to mark the site of injury.

Short segment techniques have been described for the median nerve at the carpal tunnel, ulnar nerve at the elbow and peroneal nerve at the fibular head (11–14). The pros and cons of short segment vs. traditional studies have recently been debated (15).

Autonomic Function Testing

Dysfunction of the autonomic nervous system can be a feature of numerous neurologic conditions, including multi-system atrophy, primary autonomic failure, degenerative disorders, and particularly peripheral neuropathies of many different types. Many different procedures have been developed to test the sympathetic and parasympathetic nervous systems. These have been recently reviewed from a clinical neurophysiology and electrodiagnostic medicine aspect (16). Tests can be broadly grouped into those which address cardiovascular autonomic function, thermoregulatory

function, and miscellaneous tests. An approximation of an EKG tracing adequate for assessing changes in heart rate can be done on an EMG machine by placing the active and reference leads on the precordium, using a low frequency filter of 1–5 Hz, a high frequency filter of 500 Hz, and a very slow sweep speed.

Assessments of orthostatic changes in blood pressure and heart rate are basic tests of cardiovascular autonomic function. The expiratory to inspiratory ratio quantitates the variability in heart rate on deep breathing. The Valsalva ratio is the ratio of the longest R-R interval during phase IV of the Valsalva maneuver to the shortest R-R interval during phase II. The sustained hand grip, mental stress, and cold pressor tests all look for increases in blood pressure in response to peripheral vasoconstriction induced respectively by isometric hand exercise, mental arithmetic, or immersion of the hand in cold water.

The sympathetic skin response (SSR) is used to assess peripheral sympathetic function by detecting changes in skin resistance in response to sudomotor discharges. The SSR is mediated by slowly conducting, unmyelinated C fibers, and is a low frequency, slowly evolving response. It occurs several seconds after the invoking stimulus. A low frequency filter in the range of 0.1–0.5 Hz, a high frequency filter of 500–1,000 Hz, a gain of 0.5–3.0 mV, and a very slow sweep speed are used. The active electrode is placed on either the palm or the sole and the reference over the dorsum of either the hand or foot. The response is elicited by a deep breath, or by an electrical shock remote from the area of recording. The response is all or none; latency and amplitude are not assessed and the SSR is judged as either present or absent.

Other tests of sudomotor function such as the QSART (Quantitative Sudomotor Axon Reflex Test) and the thermoregulatory sweat test require special equipment not available in most laboratories.

Intraoperative Electrodiagnosis

Intraoperative neurophysiologic monitoring has grown in popularity in recent years. It serves a variety of functions, all of which have in common the theme of avoiding postoperative neurologic deficits. Monitoring is used primarily in posterior fossa, spine and peripheral nerve surgery (17,18). Preservation of cranial nerve function and avoidance of iatrogenic injury is an important issue in surgery of the posterior fossa and skull base.

Intraoperative monitoring techniques using nerve stimulation, evoked potentials, and needle electromyography have been developed to facilitate surgery on the facial, cochlear, and lower cranial nerves (19). Stimulation of the nerve helps to locate and map the nerve in relation to the tumor and can help clarify distorted anatomy. Mechanical stimulation of a nerve, such as from traction or pressure, produces neuromyotonic discharges that can be detected by a needle electrode monitoring one or more muscles innervated by the nerve at risk. Bursts of activity provoked by specific surgical maneuvers help avoid trauma to the nerve. Monitoring expedites safe and rapid identification of motor nerves during dissection and provides the surgeon with ongoing feedback regarding the status of the nerve. Sustained discharges may indicate significant neural damage. Retained ability to obtain an M wave after tumor removal provides a reasonable prognostic indicator of postoperative nerve function. Monitoring has proven especially useful in acoustic neuroma surgery. It also lessens postoperative nerve deficits, and shortens operating time. In microvascular decompression for hemifacial spasm, monitoring can facilitate identification of the offending vessels.

Monitoring is useful in spine surgery to help avoid spinal cord injury during spinal instrumentation, nerve root injury during repair of tethered cords and other dysraphic states, in resection of tumors and vascular malformations, and in selective posterior rhizotomy for relief of spasticity (20,21). Commonly used techniques include evoked potentials (both sensory and motor), nerve root stimulation and recording, and needle EMG.

Peripheral nerve monitoring is used to help guide the surgeon in determining the precise site of pathology and in detecting neuromyotonic discharges that may signal impending damage during nerve manipulation. Any peripheral nerve can be monitored, but the greatest experience has been with the ulnar nerve at the elbow. Intraoperative electroneurography can assist in making the decision whether to perform a simple release or transposition procedure (17,22).

Evaluation of the Respiratory System

Evaluation of patients with failure to wean from the ventilator using clinical neurophysiologic methods is increasingly common. Although CNS and systemic cardiopulmonary dysfunction is the underlying etiology in many patients, a surprising number prove to have some neuromuscular disorder, such as amyotrophic lateral sclerosis, critical illness polyneuropathy,

Guillain-Barré syndrome, unilateral or bilateral phrenic nerve palsy, a neuromuscular transmission disorder, a primary myopathy, or an abnormality of central drive (23). Electrophysiological methods available for evaluation of the respiratory system include phrenic nerve conduction studies and needle electromyography of the limbs, chest wall, and diaphragm (24,25).

Special Needle Electrode Examination Methods

Single fiber EMG (SFEMG) employs a special needle with a very small recording surface and a 500 Hz low frequency filter. The main spike of the MUAP as recorded with a standard CNE or MNE is made up of the potentials from 10–15 muscle fibers. In SFEMG, the small recording surface and elevated LFF eliminate activity from all but a tiny circumscribed area, allowing the detection of the action potentials from 1–4 fibers belonging to the same motor unit. SFEMG techniques examine the time relationship between the discharges of the fibers. SFEMG is used primarily in the evaluation of neuromuscular transmission disorders, and is discussed in more detail in Chapter 18.

Quantitative EMG (QEMG) is a method for quantitating the durations of MUAPs by analyzing a number of MUAPs isolated with a trigger and delay line (26). It is primarily used when the routine needle examination suggests but does not clearly define an abnormality, such as in a minimal myopathy. The duration of a MUAP is its most robust and stable parameter, whereas amplitude is dependent on other factors, most prominently needle position. QEMG is performed by isolating MUAPs with a short rise time, using some method to capture the waveform, and measuring the duration of the unit from the initial departure to the final return to the baseline. The mean duration of 20 MUAPs is then compared to reference values for that particular muscle in a patient of that age. Reference values usually employed are those of Buchthal and colleagues, which have been reproduced a number of times and are readily available (6). Some have suggested an even larger sample size so as to avoid spurious increases in the mean duration by the inclusion of polyphasic units (27).

QEMG is tedious and time consuming and is not used routinely. One study looked at the question of sample size and compared the feasibility of analyzing only 5 MUAPs rather than the usual 20 (28). The diagnostic utility was significantly degraded with the smaller sample. Automated methods have been developed to ease the chore of analysis, but are obviously of no help in locating and capturing the MUAPs (29). Decomposition methods that can extract individual MUAPs from an interference pattern are promising but not widely available (30). Analysis of outlier potentials may provide equivalent sensitivity with less effort than calculation of mean durations (31).

Turns-amplitude analysis evaluates the overall amplitude of an envelope of active MUAPs and compares it to the number of turns that occur during the same time interval. Small, polyphasic units in myopathies would be expected to have a high number of turns in relation to amplitude, while large neuropathic units would have a low number of turns in relation to amplitude (32). Such programs are featured on some top line EMG machines.

Macro EMG provides a panoramic view of a motor unit by using the cannula of a needle electrode to capture a large number of muscle fiber potentials, rather than the handful recorded with the ordinary CNE or MNE. The needle is inserted perpendicular to the muscle so as to capture the potentials from all or most of the fibers in the unit. A single-fiber port is used to trigger from one fiber of the MUAP, as the cannula records the potentials of all the fibers that are firing in a time-locked relationship to the triggering fiber. The macro area, amplitude, and duration are compared with reference values. Electrodes have been developed that combine macro and concentric recording surfaces (33).

Scanning EMG is similar to macro EMG and employs a single fiber electrode to detect muscle fibers firing in time-locked synchrony, with a standard CNE inserted nearby. An apparatus slowly withdraws the CNE from the muscle, pausing to sample the fibers of the motor unit at a number of discrete locations along a sampling corridor (34). The technique produces a series of rastered sweeps that provide a topographic map of the motor unit's territory. Scanning EMG helps characterize the changes in motor unit architecture that occur in neuromuscular disease.

Key Points

- The blink reflex (BR) evaluates the trigeminal and facial nerves by recording from the orbicularis oculi or nasalis muscle after stimulation of the supraorbital nerve ipsilaterally and contralaterally. Elicitation of the BR should usually be preceded by conduction studies of the facial nerve to ensure normality of the peripheral motor pathways. The normal BR consists of an early ipsilateral R_1 response, with a latency of 10–13 ms and a late bilateral R_2 response, with a latency of 30–41 ms ipsilaterally and 30–44 ms contralaterally.

- Impulses that elicit R_1 travel into the brain stem via V_1 and make oligosynaptic connections in the pons with VII, generating reflex activation of facial muscles. Impulses that elicit R_2 travel into the brain stem via V_1, then ramify along complex polysynaptic pathways to make eventual connections with VII bilaterally. Impulse traffic mediating R_2 may descend far caudally into the brain stem. The BR is potentially useful in a number of clinical situations, and the pattern of BR abnormality may permit a localizing diagnosis.

- RNS consists of delivering a train of stimuli at a given frequency to a nerve, while recording the M wave from a muscle innervated by that nerve. The responses of the M wave provide information about the integrity of the peripheral nerve, neuromuscular junction (NMJ), and muscle fiber.

- RNS studies are used primarily to investigate disordered neuromuscular transmission. Pre-synaptic and post-synaptic NMT disorders produce different patterns of abnormality. Pre-synaptic disorders tend to have a low baseline M wave amplitude to single shock, as opposed to post-synaptic disorders where it is normal.

- Both pre-synaptic and post-synaptic disorders produce a decrement on repetitive stimulation at 2–3 Hz. This is the stimulation frequency at which NMT is physiologically most tenuous. In MG, brief isometric exercise repairs the decrement. In pre-synaptic disorders, brief isometric exercise not only repairs the decrement but produces marked facilitation.

- Abnormal responses to RNS can occur in a number of conditions other than NMT disorders.

- Some proximal and relatively inaccessible nerves can be studied after a fashion using proximal stimulation. This includes stimulation of nerve roots, the brachial plexus, and the lumbosacral plexus. For study of nerves arising from the brachial plexus, stimuli are delivered at Erb's point while recording the M wave from the target muscle. The lumbosacral plexus may be stimulated directly with a monopolar needle electrode. Techniques have been described for stimulation of cervical and lumbosacral nerve roots.

- The experimental error inherent in NCV determinations decreases as studies are carried out over longer distances, and the "10 cm rule" holds that conduction studies should not be done over a shorter distance because of unacceptable high experimental error. Unfortunately, experimental error and sensitivity for lesion detection are reciprocally related. Very short nerve segments, 0.5–2.0 cm, have been studied reliably and successfully, both percutaneously and intraoperatively and can often help in the evaluation of focal neuropathies. Short segment techniques have been described for the median nerve at the carpal tunnel, ulnar nerve at the elbow and peroneal nerve at the fibular head.

- Dysfunction of the autonomic nervous system can be a feature of numerous neurologic conditions, including multi-system atrophy, primary autonomic failure, degenerative disorders, and peripheral neuropathies. Autonomic function tests include those which evaluate cardiovascular autonomic function, thermoregulatory function, and miscellaneous procedures.

- Intraoperative neurophysiologic monitoring serves a variety of functions, all of which have in common the theme of avoiding postoperative neurologic deficits. Monitoring is used primarily in posterior fossa, spine, and peripheral nerve surgery. Intraoperative monitoring techniques using nerve stimulation, evoked potentials, and needle electromyography have been developed. Monitoring has proven especially useful in acoustic neuroma surgery.

- Special needle electrode examination procedures include single fiber (SFEMG), quantitative (QEMG), macro and scanning EMG. SFEMG is used primarily in the evaluation of neuromuscular transmission disorders. QEMG is a method for quantitating the durations of MUAPs when the routine needle examination suggests but does not clearly define an abnormality. The mean duration of 20 MUAPs is compared to reference values. Macro and scanning EMG provide a panoramic overview of the motor unit and help to characterize the changes in motor unit architecture that occur in neuromuscular disease

References

1. Stevens JC, Smith BE. Cranial reflexes. In: Daube JR, ed. Clinical neurophysiology. Philadelphia: F.A. Davis, Co. 1996;321–335.

2. Harper CM, Jr. AAEM case report #21: hemifacial spasm: preoperative diagnosis and intraoperative management. Muscle Nerve 1991;14:213–218.
   Hemifacial spasm (HFS) may result from chronic compression of, or injury to, the facial nerve. Electrodiagnostic studies can help distinguish HFS from other involuntary movements of the face. A 75-year-old man developed progressive involuntary hemifacial spasm. Electrophysiologic evidence of abnormal cross-transmission between neurons of the facial nerve was demonstrated. A synkinetic response was recorded from the left mentalis muscle with stimulation of the left supraorbital nerve. The lateral spread response (LSR) is elicitation of an M wave in a muscle innervated by the facial nerve after stimulation of a different branch of the nerve. An LSR was demonstrated in this patient by recording an M wave from the left orbicularis oculi after stimulation of the ipsilateral mandibular branch of the facial nerve. During intraoperative monitoring, the LSR disappeared after adequate microvascular decompression of the facial nerve. The synkinetic spread from one facial nerve branch to another also may occur following Bell's palsy, but has slightly different characteristics from the LSR seen in HFS.

3. Keesey JC. AAEE Minimonograph #33: electrodiagnostic approach to defects of neuromuscular transmission. Muscle Nerve 1989;12:613–626.
   See Chapter 18 for summary.

4. Sanders DB. Clinical neurophysiology of disorders of the neuromuscular junction. J Clin Neurophysiol 1993;10:167–180.
   See Chapter 18 for summary.

5. DeLisa JA, Mackenzie K, Baran EM. Manual of nerve conduction velocity and clinical neurophysiology. 3rd ed. New York: Raven Press, 1994.

6. Liveson JA, Ma DM. Laboratory reference for clinical neurophysiology. Philadelphia: F.A. Davis Co. 1992;408–414.

7. Tsai CP, Huang CI, Wang V, et al. Evaluation of cervical radiculopathy by cervical root stimulation. Electromyogr Clin Neurophysiol 1994;34:363–366.
   Cervical root stimulation (CRS), conventional electromyographic (EMG) studies, nerve conduction velocity studies and F responses were compared in 32 patients with clinical symptoms and signs of cervical radiculopathy. While performing CRS, a monopolar needle was inserted into the paraspinal muscles, and the compound muscle action potentials in the biceps, triceps and abductor digiti minimi muscles were recorded. Conventional EMG was abnormal in 18 (56.2%), whereas CRS was abnormal in 25 (78.1%).

8. Ertekin C, Sirin H, Koyuncuoglu HR, et al. Diagnostic value of electrical stimulation of lumbosacral roots in radiculopathies. Acta Neurol Scand 1994;90:26–33.
   Needle electrical stimulation of the lumbosacral roots at the laminar level of the T12-L1 or L1–2 intervertebral spaces was performed in 24 normal subjects and 58 patients with lumbar radiculopathy. The root stimulation method was compared with conventional needle EMG. Lumber electrical stimulation showed root abnormalities objectively in 80% of patients while the diagnostic value of needle EMG was 65%.

9. Maynard FM, Stolov WC. Experimental error in determination of nerve conduction velocity. Arch Phys Med Rehabil 1972;53:362–372.
   See Chapter 10 for summary.

10. Brown WF, Yates SK. Percutaneous localization of conduction abnormalities in human entrapment neuropathies. Can J Neurol Sci 1982;9:391–400.
    In entrapment neuropathies the characteristic abnormalities in conduction are frequently limited to a short segment of the nerve. Recognition and precise localization of these discrete conduction abnormalities may require measurement of conduction over shorter lengths of the nerves than those lengths commonly employed in the clinical laboratory. Techniques are described for the more precise location of the primary conduction abnormalities in median, ulnar and peroneal nerve entrapments. Distinctive or atypical locations of the major conduction abnormalities may point towards different mechanisms in the pathogenesis of these localized neuropathies.

11. Campbell WW, Pridgeon RM, Sahni KS. Short segment incremental studies in the evaluation of ulnar neuropathy at the elbow. Muscle Nerve 1992;15:1050–1054.
    See Chapter 17 for summary.

12. Kanakamedala RV, Simons DG, Porter RW, et al. Ulnar nerve entrapment at the elbow localized by short segment stimulation. Arch Phys Med Rehab 1988;69:959–963.
    The ulnar nerve was studied at 2-cm intervals across the elbow in 20 normal adults and in 13 patients with suspected ulnar neuropathy at the elbow. The maximum conduction time across a 2-cm segment 0.63 ms on the right side and 0.60 ms (mean +2SD) on the left. The authors conclude that short segment stimulation of the ulnar nerve at the elbow is useful in localizing the exact site of entrapment/compression.

13. Kimura J. The carpal tunnel syndrome: localization of conduction abnormalities within the distal segment of the median nerve. Brain 1979;102:619–635.
See Chapter 17 for summary.

14. Kanakamedala RV, Hong CZ. Peroneal nerve entrapment at the knee localized by short segment stimulation. Am J Phys Med Rehabil 1989;68:116–122.
This study evaluated the usefulness of short segment stimulation (SSS) of the peroneal nerve at the knee in 18 patients with suspected peroneal nerve palsy and 28 controls. CMAPs were obtained from the extensor digitorum brevis muscle after successive supramaximal stimuli of the nerve at 2 cm intervals, starting 4 cm distal (D4 and D2) and ending 6 cm proximal (P2, P4, and P6) to the fibular head prominence (P). Fourteen patients showed statistically significant reduction in amplitude and prolongation of conduction time in one or more short segments. Three patients had prolongation of conduction time only and one patient had reduction in amplitude only. When nerve conduction of the entire 10-cm segment across the knee was tested by the conventional method, only nine showed reduction in amplitude from proximal stimulation, or slowing of motor conduction velocity across the 10-cm segment or both. The authors conclude that the SSS technique is a sensitive and reliable procedure for the detection of mild compression or entrapment of the peroneal nerve around the knee.

15. Campbell WW, Geiringer SR. The value of inching techniques in the diagnosis of focal nerve lesions. Muscle Nerve, in press.
A debate on the utility of short segment studies in the evaluation and management of focal neuropathies. Experimental error in NCV determination decreases with increasing nerve segment length, but sensitivity for focal lesion detection decreases simultaneously. Following Maynard and Stolov, most investigators and clinicians adopted a minimum 10 cm distance for studying the ulnar nerve at the elbow and the peroneal nerve at the fibular head. Maynard and Stolov found the latency measurement error made a much greater contribution to the total error than did the distance measurement error. Of the relatively small contribution of distance measurement error to total experimental error, most was due to skin movement errors rather than tape measure reading errors. Though the authors did not address this aspect, it is intuitively obvious that skin movement is more of a problem over long distances than over short distances. Modern techniques have presumably increased the accuracy of latency determinations considerably. When conduction block or differential slowing is present, the localization of a focal neuropathy is straightforward. The precise site of the pathologic process is betrayed by a loss of amplitude or change in waveform configuration between two stimulation sites. The process of remyelination with shorter and therefore more slowly conducting internodes, may relieve conduction block but leave persistent focal slowing. In the chronically compressed nerve, the most likely focal abnormality is therefore restricted slowing across the lesion, unaccompanied by loss of amplitude or major changes in waveform configuration. Methods of localization which depend on changes in waveform amplitude or configuration will unfortunately fail in the majority of cases. Short segment incremental studies can frequently help resolve clinical issues related to focal mononeuropathies.

16. Ravits JM. AAEM minimonograph #48: autonomic nervous system testing. Muscle Nerve 1997;20:919–937.
Testing and quantifying autonomic nervous system function is an important but difficult area of clinical neurophysiology. Tests of parasympathetic cardiovagal regulation include heart rate analysis during standing (the 30 : 15 ratio), heart rate variation with deep breathing, and the Valsalva ratio. Tests of sympathetic adrenergic vascular regulation include blood pressure analysis while standing, the Valsalva maneuver, sustained handgrip, mental stress, and cold water immersion. Tests of sympathetic cholinergic sudomotor function include the sympathetic skin response, quantitative sudomotor axon reflex test, sweat box testing, and quantification of sweat imprints. The available tests have various sensitivities and ease of administration. They are typically administered in a battery of multiple tests, which improves sensitivity and reliability, and allows probing of various autonomic functions. See also: Toyokura M, Murakami K. Reproducibility of sympathetic skin response. Muscle Nerve 1996;19:1481–1483.

17. Brown WF, Veitch J. AAEM minimonograph #42: intraoperative monitoring of peripheral and cranial nerves. Muscle Nerve 1994;17:371–377.
Intraoperative studies of focal neuropathies have become increasingly common both as an aid to the localization of the neuropathy and a means of monitoring the integrity of the nerve in the course of surgery. Success very often depends on careful attention to the technical problems presented by working in the operating theater. Despite these difficulties, assessment of conduction directly from the exposed nerve offers opportunities for better understanding the pathophysiology of these neuropathies and correlating these findings with conventional electrodiagnostic studies. See also: Nelson KR, Phillips LH. Neurophysiologic monitoring during surgery of peripheral and cranial nerves, and in selective dorsal rhizotomy. Semin Neurol 1990;10:141–149.

18. Prass RL. Iatrogenic facial nerve injury: the role of facial nerve monitoring. Otolaryngol Clin North Am 1996;29:265–275.
Intraoperative facial nerve monitoring has emerged as a powerful tool for facilitation of surgery involving the facial nerve. This tool must be properly applied and maintained, however, in order to avoid untoward results and to maximize its potential benefits. Facial nerve monitoring is best suited for prevention of iatrogenic injury. Once injury has become established, its value may be severely limited, especially for moderate to severe injury, in which visual assessment of injury is still the most effective means to determine the need for repair. The most valuable derivative of facial nerve monitoring is enhanced awareness of the edge of the facial nerve contour. This allows strategic alterations in surgical technique for improved facial nerve functional preservation. Although facial nerve monitoring appears to have already had a favorable influence on facial nerve preservation, further improvement seems likely over time through an ongoing process of trial and error.

19. Cheek JC. Posterior fossa intraoperative monitoring. J Clin Neurophysiol 1993;10:412–424.
Monitoring of brainstem structures is requested of the neurophysiologist for both intra-axial and extra-axial surgeries of the posterior fossa. A variety of techniques to include upper extremities somatosensory evoked potentials, short latency auditory evoked potentials, spontaneous and evoked electromyographic activity, and recordings from the cochlea and the eighth nerve are available. The indication, implementation, interpretation, efficacy and utility of these techniques is reviewed.

20. Staudt LA, Nuwer MR, Peacock WJ. Intraoperative monitoring during selective posterior rhizotomy: technique and patient outcome. Electroencephal Clin Neurophysiol 1995;97:296–309.

A study of intraoperative EMG results in patients with spastic cerebral palsy who underwent selective posterior rhizotomy. Intraoperative EMG monitoring techniques have been adopted at many centers but with variations in specific methods. Controversy has arisen about the usefulness of intraoperative monitoring. The authors describe the details of their methods for nerve rootlet testing and selection.

21. Herdmann J, Deletis V, Edmonds HL, Jr., et al. Spinal cord and nerve root monitoring in spine surgery and related procedures. Spine 1996;21:879–885.

Intraoperative neurophysiologic monitoring research has been directed at finding reliable stimulating and recording techniques and adequate anesthetic regimens applicable to spinal procedures. The aim is a comprehensive monitoring not only of afferent and efferent spinal cord pathways but also of sensory and motor nerve roots and cauda equina fibers. Conventional somatosensory evoked potentials (SEPs) are complemented by motor evoked potentials, dermatomal sensory evoked potentials, spinal cord evoked potentials, evoked electromyography, sensory and motor fiber mapping of the cauda equina, bulbocavernosus reflex testing, and neurogenic evoked potentials. This article describes the essentials of these techniques, their indications and limitations, and the influence of anesthetic management on the production and interpretation of evoked potentials.

22. Campbell WW, Sahni SK, Pridgeon RM, et al. Intraoperative electroneurography: management of ulnar neuropathy at the elbow. Muscle Nerve 1988;11:75–81.

23. Bolton CF. AAEM minimonograph #40: clinical neurophysiology of the respiratory system. Muscle Nerve 1993;16:809–818.

Disorders of nerve and muscle are frequent causes of respiratory insufficiency, but current methods often fail to adequately assess the problem. Phrenic nerve conduction and needle electromyography of the diaphragm are of great assistance in identifying the nature and site of the disorder: the various disturbances of central drive, axonal or demyelinating neuropathies of the phrenic nerves, and certain myopathies. These studies may be performed on adults, children, or infants, and in outpatient, general ward, or critical care settings.

24. Bolton CF, Grand'Maison F, Parkes A, et al. Needle electromyography of the diaphragm. Muscle Nerve 1992;15:678–681.

A method is described for performing needle electromyography of the diaphragm which is safe and causes little discomfort. It provides valuable information concerning neuropathies and myopathies which may affect the diaphragm, and complements information derived from phrenic nerve conduction studies. Firing patterns of motor unit potentials during spontaneous respiration identify upper motor neuron disorders causing respiratory insufficiency.

25. Swenson MR, Rubenstein RS. Phrenic nerve conduction studies. Muscle Nerve 1992;15:597–603.

An attempt to refine the technique of phrenic nerve conduction by studying electrode positioning and sources of chest wall artifact. Diaphragmatic compound motor action potentials (DCMAPs) were mapped at close intervals over 4 hemithoraces of two subjects, finding optimum recording sites which were then used to quantitate artifacts due to EKG, chest wall EMG, and configurational thoracic changes of respiration. Based on these findings, 20 normal subjects were studied, showing ease of application and good side-to-side agreement for DCMAP latencies; but, in contrast to prior reports, right-to-left correlation for amplitude and waveform was poor, making the unaffected side an unreliable standard in unilateral partial phrenic nerve lesions.

26. Stalberg E, Nandedkar SD, Sanders DB, et al. Quantitative motor unit potential analysis. J Clin Neurophysiol 1996;13:401–422.

A review of quantitative methods for electromyography, providing background information about motor unit anatomy, physiology, and pathology to explain some of the electrophysiological phenomena. Different aspects of quantitation, such as motor unit action potential parameters, automatic analysis methods, reference values, and findings in abnormal conditions are discussed.

27. Trojaborg W. Quantitative electromyography in polymyositis: a reappraisal. Muscle Nerve 1990;13:964–971.

A study of the manual quantitative analysis of MUAPs in 33 patients with polymyositis, 16 in the acute and 17 in the chronic stage. Contrary to common description of "myopathic potentials" as being of low amplitude, short duration, and polyphasic shape, this study revealed no difference as to amplitude of short duration MUAPs in patients and normal subjects, though short-duration MUAP and short duration polyphasic potentials were 4 and 3 times, respectively, more common in patients than in controls. Although the mean duration of MUAPs usually was significantly shorter in polymyositis than in controls, the average scatter of MUAPs' duration was the same in the 2 groups. The average incidence of polyphasic MUAPs was 4 times higher in patients than in controls, as was the incidence of those of long duration. To avoid misinterpretation of EMG findings due to an excess of polyphasic MUAPs, a greater number of individual potentials than usually recommended should be collected allowing a valid estimate of the mean duration of MUAPs of simple configuration.

28. Engstrom JW, Olney RK. Quantitative motor unit analysis: the effect of sample size. Muscle Nerve 1992;15:277–281.

A study of the influence of sample size on QEMG determined MUAP tolerance limits, intertrial variability, and diagnostic sensitivity. 20 randomly selected MUAPs were recorded from the biceps muscle twice in 21 normal subjects, and once in 10 patients with myopathy. QEMG duration results supported the presence of myopathy in 2 of 10 patients with analysis of 5 MUAPs, and 9 patients with analysis of 20 MUAPs. Although analysis of 5 potentials may be adequate for diagnosis occasionally, quantitative analysis of 20 MUAPs narrows tolerance limits, reduces intertrial variability, and improves diagnostic sensitivity.

29. Dorfman LJ, McGill KC. AAEE minimonograph #29: automatic quantitative electromyography. Muscle Nerve 1988;11:804–818.

See Chapter 8 for summary.

30. Nandedkar SD, Barkhaus PE, Charles A. Multi-motor unit action potential analysis (MMA). Muscle Nerve 1995;18:1155–1166.

An algorithm, called multi-motor unit action potential analysis (MMA), was developed to aid quantification in routine needle EMG examination. In only 5–8 min, it was possible to extract, analyze, and validate 20 MUAPs. Results are compared with measurements using manual, triggered averaging, automatic decomposition, and other MMA algorithms described in the literature.

31. Stalberg E, Bischoff C, Falck B. Outliers, a way to detect abnormality in quantitative EMG. Muscle Nerve 1994; 17:392–399.

In visual analysis of MUAPs it is common to decide abnormality by a few potentials with definitely abnormal amplitude, duration, and shape. This investigation defined the limits of normal values and compared the diagnostic yield of assessing definitely abnormal outliers, with conventional mean values of MUAP parameters. MUAPs were extracted and measured with a new decomposition method. Reference values were obtained for three commonly studied muscles. Patients with various types of neuropathies and myopathies were studied with measurement of outliers and mean values. Analyses of outliers were as sensitive as determination of mean values in neuropathies and better in myopathies. Often an increased number of outliers could already be detected after only a few MUAPs had been obtained, obviating the need to obtain all 20 MUAPs. The authors conclude the outlier method is as sensitive as mean values. Because the number of MUAPs required may be reduced, the investigation takes a shorter time and is less painful for the patient. If the degree of abnormality is to be quantified, calculation of mean values is still necessary. The combination of outliers and mean values may be the optimal way to detect and express abnormality.

32. Fisher MA. Root mean square voltage/turns in chronic neuropathies is related to increase in fiber density. Muscle Nerve 1997;20:241–243.

The number of turns is a measure of the complexity of motor unit activity. The root mean square voltage is a standard measure of electrical power (see Chapters 1 and 2). A high ratio of rms voltage to turns may be a sensitive method for detecting and quantitating chronic neurogenic motor unit potential changes.

33. Jabre JF. Concentric macro electromyography. Muscle Nerve 1991;14:820–825.

Concentric EMG electrodes record from a few (10 to 15) muscle fibers of a motor unit (MU). Macro EMG is able to record from the majority of muscle fibers in the MU. The macro EMG electrode uses a single fiber action potential on one channel to trigger the time-locked cannula (macro) response on the other channel. To study the concentric motor unit action potential, alongside the macro potential, we built a needle electrode combining concentric and macro recording surfaces. The ability to study a small and a large section of the MU simultaneously offers insights into the local or global nature of MU changes not otherwise available to the electromyographer.

34. Stalberg E, Dioszeghy P. Scanning EMG in normal muscle and in neuromuscular disorders. Electroencephalogr Clin Neurophysiol 1991;81:403–416.

The spatial distribution of motor units in normal subjects and in patients with neurogenic and myogenic conditions was studied. Normal values are presented for the brachial biceps and anterior tibial muscles. Scanning EMG verified the rearrangement of muscle fibers in abnormal muscles. The most striking finding was the presence of long polyphasic sections in abnormal muscles. However, this parameter did not differentiate neurogenic from myogenic cases. The length of the motor unit cross-section did not differ significantly in the abnormal muscles compared to normal. Thus, the size of motor unit territory does not seem to be a useful parameter to detect pathology. Scanning EMG gives a new dimension to exploring the motor unit characteristics not attainable by conventional methods and provides important information toward a better understanding of concentric needle EMG. Examples are shown from healthy subjects and from patients with neuromuscular diseases.

10

Tips, Tricks, and Traps in Electrodiagnostic Medicine

Many of the principles of electrodiagnostic medicine are conceptually straightforward, but everyday practice is a constant battle against the threat of misstep. Difficulties can arise from a multitude of technical, physiologic, and anatomic factors, ranging from shock artifact to anomalous innervation to the statistical methods used to derive the reference values. Dealing with the effects of volume conduction and temperature effects are everyday problems in clinical electrodiagnosis (1,2). Kimura's classic 1984 paper reviews the pitfalls of nerve conduction studies (3). Dumitru's text nicely summarizes pitfalls in general, as well as the potential electrodiagnostic medicine consultation errors related to specific clinical problems (4). Realizing the greatest clinical utility of electrodiagnostic medicine depends not only on understanding the principles involved but also on recognizing and avoiding the traps and errors leading to misinterpretation. This chapter will review some of the more common methodologic pitfalls in electrodiagnosis. Many of the details are elaborated in Chapters 7–9.

Nerve Conduction Studies

There is an inherent variability in nerve conduction studies. In numerous studies comparing results done on the same individual at time intervals from several hours to several weeks, the coefficient of variation (the standard deviation as a percentage of the mean) for nerve conduction velocities and latencies has ranged from 2–9%, even higher for amplitudes (5). Only about half of the variation is due to true biologic variability (6). To minimize variability, avoidance of myriad technical and methodologic pitfalls is necessary. Potential sources of error in nerve conduction studies include the stimulating current, factors related to the active and recording electrodes, distance measurements, latency measurements, and failure to recognize innervation anomalies, artifacts, and other technical faults (Table 10.1).

STIMULATION PITFALLS

Conventional nerve conduction techniques presume delivery of a supramaximal cathodal stimulus to activate all the fibers in the nerve. When the stimulus is not supramaximal, the amplitude of the evoked M wave is decreased and the conduction velocity slowed. One must constantly guard against submaximal stimulation, particularly when stimulating the median nerve at the elbow, the ulnar nerve at the below elbow site or the tibial nerve at the knee. If the anode and cathode are inadvertently reversed, the distance measurement will be off by an increment equal to the stimulator's interelectrode distance. Anodal block

TABLE 10.1
Some Sources of Error in Nerve Conduction Studies

Stimulation errors
  Not located directly over nerve
  Cathode/anode reversal
  Submaximal
  Excessivly supramaximal with distal migration of the
    virtual cathode
  Spread to nearby nerves
Recording errors
Measurement errors
  Latency errors
  Amplitude errors
  Distance errors
    Skin movement
    Tape measure misreading
    Nonlinear nerve courses (radial, ulnar, peroneal, brachial plexus)
    Limb position (primarily the elbow)
      Different from that used to obtain reference
        values
      Changing during course of examination
Instrumentation errors
  Using filter, gain, or sweep settings different from
    those used to obtain reference values
  Changing gain or sweep speed between two stimulation sites along the same nerve
Physiologic variables
  Temperature
  Height
  Age
  Anomalous innervation

causing hyperpolarization between the cathode and the recording electrode is more a theoretical than practical consideration (7). The stimulus should be delivered directly over the nerve; lateral misplacement can increase the latency. A difference of up to 0.4 ms in latency can occur when the stimulus is delivered 1–5 cm perpendicular to the nerve (5). Although supramaximal stimulation is important, an excessively supramaximal stimulus introduces new possibilities for error. With increasing stimulus intensity, the effective cathode may migrate distally, spuriously shortening the latency. Supramaximal is customarily defined as 20–50% above maximal, no more. Precise control of stimulus intensity is especially important in short segment and intraoperative studies. Even reasonably supramaximal stimuli may spread to adjacent nerves and produce inadvertent, unwanted, sometimes unrecognized activation (vida infra).

Stimulus delivery always produces shock (stimulus) artifact (Fig. 10.1). Because of the amplitude discrepancy, shock artifact seldom troubles an M wave. But, large shock artifact can significantly obscure sensory potentials, especially those done over relatively short distances, such as palmar studies. Because of the short distance and relatively low amplitude, shock artifact is usually most problematic with ulnar palmar sensory potentials. The artifact occurs because some amount of current is conducted directly over the skin surface from the stimulating to the active recording electrode. This transcutaneous current flow is virtually instantaneous, far more rapid than conduction through tissue and along nerve trunks. When the surface current flow is minimized, shock artifact is usually easily controlled. When conditions favor transcutaneous spread, the shock artifact can overwhelm the nerve action potential. The most favorable conditions for trouble free recording are when the electrode impedances are low and equal, skin impedance is high and the ground is located between the stimulating and recording electrodes.

Assuming otherwise good technique, the quickest and simplest way to control shock artifact is to rotate the anode about the cathode in search of the spot at which the shock artifact changes direction; near that point the shock artifact will have its lowest amplitude (8). This works because the anode and cathode of the stimulator create a dipole with isopotential lines forming a figure 8, which radiates outward to the recording electrodes (see Chapter 4). If the active and recording electrodes lie on the same isopotential line, the stimulus artifact becomes a common mode signal and is maximally attenuated by the differential amplifier. Rotating the anode about the cathode is an empiric manipulation of the stimulator's isopotential

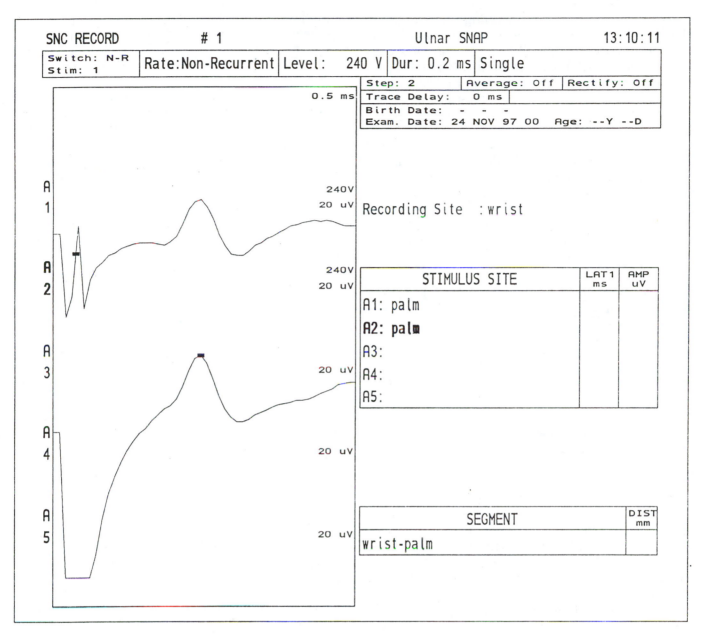

FIGURE 10.1. An ulnar palmar sensory potential, demonstrating the variability of shock artifact depending on conditions. Both SNAPS were obtained at the same distance and with the same stimulus intensity. In the top tracing, the field is dry and clean and the stimulus artifact is under reasonable control. In the bottom tracing, the exact same conditions were present, including the position of the anode, but a conductive material was smeared between the stimulating and recording electrodes. Now the shock artifact is of much larger amplitude and longer duration, interfering with the initial portion of the SNAP.

lines in hope of happening upon one which links the recording electrodes. The same effect could theoretically be achieved, with far more effort, by holding the stimulator still and rotating G_2 about G_1.

The other major source of interference in electrodiagnosis is 60 Hz AC power line artifact. This can arise from any number of sources both intrinsic and extrinsic to the equipment. Electrode wires are commonly braided, for two reasons. The spiral winding creates twin coils and takes advantage of the property of inductance. Current (emf) flowing in a wire can induce a current in an adjacent wire, the counter emf (cemf). The cemf always acts to oppose the emf that produced it (Lenz's law). The inductance of the twin coils lessens power line interference by resisting the flow of AC; the cemf in one wire counteracts the current flow in the other wire. Braiding also keeps the wires close together so that interference will impinge on each equally, maximizing common mode rejection. One can sometimes take advantage of these properties and reduce troublesome interference by creating rudimentary coils: wadding electrode wires into a loose ball, or tying wires or cables into loose knots. Interference can also come from stray capacitance and stray inductance. Stray capacitance increases as length of wire increases, so keeping wires and cables at the shortest feasible length decreases this source of interference. Some measures to minimize shock artifact, 60 Hz and other types of interference, are summarized in Table 10.2.

RECORDING ELECTRODE PLACEMENT PITFALLS: DIPS AND PSEUDODIPS

For motor nerve conduction studies, the active recording electrode must be placed directly over the motor point of the muscle to obtain a clean, initially negative deflection that reflects depolarization of the muscle end plate immediately subjacent to the electrode. As discussed in Chapter 4, an action potential propagating toward the active electrode is detected at a distance through the volume conductor and produces an initial positive deflection, followed by a negative deflection as the main wave of negativity arrives beneath the electrode. An initial positive deflection is a normal feature of a nerve action potential recorded in a good volume conductor. In motor conduction studies, however, an initial positive deflection, a "dip," signifies that the recorded depolarization has taken place remote from the electrode and is propagating toward it. The usual reason for an initial dip is that the active electrode is off the motor point, and the duration of the dip is proportional to the distance from the motor point (Fig. 10.2). When this occurs, the active electrode should be moved about over the surface to find the location that produces an initially negative deflection. When the motor point proves difficult to find, it is useful to create an insulating "handle" with which to move the electrode about rather than having to retape it at each prospective site (Fig. 10.3).

There are other reasons for a dip. If the stimulating current is too robust, an adjacent nerve may be activated which conducts more quickly than the nerve under study (Fig. 10.2). The active electrode then records the negativity at a distance from the motor point of the inadvertently stimulated nerve; G_1 is effectively off the motor point, but because of a stimulation error,

TABLE 10.2
Techniques to Minimize Shock Artifact and Other Interference

Routine measures

Keep stimulating and recording electrode impedances low and equal; if necessary abrade the skin; keep electrodes well secured (especially for repetitive stimulation studies).

Use the minimal necessary amount of electrode gel.

Keep the skin dry and free of perspiration and excessive electrode gel.

Avoid excessive stimulus intensity.

Place the ground between the stimulating and recording electrodes, keep the ground connecting wire of the shortest feasible length.

Use braided electrode wires of the shortest feasible length or shielded cables.

Attach the recording electrodes so that their wires trail away from the stimulation site, and keep the stimulator cable well separated from the recording electrode connections.

Unplug, don't merely turn off, any extraneous electrical equipment in the room.

Turn off the fluorescent lights.

Keep all electrical cables (monitor, printer, etc) tightly coiled and of the shortest possible length.

Rotate the anode.

During monopolar needle EMG keep the reference electrode near the active.

Special tactics

Bundle the electrode wires into a loose ball, and place the preamplifier as close as possible to the recording site.

Bundle the ground wire.

Use needle stimulation.

Increase the distance between G_1 and stimulating cathode—must be supported by reference values.

Desperation efforts

Tie a knot(s) in, coil, loop, and shorten the power cable.

Activate the notch filter.

Increase the LFF—will lower the amplitude of any waveform, may decrease the peak latency of a SNAP, will shorten the duration of a MUAP and may induce polyphasia.

not because of misplacement. This occurs most often when stimulating the median nerve at the wrist, especially in patients with small wrists. At maximal intensity the median is stimulated, but when the current is increased to ensure a supramaximal stimulation, it

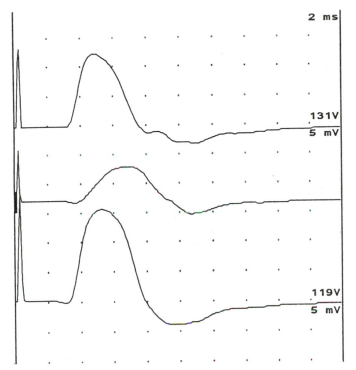

FIGURE 10.2. Recording from the APB with stimulation of the median nerve at the wrist. In the top tracing, the active electrode is in acceptable position over the motor point and there is a clean, initially negative takeoff. In the second tracing, the active electrode is off the motor point and the initial deflection is positive, a "dip." In the third tracing, the active electrode is in proper position over the APB motor point, but the stimulating current has spread to the ulnar nerve producing a dip because the active electrode detects volume conducted potentials from ulnar innervated muscles whose depolarization precedes that of the APB.

spreads medially and activates the ulnar nerve. The active electrode over the motor point of the APB then detects the volume conducted depolarization of nearby ulnar innervated muscles such as the adductor pollicis or first dorsal interosseous (FDI). The unwanted current spread can often be eliminated, while retaining the supramaximal intensity, simply by rotating the anode toward the radial aspect of the wrist. Inadvertent spread of the stimulating current to the ulnar at the wrist is one of the most common sources of error in performing nerve conduction studies. It may be particularly problematic when the median nerve is diseased, the M wave amplitude is low, and the examiner increases the stimulus intensity attempting to overcome presumed submaximal stimulation, inducing stimulus spread which activates the ulnar, causing a "normal" M wave to appear (although perhaps with an intractable dip). Thus, major median nerve pathology may be totally missed.

Unwanted spread of the stimulating current is also a common problem when studying the facial nerve, the peroneal nerve at the above fibular head site, or nerves in the upper arm, axilla or at Erb's point, and especially during intraoperative studies. During blink reflex studies, stimulus spread can occasionally evoke an ersatz contralateral R1 (see Fig. 9.1). A dip on stimulation of the median nerve at the elbow not present on stimulation at the wrist has particular significance, which is discussed in the section on anomalous innervation.

By and large, dips are bad, but not invariably. A "pseudodip" is an initially positive deflection that does not signify anything amiss. Routinely, when doing peroneal nerve motor conduction studies, a long duration, gentle positive downslope occurs prior to the M wave on proximal stimulation which is not present on distal stimulation (Fig. 10.4). The initial positivity is a normal phenomenon that occurs because the active electrode over the EDB detects the preceding volume conducted depolarization of the tibialis anterior and other foreleg muscles. The initial positivity can sometimes take on a sharper contour that can be mistaken for a real dip. However, a true, off-the-motor-point dip should be present on distal as well as proximal stimulation.

Another form of pseudodip can occur when an intramuscular nerve action potential, or premotor potential, causes a ripple in the baseline immediately

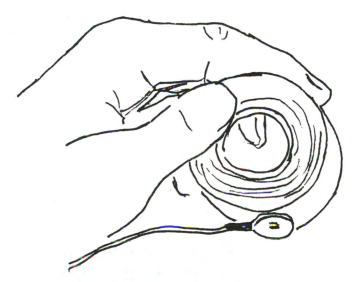

FIGURE 10.3. The sharp post on the back of the active electrode has been impaled into the edge of a roll of tape. The tape serves as an implement useful for quickly scouting for points that will produce a clean, negative deflection. Once the motor point is located, the electrode is taped in place in the usual fashion.

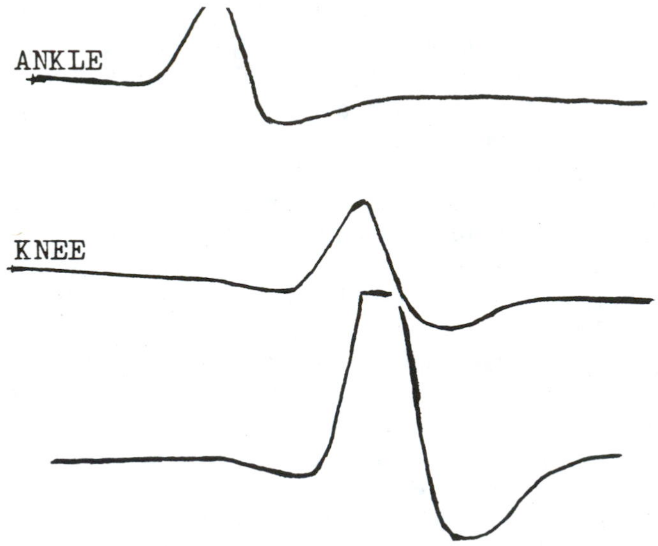

ANKLE

KNEE

FIGURE 10.4. The M wave recorded from the EDB on ankle stimulation (top tracing); there is an initial negative deflection. The M wave on knee stimulation at normal gain (middle tracing) and high gain (bottom tracing); the initial positivity is the volume-conducted potential arising from the pretibial muscles, a normal feature.

preceding the M wave (Fig. 10.5). Premotor potentials are most often seen during median conduction studies and can be recognized by increasing the gain, amplifying the initial portion of the waveform to recognize the small, negative potential that precedes the main deflection (9). Failure to recognize the presence of a premotor potential may cause taking the latency too early, at the start of the pseudodip, resulting in a falsely short distal motor latency. The initial positivity of a nerve action potential is of course a normal phenomenon and should not be mistaken for a technical error; this confusion would arise only when taking the onset latency of a nerve action potential when performing sensory nerve conduction studies.

The reference electrode, G_2, in the belly-tendon method for motor nerve conduction studies, is hypothetically located over an electrically inert distal point. However, the tendon sites are not nearly so inactive as often assumed (10,11). Moving G_2 to different locations can have a significant effect on the amplitude and configuration of the M wave (Fig. 10.6). The position of the ground electrode does not affect the waveform per se, but can influence the size of the shock artifact and the ease of recording (Fig. 10.7). The distance between G_1 and G_2 for antidromic sensory studies should be 3–4 cm. Shorter and longer distances may introduce an amplitude error or cause increased noise (12). Because of the shorter interelectrode dis-

tance, orthodromically potentials recorded with a bar electrode, with an interelectrode separation of 3.0 cm, may have a slightly shorter latency than the counterpart antidromic potentials with ring electrodes separated by 4 cm (13).

Volume Conduction

As discussed in the Chapter 4, the body is an excellent volume conductor and electrical events ramify widely within it (1). Stimulating current can readily activate nearby nerves, and potentials arising at a distance may be detected by the recording electrodes. The examiner must always be aware of the possibility that the waveform on the screen may have arisen from some site other than the one assumed (Fig. 10.8).

Gains, Sweeps, and Filters

The gain and filter settings used for recording have a significant effect on the waveforms. Most modern machines take the latencies automatically, but always with the option of manual override. The equipment uses objective rate-of-rise criteria to detect the onset of the waveform. The human eye is more easily fooled. When normal amplification is used there is a tendency not to visually detect the initial deflection from the baseline until after it has already begun. Thus, the latencies taken by visual inspection at high amplification are shorter than those taken at normal gain, and the higher the gain, the shorter the latency (Fig. 10.9).

Changing the sweep speed has the same effect. Very fast sweep speeds spread out the potential, allowing better appreciation of the details of the initial deflection; slow sweeps cram the waveform into a more compact space on the screen, obscuring subtleties. As long as these errors are made consistently, the effect is nullified. A problem can arise when the examiner uses different gains and sweeps than were used to determine the reference values. Before depending on a reference value, all the variables should match the experimental conditions precisely, including temperature, distance, electrode placement, and instrument settings. Theoretically, reference values obtained using visual inspection to determine latencies might change if using computerized equipment, but in fact there is usually good agreement in the uncomplicated instance between the visual and digital information.

An even greater problem occurs when different gains and sweeps are used to take the latencies at different stimulation sites along the same nerve. Every

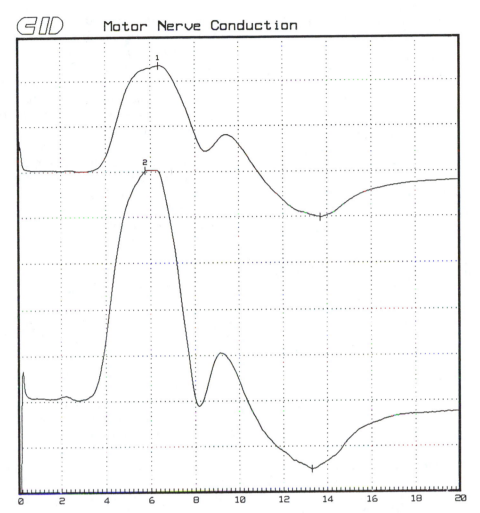

FIGURE 10.5. Median M wave on wrist stimulation demonstrating a premotor potential, or intramuscular nerve action potential, at normal gain (top tracing), and the same premotor potential at high gain (bottom tracing). The perturbation in the baseline preceding the M wave can be mistaken for a dip.

machine setting in electrodiagnosis is a compromise. The gain should be high enough to maximally appreciate the details of the baseline, but low enough that the entire potential is captured without blocking. The sweep should be the fastest that will allow capture of the entire waveform with stimulation at the proximal site. Seeing the entire waveform at all stimulus sites is important in assuring the M wave does not change amplitude or configuration, which can be a sign of inadvertent spread to an adjacent nerve, submaximal stimulation, or focal nerve pathology. Using a fast sweep and glimpsing only enough of a nubbin of the M wave to determine the proximal onset latency is terrible technique. The best compromise sweep for upper extremity motor conduction studies with velocities in the near normal range is 2 ms/division. The best compromise for lower extremity motor conduction

studies is 3 ms/division, a setting possible on the previous generation of equipment. For the current EMG machines, 5 ms/division is most suitable. The cardinal rule is: *never change the gain or sweep settings during the course of studying a given nerve.* Latency and amplitude determinations should be done using the same machine parameters at all sites studied.

Filter settings are also a compromise. The bandpass is set to eliminate unwanted high and low frequency components of the waveform(s), the noise, but with the realization that some biologically meaningful frequencies, the signal will be unavoidably attenuated as well. Filters optimize the signal to noise ratio, but cannot totally eliminate the noise without some effect on the signal. For instance, the tradeoff necessary for adequate noise reduction in sensory studies is a 10–15% decrease in SNAP amplitude (14,15). Reference

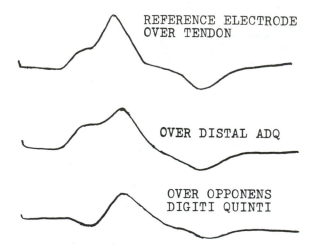

REFERENCE ELECTRODE
OVER TENDON

OVER DISTAL ADQ

OVER OPPONENS
DIGITI QUINTI

FIGURE 10.6. An M wave recorded from the ADQ after ulnar nerve stimulation at the wrist; the active recording electrode (G₁) is located over the motor point. In the top tracing G₂ is located over the tendon in the usual fashion. In the second tracing G₂ is positioned more proximally, over the distal part of the ADQ. In the third tracing, G₂ is positioned about 1 cm medial to its placement in trace 2. The position of the reference electrode can have a significant effect on the amplitude and configuration of the M wave.

values are obtained at empirically determined filter settings that reflect this compromise. If the filter settings are changed, the latency, amplitude, configuration or any other attribute of a waveform may change as well (14–16) (Table 10.3, Fig. 10.10). For example, if either the high frequency filter (HFF) or low frequency filter (LFF) is widened to expand the bandpass, the amplitude and area of the waveform will increase because more frequencies are included; there is an increase in the amount of information. Conversely, narrowing the bandpass will decrease the amplitude.

The onset of the rapidly rising, steep, negative portion of a potential represents the highest frequencies comprising the waveform; the trailing components contain the lower frequency components. Closing down the HFF (by lowering the filter setting, e.g., from 10 kHz to 1 kHz), constricts the bandpass, eliminating some high frequency components, attenuating the onset and effectively prolonging the latency. Raising the high frequency cutoff widens the bandpass and will allow detection of more high frequency components, shortening the latency. Changing the LFF has little effect on the onset latency, as there are few low frequency components at the inflection points, but a greater effect on amplitude, duration, and area. Abrupt changes in baseline direction are high frequency events, and increasing the proportion of high fre-

quency components in the waveform, by either closing down the LFF or opening up the HFF, will increase the number of turns or phases. Changing the HFF will have a greater effect on SNAPs since they are made up of higher frequencies than the M wave; conversely for the LFF. Changing the LFF has its greatest effect on the low frequency leading and trailing components of MUAPs; changing the HFF has its greatest effect on the rise time and peak amplitude (14,15). The effects are slightly different for monopolar and concentric electrodes (17). Because of these effects of filtering, the bandpass used for performing any electrodiagnostic procedure should be as close as possible to that used for obtaining the reference values.

Measurement Errors

In the course of nerve conduction studies, multiple measurements are obtained: latencies, amplitudes, and distances. In the course of needle electromyography, semi-quantitative and occasionally precisely quantitative measurements are made of amplitudes, durations, firing frequencies, recruitment level and other parameters of both normal and abnormal waveforms. Inaccuracies in any of these measurements can result in misinterpretation of the study. Some of the sources of measurement error in nerve conduction studies are listed in Table 10.1.

In nerve conduction studies, latency and amplitude measurements taken of the same waveform by different examiners, or by the same examiner at different times, will vary at least slightly, even assuming that all controllable variables are held constant. Similarly, determination of the distance between two skin points may vary because of skin movement, slight differences in tape measure reading or other factors. Experimental error is additionally related to the magnitudes of the distances and conduction times (6). These variables introduce an irreducible minimum of experimental error into conduction studies, such that true biologic variation may account for only about half of the variability in nerve conduction velocity reported in the literature (6).

Maynard and Stolov found that 89% of the error was related to latency measurement and only 11% to distance measurement. The greatest error was found reading distal latencies at high amplification. Distance error was related primarily to skin movement rather than tape measure reading errors. Experimental error was greater with shorter interstimulus distances and with slower conduction velocities (6). However, Ki-

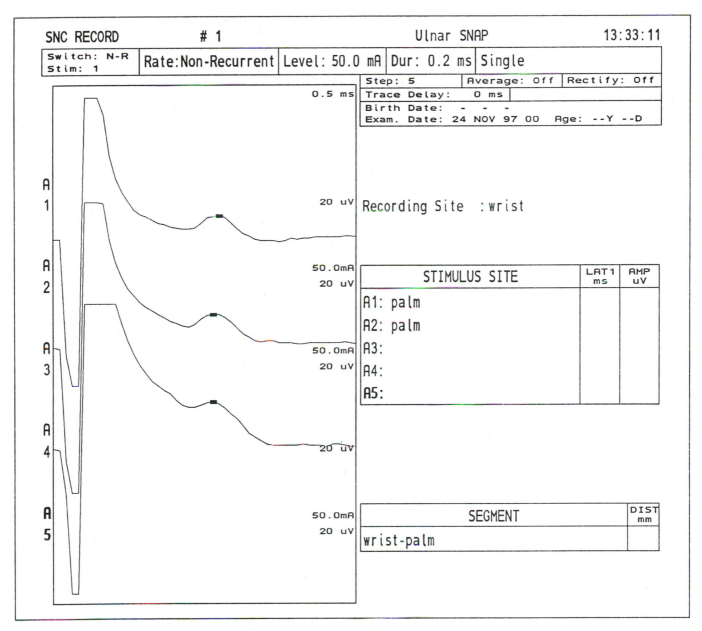

FIGURE 10.7. An orthodromic ulnar digital SNAP recorded from the wrist after stimulation of the small finger, using different ground electrode locations. The stimulus intensity and duration and electrode positions are the same for each tracing. In the top tracing, the ground is located on the palm of the hand between the stimulating and recording electrodes, in the middle tracing, on the back of the hand, and in the bottom tracing, on the volar forearm proximal to the recording electrodes. The best control of shock artifact is in the top tracing.

mura states that larger errors occur in measuring distance than latency (3).

Physiologic Factors

A number of physiologic factors may influence electrodiagnostic testing, including age, height, limb length, and temperature, as discussed in the following sections.

TEMPERATURE

Temperature has important effects on nerve conduction velocity, and on action potential amplitude and

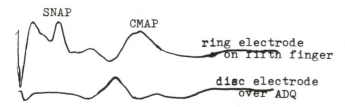

FIGURE 10.8. Volume-conducted motor potentials can interfere with the recording of sensory potentials, especially when using an antidromic technique. In the top tracing, an antidromic ulnar sensory potential is recorded with ring electrodes from the fifth finger; the trailing deflections are due to volume conducted motor activity from the hypothenar muscles. In the lower tracing, a disc electrode over the hypothenar muscles records the motor activity, which is simultaneous with the late components of the top tracing. When the SNAP is low amplitude, absent or lost in shock artifact, such volume-conducted motor potentials may be mistaken for the sensory potential.

duration (Table 10.4). Failure to recognize and deal with decreased temperature is likely the most common and important error in clinical electrodiagnosis. The effects of generalized and local cooling differ in some details. The EMGer mainly has to cope with generalized cooling of body regions, primarily the hands and feet, and such cold extremities are probably the most frequent cause of misdiagnosis in electrodiagnostic medicine (2).

The primary effect of cold is prolonging the recovery phase of the action potential by slowing the inactivation of Na+ channels and blunting the increase in K+ conductance, increasing the duration, amplitude and refractory period of the action potential and slowing its conduction. Nerve conduction velocity varies linearly with temperature within the physiologic range. At extremely low temperature (estimated at about 9.1° C), conduction fails (2). Conduction velocity then increases by about 2 m/s, or 5%, per degree up to a maximal temperature at which conduction slows slightly and then fails (the blocking temperature). In experimental demyelination, the blocking occurs at a lower than normal temperature. With CNS demyelination, blocking can develop within the physiologic temperature range; this effect was the basis for the old hot tub test for the diagnosis of MS. Temperature effects in peripheral nerve demyelination has been less well studied. In patients with neuropathy and a cold hand or foot, we have occasionally observed a prolonged latency sensory potential become unobtainable after warming (the "cold slow/warm gone phenomenon").

Distal latencies decrease by about 0.2 ms/°C below

30–32°. The generally accepted minimum surface temperature for nerve conduction studies is 31–32° C, but the temperature for clinical studies should ideally reflect that at which the reference values were obtained. Formulas have been developed to correct for temperature effects, but may not be accurate for diseased nerves (18). The best approach is to warm the extremity to the reference range and resort to corrective formulas only when warming attempts fail.

Temperature has very profound effects on neuromuscular transmission, such that safety factor is increased and transmission facilitated in the cold. Awareness of these changes is very important when performing electrodiagnostic evaluation of neuromuscular transmission disorders (see Chapter 18).

AGE

Nerve conduction velocity varies with age. The conduction velocities mirror gestational age reliably enough to help distinguish premature from low birth weight term infants. Normal newborns have nerve conduction velocities approximately half adult normal values. H-reflexes may be elicited from many muscles until about 1 year of age, after which they retreat into the normal restricted adult distribution. Nerve conduction velocities increase from birth until about age 20, reaching the adult range by about age 5. Between the ages of 20 and 60, conduction velocities decrease by about 1 m/s/decade; after age 60 by about 3 m/s/decade. For this reason, many reported reference values are grouped by decade, although in pragmatic terms the age decline seldom has clinical significance until after age 60. F response latencies also gradually increase with age, and M wave and SNAP amplitudes may decline. Some contend H-reflexes may disappear with normal aging, but this belief has been challenged (19). Conventional wisdom holds that sural potentials may be unobtainable in normal individuals after age 60, although many patients in the 9th and 10th decades have robustly normal surals. Taylor found many conduction parameters exhibited a parabolic rather than a linear decline with age and offered corrective formulas (20).

Attrition of anterior horn cells with subsequent motor unit remodeling leads to an increase in MUAP amplitude, duration and polyphasia in older patients. Reference data for quantitative electromyography is stratified by decade and shows a progressive increase in MUAP duration over the lifespan. In single fiber EMG, fiber density and jitter also increase with age, and reference values must be adjusted accordingly, especially after age 60 (21). In some muscles, especially the tibi-

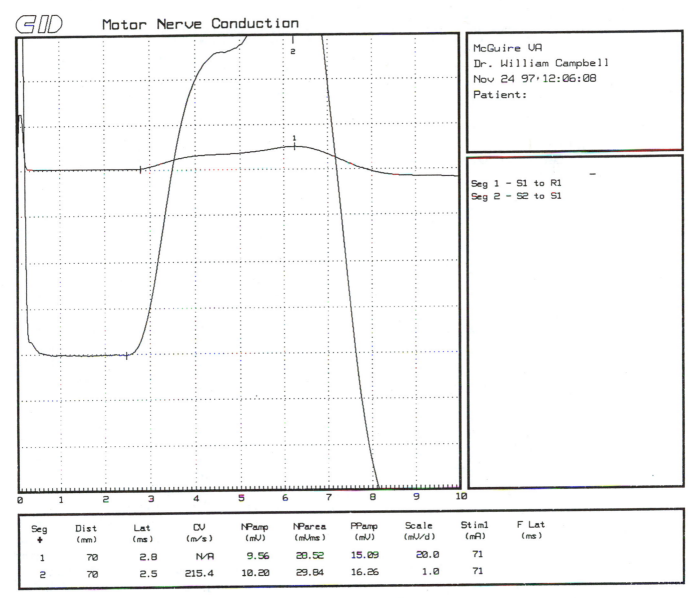

Motor Nerve Conduction

McGuire VA
Dr. William Campbell
Nov 24 97,12:06:08
Patient:

Seg 1 - S1 to R1
Seg 2 - S2 to S1

Seg +	Dist (mm)	Lat (ms)	CV (m/s)	NPamp (mV)	NParea (mVms)	PPamp (mV)	Scale (mV/d)	Stim1 (mA)	F Lat (ms)
1	70	2.8	N/A	9.56	28.52	15.09	20.0	71	
2	70	2.5	215.4	10.20	29.84	16.26	1.0	71	

FIGURE 10.9. An ulnar M wave recorded from the ADQ on wrist stimulation. The top tracing was obtained at an amplification of 20 mV/division and the visually determined latency was 2.8 ms. The same potential analyzed at an amplification of 1.0 mV/division produced a latency of 2.5 ms. The gain is an important variable in visually determining the onset latency, with the latency appearing shorter and shorter as the amplification is increased.

alis anterior and extensor digitorum brevis, increased jitter values are found even before age 60.

HEIGHT AND LIMB LENGTH

It was recognized early in the development of clinical electrodiagnostic medicine that nerve conduction velocities were faster in the arms than legs, faster through proximal nerve segments than distal, and faster in women than men. Later it was appreciated than lower extremity nerve conduction velocities varied inversely with height, with taller subjects having significantly slower velocities than shorter subjects (22). The initial assumption that the variability was due to temperature differences was not borne out (22–24). The influence of gender on nerve conduction velocity disappears when corrected for height differences, although women may still have higher amplitude digital sensory potentials related to small finger circumference. With one dissent (25), multiple investigations

TABLE 10.3
Effects of Changes in the High and Low Frequency Filter Settings on Waveforms

	Amplitude	*Latency*	*Phases*
Widen LFF (decrease the setting)	Increase	Little change	Decrease
Narrow LFF (increase the setting)	Decrease	Little change	Increase
Widen HFF (increase the setting)	Increase	Decrease	Increase
Narrow HFF (decrease the setting)	Decrease	Increase	Decrease

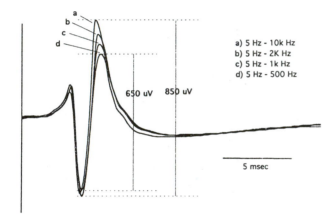

a) 5 Hz - 10k Hz
b) 5 Hz - 2K Hz
c) 5 Hz - 1k Hz
d) 5 Hz - 500 Hz

650 uV   850 uV

5 msec

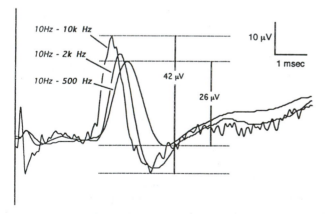

10Hz - 10k Hz
10Hz - 2k Hz
10Hz - 500 Hz

10 µV

1 msec

42 µV

26 µV

FIGURE 10.10. The effect of decreasing the high frequency filter on a motor unit action potential (top) and a sensory nerve action potential (bottom). Narrowing the bandpass results in loss of amplitude. Lowering the high frequency cutoff selectively removes high frequency components from the waveform, blunting the rise time and prolonging the inflection points at which the baseline changes direction. See text and Table 10.3 for further discussion.

have confirmed the height effect, and some studies even suggest the possibility that the susceptibility to develop some neuropathies is increased in tall patients (22–24,26) The height effect is sufficient that some tall subjects (more than about 1.9 m) may have lower extremity nerve conduction velocities in the mildly abnormal range. Though less well documented as a clinical problem, short patients with mild neuropathy could have velocities in the normal range. Wilbourn has noted an "athlete's neuropathy": large men with slightly slow nerves and slightly low sensory amplitudes but no clinical evidence of neuropathy, which is probably an artifact of the height effect plus large hands and feet (Wilbourn, personal communication).

Although the origin of the height effect is not known, the best hypothesis is that it results from progressive tapering of axons as they travel distally, with the longer length of leg allowing more opportunity to taper (Fig. 10.11). Other possibilities include shorter internodes or thinner myelin distally. These alternatives are not mutually exclusive. Per the preponderance of current evidence, the height effect is genuine and is not explained by temperature.

The complex interplay of the physiologic variables, compounded by the inherent variability in conduction studies can lead to significant misinterpretation. Rivner has developed formulas that concurrently correct for the effects of height, age, and temperature (23). Late response latencies are also obviously related to height and limb length, and corrective formulas are usually readily available.

ANATOMICAL ANOMALIES

Normal anatomical variants frequently come into play in electrodiagnostic medicine. These range from anomalous communications between nerves, to the presence of anomalous muscles, bands or blood ves-

TABLE 10.4
Effects of Reduced Temperature in Electrodiagnostic Medicine

M wave amplitude, duration and latency	Increased
SNAP amplitude, duration and latency	Increased
Nerve conduction velocity	Decreased
Motor unit action potentials	Increased duration and polyphasia
Fibrillation potentials and positive sharp waves	Amplitude increased, but frequency decreased and may disappear completely
Fasciculations	???
Myotonic discharges, generally	Likely increase in intensity, although documentation scanty
Myotonic discharges in paramyotonia congenita	Decreased
Refractory period	Prolonged

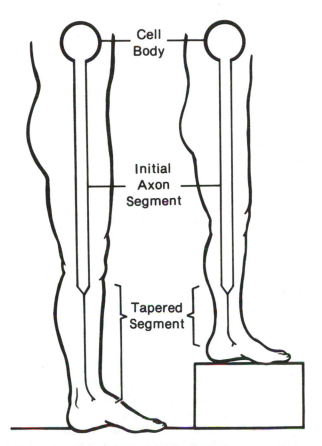

FIGURE 10.11. An exaggerated schematic illustrates the proposed abrupt mode of axonal tapering. If tall and short individuals have cell bodies and initial axonal segments of similar size, an abrupt tapering at an equivalent distance from the cell body leaves the tall individual with a greater proportion of distal nerve segment composed of smaller axons, thus lowering the average conduction velocity distally. Proximal conduction velocity would remain the same.

sels causing compressive neuropathies. Anomalous communications between nerves are common. For EMG purposes, the most relevant are the Martin-Gruber anastomosis, a crossover of median fibers to the ulnar nerve in the forearm, and the accessory peroneal nerve, a branch of the superficial peroneal which runs posterior to the lateral malleolus to innervate the lateral portion of the EDB (27).

The presence of an anomaly is usually betrayed by failure to find the expected distal to proximal decrement of M wave amplitude. Because of normal temporal dispersion, the M wave amplitude on proximal stimulation should always be of lower amplitude than on distal stimulation. If the proximal amplitude is higher, or even the same, an anomaly may be present.

The accessory peroneal anomaly seldom causes a major clinical problem in terms of misinterpretation of a study. Occasionally, submaximal stimulation at the ankle due to a deep peroneal branch at the ankle running more laterally than normal may simulate the anomaly. Stimulation behind the lateral malleolus will quickly confirm or exclude the possibility. On very rare occasion, the entire innervation of the EDB is via the accessory branch and no M wave can be elicited from the usual peroneal ankle site.

The median-to-ulnar forearm anastomosis is far more problematic, particularly when it occurs in a patient with carpal tunnel syndrome or an ulnar neuropathy at the elbow. The usual clue is a higher amplitude median nerve M wave at the elbow than the wrist. The higher amplitude at the elbow results from stimulation of anomalous ulnar fibers travelling with the median nerve. These activate the FDI and ulnar innervated thenar muscles (adductor pollicis and ulnar head of the flexor pollicis brevis), whose depolarization is volume conducted to the active electrode on the APB. The resulting summated M wave (APB +

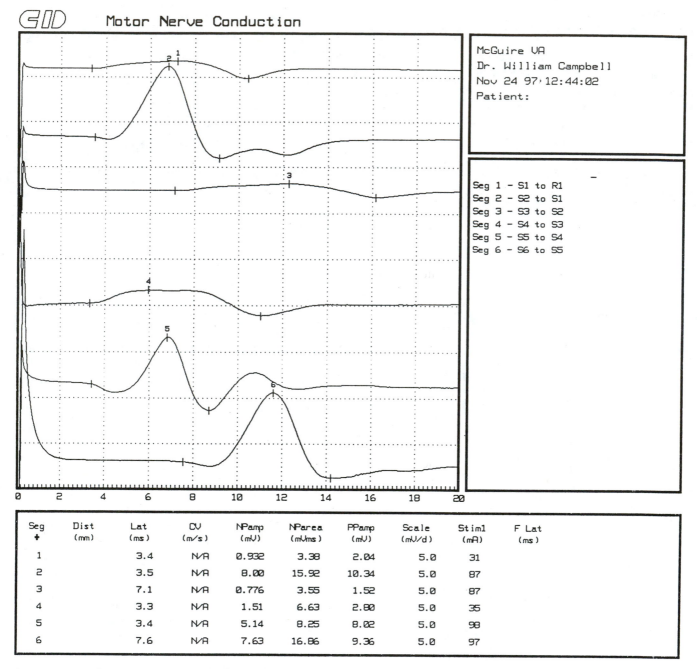

Motor Nerve Conduction

McGuire VA
Dr. William Campbell
Nov 24 97,12:44:02
Patient:

Seg 1 - S1 to R1
Seg 2 - S2 to S1
Seg 3 - S3 to S2
Seg 4 - S4 to S3
Seg 5 - S5 to S4
Seg 6 - S6 to S5

Seg #	Dist (mm)	Lat (ms)	CV (m/s)	NPamp (mV)	NParea (mVms)	PPamp (mV)	Scale (mV/d)	Stim1 (mA)	F Lat (ms)
1		3.4	N/A	0.932	3.38	2.04	5.0	31	
2		3.5	N/A	8.00	15.92	10.34	5.0	87	
3		7.1	N/A	0.776	3.55	1.52	5.0	87	
4		3.3	N/A	1.51	6.63	2.80	5.0	35	
5		3.4	N/A	5.14	8.25	8.02	5.0	98	
6		7.6	N/A	7.63	16.86	9.36	5.0	97	

FIGURE 10.12. The top three tracings are normal, the bottom three demonstrate a Martin-Gruber anastomosis. The active electrode is over the FDI. The three tracings in each set have been obtained with stimulation of 1) the median nerve at the wrist; 2) the ulnar nerve at the wrist; and 3) the median nerve at the elbow. Stimulating the median at the wrist indicates the degree to which volume conducted transmission of potentials arising from median innervated thenar muscles will be detected by the electrode over the FDI. Stimulating the ulnar at the wrist demonstrates the expected potential from ulnar stimulation. Stimulation of the median at the elbow will then have one of two outcomes: in normals, it will resemble the response obtained on median wrist stimulation (top tracing in each set); in patients with a crossover it will resemble the response obtained on ulnar wrist stimulation (middle tracing in each set).

TABLE 10.5

Steps to Follow to Confirm Martin-Gruber Anastomosis

1. Place a recording electrode over the FDI.
2. Stimulate the median nerve at the wrist. Ensure that the stimulation is just supramaximal, and not spreading to the ulnar; rotating the anode radially is wise. The resulting waveform represents the volume conducted response from the APB as recorded by the electrode over the FDI, and will usually be low amplitude and irregular.
3. Stimulate the ulnar nerve at the wrist. This should produce a robust M wave from the FDI.
4. Stimulate the median nerve at the elbow, just supramaximally so as not to spread to the ulnar. If the resulting M wave resembles that in step 3, a crossover is present. If it resembles the M waveform in step 2, a crossover is not present.

Caveat: the majority of crossover fibers innervate the FDI. If the above steps do not clarify the issue and clinical suspicion remains, follow the same procedure recording from the hypothenar muscles.

FDI + adductor pollicis + flexor pollicis brevis) is larger than that which is produced by the APB alone on purely median wrist stimulation. In a patient with a complete ulnar lesion at the elbow, sparing of muscles innervated via the crossover may lend the false impression that the lesion is incomplete. The easiest way to confirm a crossover is outlined in Table 10.5 and demonstrated in Figure 10.12.

Interesting waveforms occur when a crossover exists in a patient with CTS. Median wrist stimulation produces a clean, initially negative deflection; the distal motor latency may be normal or prolonged, depending on severity. On elbow stimulation one of two patterns may emerge. Most commonly, a dip occurs which was not present on wrist stimulation. The initial positivity is due to activation of the FDI and ulnar innervated thenar muscles via the crossover. Their depolarization occurs first because the median fibers to the APB have been pathologically delayed traversing the carpal tunnel. The recording electrode over the APB then detects the volume-conducted M waves from the ulnar innervated muscles (is effectively off the motor point), hence the dip. More rarely, a prolonged distal motor latency with a spuriously fast (80+ m/s) median nerve conduction velocity occurs because the crossover fibers reach the thenar muscles far ahead of the normal median fibers, but do not produce a dip. Because of the prolonged distal motor latency, the elbow to wrist latency difference is falsely short for the distance and the conduction velocity thus

falsely fast. The presence of either of these, a dip on median elbow stimulation not present on wrist stimulation or an unrealistically fast median forearm conduction velocity, may signify the presence of CTS even when routine studies remain normal (28). In the face of CTS and a crossover, reliable median forearm nerve conduction velocity cannot be calculated.

Another crossover-related error can lead to frank

TABLE 10.6

Traps and Potential Sources of Error in the Needle Electrode Examination

Incorrect filter settings (may change amplitude, duration and configuration of MUAPs, or mask spontaneous activity); use of a notch filter

Use of CNE reference values when examining with a MNE, or vice versa

Improper needle for the task (e.g., trying to get by with a 37 mm electrode when the situation calls for a 50 mm)

Anatomical mislocalization (e.g., needling the first lumbrical instead of the first dorsal interosseous, and thinking a patient with CTS also has ulnar nerve pathology)

Elicitation of maximal contraction with the needle intramuscular (pain, bent needles)

Inefficient probing for insertional activity (using in/out or jiggle motion rather than thrust and hold; see Chapter 8); insufficient pauses between needle movements

Too cursory, or too extensive, an examination than necessary to answer the clinical question; unfocused searching and rote information gathering

Failure to recognize artifacts, e.g. pacemaker spikes mistaken for fibrillation potentials

Examination of muscles that are too cool, masking fibrillations (see case report in reference 2)

Mistaking of other electrical activity for fibrillation potentials (end plate spikes, positively configured MUAPs, cannula potentials from a CNE)

Mistiming of the examination (usually done too early for changes to have appeared, sometimes too late after changes have resolved)

Failure to appreciate the limitations of the needle examination in distinguishing myogenic from neurogenic processes (see Chapter 8)

Overinterpretation of dramatic but normal variants (EMG disease; snap, crackle, pop; CRDs in the iliopsoas)

Failure to observe universal precautions

misdiagnosis of ulnar neuropathy at the elbow. Physiologic temporal dispersion does not normally lead to more than about a 20% loss of amplitude between wrist and elbow. When many ulnar fibers are participating in a crossover, they are not in their normal location in the ulnar groove. Elbow stimulation may then show a greater than expected distal to proximal amplitude decrement mimicking a neurapraxic lesion involving the ulnar nerve at the elbow. Lack of other evidence of ulnar neuropathy (slow conduction velocity, abnormal sensory potential, abnormal needle examination) should be a clue to the anomalous innervation, which can then be confirmed by following the steps in Table 10.5.

Pitfalls of Needle Electrode Examination (NEE)

Many NEE errors are simple oversight, such as assessing voluntary activity at 1 mV per division, and forgetting to change the gain when moving to insertional and spontaneous activity. On manual machines, failure to properly adjust the filters can significantly alter the waveforms. The examiner must always be certain to apply the proper reference values for the type of electrode in use. Abnormalities on NEE evolve in dynamic fashion, and proper timing of the examination in relation to the evolution of the disease process is critical (see Chapter 8). Some of the errors and potential problems related to the NEE are summarized in Table 10.6.

Key Points

- The everyday practice of electrodiagnostic medicine is a constant battle against the threat of misstep. Difficulties can arise from a multitude of technical, physiologic and anatomic factors: shock artifact, volume conduction, temperature effects, and anomalous innervation.

- There is an inherent variability in nerve conduction studies, with a coefficient of variation of 2–9%; only half due to true biologic variability.

- Potential sources of error in nerve conduction studies include the stimulating current, factors related to the active and recording electrodes, distance measurements, latency measurements and failure to recognize innervation anomalies, artifacts, and other technical faults.

- Conventional techniques require a supramaximal stimulus, and submaximal stimulation is a common source of error. An excessively supramaximal stimulus may cause the effective cathode to migrate distally, spuriously short-

ening the latency or produce inadvertent, unwanted, activation of adjacent nerves.

- Stimulus artifact occurs because current is conducted directly over the skin surface from the stimulating to the active recording electrode. When conditions favor transcutaneous spread, the shock artifact can overwhelm the nerve action potential.

- The most favorable conditions for trouble free recording are: electrode impedances low and equal, skin impedance high and ground located between the stimulating and recording electrodes. Usually, the quickest and simplest way to control shock artifact is to rotate the anode. The other major source of interference in electrodiagnosis is 60 Hz AC power line artifact.

- For motor NCS, the active recording electrode must be directly over the motor point. An initial positive deflection, a "dip," usually signifies that the active electrode is off the motor point. A "pseudodip" is an initially positive deflection that does not signify anything amiss and can occur for several reasons.

- The gain and sweep settings can have a significant effect on the visual determination of latencies. A problem can arise when the examiner uses different gains and sweeps than were used to determine the reference values or uses different gains and sweeps at different stimulation sites along the same nerve.

- Filter settings are also a compromise. The bandpass is set to optimize the signal to noise ratio with the realization that some signal will be unavoidably attenuated. Reference values are obtained at empirically determined filter settings that reflect this compromise. If the filter settings are changed, the latency, amplitude, configuration or any other attribute of a waveform may change as well. The bandpass used for performing any electrodiagnostic procedure should be as close as possible to that used for obtaining the reference values.

- The primary effect of decreased temperature is to prolong the recovery phase of the action potential, increasing its duration, amplitude and latency and slowing its conduction.

- Nerve conduction velocity decreases by about 2 m/s per degree C, and distal latencies increase by about 0.2 ms/° C below the accepted minimum surface temperature for nerve conduction studies of 31–32°. Formulas have been developed to correct for temperature effects, but may not be accurate for diseased nerves. The best approach is to warm the extremity to the reference range and resort to corrective formulas only when warming attempts fail. Nerve conduction velocity also varies with age. Normal newborns have nerve conduction velocities approximately half of adult normal values, which reach the adult range by about age 5. Between the ages of 20 and 60, conduction velocities decrease by about 1 m/s/decade; after age 60 by about 3 m/s/decade.

- Sural potentials may be unobtainable in normal individuals after age 60.

- Attrition of anterior horn cells with subsequent motor unit remodeling leads to an increase in MUAP amplitude, duration, and polyphasia in older patients.

- Some nerve conduction velocities vary inversely with height, with taller subjects having significantly slower velocities than shorter subjects, possibly due to tapering of axons as they travel distally.

- Anatomical anomalies are a common problem. For EMG purposes, the most relevant is the Martin-Gruber anastomosis, a crossover of median fibers to the ulnar nerve in the forearm, usually detected by finding a higher M wave amplitude on proximal than distal stimulation, the reverse of the normal gradient. The presence of a dip on median elbow stimulation not present on wrist stimulation, or an unrealistically fast median forearm conduction velocity, may signify the presence of CTS in the face of a crossover, even when routine studies remain normal. An unrecognized crossover can lead to frank misdiagnosis of ulnar neuropathy at the elbow.

References

1. Dumitru D, DeLisa JA. AAEM Minimonograph #10: volume conduction. Muscle Nerve 1991;14:605–624.
   See Chapter 4 for abstract.

2. Denys EH. AAEM minimonograph #14: The influence of temperature in clinical neurophysiology. Muscle Nerve 1991;14:795–811.
   See Chapter 7 for abstract.

3. Kimura J. Principles and pitfalls of nerve conduction studies. Ann Neurol 1984;16:415–429.
   See Chapter 7 for abstract. See also: Gassel MM. Sources of error in motor nerve conduction studies. Neurology 1964; 14:825–835; Simpson JA. Fact and fallacy in measurement of conduction velocity in motor nerves. J Neurol Neurosurg Psychiat 1964;27:381–385; Kimura J. Facts, fallacies, and fancies of nerve conduction studies: twenty-first annual Edward H. Lambert Lecture. Muscle Nerve 1997;20:777–787.

4. Dumitru D. Electrodiagnostic medicine. Philadelphia: Hanley & Belfus, 1995.

5. Oh SJ. Clinical Electromyography: Nerve Conduction Studies. 2nd ed. Baltimore: Williams and Wilkins, 1993.

6. Maynard FM, Stolov WC. Experimental error in determination of nerve conduction velocity. Arch Phys Med Rehabil 1972;53:362–372.
   A study of 20 EMGers reading latencies and measuring distance. Mathematical determinations of experimental error were dependent not only on the measurement errors but on the magnitude of the distance and conduction time as well. Families of curves describing error as a function of NCV were constructed. Majority of error came from measuring latency. Largest error is at slow NCV. True biologic variation may account for only half of total variability reported in NCVs.

7. Dreyer SJ, Dumitru D, King JC. Anodal block v. anodal stimulation. Fact or fiction. Am J Phys Med Rehabil 1993;72:10–18.
   Anodal block and stimulation are poorly documented electrophysiologic phenomena. Based on the findings in this investigation, anodal block does not appear to occur during routine nerve conduction studies.

8. Kornfield MJ, Cerra J, Simons DG. Stimulus artifact reduction in nerve conduction. Arch Phys Med Rehabil 1985;66:232–235.
   Techniques recommended to reduce stimulus artifact (SA) include modifications of electrodes, electrode contact, and stimulus circuitry. Twenty-two subjects were studied to evaluate two electrode positioning techniques to reduce the SA in sensory nerve conduction velocity recordings. In 16 normal subjects, rotating the stimulator anode around the cathode 70–105 degrees flattened the baseline and permitted recording a clear take-off of the sural evoked response. In the remaining six subjects, other angles were optimal. Reconfiguring location of the reference and ground electrodes to increase common mode rejection was not consistently effective in reducing the SA in the eight patients tested. Isopotential lines produced by the stimulator electric dipole are described to explain the findings. This technique is simple and effective in reducing SA.

9. Dumitru D, Walsh NE, Ramamurthy S. The premotor potential. Arch Phys Med Rehabil 1989;70:537–540.
   A small waveform precedes the thenar CMAP with median nerve stimulation with high amplifier gains. This potential is believed to emanate from fibers destined to innervate the volar aspect of the first digit. It has been suggested recently that the source of the premotor potential is the palmar cutaneous branch of the median nerve. In this study, the palmar cutaneous branch of the median nerve was blocked at the wrist. A localized zone of anesthesia was observed over the proximal midpalm, not the thenar eminence, and the premotor response remained unchanged as did a midpalmar potential. The median nerve was then blocked at the base of the thenar eminence; only then did the premotor potential disappear. The palmar cutaneous branch of the medial nerve innervates only a small portion of the medial aspect of the thenar eminence and does not produce the thenar premotor potential.

10. Kincaid JC, Brashear A, Markand ON. The influence of the reference electrode on CMAP configuration. Muscle Nerve 1993;16:392–396.
    See Chapter 7 for abstract.

11. Brashear A, Kincaid JC. The influence of the reference electrode on CMAP configuration: leg nerve observations and an alternative reference site. Muscle Nerve 1996;19:63–67.
    See Chapter 7 for abstract.

12. Walker FO, Gitter AJ, Stolov WC. Optimal interelectrode recording distances. Muscle Nerve 1996;19:536–538.

13. Cohn TG, Wertsch JJ, Pasupuleti DV, Loftsgaarden JD, Schenk VA. Nerve conduction studies: orthodromic vs antidromic latencies. Arch Phys Med Rehabil 1990; 71:579–582.
    There is debate concerning the effect of orthodromic vs antidromic stimulation on the latency of the SNAP. This question was studied with the same methodology of those who reported a difference between antidromic and orthodromic latencies, but with control of the interelectrode distance. The median and ulnar digital nerves were analyzed both orthodromically and antidromically in 25 normal hands. There was careful control of interelectrode distance, which was the same for both

the recording and stimulating electrodes. Studies were done with both a 3-cm and 4-cm interelectrode distance. Extensive statistical analysis was performed for all parameters. No differences were found between antidromic and orthodromic studies when the interelectrode distance was the same.

14. Gitter AJ, Stolov WC. AAEM minimonograph #16: instrumentation and measurement in electrodiagnostic medicine—Part I. Muscle Nerve 1995;18:799–811.
   See Chapter 2 for abstract.

15. Gitter AJ, Stolov WC. AAEM minimonograph #16: instrumentation and measurement in electrodiagnostic medicine—Part II. Muscle Nerve 1995;18:812–824.
   See Chapter 2 for abstract.

16. Dumitru D, Walsh NE. Practical instrumentation and common sources of error. Am J Phys Med Rehabil 1988;67:55–65.
   A thorough comprehension of electrodiagnostic equipment is essential to consistently obtain accurate and reproducible data. Unreliable waveform latencies or morphologies may result from inappropriate filter settings, sensitivity comparisons, sweep speeds, interelectrode separation, cathode/anode reversals and stimulus artifact. A low frequency filter with too high a frequency limit may decrease amplitude, shorten peak latency, decrease the negative spike duration, add a phase and increase total waveform duration. A high frequency filter with too low a cut-off may decrease amplitude and prolong onset and peak latencies. Increasing the amplifier's sensitivity may shorten the onset latency of a response. Sweep speeds that are too slow may omit phases, turns or entire potentials when using digital equipment. If the interelectrode separation is inadequate, waveform morphology and amplitude can be altered. Reversing cathode and anode placement affects latency and velocity determinations. Stimulus artifact may obscure a response and its reduction must be understood. Comparing latencies and amplitudes at different instrument settings is never appropriate and can lead to serious errors and misdiagnoses. A naive approach to instrumentation, therefore, is indefensible.

17. Chu J, Chen RC. Changes in motor unit action potential parameters in monopolar recordings related to filter settings of the EMG amplifier. Arch Phys Med Rehabil 1985;66:601–604.
   A study of the effect of different EMG amplifier settings on various parameters of MUAP as recorded by the monopolar needle. Of the four filter settings used (2Hz-10kHz, 20Hz-10kHz, 20Hz-2kHz and 500Hz-10kHz) 2Hz-10kHz yielded longest duration recordings. Reductions of all parameters of the MUAP except for phases and turns were demonstrated with the 500Hz-10kHz filter. No significant differences were noted between recordings obtained with 20Hz- 10kHz and 20Hz-2kHz filters. Frequencies below 500Hz were more significant in determining the various parameters of the MUP than were those above 2kHz. Most suitable filter settings for recording MUPs were 2Hz-10kHz and 20Hz-10kHz. Measurements of MUPs were shown to be specific for a given filter setting. See also: Chu J, Chan RC, and Bruyninckx F. Effects of the EMG amplifier filter settings on the motor unit action potential parameters recorded with concentric and monopolar needles. Electromyogr Clin Neurophysiol 1986;26:627–639.

18. Ashworth NL, Marshall SC, Satkunam LE. The effect of temperature on nerve conduction parameters in carpal tunnel syndrome. Muscle Nerve, in press.
   See Chapter 7 for abstract.

19. Falco FJ, Hennessey WJ, Goldberg G, et al. H reflex latency in the healthy elderly. Muscle Nerve 1994;17:161–167.
   The H reflex was recorded bilaterally in 92% of 103 carefully screened individuals aged 60–88 years. The mean H reflex latency was 30.8 (SD = 2.6) and 30.7 (SD = 2.6) ms for right and left legs, respectively. A high correlation (r = 0.55, P < 0.05) was present between H reflex latency and leg length. No significant correlation existed for H reflex latency and age but there was an increase in the between-leg latency variability. This greater difference must be taken into account when using side-to-side H reflex latency comparison to detect unilateral pathology in the elderly.

20. Taylor PK. Non-linear effects of age on nerve conduction in adults. J Neurol Sci 1984;66:223–234.
   The effects of age on conduction and amplitude in median and ulnar (motor and sensory), superficial radial, sural and common peroneal (motor) nerves of adults were prospectively investigated. Four routinely recorded parameters, including conduction velocity, amplitude and duration, were considered for each sensory nerve and measurements of conduction velocity, terminal motor latency and amplitude were made for each motor nerve. The resulting 25 sets of data were analyzed using both linear and quadratic regression. The three sets of terminal motor latency data showed no age dependence while in six other instances there was a linear relationship with age (three of these being motor amplitude). The remaining 16 sets of data were statistically best represented by quadratic analysis. The shapes of the paraboli were remarkably similar, reaching a maximum (conduction velocity and amplitude) or minimum (duration) value in the fourth decade and thereafter declining or rising respectively at an accelerating rate. With only one exception, quadratic curves of the same parameter were shown to be parallel. Tables of normal data which make accurate adjustments for the aging effect can be constructed from this analysis for use in routine clinical investigation.

21. Gilchrist JM, et al. Single fiber EMG reference values: a collaborative effort. Ad Hoc Committee of the AAEM Special Interest Group on Single Fiber EMG. Muscle Nerve 1992;15:151–161.
   The normal values of SFEMG measurements of fiber density and jitter for most muscles and age groups are not well documented in the literature. This study reports a multicenter collection of SFEMG jitter and fiber density data from control subjects obtained for the purpose of defining reference values for many muscles and different ages. See also: Bromberg MB, Scott DM, et al. Single fiber EMG reference values: reformatted in tabular form. Muscle & Nerve 1994;17:820–821.

22. Campbell WW, Ward LC, Swift TR. Nerve conduction velocity varies inversely with height. Muscle Nerve 1981;4:520–523.
   Even when all known factors affecting the determination of nerve conduction velocity are controlled, large individual variations persist. In 40 normal controls, the peroneal and sural conduction velocities varied inversely with body height (p < 0.001). This height effect is not due to temperature differences, and it explains almost 50% of the intersubject variability in conduction velocity. The height influence may reflect abrupt, rather than gradual, tapering of axons distally. This mode of tapering may help explain the decrements in conduction velocity from proximal to distal nerve segments and from upper to lower extremities, which have long been observed in clinical electromyography. Clinical recognition of this height effect is important lest one label as abnormal an individual with mildly

slowed peripheral nerve conduction velocity solely related to large stature. See also: Soudmand R, Ward LC, Swift TR. Effect of height on nerve conduction velocity. Neurology 1982;32:407–410.

23. Rivner MH, Swift TR, Crout BO, et al. Toward more rational nerve conduction interpretations: the effect of height. Muscle Nerve 1990;13:232–239.

One hundred and four normal subjects ranging in age from 17 to 77 years and in height from 115 to 203 cm underwent nerve conduction studies of sural, peroneal, tibial, and median nerves. Foot temperature was measured in each patient. A strong inverse correlation was found between height and sural (r = −0.7104), peroneal (r = −0.6842), and tibial (r = −0.5044) conduction velocities. These correlations were significant at the P less than 0.001 level. Median conduction velocity was not correlated with height. Height was correlated with the distal latencies of all nerves studied (sural r = 0.6518, peroneal r = 0.4583, tibial r = 0.7217, median r = 0.5440). These correlations were significant at the P less than 0.001 level. Age was inversely correlated with both tibial (r = −0.4071) and median (r = −0.3464) nerve conduction velocities but not with sural and peroneal conductions. There were no correlations between distal latencies and age. If the variation in conduction velocity accounted for by the linear relationship with height was removed, then age would be inversely correlated to all conduction velocity measurements with the exception of the sural. Temperature is inversely correlated with the sural (r = −0.2233), peroneal (r = −0.2102), and tibial (r = −0.2710) distal latencies. In all instances, the effects of age and temperature were minor determinants when compared with the effects of height. Diagnostic conclusions made from nerve conduction data without correcting for height may be invalid in patients taller and shorter than normal.

24. Robinson LR, Rubner DE, Wahl PW, et al. Influences of height and gender on normal nerve conduction studies. Arch Phys Med Rehabil 1993;74:1134–1138.

A study of the effects of gender on nerve conduction results in healthy subjects. Fifty-four men, mean age 60.2 years and mean height 167 cm, were compared with 62 women, mean age 62.2 years and mean height 153 cm. After adjustment of the data for height, most statistically significant differences in conduction velocity disappeared.

25. Trojaborg WT, Moon A, Andersen BB, et al. Sural nerve conduction parameters in normal subjects related to age, gender, temperature, and height: a reappraisal. Muscle Nerve 1992;15:666–671.

Failure to take body height into consideration in the evaluation of nerve conduction velocities (CV) has recently been deemed unacceptable. This statement prompted the present study. Besides height, the influence of age, gender, and temperature was studied in 92 normal subjects, half of whom were females. The CV decreased 0.9 m/s per 10 years increase in age, the same in women and men aged 15 to 44 years. Mean temperature between distal and proximal ends of the nerve segment examined increased 6.1 +/− 0.3 degree C after heating followed by a CV increase of 7.0 +/− 0.5 m/s. The CV decreased 0.15 m/s per 100-mm increase in height. When considering 37 individuals aged 25 to 34 years only, the CV increased 0.34 m/s per 1-m increase in height. In both instances, the changes were within the experimental error (2.3%) of the method.

26. Gadia MT, Natori N, Ramos LB, et al. Influence of height on quantitative sensory, nerve conduction, and clinical indices of diabetic peripheral neuropathy. Diabetes Care 1987;10:613–616.

A study of the associations between height and quantitative sensory, nerve-conduction, and clinical indices of diabetic peripheral neuropathy in adult diabetic patients. Vibratory sensitivity was strongly related to height; however, there was no relation between thermal sensitivity and height. The peroneal and posterior tibial motor NCVs were inversely related to height (P < .05 for both). When age and diabetes duration were included as variables in multiple regression analyses, the associations with height became stronger. Clinical indices of peripheral neuropathy were also related to height in these analyses. These data indicate that height has a marked influence on quantitative sensory, nerve-conduction, and clinical indices of diabetic peripheral neuropathy.

27. Gutmann L. AAEM minimonograph #2: important anomalous innervations of the extremities. Muscle Nerve 1993;16:339–347.

Anomalous innervations of the extremities are common and can significantly influence the interpretation of electrodiagnostic studies in various conditions. The Martin-Gruber anastamosis or crossover, consists of a subpopulation of median nerve motor axons, usually arising from the anterior interosseous branch, which cross in the upper forearm to run distally with the ulnar nerve. Anomalous fibers most often innervate the FDI or adductor pollicis, occasionally the hypothenar muscles. The reported incidence of this anomaly ranges from 15% to 30%. Rarely, sensory fibers may participate in the usual crossover or communications may run from the ulnar to the median. The Riche-Cannieu anomaly consists of communications between the median motor and deep palmar ulnar branches in the radial aspect of the palm; it is of equivocal clinical significance. The accessory peroneal nerve is an anomalous branch arising from the superficial peroneal which passes behind the lateral malleolus to innervate the lateral aspect of the EDB in 20–30% of individuals. See also: Santoro L, Rosato R, Caruso G. Median-ulnar nerve communications: electrophysiological demonstration of motor and sensory fibre cross-over. J Neurol 1983;229:227–235; Dumitru D, Walsh NE, Weber CF. Electrophysiologic study of the Riche-Cannieu anomaly. Electromyogr Clin Neurophysiol 1988;28:27–31; van Dijk JG, Bouma PAD. Recognition of the Martin-Gruber anastomosis. Muscle Nerve 1997;20:887–889.

28. Gutmann L, Gutierrez A, Riggs JE. The contribution of median-ulnar communications in diagnosis of mild carpal tunnel syndrome. Muscle Nerve 1986;9:319–321.

In six patients with characteristic symptoms of carpal tunnel syndrome, electrophysiologic studies were normal, except for an initial positive deflection of the thenar muscle action potential with median nerve stimulation at the elbow but not at the wrist. This phenomenon is only seen with coexistent carpal tunnel syndrome and median to ulnar nerve communication and suggests carpal tunnel syndrome is present in these patients. As normal electrophysiologic studies occur in carpal tunnel syndrome (up to 8%) and median to ulnar communications are common (15%–31%), this observed finding is of practical clinical importance in the diagnosis of mild carpal tunnel syndrome despite otherwise normal electrophysiologic studies.

11

An Overview of Electrodiagnostic Findings in Neuromuscular Disorders

Neuromuscular diseases can be broadly classified into neurogenic, myopathic, and neuromuscular transmission disorders. One of the fortes of electrodiagnostic medicine is its ability to sort out these various etiologic categories of disease. But there is significant overlap in the findings in different types of disease, especially on the needle electrode examination (NEE).

Myopathies may have features more typically associated with neurogenic disease, and vice versa. For instance, fibrillation potentials were first described in neurogenic disease and were called "denervation potentials" for many years before it was recognized that many myopathies could also be associated with abnormal spontaneous activity. It is the ability to recognize these exceptions and quirks that marks the proficient electrodiagnostic medicine consultant. The picture on NEE in both neurogenic and myopathic disease depends in large measure on the time course of the process. Acute, subacute, chronic and very indolent conditions produce different patterns of abnormality.

Neurogenic diseases include neuronopathies, radiculopathies, plexopathies, and peripheral neuropathies. All are discussed in detail in the respective chapters covering these conditions. The following section provides a brief overview of the electrodiagnostic medicine findings typical of the more common neuromuscular disorders.

Neuronopathy

Neuronopathies are conditions that affect neurons, either motor neurons as in poliomyelitis, spinal muscular atrophy or amyotrophic lateral sclerosis (ALS), or sensory neurons as in carcinomatous sensory neuropathy. ALS, the most common neuronopathy by far, is characterized electrodiagnostically by evidence of acute and chronic denervation with reinnervation (1). Denervation produces decreased recruitment and fibrillation potentials. Reinnervation results in large amplitude, long duration, complex, unstable, polyphasic MUPs (2). Fasciculations are usually prominent. These abnormalities should be demonstrated in a widespread distribution to document the diffuseness of the process. One common criterion employed is that typical changes involve at least three extremities in a multinerve, multiroot distribution, with the bulbar muscles and the thoracic paraspinals counting as extremities. Atypical features can occur in patients with rapidly progressive disease or far advanced disease, or in the face of ineffective reinnervation. Thus low amplitude or short duration motor unit action potentials (MUAPs) may occasionally be seen (3). Modified SF studies may show abnormal "jiggle."

Motor nerve conduction studies are normal, or show loss of M wave amplitude and mild slowing due to axon loss. This is not so straightforward a statement as it might at first appear. The complex subject of nerve conduction abnormalities in motor neuron disease is covered in detail in the chapter on neuronopathies. Sensory potentials should always be normal, barring some complication or technical misstep.

Reviews on various neuronopathies have been published under the auspices of the American Association of Electrodiagnostic Medicine (AAEM) (1,4–6).

Radiculopathy

The general electrodiagnostic picture in radiculopathy includes normal motor and sensory conduction studies, with the NEE disclosing abnormalities in a myotomal distribution, including the paraspinal muscles. Motor conduction abnormalities should reflect only axon loss, and even this is usually minimal. Sensory studies should be normal.

The diagnosis of radiculopathy is based primarily on the NEE, and primarily on the presence of fibrillation potentials. Normal muscles may contain complex or polyphasic potentials, and it is hazardous to diagnose radiculopathy on MUAP changes in isolation unless there are flagrant abnormalities in a myotomal distribution, in which case fibrillation potentials will usually be present as well. For confident diagnosis, the abnormalities should involve at least two muscles sharing the same myotomal but different peripheral nerve innervations. The examination must be extensive enough to exclude a diffuse process (7).

The timing of the study in relation to the onset of symptoms is pivotal. It usually requires 7–10 days for fibrillation potentials to appear in the paraspinal muscles and 2–3 weeks in limb muscles. Reinnerva-

tion with disappearance of fibrillation potentials occurs in the same sequence after a variable delay. Thus, depending on the duration of the process, fibrillations could be found in any combination of limb and paraspinal muscles. The paraspinal findings are critical in the evaluation of radiculopathy patients, and it is important to specifically examine the muscles of the multifidus compartment (8). There are clear limitations of EMG in the diagnosis of radiculopathy, related to the multiple root innervation of most muscles, the variable relationship between the root level and the vertebral level of injury, the potential for reinnervation by collateral sprouts, the severity of the radicular lesion and whether it involves axon loss or only demyelination. A normal study does not exclude radiculopathy.

Plexopathy

From a clinical and electrodiagnostic standpoint the most common exercise is distinguishing plexopathy from radiculopathy. The NEE is the mainstay of diagnosis and localization, although sensory (more so than motor) conduction studies, late responses, and SEPs can sometimes provide helpful information. The key feature is abnormalities in the distribution of some plexus component, a trunk or a cord, sparing the paraspinals. The status of the sensory potentials is critical for distinguishing plexopathy from radiculopathy. In radiculopathy, the sensory potentials are normal, in plexopathy they are frequently absent or low in amplitude.

Neuralgic amyotrophy produces a stereotyped clinical syndrome, a spotty axon loss pattern on EMG and abnormal sensory nerve action potentials (9). Myokymia, and the absence of pain suggest radiation plexopathy in the patient with a history of cancer and radiotherapy. Traumatic plexopathies can follow stretch, external pressure, and penetrating wounds; lower trunk lesions occur in 5–10% of patients undergoing coronary artery bypass grafts. Electrodiagnosis can help determine the pathophysiology, distribution, and completeness of the lesion and rule out root avulsion. True neurogenic thoracic outlet syndrome has a characteristic clinical and electrodiagnostic picture. The disputed neurogenic form of TOS is muddy clinically and electrodiagnostically.

Diabetic amyotrophy, the most common condition affecting the lumbosacral plexus, has a characteristic clinical presentation (10). The primary alternative diagnostic possibility is high lumbar radiculopathy. Unfortunately for diagnostic localization purposes, diabetic amyotrophy commonly produces paraspinal fibrillations.

Neuropathy

The electrodiagnostic evaluation attempts to place a peripheral neuropathy into one of several categories that have pathophysiologic, etiologic and therapeutic significance. The process may be generalized, focal, or multifocal; axonal or demyelinating; motor, sensory, or mixed; with or without autonomic dysfunction; acute or chronic; progressive, stable or resolving; hereditary or acquired.

For incompletely understood reasons, neuropathies may have a predilection for certain types and sizes of fibers, a tendency that can sometimes be exploited to diagnostic advantage. Demyelinating neuropathies typically produce slowing of CV with preservation of distal amplitudes; axonopathies typically produce marked loss of distal M wave and sensory potential amplitudes with relative preservation of CV. Axonopathies tend to demonstrate a proximal to distal gradient of increasing neuropathic abnormality on needle examination; myelinopathies are more likely to exhibit a paucity of denervation and no proximal to distal gradient. Myelinopathies may cause uniform, diffuse demyelination, or segmental, multifocal demyelination; the likely etiologies of these two patterns are quite different. Conduction block and temporal dispersion are hallmarks of acquired demyelination and help to distinguish acquired from hereditary neuropathies. Numerous helpful reviews on the subject of generalized neuropathies are available (11–16).

The electrodiagnostic profile in focal and multifocal neuropathies may include a complicated amalgam of conduction block, focal slowing, and axon loss. Large nerve fibers are more susceptible to pressure than small, and peripheral fibers more vulnerable than central ones. Selective fascicular involvement is common, underappreciated, and may seriously complicate the clinical and electrodiagnostic evaluation. In some focal neuropathies, almost any combination of demyelination and axon loss can involve any of the target muscles to different degrees. The vulnerable nerve syndrome describes patients with generalized polyneuropathies who are at increased risk of developing a superimposed compression neuropathy.

The electrodiagnostic evaluation of focal neuropathy is simplified when the location of the lesion permits stimulation or recording proximal and distal to the lesion. Abnormalities of the nerve action potential are a sensitive indicator of peripheral nerve damage, but are often nonlocalizing. Motor conduction abnormalities, although less sensitive, are usually more localizing. Conduction block or asynchronous focal slowing are the most helpful features allowing precise localization of a focal neuropathy. Axon loss can produce confusing secondary slowing of CV.

Reviews on most of the common, and some not so common, focal neuropathies have been published under the auspices of the AAEM (17–29).

Neuromuscular Transmission (NMT) Disorders

Electrodiagnostically, NMT disorders produce characteristic changes that allow them to be distinguished from diseases of nerve and from diseases of muscle. The vast oversupply of acetylcholine and acetylcholine receptors beyond the minimum required for depolarization is referred to as the safety factor for NMT. One of the hallmarks of NMT disorders is diminution in this safety factor. Presynaptic and postsynaptic NMT disorders alter the safety factor through different mechanisms and produce different patterns of abnormality on repetitive stimulation studies. The two most common NMT disorders are myasthenia gravis and the Lambert-Eaton syndrome, both due to autoantibodies (30–33). In both, safety factor declines because of a decreased number of ligand-receptor interactions, because of a lack of acetylcholine receptors in myasthenia and a lack of acetylcholine molecules in Lambert-Eaton syndrome.

Single fiber EMG abnormalties, while the most sensitive indicator of transmission disorders, are nonspecific (34). Repetitive nerve stimulation (RNS) studies are less sensitive, but more specific for localizing a disorder to the postsynaptic or presynaptic membrane and are less technically demanding. Presynaptic and postsynaptic NMT disorders produce RNS abnormalities that have some features in common and some features that are different. Decremental responses are most likely to be seen in either type with stimulation at 2–3 Hz, the frequency at which safety factor is lowest. The responses to rapid stimulation or brief, isometric exercise are different with presynaptic and postsynaptic disorders. Routine needle examination in most patients with a NMT disorder is normal, or shows a beat to beat variability in the amplitude or configuration of a MUAP due to transmission failures involving some fibers. Impulse blocking on single fiber studies correlates best with MUAP variability on NEE, a decremental response on RNS, and with clinical weakness and fatiguability.

Myopathy

Wilbourn has written a comprehensive review of the electrodiagnosis of myopathies (35). The topic is considered further, and the specific findings in various diseases are discussed in detail in Chapter 19. Electrodiagnosis is an invaluable adjunct in the clinical evaluation of patients with suspected myopathy, but has clear limitations. The EMG permits a wide sampling of muscles and can guide the choice of muscle for biopsy. Although no specific etiologic diagnosis is usually possible, the EMG can place the process into a broad category of likely causes and help exclude other conditions that mimic myopathy.

Unfortunately, the electodiagnostic findings typical of myopathy are not specific for primary muscle disease. Abnormalities may involve the MUAP or produce abnormal insertional or spontaneous activity, in various combinations. The spectrum of possible electrodiagnostic findings ranges from no detectable abnormality to flagrantly abnormal "myopathic" MUAPs with accompanying fibrillation potentials, to long-duration polyphasic units easily confused with neurogenic disease.

Typical features on NEE in myopathy include short duration, low amplitude, polyphasic units, and abnormal recruitment. A MUAP that is polyphasic, yet still of overall short duration is particularly suspicious. A reduction in MUAP duration is the most sensitive indicator of myopathy, and units may be of short duration, yet retain normal amplitude (36). At minimal levels of muscle contraction, it should be possible to discern different MUAPs, to recognize different waveforms, and to estimate the firing rates. Normal patients should be able to recruit and control the discharge of 1–2 units with a finely graded minimal contraction. If this cannot be done, if individual units cannot be identified, or if ≥ 3 MUAPs are activated with a barely perceptible contraction, early recruitment may be present (37). Increased recruitment is a reliable indicator of myopathy, but does not usually appear until late in the course when there has been extensive muscle fiber drop out. It should never be the inital or only finding; by the time it is evident, major changes in MUAP amplitude, duration and configuration should be obvious (35). In late stage myopathies, recruitment may appear decreased (38).

The distribution of abnormalites on NEE may be very restricted. Although most muscle disorders primarily affect proximal muscles, some myopathies are distal. The highest yield of abnormality is in clinically weak muscles. With proximal myopathies, abnormalities are most often seen in the iliopsoas, glutei, spinati and paraspinals (35). Primary muscle disorders may cause anything from minimally abnormal MUAPs in isolation, to blatantly abnormal MUAPs accompanied by spontaneous and increased insertional activity, fibrillation potentials alone, myotonic discharges with or without abnormal MUAPs, or no changes at all. A useful scheme is to group muscle diseases into bland myopathies, myonecrotic myopathies, and the myotonic disorders.

Bland myopathies are those which either produce no detectable electrodiagnostic abnormality, or cause abnormal MUAPs alone, without any accompanying spontaneous or increased insertional activity. The MUAP abnormalities may range from so minimal as to require quantitative EMG to distinguish them from normal, to frank small amplitude, short duration polyphasics. When assessing MUAP duration, it is important to analyze only simple potentials, excluding any long duration polyphasics to avoid spuriously increasing the mean duration (39). Recruitment may range from normal, to subtly increased, to a shower of small, short units producing a complete interference pattern on minimal contraction. Most congenital, metabolic, mitochondrial and endocrine myopathies are bland.

Myonecrotic myopathies are those which not only cause MUAP abnormalities, but also produce muscle membrane instability with fibrillation potentials, positive sharp waves and complex repetitive discharges. The inflammatory myopathies and muscular dystrophies are particularly likely to produce muscle fiber necrosis.

The myotonic disorders include myotonic dystrophy, and several other disorders which are due to abnormal channel function. The defining electrodiagnostic characteristic is myotonic discharges. Myotonic dystrophy also produces the other abnormalities typical of a myonecrotic myopathy

Fibrillation potentials in myonecrotic myopathies may be more difficult to detect than usual. They are frequently of low amplitude, arising from an atrophic or diseased muscle fiber. They may begin to discharge at a very slow rate, then gradually speed up. When examining a patient with suspected myopathy, increase the gain to 50 μV per division and increase the length of the pauses between needle movements. Probing should be slow and deliberate. Fibrillation potentials in myopathy may be patchy and variable in distribution, both between and within muscles. Some believe they are more common at the periphery of the fascicles, and advocate turning on the preamp before inserting the needle. It is particularly important to examine the paraspinal muscles in suspected myopathies. In contrast to the situation in radiculopathy, it is not necessary to specifically probe the multifidus compartment, as the abnormal spontaneous activity is just as readily seen in the more superficial layers.

Continuous Motor Unit Activity (CMUA) Syndromes

Conditions associated with CMUA produce more or less continuous MUAP activity, which is not under the patient's voluntary control (40). Nerve conduction studies are normal. The NEE shows normal appearing MUAPs, often firing as multiplets, but the patient is unable to relax and the activity can never be made to totally disappear. The failure to relax is not deliberate. The motor units are discharging on autopilot, not at the patient's behest. CMUA syndromes include the stiff man syndrome and Issac's syndrome (which goes by a number of other names). In addition to the continuously firing MUAPs, patients with Isaac's syndrome may have spontaneous activity in the form of neuromyotonic, myokymic, and cramp discharges.

Key Points

- Neuromuscular diseases include neuropathic, myopathic, and neuromuscular transmission (NMT) disorders. Neuropathic diseases include neuronopathies, radiculopathies, plexopathies, and peripheral neuropathies. Myopathies may be classified as bland, myonecrotic, or myotonic. NMT disorders are either presynaptic or postsynaptic. Although there may be significant overlap in the clinical neurophysiologic features, electrodiagnostic medicine consultation usually can distinguish between these various conditions and provide localizing and prognostic information.

- Neuronopathies are conditions that affect neurons, either motor or sensory. ALS is the archtypal neuronopathy, producing a picture of widespread acute and chronic denervation with reinnervation, with prominent fasciculations. Motor conduction studies are normal or show loss of M wave amplitude and variable slowing due to axon loss; sensory studies should be normal.

- Radiculopathies may produce abnormalities on the needle electrode examination in a myotomal distribution, including the paraspinal muscles, with no abnormality of motor or sensory conduction studies. The timing of the study is critical, as findings evolve in a dynamic fashion. Fibrillation potentials typically appear in the paraspinal muscles in 7–10 days and in limb muscles in 2–3 weeks, followed by reinnervation. Depending on the duration of the process, fibrillations could be found in any combination of limb and paraspinal muscles.

- The typical electrodiagnostic picture in plexopathy includes abnormal sensory potentials, normal motor conduction studies except for changes due to axon loss, and a needle examination demonstrating abnormalities in the distribution of some plexus component, a trunk or a cord, sparing the paraspinals. Neuralgic amyotrophy, which involves the brachial plexus, and diabetic amyotrophy, which involves the lumbosacral plexus, are the two most common plexopathies. Both produce a spotty axon loss pattern on EMG.

- Peripheral neuropathies may follow one of several electrodiagnostic patterns. The electrodiagnostic medicine evaluation helps to characterize a neuropathy neurophysiologcically, which can provide important insights into possible etiologies, therapeutic approaches, and ultimate prognosis.

- Demyelinating neuropathies typically produce marked slowing of CV with preservation of distal amplitudes. The pattern may be one of uniform, diffuse or segmental, multifocal demyelination, with or without conduction block or temporal dispersion. The likely etiologies of these two patterns are quite different.

- Axonopathies typically produce marked loss of distal M wave and sensory potential amplitudes with relative preservation of CV.

- The electrodiagnostic profile in focal and multifocal neuropathies may include a complicated amalgam of conduction block, focal slowing, and axon loss.

- Presynaptic and postsynaptic NMT disorders produce characteristic electrodiagnostic changes that allow them to be distinguished from each other, and from diseases of nerve or muscle. The two most common NMT disorders are myasthenia gravis (postsynaptic) and the Lambert-Eaton syndrome (presynaptic). Single fiber EMG changes are sensitive but nonspecific indicators of NMT disorders. Repetitive nerve stimulation studies are less sensitive, but more specific for localizing a disorder to the postsynaptic or presynaptic membrane. Decremental responses are most likely to be seen in either type with stimulation at 2–3 Hz. Rapid stimulation or brief, isometric exercise produces different responses in presynaptic and postsynaptic disorders.

- Electrodiagnosis is an invaluable adjunct in the clinical evaluation of patients with suspected myopathy. Although no specific etiologic diagnosis is usually possible, the EMG can place the process into a broad category of likely causes, as well as help exclude other conditions that can mimic myopathy.

- The spectrum of possible electrodiagnostic findings is wide, and may include anything from minimally abnormal MUAPs in isolation, to blatantly abnormal MUAPs accompanied by spontaneous and increased insertional activity, fibrillation potentials alone, myotonic discharges with or without abnormal MUAPs, or no changes at all.

- Motor unit potentials in myopathy are typically short duration, low amplitude, polyphasic units. A MUAP that is both polyphasic and short duration is particularly suspicious. A reduction in MUAP duration is the most sensitive indicator of myopathy. Increased recruitment is a very reliable indicator of myopathy, but does not usually appear until late in the course. In late stage myopathies, recruitment may in fact be decreased and motor units may be long duration and polyphasic. The highest yield of abnormality is in clinically weak muscles.

- It is helpful for diagnostic purposes to broadly group myopathies into bland, myonecrotic, and myotonic categories. Bland myopathies cause either no detectable electrodiagnostic abnormality, or abnormal MUAPs alone. Myonecrotic myopathies cause MUAP abnormalities accompanied by muscle membrane instability with fibrillation potentials, PSWs and CRDs. The inflammatory myopathies and muscular dystrophies are particularly likely to produce muscle fiber necrosis. The myotonic disorders include myotonic dystrophy and other disorders that are due to abnormal channel function. The defining electrodiagnostic characteristic is myotonic discharges.

References

Summaries are not provided for this chapter, as most of these references are abstracted in the relevant chapters on the different disease entities.

1. Denys EH. AAEM case report #5: Amyotrophic lateral sclerosis. Muscle Nerve 1994;17:263–268.
2. Lambert EH. Electromyography in amyotrophic lateral sclerosis. In: Norris FH, Kurland LT, eds. Motor neuron diseases: research on amyotrophic lateral sclerosis and related disorders. New York: Grune & Stratton, 1969.
3. Daube JR. AAEM minimonograph #11: Needle examination in clinical electromyography. Muscle Nerve 1991;14:685–700.
4. So YT, Olney RK. AAEM case report #23: acute paralytic poliomyelitis. Muscle Nerve 1991;14:1159–1164.
5. Donofrio PD. AAEM case report #28: monomelic amyotrophy. Muscle Nerve 1994;17:1129–1134.
6. Pourmand R, Maybury BG. AAEM case report #31: paraneoplastic sensory neuronopathy. Muscle Nerve 1996;19:1517–1522.
7. Wilbourn AJ, Aminoff MJ. AAEE minimonograph #32: the electrophysiologic examination in patients with radiculopathies. Muscle Nerve 1988;11:1099–1114.
8. Haig AJ, Moffroid M, Henry S, et al. A technique for needle localization in paraspinal muscles with cadaveric confirmation. Muscle Nerve 1991;14:521–526.
9. Subramony SH. AAEE case report #14: neuralgic amyotrophy (acute brachial neuropathy). Muscle Nerve 1988;11:39–44.
10. Chokroverty S, Sander HW. AAEM case report #13: diabetic amyotrophy. Muscle Nerve 1996;19:939–945.
11. Albers JW. Clinical neurophysiology of generalized polyneuropathy. J Clin Neurophysiol 1993;10:149–166.
12. Albers JW. AAEE case report #4: Guillain-Barré syndrome. Muscle Nerve 1989;12:705–711.
13. Chad DA. AAEE case report #20: hereditary motor and sensory neuropathy, type I. Muscle Nerve 1989;12:875–882.
14. Parry GJ. AAEM case report #30: multifocal motor neuropathy. Muscle Nerve 1996;19:269–276.
15. Donofrio PD, Albers JW. AAEM minimonograph #34: polyneuropathy: classification by nerve conduction studies and electromyography. Muscle Nerve 1990;13:889–903.
16. Olney RK. AAEM minimonograph #38: neuropathies in connective tissue disease. Muscle Nerve 1992;15:531–542.
17. Miller RG. AAEM case report #1: ulnar neuropathy at the elbow. Muscle Nerve 1991;14:97–101.
18. Ross MA, Kimura J. AAEM case report #2: the carpal tunnel syndrome. Muscle Nerve 1995;18:567–573.
19. DeLisa JA, Saeed MA. AAEE case report #8: The tarsal tunnel syndrome. Muscle Nerve 1983;6:664–670.
20. Wilbourn AJ. AAEE case report #12: Common peroneal mononeuropathy at the fibular head. Muscle Nerve 1986;9:825–836.
21. Olney RK, Hanson M. AAEE case report #15: ulnar neuropathy at or distal to the wrist. Muscle Nerve 1988;11:828–832.
22. Campbell WW. AAEE case report #18: Ulnar neuropathy in the distal forearm. Muscle Nerve 1989;12:347–352.
23. Wertsch JJ. AAEM case report #25: anterior interosseous nerve syndrome. Muscle Nerve 1992;15:977–983.
24. Gilchrist JM. AAEM case report #26: seventh cranial neuropathy. Muscle Nerve 1993;16:447–452.
25. Brown WF, Watson BV. AAEM case report #27: acute retrohumeral radial neuropathies. Muscle Nerve 1993;16:706–711.
26. Kincaid JC. AAEE Minimonograph #31: The electrodiagnosis of ulnar neuropathy at the elbow. Muscle Nerve 1988;11:1005–1015.
27. Stevens JC. AAEE minimonograph #26: The electrodiagnosis of carpal tunnel syndrome. Muscle Nerve 1987;10:99–113.
28. Jablecki CK, Andary MT, So YT, et al. Literature review of the usefulness of nerve conduction studies and electromyography for the evaluation of patients with carpal tunnel syndrome. AAEM Quality Assurance Committee. Muscle Nerve 1993;16:1392–1414.
29. Campbell WW, Greenberg MK, Krendel DA, et al. Literature review of the usefulness of nerve conduction studies and electromyography in the evaluation of patients with ulnar neuropathy at the elbow. Muscle Nerve, in press.
30. Jablecki CK. AAEM case report #3: myasthenia gravis. Muscle Nerve 1991;14:391–397.
31. Keesey JC. AAEE Minimonograph #33: electrodiagnostic approach to defects of neuromuscular transmission. Muscle Nerve 1989;12:613–626.
32. Sanders DB. Clinical neurophysiology of disorders of the neuromuscular junction. J Clin Neurophysiol 1993;10:167–180.
33. Howard JF, Jr., Sanders DB, Massey JM. The electrodi-

agnosis of myasthenia gravis and the Lambert-Eaton myasthenic syndrome. Neurol Clin 1994;12:305–330.

34. Sanders DB, Stalberg EV. AAEM minimonograph #25: single-fiber electromyography. Muscle Nerve 1996;19: 1069–1083.

35. Wilbourn AJ. The electrodiagnostic examination with myopathies. J Clin Neurophysiol 1993;10:132–148.

36. Trojaborg W. Quantitative electromyography in polymyositis: a reappraisal. Muscle Nerve 1990;13:964–971.

37. Petajan JH. AAEM minimonograph #3: motor unit recruitment. Muscle Nerve 1991;14:489–502.

38. Dorfman LJ, Howard JE, McGill KC. Motor unit firing rates and firing rate variability in the detection of neuromuscular disorders. Electroencephalogr Clin Neurophysiol 1989;73:215–224.

39. Uncini A, Lange DJ, Lovelace RE, et al. Long-duration polyphasic motor unit potentials in myopathies: a quantitative study with pathological correlation. Muscle Nerve 1990;13:263–267.

40. Auger RG. AAEM minimonograph #44: diseases associated with excess motor unit activity. Muscle Nerve 1994;17:1250–1263.

12

The Electrodiagnostic Medicine Consultation

"There are only two sorts of doctors: those who practise with their brains and those who practise with their tongues."

Sir William Osler

Patients are referred to the EMG laboratory with sundry problems: neck and arm pain, back and leg pain, suspected carpal tunnel syndrome, suspected peripheral neuropathy, weakness, wasting, cramps, fatigue, nerve injuries and numerous others. The electrodiagnostic medicine consultation is requested to help sort out these problems, establish the etiology, assess severity, and sometimes to provide some objective prognostic information (1). In general, neuromuscular disease has a limited repertoire of clinical presentations; the most salient symptoms are pain, weakness, and disturbances of sensation.

Principles of Clinical Reasoning

Patients are sent to the electrodiagnostic medicine laboratory in search of a diagnosis that explains some clinical complaint. Establishing an accurate diagnosis often makes the difference between truly effective therapy and empirically muddling through. Epistemologic studies have helped to gain an understanding of clinical thinking (2). The precepts of diagnostic reasoning in electrodiagnostic medicine are no different than in the wider clinical arena (3). There are two components to making a diagnosis: information gathering and hypothesis testing. As medical students we learned to gather information *ad nauseam*—the complete history and physical—but were at a loss for what to do with it. An experienced clinician may gather much less information but rapidly arrive at an accurate diagnosis.

The accomplished clinician employs a multi-faceted diagnostic process: gathering information, or searching for clues, using the clues to generate hypotheses that may explain the clinical facts, and testing the hypotheses to see which best matches clinical reality, rejecting those which do not until finally coming to closure by arriving at one best-fit hypothesis which becomes the diagnosis (4). The generation and testing of hypotheses approach is a mark of experience and intimate familiarity with the subject. The inexperienced tend to gravitate to rote information gathering, in hopes the diagnosis will magically emerge at some point. The nonselective search-and-seek strategies that nonexperts tend to use are weak in generating specific hypotheses (5). The more experienced often eschew the gathering of information that will not aid in either generating or testing some hypothesis; less is more. Experts focus on a problem by recognizing patterns and gathering data relevant to a solution to a formulated problem (5). Experts are also more flexible in modifying their initial diagnostic assumptions (6). Whenever confronted with a novel situation, the natural tendency is to fall into that which we know how to do: gather information. Rarely, a characteristic and unmistakable clinical phenomenon permits an instantaneous diagnosis "at a glance," the phenomenon of augenblickdiagnose (7).

The list of hypotheses produced from information gathering is the differential diagnosis. Each hypothesis should be testable, and disprovable or falsifiable. The differential diagnosis is therefore a list of falsifiable hypotheses (3). Some test is then employed in an attempt to falsify the hypothesis, ideally a test whose results definitively exclude one of the diagnostic possibilities. Differential diagnosis is commonly considered in order of probability: Sutton's law ("Why do you keep robbing banks, Willie?". . ."Because that's where the money is") (3). The precepts of Bayes' theorem, which takes into account the prevalence of the disease in the population and the results of prior tests, are often considered intuitively if not formally. Occam's razor, or the principle of parsimony, first articulated by William of Occam, states that the most likely solution is the simplest. In terms of medical diagnosis, it says that the least complex diagnosis is most likely to be correct, or never make two diagnoses when one will do. Usually valid, Occam's razor must be tempered in older patients, who may very well have more than one diagnosis. Another very useful diagnostic aphorism is the so-called barking dog rule (3). Derived from a Sherlock Holmes' story in which a dog did not

TABLE 12.1
Selection of Axioms Relevant to Clinical Reasoning and Diagnostic Principles (3,4,8)

Fisher's rules

- In arriving at a clinical diagnosis, think of the five most common findings (historical, physical findings, or laboratory) found in a given disorder. If at least three of these five are not present in a given patient, the diagnosis is likely to be wrong.
- Resist the temptation to prematurely place a case or disorder into a diagnostic cubbyhole that fits poorly. Allowing it to remain unknown stimulates continuing activity and thought. (Also known as premature closure) (22)
- The details of a case are important; their analysis distinguishes the expert from the journeyman.
- Pay particular attention to the specifics of the patient with a known diagnosis; it will be helpful later when similar phenomena occur in an unknown case.
- Fully accept what you have heard or read only when you have verified it yourself.
- Maintain a lively interest in patients as people.

Other

- When test results are equivocal, the best step is to repeat the testing later ("Susann's Law" from the book *Once is Not Enough* by Jacqueline Susann) (3).
- When the diagnosis is in doubt, take another history.
- Know the limits of the diagnostic tests; it is essential to know the likelihood of a false negative test when interpreting the data (see statistics chapter).
- If a diagnosis is not considered, it is not likely to be made: expand the differential diagnosis
- Diagnosis by exclusion is treacherous if the differential diagnosis is incomplete.
- Uncommon manifestations of common diseases are much more common than common manifestations of uncommon diseases.

bark when a horse was stolen in the night, implying that the thief was someone the dog knew well; it refers to a phenomenon most significant by its absence, e.g., lack of fasciculations is a strong point against the diagnosis of ALS. "Fisher's rules" are clinical maxims collected by Caplan from his observations of C. Miller Fisher, a clinician of legendary diagnostic acumen, some of which are particularly helpful to bear in mind (8). Table 12.1 summarizes these and some other maxims useful from a clinical reasoning perspective. Efforts to emulate clinical electrodiagnostic reasoning with computer programs have had at best mixed success (9).

Errors in clinical reasoning can lead to a variety of adverse consequences. Kassirer and Kopelman found that the two most common sources of error lay in faulty triggering (failure to recognize a possible diagnostic hypothesis) and in faulty information gathering and processing (10). In the latter category, the most common errors related to faulty estimation of disease prevalence (the dictates of Bayes' theorem) and faulty data interpretation. It is important to realize that when the prevalence of a disease is low, a positive test result is likely to be a false-positive unless the test has very high specificity. Among neurologic diagnoses, some of the highest error rates occur when dealing with neuromuscular diseases such as myasthenia gravis and Guillain-Barre syndrome (11). Unfortunately, experience is no guarantee against poor diagnostic reasoning in neurologic patients (12). Some measures to avoid diagnostic errors have been recently reviewed (13).

Principles of Electrodiagnostic Reasoning

There is uniform agreement that electrodiagnostic medicine evaluations are most appropriately done as a high tech extension of a basic history and physical examination (HPE). Only with a preceding HPE can the proposed electrodiagnostic evaluation be adequately planned and placed in proper clinical context. There are two fundamental, slightly contradictory, approaches to performing the electrodiagnostic medicine consultation. The philosophical difference lies in the extent of the preliminary clinical evaluation, and in making recommendations. Some advocate an extensive clinical evaluation prior to the EMG, and a consultation complete with treatment recommendations (14,15). Dumutri formulates two separate impressions, one clinical and the other electrodiagnostic (15). There are countervailing arguments against doing a detailed clinical assessment before the electrodiagnostic study. The electrodiagnostic evaluation should stand as an independent, objective assessment of the clinical problem. Too detailed a clinical assessment runs the potential risk of creating subjective prejudice that might affect the outcome of the electrodiagnostic study. A detailed consult may needlessly duplicate time and effort already spent by the referring MD.

The minimal amount of HPE is that which will suffice at least to plan the examination and to recognize when the problem is not neuromuscular. One should do enough, for instance, to recognize the possibility of a neuromuscular transmission disorder and the need to do repetitive stimulation studies, even if this possibility was not recognized by the referring physician. One should do enough examination to detect weak muscles as they have the greatest yield on needle examination, and to find abnormal reflexes, as they may point to a specific root needing focused evaluation, or signal upper motor neuron dysfunction. Weakness is usually assessed using the MRC scale, in which 5 is normal and 0 is paralyzed. Dr. John K. Wolf has described some elegant techniques for the clinical evaluation of strength (16). Some of the most germane elements of the clinical evaluation are summarized in Table 12.2. A problem-oriented approach is often used, with a more or less standardized set of initial tests done in common, defined clinical situations: neck and arm pain, back and leg pain, suspected CTS, and so forth (15,17). Findings uncovered on this initial screen determine the extent of further testing.

Does one turn every EMG into a formal consultation, requested or not, and charge for it? As physicians, we labor under perverse incentives in almost every situation. Under managed care and capitation, there is an incentive to omit anything of marginal utility, and even not to do things that are clearly

TABLE 12.2

Relevant Aspects of the History and Physical Examination in Patients Presenting for Electrodiagnostic Medicine Consultation

Weakness
  Symmetric
    Generalized
    Proximal
    Distal
  Asymmetric
    Focal
      Peripheral nerve field
      Myotome
    Regional
Facial and other bulbar weakness
Atrophy or hypertrophy
Reflex changes
Sensory loss
Pes cavus and other skeletal deformities
Grip or percussion myotonia
Fasciculations
Abnormalities of eye movement
Pain, tenderness, limitation of motion
Gait
Status of heel cords, EDB muscle bulk
History of infectious disease or anticoagulation

needed. Under fee for service, there is a temptation to do too much. In the end, the best approach is to do whatever is clinically appropriate, to maintain a high quality service, and to resist the pull of perverse incentives.

Referring physicians are not all the same. Some are sophisticated consumers of electrodiagnostic information who are seeking very specific answers to resolve important clinical issues. In our laboratory, a needle examination of the posterior belly of the digastric was recently requested to help decide whether a facial nerve lesion was intra- or extra-canalicular in a patient with a massive laceration of the face and ear, and a fracture of the mastoid. The electrodiagnostic information dictated the surgical approach. To perform a detailed consultation in such a circumstance is ludicrous, to bill for it even more so. An endocrinologist referring a diabetic to assess the severity of neuropathy, or a good orthopedist referring a patient with suspected cervical radiculopathy, is not requesting a detailed clinical assessment. One need only do, for instance, as much as necessary to identify the suspect root and decide whether to do a generic root screen or to focus on one particular root. More than this is not appropriate. On the other hand, a primary care physician referring a patient with generalized weakness when the working clinical diagnosis is obviously fuzzy, is usually seeking all available help. Flexibility is needed.

Dr. Homer Wells, the main character in John Irving's *Cider House Rules* had as his goal in life "to be of use." We should adopt this philosophy and have as our goal to make a clinical contribution to the care of the patient, not do a test. In the final analysis, the patient should be better off for having been to the lab, whether they have only an electrodiagnostic medicine consultation, a separate formal clinical consultation, or both.

There are also two conceptually different diagnostic strategies in performing an electrodiagnostic evaluation. In one, all possibly relevant information is gathered, then analyzed and considered. In the other, hypothesis testing begins early and continues as the study unfolds; the consultant thinks on his or her feet. Unexpected findings may lead to procedures not initially considered, other nerves run, other muscles examined. The process is dynamic, not rote. In one instance, the approach is get the data and think about it later; in the other, it is think about what data is needed; shotgunning vs. focused searching. The former runs the risk of overtesting, the latter the risk of failing to obtain some bit of information that might in retrospect have proven useful. Hypothesis testing tends to lead to efficient accumulation of data and

interpretation of findings as they arise. Stereotypical data collection with analysis after the fact is relatively inefficient (12).

Other Considerations

Communication with the patient in reassuring and understandable layman's language prior to the study is important. Some electrodiagnostic medicine consultants (EMCs) use printed information forms or pamphlets. Although patients certainly are entitled to an explanation of the procedure and the risks, benefits and alternatives, there is some risk of "overconsenting" to the point of frightening the patient out of undergoing a potentially useful study in which the risks of any serious complication are in fact trivial. The vast majority of patients find electrodiagnostic testing only mildly painful, not as bad as expected, and would undergo the procedure again if necessary (18).

One of the most important precepts of electrodiagnostic medicine is to define a distribution of findings, to "surround abnormality with normality." Only in this way can one avoid missing a widespread process. Each study must document normality in some nerves, muscles, or limbs to prove the process is limited to a certain distribution (the field of a root, a plexus, a peripheral nerve, etc), or else conclude that the condition is generalized (such as a myopathy or anterior horn cell disease). This may necessitate examining asymptomatic and clinically uninvolved limbs.

When faced with a patient with an obvious neuromuscular disease, such as generalized neuropathy from well-established diabetes, and an additional focal complaint, such as unilateral hand numbness, it is often helpful to gain perspective by initially screening an asymptomatic region, or at least one that is not involved in the presenting complaint. This helps to lay a backdrop against which to judge any abnormalities involving the focally symptomatic area.

Because of the problems on the one hand of detecting abnormality when electrodiagnostic changes are mild, and on the other hand of interpreting the sometimes confusing changes of endstage disease, it is best to decide where to begin the examination based on the severity of involvement. For instance, with a severe, generalized polyneuropathy, it is best to begin the examination with the least involved areas, as the most involved nerves may well not respond to electrical stimuli, or decreased M wave amplitude may make interpretations of conduction velocity changes difficult. When the neuropathy is mild, the least involved areas may well be normal and it is then best to begin with the most involved areas. As a general approach, study the most involved muscle or nerve when the process is mild and the least involved one when the process is severe.

Situations commonly arise in which the study results are equivocal or borderline. Examples include a nerve conduction parameter just at the limit of normal, minimally increased insertional activity with a few, brief runs of unsustained positive sharp waves, or a borderline decrement on repetitive nerve stimulation. Should the EMC report the study to the referring physician as normal, abnormal or equivocal? In general, it is best to undercall abnormalities. The EMC should recognize the limitations of electrodiagnostic testing in terms of pathophysiology, timing, statistics and other factors that might result in a false-positive (type I error). One of the strengths of electrodiagnosis is its low incidence of false positives, which should not be undermined by overcalling minor changes. As a broad generalization, false-negatives are preferable to false-positives. Language such as "trivial abnormalities of uncertain clinical significance; clinical correlation required" are useful under such circumstances.

Patients may be referred to the lab to "rule out" a particular problem, such as carpal tunnel syndrome. Faced with normal median motor and sensory conduction studies the EMC can adopt either of two approaches: stop the study, having ruled out carpal tunnel as requested, or make an effort (clinical or electrodiagnostic) to "rule in" some other entity that might explain the patient's symptomatology. The latter is always preferable. The "rule in" approach is much more likely to provide a helpful service to the patient and the referring physician than the "rule out" approach.

The EMC must always bear in mind that a normal study does not exclude disease, for a variety of reasons. Electrodiagnostic abnormalities evolve in a dynamic fashion related to the pathophysiologic sequence of events which disease or injury produces. Other limitations include sampling error and the sensitivity of different procedures. When clinically indicated, a repeat examination several weeks later will often disclose abnormalities not detected initially.

The Unindicated Study

Patients are sometimes sent to the lab for inappropriate reasons. EMCs are often skilled neuromuscular clinicians with unique expertise in caring for particular patients. In some situations it may be easier to obtain an EMG than a neurologic or physiatric consultation and referring physicians may succumb to the temptation of substituting the one for the other.

On the other hand, patients are sometimes sent for electrodiagnostic medicine consultation who clearly do not need it. The preliminary clinical evaluation reveals a mild, spastic hemiparesis or an impingement syndrome of the shoulder, or a patient with radiculopathy presents 3 days after the onset of symptoms. Does one proceed with the study as requested, perform some token evaluation, or send the patient away? It is best, if possible, to discuss the situation with the referring physician and diplomatically give him or her the option of canceling or rescheduling the study. If this is not possible and the study is not done, a explanation to the referring physician is called for. On a few occasions I have refused to do a study: in a child with congenital absence of a pectoral muscle, a patient with referred shoulder pain from liver metastases, another with Dupuytren's contracture mistaken for an ulnar griffe. By not doing a study which is not indicated, more patients who really need electrodiagnostic evaluation may be referred in the future.

Reports

Physicians refer patients to the electrodiagnostic medicine laboratory for evaluation, and the EMC in turn renders a report that summarizes the results of the study and concludes with a diagnostic impression, and sometimes with recommendations.

EMG reports may be done in a number of different ways, but the two broad report categories are tabular and narrative. In a tabular report, the numeric data are summarized in a graphic format of some design, followed by a summary and/or an impression. In a narrative report, the study, including the numeric information, is dictated. The tabular format is vastly preferable. It is very difficult to extract information from a narrative report, and they should be avoided whenever possible. A verbose and lengthy report runs the risk of being skimmed or not read at all. Arcane terminology should be avoided. For instance, most of the world knows the entity of carpal tunnel syndrome by that specific name. To insist on calling it "median neuropathy at the wrist" is not only anatomically incorrect, as the lesion is actually in the hand, but may be frankly obfuscatory to the referring physician. On the other hand, such terms as tardy ulnar palsy and cubital tunnel syndrome are used with such variability and imprecision they should be avoided.

Only a few referring physicians will understand the intricacies and esoterica of an electrodiagnostic medicine report. Most will read only the final summary and impression. It is important to be brief and clear, trying to convey the essential information in an understandable way. The reader of the EMC's report should come away with clinically helpful information, succinctly and unambiguously presented.

Rarely, a referring physician may object to the EMC telling the patient the results of their study. This is idiosyncratic and by and large inappropriate. As a general rule, the patient is entitled to know in layman's terms what was found. However, recommendations regarding clinical management should be made directly to the referring physician. The AAEM ethics guidelines expressly caution against discussing clinical management issues directly with the patient unless the referring physician has requested the EMC participate in clinical management.

Ethics

The AAEM has outlined some principles of medical ethics for the practice of electrodiagnostic medicine (19). A later publication by the AAEM Ethics and Peer Review Committee discusses these issues in greater detail (20). The EMC must not decline to care for a patient because of their ethnic origin, gender or known medical diagnosis. The consultant has a duty to communicate with the patient. Consultations should only be performed which are within the scope of the practitioner's training, experience and professional competence. This admonition is particularly appropriate for nonphysicians attempting to practice electrodiagnostic medicine. Competency, education and training issues are elaborated on in the Guidelines (19). In training situations, the new HCFA Teaching Physician regulations require the attending consultant to be physically present during the key portions of the examination. Miller and Nora have recently debated the issue of informed consent in electrodiagnostic testing (21).

Key Points

- The accomplished clinician employs a multi-faceted diagnostic process: gathering information, or searching for clues, using the clues to generate hypotheses that may explain the clinical facts, and testing the hypotheses to see which best matches clinical reality, rejecting those which do not until finally coming to closure by arriving at one best-fit hypothesis that becomes the diagnosis. The generation and testing of the hypotheses approach is a mark of experience and intimate familiarity with the subject.

- The differential diagnosis is therefore a list of falsifiable hypotheses. Differential diagnosis is commonly considered in order of probability.

- Occam's razor, or the principle of parsimony, says that the least complex diagnosis is most likely to be correct, or never make two diagnoses when one will do. The barking dog rule refers to a phenomenon most significant by its absence, e.g., lack of fasciculations is a strong point against the diagnosis of ALS. "Fisher's rules" are clinical maxims helpful to bear in mind in diagnostic reasoning.

- Common sources of diagnostic error are recognizable. Some of the highest error rates occur when dealing with neuromuscular diseases such as myasthenia gravis and Guillain-Barre syndrome.

- There is uniform agreement that electrodiagnostic medicine evaluations are most appropriately done as an extension of a basic history and physical.

- There are two fundamental, slightly contradictory, approaches to performing the electrodiagnostic medicine consultation. The philosophical difference lies in the extent of the preliminary clinical evaluation and in making recommendations. The minimal amount of HPE is that which will suffice at least to plan the examination and to recognize when the problem is not neuromuscular.

- Referring physicians are not all the same. Some are sophisticated consumers of electrodiagnostic information who are seeking very specific answers to resolve important clinical issues. Other are seeking all available help.

- We should have as our goal to make a clinical contribution to the care of the patient, not do a test.

- There are also two conceptually different diagnostic strategies in electrodiagnostic medicine. In one, all possibly relevant information is gathered, then analyzed and considered. In the other, hypothesis testing begins early and continues as the study unfolds. In one instance, the approach is get the data and think about it later; in the other, it is think about what data is needed.

- Communication with the patient before the study is important. There is some risk of "overconsenting" to the point of frightening the patient out of undergoing a potentially useful study in which the risks of any serious complication are in fact trivial. The vast majority of patients find electrodiagnostic testing only mildly painful, not as bad as expected, and would undergo the procedure again if necessary.

- One of the most important precepts of electrodiagnostic medicine is to define a distribution of findings, to "surround abnormality with normality." Only in this way can one avoid missing a widespread process. Study the most involved muscle or nerve when the process is mild and the least involved one when the process is severe.

- Situations not uncommonly arise in which the study results are equivocal or borderline. As a broad generalization, false-negatives are preferable to false-positives.

- The "rule in" approach to EMG is much more likely to provide a helpful service to the patient and the referring physician than the "rule out" approach.

- The electrodiagnostic medicine consultant must always bear in mind that a normal study does not exclude disease, for a variety of reasons.
- Dealing with patients who are sometimes sent to the lab for inappropriate reasons is a delicate matter.
- EMG reports may be done in a number of different ways, but the two broad report categories are tabular and narrative. The tabular format is vastly preferable. The reader of the electrodiagnostic medicine consultant's report should come away with clinically helpful information, succinctly and unambiguously presented.* The AAEM has outlined some principles of medical ethics for the practice of electrodiagnostic medicine.

References

1. Campbell WW. Entrapment neuropathies. In: Gilchrist JM, ed. Prognosis in Neurology. Boston: Butterworth-Heinemann, 1998.

2. Gifford DR, Mittman BS, Vickrey BG. Diagnostic reasoning in neurology. Neurol Clin 1996;14:223–238.
   Studies examining physicians' clinical decisions have demonstrated considerable variation in decisions and practices and identified numerous challenges to effective, efficient, and accurate decision making. Although use of the decision aids and tools described in this article may help overcome many of these challenges, greater self-awareness of the diagnostic reasoning process and the factors influencing decisions also should help improve clinical decisions and reduce variation, irrespective of the use of these tools. Continued research into the determinants and nature of the diagnostic reasoning process will provide additional insights that can be used to develop and apply improved decision aids and corrective procedures to overcome persistent problems.

3. Sapira JD. The art and science of bedside diagnosis. Baltimore: Urban & Schwarzenberg, 1990.529–540.

4. DeGowin RL. DeGowin & DeGowin's beside diagnostic examination. New York: McGraw-Hill, 1993.1–48.

5. Kassirer JP. Diagnostic reasoning. Ann Intern Med 1989;110:893–900.
   Research in cognitive science, decision sciences, and artificial intelligence has yielded substantial insights into the nature of diagnostic reasoning. Many elements of the diagnostic process have been identified, and many principles of effective clinical reasoning have been formulated. Three reasoning strategies are considered here: probabilistic, causal, and deterministic. Probabilistic reasoning relies on the statistical relations between clinical variables and is frequently used in formal calculations of disease likelihoods. Probabilistic reasoning is especially useful in evoking diagnostic hypotheses and in assessing the significance of clinical findings and test results. Causal reasoning builds a physiologic model and assesses a patient's findings for coherency and completeness against the model; it functions especially effectively in verification of diagnostic hypotheses. Deterministic reasoning consists of sets of compiled rules generated from routine, well-defined practices. Much human problem solving may derive from activation and implementation of such rules. A deeper understanding of clinical cognition should enhance clinical teaching and patient care.

6. Arocha JF, Patel VL, Patel YC. Hypothesis generation and the coordination of theory and evidence in novice diagnostic reasoning. Med Decis Making 1993;13:198–211.
   This study investigates hypothesis generation and evaluation in clinical problem solving by medical trainees. The study focuses on 1) directionality of reasoning and 2) use of confirmation and disconfirmation strategies in generating and evaluating hypotheses. Two clinical problems were divided into segments of information containing presenting complaint, past history, and physical examination. The initial information indicated a typical myocardial infarct but subsequent information contradicted it. The results showed that the participating students predominantly used forward reasoning and confirmation strategies. When faced with contradictory evidence: 1) second-year students ignored cues in the problem or reinterpreted them to fit the hypothesis; 2) third-year students generated concurrent hypotheses to account for different sets of data; and 3) fourth-year students generated several initial hypotheses and subsequently narrowed the hypothesis space by generating a single coherent diagnostic explanation. The results are discussed in terms of coordination of clinical evidence and its relationship to scientific reasoning.

7. Campbell WW. Augenblickdiagnose. Semin Neurol 1998;18:169–176.

8. Caplan LR. Fisher's Rules. Arch Neurol 1982;39:389–390.
   C. Miller Fisher is a clinician whose methods and style deserve the same attention given his accomplishments. The 17 "rules" presented summarize some of the basic principles he has followed in the practice of medicine.

9. Vingtoft S, Fuglsang-Frederiksen A, Ronager J, et al. KANDID—an EMG decision support system—evaluated in a European multicenter trial. Muscle Nerve 1993;16:520–529.
   KANDID is an advanced EMG decision support system dedicated to the support of the clinical neurophysiologist during EMG examinations. It has facilities for test planning, automatized and structured data interpretation, EMG diagnosis, explanation, and reporting. In a prospective trial, the agreement levels between clinical neurophysiologists and KANDID's diagnostic statements were measured under ordinary clinical EMG practice. The diagnostic agreement with KANDID was, on average, 61%. A pronounced interexaminer variation in the agreement level related to the different EMG centers was observed.

10. Kassirer JP, Kopelman RI. Cognitive errors in diagnosis: instantiation, classification, and consequences. Am J Med 1989;86:433–441.
    A study of diagnostic errors caused by faulty clinical cognition by analysis of transcripts of problem-solving exercises published in a pedagogic series of clinical reasoning. The analysis disclosed multiple errors in cognition and produced a provisional classification of these errors based on a framework derived from cognitive science. Faults in cognition were identified in all steps of the diagnostic process, including triggering, context formulation, information gathering and processing, and verification. Detailed specific examples of each type of error is provided, and the consequences of each error identified. A classification of cognitive errors is a step toward a deeper understanding of the epidemiology, causes, and prevention of diagnostic errors.

11. Wei SC, Tsai JJ. Bedside diagnosis for neurological residents in neurological emergencies: a retrospective analy-

sis. Chung Hua I Hsueh Tsa Chih (Taipei) 1994;53: 331–337.

This study examined the common errors of daily practice among neurological residents. The overall rate of diagnostic error and the frequency of diagnostic inaccuracy in various disease entities were evaluated. The reason for the diagnostic error was determined by reviewing the records regarding the entire diagnostic process. In 1336 consecutive patients the initial bedside diagnosis was correct in 901 (67%) patients. The diagnoses were incorrect in 266 (20%) patients. The highest rate of inaccuracy was found in the diagnosis of subdural hematoma (56%). The other common diseases of high rate of diagnostic inaccuracy were myasthenia gravis (50%), subarachnoid hemorrhage (42%), Guillain-Barre syndrome (40%), traumatic disorders (39%), herniation of intervertebral disc (33%), metabolic encephalopathy (30%), infection of central nervous system (30%), intracranial neoplasm (24%), drug overdose or intoxication (22%), and mixed neurological and metabolic encephalopathy (21%). The explored reasons for diagnostic inaccuracy were errors of reasoning (38%), inadequate data base (35%), and inadequate fund of knowledge (27%).

12. Chimowitz MI, Logigian EL, Caplan LR. The accuracy of bedside neurological diagnoses. Ann Neurol 1990; 28:78–85.

The accuracy of bedside diagnoses was prospectively studied in patients admitted to a neurology service. Each patient was evaluated independently by a junior resident, a senior resident, and a staff neurologist, who were required to make an anatomical and etiological diagnosis based solely on the history and physical examination. In a series of 86 patients, it was possible to confirm anatomical and etiological diagnoses in 40 by matching the clinical syndromes with highly specific laboratory findings. In 40 patients with laboratory confirmed final diagnoses, the clinical diagnoses of the junior residents, senior residents, and staff neurologists were correct in 26 (65%), 30 (75%), and 31 (77%), respectively. There was a trend for error rates to be higher among junior residents than staff ($p = 0.06$). The errors by the junior residents, <senior residents>, (staff) were attributed to incomplete history and examination in 4 <1> (0), inadequate fund of knowledge in 4 <3> (3), and poor diagnostic reasoning in 6 <6> (6). These results indicate that technology is not a-panacea for our diagnostic difficulties and that there is room for improvement in our clinical skills, especially diagnostic reasoning.

13. Staiger T, Paauw DS. Strategies for reducing diagnostic errors. Res Staff Phys 1996;42:55–63.

Errors are an inevitable aspect of caring for patients. Clinical practice is too complex to expect that they can be eliminated entirely, but there are strategies that may allow serious errors to be reduced. The authors present some techniques to reduce diagnostic errors. 1) When the diagnosis is in doubt, take another history. 2) A careful physical examination will often provide clues to the presence or absence of a serious condition. 3) Know the limits of the diagnostic tests. 4) If a diagnosis is not considered, it is not likely to be made; expand the differential diagnosis. 5) If the diagnosis remains in doubt of a condition that may present a significant health risk, seek the advice of a colleague or a consultant. 6) Beware of overinterpretation and premature closure. 7) A knowledge of the natural history of the symptoms and the diagnoses can be a key diagnostic tool. 8) Remember that psychosocial factors can generate or magnify symptoms. 9) A reminder of the famous maxim, "the secret of the care of the patient is caring for the patient."

14. Murray SA, Johnson EW, Pease WS. Quality improvement for the electrodiagnostic consultation. In: Johnson EW, Pease WS, eds. Practical electromyography. 3rd ed. Baltimore: Williams and Wilkins, 1997.15–40.

15. Dumitru D. Electrodiagnostic medicine. Philadelphia: Hanley & Belfus, 1995.

16. Wolf JK. Segmental neurology: a guide to the examination and interpretation of sensory and motor function. Baltimore: University Park Press, 1981.

See chapter 3 for abstract.

17. Daube JR. Application of clinical neurophysiology: assessing symptom complexes. In: Daube JR, ed. Clinical neurophysiology. Philadelphia: F.A. Davis, Co. 1996. 473–498.

18. Kothari MJ, Preston DC, Plotkin GM, et al. Electromyography: do the diagnostic ends justify the means? Arch Phys Med Rehabil 1995;76:947–949.

The results of two separate surveys on 126 and 100 consecutive patients referred to an EMG laboratory to determine if EMG/NCS was beneficial to the referring physician and to compare the level of anxiety experienced by patients before the study with the pain actually experienced during the study. The electrodiagnosis was discordant from the referring diagnosis in 39% of the patients with an abnormal EMG/NCS. Pretest anxiety levels were low in 59% of the patients, medium in 27%, and high in 14%. After the tests, 82% of the patients said that the test was not as bad as expected, and was generally only mildly painful. Ninety-three responded that they would have the test performed again. The authors conclude that EMG/NCS often suggest alternative diagnoses, and the actual pain experienced during an EMG/NCS study is significantly less than expected.

19. Guidelines in electrodiagnostic medicine. American Association of Electrodiagnostic Medicine. Muscle Nerve 1992;15:229–253.

20. The AAEM Ethics and Peer Review Committee. Guidelines for ethical behavior relating to clinical practice issues in electrodiagnostic medicine. American Association of Electrodiagnostic Medicine. Muscle Nerve 1994; 17:965–967.

Guidelines for ethical behavior relating to clinical practice issues in electrodiagnostic medicine were developed to formalize the standards of professional behavior for electrodiagnostic medical consultants. The guidelines are modeled after the Code of Professional Conduct of the American Academy of Neurology and are consistent with the Guidelines in Electrodiagnostic Medicine of the AAEM and Principles of Medical Ethics as adopted by the American Medical Association. Topics covered include the patient-consultant relationship, general principles of electrodiagnostic medicine consultation (professional competence, confidentiality, record keeping, fees, and appropriateness of services), personal conduct, conflicts of interest, relationships with other professionals, relationships with the public and community, and clinical research.

21. Miller RG, Nora LM. Written informed consent for electrodiagnostic testing: pro and con. Muscle Nerve 1997; 20:352–356.

Dr. Miller argues proposes a number of reasons to consider obtaining written informed consent for electrodiagnostic studies. Dr. Nora counters that written informed consent is currently not proscribed but also not mandated, and that this standard should not be changed without demonstrating that the proposed alternative will result in improved patient care.

22. McSherry D. Avoiding premature closure in sequential diagnosis. Artif Intell Med 1997;10:269–283.

An important aspect of diagnostic reasoning is the ability to recognize when there is sufficient evidence to enable a working diagnosis to be made and thus avoid the unnecessary risks and costs of further testing. On the other hand, the reasoner must be careful to avoid the error, known as premature closure, of accepting a diagnosis before it is fully verified. In the absence of a more rigorous approach to verification, a pragmatic approach adopted in many programs for sequential diagnosis is to discontinue testing when the probability of the leading hypothesis reaches an arbitrary threshold. Experimental results are presented to illustrate the potential unreliability of this approach. A more reliable way to avoid premature closure is to discontinue testing only when the lower bound for the probability of the leading hypothesis reaches an acceptably high level. A termination strategy informed by upper and lower bounds for the probability of the leading hypothesis may help to avoid both premature closure and undue prolongation of the testing process. Based on the independence Bayesian framework, the theory presented extends a probabilistic model of hypothetico-deductive reasoning designed to enable programs for sequential diagnosis in medicine to emulate the reasoning processes of human diagnosticians. See also: Dubeau CE, Voytovich AE, Rippey RM. Premature conclusions in the diagnosis of iron-deficiency anemia: cause and effect. Med Decis.Making 1986;6:169–173; and Voytovich AE, Rippey RM, Suffredini A. Premature conclusions in diagnostic reasoning. J Med Educ 1985;60:302–307.

P A R T

CLINICAL APPLICATIONS

C H A P T E R

13

Neuronopathies

The term neuronopathy refers to disease affecting the nerve cell body, either the motor neuron in the ante-rior horn or cerebral cortex, or the sensory neuron in the dorsal root ganglion. Neuronopathies occur in many forms. Most are acquired disorders, but heredi-tary forms are common, usually presenting in infancy or childhood as one of the varieties of spinal muscular atrophy (SMA). Motor neuronopathies are much more common than sensory neuronopathies. Amyotrophic lateral sclerosis (ALS) and its variants and the heredi-tary SMA syndromes account for the overwhelming majority of motor neuronopathies.

Motor Neuronopathy

Motor neuronopathies result in degeneration of motor neurons, either in the spinal cord or in the cerebral cortex, or both. Curiously, the motor neurons supply-ing the eye muscles and the bladder usually escape. Rarely, minimal sensory dysfunction accompanies the motor system devastation.

Different combinations of involvement result in a variety of clinical syndromes. Acquired motor neuron-opathies most often produce involvement of both the upper motor neuron (UMN) and lower motor neuron (LMN), resulting in the characteristic syndrome of classical ALS. Pure UMN dysfunction produces spas-ticity without amyotrophy, the rare syndrome of pri-mary lateral sclerosis. Pure LMN dysfunction pro-duces amyotrophy without spasticity, the common syndrome of acquired SMA or LMN ALS. Progressive bulbar palsy refers to LMN dysfunction beginning in bulbar muscles, and carries a dire prognosis. The most common syndrome by far is classic ALS, with both amyotrophy and spasticity. Even patients with seemingly pure LMN involvement often have abnormalities of the corticospinal tracts at autopsy, suggesting subclinical UMN involvement.

ALS runs its course in 3–4 years in most patients (1). About 15–20%, most often those with predominant LMN dysfunction, run a more benign clinical course with prolonged survival. Some of these seem to go into a remission of sorts, with no or only minimal progression for long periods of time (2,3). The British physicist, Steven Hawking, has had ALS for many, many years.

Hereditary motor neuronopathies are usually restricted to the LMN. Most common are the various SMA syndromes, which are separated into different types depending on the age of onset and clinical course: SMA I (Werdnig-Hoffman disease), SMA II (the intermediate form, or chronic infantile form), SMA III (Kugelberg-Welander disease, or the juvenile form) and SMA IV (the adult form).

The electrophysiologic diagnosis of motor neuronopathy requires the demonstration of diffuse neuropathic abnormalities without other explanation. Neuropathy, plexopathy and radiculopathy must be excluded. Generally, motor NCV is normal but loss of axons in the peripheral nerve due to degeneration of motor neurons can produce some slowing of CV, especially when recording from a muscle where there is severe weakness and atrophy. The degree of slowing still consistent with motor neuron disease is debatable, but slowing in the demyelinating range clearly suggests the presence of another disease process. Marked slowing in the indeterminant range between clear demyelination and clear axon loss becomes quite problematic when evaluating patients who may have an ALS mimicker, such as multifocal motor neuropathy, which can resemble the LMN form of ALS. Sensory conduction studies should be normal.

Before making a diagnosis of motor neuronopathy, needle examination should demonstrate characteristic abnormalities in a diffuse distribution. These are chronic, progressive denervating syndromes, and the electrodiagnostic picture is typically a combination of denervation and compensatory reinnervation. The characteristic abnormalities are very large amplitude, usually 4–10x normal, and long duration MUAPs (due to reinnervation), fibrillation potentials (due to ongoing denervation) and fasciculations (4). The large amplitude, long duration MUPs are sometimes called giant units, though exactly how large a unit must be to qualify for this designation is not precisely defined. Reinnervation also leads to complexity of the MUPs with polyphasicity, increased fragmentation and turns, and frequently late components or satellite potentials. Occasional patients with rapidly progressive

disease may not demonstrate evidence of reinnervation. Sometimes, small amplitude highly polyphasic "pseudomyopathic" MUAPs appear, particularly in the SMA syndromes. A combination of large and small fibrillation potentials may arise from the mixture of recently and remotely denervated muscle fibers. Only rarely does a patient with ALS fail to demonstrate impressive fasciculations, but in some of the hereditary SMA conditions fasciculations may be minimal or absent.

The characteristic abnormalities should be demonstrated in a multi-nerve, multi-root distribution in at least three limbs, with the head and the thoracic paraspinals counting as "limbs." The best bulbar muscle to examine is the genioglossus; abnormalities there, especially fibrillations, convincingly affirm the diffuseness of the process. The electrodiagnostic findings expected in motor neuronopathy are listed in Table 13.1.

AMYOTROPHIC LATERAL SCLEROSIS (ALS)

ALS is most often a sporadic disease, but about 5–10% of cases are familial. In about 20% of familial cases, a mutation has been identified in the gene that codes for superoxide dismutase (SOD). The precise mechanism by which this abnormality produces motor neu-

TABLE 13.1
Electrodiagnostic Findings Typical of Motor Neuronopathies

Normal motor NCVs, or slowing in proportion to axon loss
Decreased M wave amplitude in proportion to muscle atrophy
Normal sensory potentials
Motor unit action potential abnormalities
   Decreased recruitment
   Decreased number of MUAPs
   Fast firing
   Increased amplitude and duration
   Increased complexity
      Increased turns
      Polyphasicity
      Late components
Fibrillations and positive sharp waves
Fasciculations
Needle examination abnormalities in a diffuse distribution
   Multinerve/multiroot
   At least 3 limbs and associated paraspinals
   Head and thoracic paraspinals may count as limbs

ron disease remains unclear, nor is there any explanation for the majority of patients with familial ALS who have no SOD defect.

The etiology of the sporadic form and of the familial cases without the SOD mutation remains elusive. The many etiologic possibilities considered over the years have not panned out, and numerous trials to find effective therapy have failed. Currently, it seems most likely the disease is multifactorial; somehow related to excitotoxicity, probably driven by glutamate, under the influence of genetic and environmental factors and possibly contributed to by oxidative stress and free radical formation (5,6) The glutamate antagonist, riluzole, has been proven effective but only slows the disease slightly (7). Gabapentin, neurotrophic factors, antioxidants and drug combinations continue to be explored as treatments. The disease produces a steady but variable rate of decline, and rarely may spontaneously remit (1–3).

The electrophysiologic hallmark of ALS is diffuse acute and chronic denervation with reinnervation (8). As the disease begins, motor neurons degenerate, leaving denervated muscle fibers. These are reinnervated by surviving motor neurons. This reinnervation produces chronic neurogenic MUAP changes: decreased recruitment and large amplitude, long duration, complex, polyphasic MUAPs. The mean increase in amplitude is 4x normal and the mean increase in duration is 35% (4). The more chronic the disease process the larger the amplitude, the longer the duration, and the greater the complexity. Early in the disease, if reinnervation is efficient, spontaneous activity may be sparse or lacking. As motor neurons continue to degenerate, reinnervation can no longer keep pace with denervation. Weakness and atrophy progress, and fibrillations appear. Well-established disease thus typically demonstrates a combination of chronic neurogenic MUAP changes and fibrillations. The fibrillations are often a mixture of large and small because of acute superimposed on chronic denervation. The small fibrillations arise from atrophic fibers where denervation is long standing, and the large fibrillations from more recently denervated fibers. The intensity and distribution of fibrillations and the CMAP amplitudes provide the best prognostic information (9).

Fasciculations are also characteristic of motor neuron disease, although their exact mechanism remains debatable. For many years, fasciculations were thought to represent the dying gasps of sick motor neurons. Current evidence indicates they more likely arise much more distally in the neuron, perhaps in immature, unstable peripheral sprouts (10). Whichever is the case, they serve as a very useful marker for ALS. The diagnosis should always remain circumspect when fasciculations are not demonstrable.

Typical needle exam abnormalities are more often demonstrable in clinically weak muscles. The EMG should therefore be preceded by a careful clinical examination in order to test the muscles of greatest potential yield. Denervation changes are characteristically widespread. Most EMGers require the demonstration of denervation in at least three extremities in order to state that the patient meets criteria for the diagnosis. The thoracic paraspinals and the bulbar muscles may count as an extremity. The thoracic paraspinals are particularly useful because they are often involved in ALS, and seldom involved in spondylosis (11). In the arms and legs, abnormalities should be demonstrated in at least two muscles which do not share the same peripheral nerve or nerve root innervation. Denervation in bulbar muscles is difficult to demonstrate except in advanced cases. The bulbar muscle most often examined is the genioglossus, and its evaluation is usually hampered by poor relaxation, making fibrillations and fasciculations difficult to appreciate. Patients with rapidly progressive disease and inefficient reinnervation may occasionally lack the large amplitude chronic neurogenic MUAPs which otherwise typify the disease. Patients with very early, rapidly progressive or far advanced disease may occasionally have low amplitude, polyphasic "nascent" units which simulate myopathy. The clinical picture usually suffices to make the distinction.

Sensory nerve conduction studies should be normal in ALS although trivial abnormalities of uncertain pathogenesis have been reported (12). Apparent sensory abnormalities may be due to cold temperature in a wasted, flaccid extremity. An occasional ALS patient may have a coincidental entrapment syndrome.

Motor conduction studies are usually normal. However, due to axon loss and random (maybe even preferential) involvement of large diameter fibers, some slowing of maximal motor CV can clearly occur in ALS. The question is, how much slowing is permissible? The degree of CV slowing is related to loss of M wave amplitude. The CV when recording from relatively unaffected muscles should be normal, or very nearly so. When recording from extremely atrophic muscles, the CV may be unreliable (12). The Lambert criteria state that slowing should not be below 70% of the average normal (4). Most labs do not know their average normal, and typically make decisions according to the lower limit of normal. As an approximation, 80–85% of the lower normal limit approximates 70% of the average normal value. In ALS, the motor NCV rarely falls to <80% of the lower limit of normal (13). The CNTF study criteria state that CV

TABLE 13.2
Lambert Criteria for the Diagnosis of ALS (4)

1. Fibrillation and fasciculation potentials in muscles of the lower and the upper extremities, or the extremities and the head
2. Reduction in number and increase in amplitude and duration of motor unit potentials
3. Normal electrical excitability of the remaining fibers of motor nerves, and motor fiber CV within the normal range in nerves of relatively unaffected muscles, and not less than 70 per cent of the average normal value according to age in nerves of more severely affected muscles.
4. Normal excitability and CV of afferent nerve fibers even in severely affected extremities

should be normal when M wave amplitude is >50% of the lower normal limit, and that CV is generally ≥80% of the lower normal limit when M wave amplitude is <50% (14). Thus, slowing to less than 80–85% of the lower limit of normal should be viewed with suspicion and suggests the possibility of an alternative diagnosis. Conduction block or significant temporal dispersion at a site not normally prone to compression should also cast suspicion on the diagnosis.

There are several electrophysiologic curiosities that occasionally occur. H-reflexes may appear outside their usual distribution because of upper motor neuron involvement. Sometimes CRDs are prominent. Myotonia has been reported, but true myotonic discharges must be exceedingly rare. Reinnervating axonal sprouts may have immature unstable neuromuscular junctions, and precarious neuromuscular transmission at these immature junctions can produce findings associated with neuromuscular transmission disorders: a decremental response on repetitive nerve stimulation; jitter and blocking on single fiber EMG (4,15). Because of these secondary neuromuscular transmission defects patients are sometimes treated symptomatically with anticholinesterase agents, particularly to improve swallowing. The pattern of abnormality on repetitive nerve stimulation (RNS) can simulate that seen in myasthenia gravis. The clinical picture usually, but not always, suffices to make the distinction. Neuromuscular transmission abnormalities are more common in active, progressive disease and imply a poor prognosis.

A large ALS clinic reported confirmation of an initial impression of ALS in 95% of cases, but clinicians who do not see ALS patients frequently may struggle with the diagnosis (16). About 40% of patients are initially misdiagnosed; patients frequently undergo unnecessary tests and occasionally undergo unnecessary surgery. The two sets of diagnostic criteria in common use are the Lambert criteria (Table 13.2) and the World Federation of Neurology (WFN or El Escorial) criteria (Table 13.3) (4,17). The El Escorial criteria have been validated (18). Another set of criteria was used for the CNFT study (14). A significant proportion of patients may not fulfill strict neurophysiologic criteria for the diagnosis on initial testing (12).

There are several regularly recurrent problem scenarios in the evaluation of patients with suspected ALS. These conditions are discussed in more detail in their respective chapters, the emphasis here is on the differential diagnosis with ALS. Modern imaging stud-

TABLE 13.3
World Federation of Neurology, or El Escorial, Criteria for the Diagnosis of ALS (17)

Clinical features required for the diagnosis
(1) Signs of lower motor neuron degeneration (weakness, wasting and fasciculation in one or more of the four regions (bulbar, cervical, thoracic, lumbosacral)
(2) Signs of upper motor neuron degeneration (increased or clonic tendon reflexes, spasticity, pseudobulbar features, Hoffman reflexes and extensor plantar response) in one or more of the four regions
(3) Progression

Clinical features that support the diagnosis include
(1) Fasciculations in one or more regions
(2) Abnormal pulmonary function not explained by other causes
(3) Abnormal speech studies not explained by other causes
(4) Abnormal swallowing studies not explained by other causes
(5) Abnormal larynx function studies not explained by other causes
(6) Abnormal isokinetic or isometric strength tests in clinically uninvolved muscles
(7) Abnormal muscle biopsy with evidence of denervation

Clinical findings inconsistent with the diagnosis include one or more of the following not explained by physiological changes associated with aging or other disease processes
(1) Sensory dysfunction
(2) Sphincter abnormalities
(3) Autonomic nervous system dysfunction
(4) Anterior visual pathway abnormalities
(5) Parkinson's disease
(6) Alzheimer's disease

ies can help greatly. Not only may MRIs of the cervical or lumbar spine disclose structural abnormalities, but altered signal intensity in the motor cortex and corticospinal tracts on head MRI has been reported as a feature of ALS (19,20). Selective corticospinal tract degeneration through the internal capsule and cerebral peduncles is seen in no other disease process. The regularly recurrent differential diagnostic exercises include:

1. *ALS vs. benign fasciculations.* About 70% of the population, especially health care workers, have occasional fasciculations. Some patients, most often older men, have prominent fasciculations without other abnormality. These most often occur in the calves, and the patients are quite aware of the movements, whereas most patients with ALS seem surprisingly oblivious to their fasciculations. The clinical examination is otherwise normal, and the EMG is normal except for the fasciculations. The problem is that the EMG in unaffected muscles early in the course of motor neuron disease may show at best subtle abnormalities (12). There is no infallible way to distinguish benign from malignant fasciculations from the fasciculating discharge itself; judgment is made by the company they keep. A non-progressive course over time is more reassuring than a single normal electrodiagnostic evaluation. Of 121 patients with benign fasciculations followed up to 32 years, none developed ALS (21). In another report, 6.7% of ALS patients had fasciculations as an isolated, initial manifestation of the disease (22).

2. *ALS vs. ulnar neuropathy.* ALS commonly begins asymmetrically, often with painless weakness and wasting of one hand. Patients with ulnar neuropathy may present similarly, except that they usually have ulnar distribution sensory complaints and sensory loss as well. A focal ulnar demyelinating lesion produces characteristic conduction abnormalities, but a pure axon loss lesion can produce a motor nerve conduction picture similar to that seen in ALS. An abnormal ulnar sensory potential strongly favors ulnar neuropathy. Needle exam abnormalities in ALS are not restricted to the ulnar distribution. Lesions of the ulnar nerve at the wrist are more difficult to distinguish from ALS because they may not cause sensory loss and because the electrodiagnosis is trickier. Early clinicians thought focal hand atrophy in gold polishers was a restricted form of motor neuron disease until Ramsay Hunt deduced that it was due to compression of the

deep palmar branch from the tools used for polishing.

3. *ALS vs. C8 radiculopathy.* This is more problematic than ulnar neuropathy because of the more widespread weakness and wasting, and the absence of an abnormal sensory potential in radiculopathy. Patients usually have clinical sensory complaints. A depressed triceps jerk favors a radiculopathy; increased reflexes in the affected extremity favor ALS. Neck pain, limited cervical spine range of motion and positive root compression signs favor radiculopathy. Obeying the dictum to always surround abnormality with normality helps avoid misinterpretation (Chapter 12).

4. *ALS vs. true neurogenic thoracic outlet syndrome (TOS).* Neurogenic TOS is rare and generally occurs in patients much younger than those affected by ALS. Either the ulnar or the medial antebrachial cutaneous sensory potential, or both, are usually abnormal in TOS, and needle exam abnormalities are restricted to the distribution of the lower trunk of the brachial plexus. Weakness and wasting in TOS is often limited to the thenar muscles. Other brachial plexus pathology, e.g., Pancoast tumor, is usually signaled by accompanying pain and Horner's syndrome.

5. *ALS vs. cervical spondylosis.* This is a very frequent differential diagnostic conundrum. Both diseases are common and may coexist in some patients. Cervical spondylotic radiculomyelopathy produces LMN abnormalities in the upper extremities due to radiculopathy and UMN signs in the lower extremities due to myelopathy. It frequently causes fasciculations in the upper extremities, especially across the shoulders and chest. Trying to distinguish cervical spondylosis from ALS can be maddening and sometimes impossible; patients occasionally have decompressive surgery because of the inability to be certain. Patients with both cervical and lumbar spondylosis may also have lumbosacral radiculopathies, adding LMN findings in the legs to the picture and further simulating motor neuron disease. Most helpful are the depressed reflexes in the upper extremities, neurogenic bladder symptoms, occasional posterior column dysfunction, limited neck motion and lack of bulbar symptoms in spondylosis patients. Quick reflexes in the arms, widespread fasciculations, lack of bladder or sexual dysfunction and bulbar involvement suggest ALS. Electrodiagnostically, huge MUAPs (3–5x normal amplitude and very long duration),

very active and diffuse fasciculations, and fibrillations in the thoracic paraspinals or bulbar muscles favor ALS. When present, corticospinal tract degeneration on head MRI resolves any doubt.

6. *ALS vs. peroneal neuropathy.* Patients with ALS often present with painless foot drop, and patients with peroneal neuropathy may present similarly. Patients with peroneal neuropathy typically have an abnormal superficial peroneal sensory response and needle exam abnormalities are limited to the peroneal distribution. Conduction abnormalities may be difficult to demonstrate. Sometimes conduction block or conduction slowing is apparent when recording from the tibialis anterior or peroneus longus when it is not apparent recording from the usual EDB site.

7. *ALS vs. L5 radiculopathy.* Patients with L5 radiculopathy may also present with foot drop, but it is most often accompanied by low back pain and ipsilateral radicular leg pain. Peroneal motor conduction studies may show diffuse conduction slowing due to axon loss, but no focal abnormalities at the fibular head. The superficial peroneal sensory response should be normal, and needle examination abnormalities should be limited to the L5 myotome and ipsilateral lumbosacral paraspinal muscles.

8. *ALS vs. multifocal motor neuropathy (MMN) (23).* Very long-standing insidiously progressive weakness involving the upper extremities asymmetrically is the typical presentation of MMN. Involvement is occasionally limited initially to the distribution of one peripheral nerve. Wasting is variable, and in many patients the absence of wasting consonant with the degree of weakness and the chronicity of the process is a clue to the presence of MMN. About 40% of MMN patients have sensory complaints or sensory abnormalities on exam, but invariably have normal sensory conduction studies. Fasciculations can occur in MMN and reflexes are occasionally brisk, but clear-cut upper motor neuron signs are not a feature. The clinical resemblance to ALS is usually only superficial. The condition is characterized electrophysiologically by conduction block which involves motor but not sensory fibers. The conduction block usually appears with stimulation at the knee or elbow, and is not generally difficult to demonstrate. Heroic efforts at extremely proximal stimulation are seldom rewarded. Not uncommonly, there is also marked slowing, in the demyelinating range, of one or more nerves. De-

termination of antiganglioside antibodies has not proven as helpful as anticipated.

9. *ALS vs. bulbar myasthenia gravis (MG).* The progressive bulbar palsy form of ALS and myasthenia gravis (MG) may both present with progressive dysarthria and dysphagia. In a young patient, particularly a woman, the diagnosis will almost always be MG. In the elderly, the differential diagnosis can be difficult in the early stages. Patients with ALS can have abnormal RNS studies and abnormal single-fiber EMG due to the secondary neuromuscular transmission disturbances (15). Denervation changes in early bulbar ALS may be difficult to demonstrate. Subclinical electrical abnormalities may be demonstrated in non-weak muscles, but only in a minority of cases. The Tensilon test can be positive in either condition, but the response is more dramatic in MG. Positive antiacetylcholine receptor antibodies and corticospinal tract degeneration on head MRI clinch the diagnosis when present.

10. *ALS vs. monomelic motor neuron disease (24).* Patients with monomelic motor neuron disease are usually young men with insidiously progressive weakness and wasting of one extremity, most often a distal arm. Chronic denervation changes are usually widespread in the affected extremity, and may be present to a less impressive degree even in extremities that are not clinically involved. Active fibrillations are seen in fewer than half the patients. The disease lays waste to the affected extremity over 1–2 years, but then progresses little if at all over many years. There is often curious sparing of the brachioradialis, which may remain as an island of muscle in a sea of atrophy. Distinguishing monomelic motor neuron disease from early ALS may be impossible at the outset, and the diagnosis is usually made in retrospect following a benign course.

11. *ALS vs. polymyositis (PM).* Patients with ALS frequently develop elevated CK, up to 10–20X normal, along with their generalized weakness (25). Patients with PM likewise have generalized weakness and an elevated CK. Spectacular CK elevations strongly favor PM. Occasional PM patients have prominent distal weakness. Inclusion body myositis is especially prone to have distal involvement and accompanying neurogenic features (26). Both inflammatory myopathies and ALS may produce dysphagia, and both may be associated with widespread fibrillations on needle exam. Occasional ALS patients may lack the typical large MUAPs and may even have small, poly-

phasic "pseudomyopathic" MUAPs, further compounding the confusion. Muscle pathology usually resolves the issue, but the biopsy in ALS can show myopathic changes admixed with neurogenic abnormalities; these myopathic changes correlate with the CK elevation (27). Neither condition causes sensory loss.

12. *ALS vs. postpolio syndrome.* For many years there has been an interest in the relationship between paralytic poliomyelitis early in life and the development of motor neuron disease later in life. Some patients develop new symptoms many years after a bout of polio (28). Typical complaints include weakness, fatigue, muscle pain, joint pain and depression—the postpolio syndrome. The concern was that chronically overworked surviving motor neurons carrying a heavy burden of collateral sprouts could begin to die prematurely, producing progressive weakness and an ALS like syndrome. In fact, there have been very few reports of classical ALS developing in patients with remote polio, so few as to raise the question of whether old polio might in fact somehow protect against later ALS (29). Despite extensive research, no electrodiagnostic or pathologic features have emerged which distinguish patients with postpolio syndrome from those with stable old polio. Many of the complaints in postpolio syndrome are likely musculoskeletal in origin, and the condition seldom shows significant progression (30).

13. *ALS in the ICU.* Many patients in an ICU, especially those with sepsis and multiorgan failure, develop neuromuscular weakness (31,32). This complication often comes to light as a failure to wean from the ventilator. Previously undiagnosed ALS is occasionally but not often the final diagnosis under these circumstances (33). More often the problem is due to some other process. Some of the possibilities include: critical illness polyneuropathy, prolonged effect of neuromuscular blocking agents, acute myopathy related to blocking agents and/or steroids (thick filament or myosin deficient myopathy), necrotizing critical illness myopathy, hypophosphatemia, electrolyte imbalance, rhabdomyolysis, septic encephalopathy, and unrecognized spinal cord pathology (34).

SPINAL MUSCULAR ATROPHY (SMA)

SMA syndromes affect only the lower motor neuron, producing muscular weakness and wasting without any element of upper motor neuron involvement. Oc-

casional patients with sporadic ALS have a predominantly LMN form of the disease, an acquired form of SMA, but most patients with SMA have a hereditary disorder. The hereditary forms are now thought to result from genetically based derangements in the normal mechanisms of apoptosis, or preprogrammed cell death. All seem to be variations on a gene defect at the same locus on chromosome 5 (35). Two genes may be involved (36). Patients with SMA may present in infancy, childhood, adolescence or rarely adulthood (37). The most common form is SMA I, or Werdnig-Hoffman disease, in which generalized, symmetric weakness is noted in the first 6 months of life and often at birth. Patients rarely survive more than 12–18 months before succumbing to respiratory failure. SMA I is a prominent consideration in the differential diagnosis of infantile hypotonia, or the floppy baby syndrome (38). About 80% of floppy babies have a central origin of their hypotonia. About half of the remainder have SMA I. Entities to be excluded include such things as infantile botulism, congenital muscular dystrophy, neonatal myotonic dystrophy, congenital myopathies, metabolic and mitochondrial myopathies, neonatal myasthenia gravis, congenital myasthenia gravis, peripheral nerve disorders, and benign congenital hypotonia. The electrodiagnostic picture, sometimes coupled with muscle pathology, usually can make the correct diagnosis (39).

The electrodiagnostic evaluation in SMA I typically discloses normal SNAPs and normal or near normal motor NCVs for age. Some MNCV slowing can occur; the debate about permissible limits is the same as for adult ALS, compounded by consideration of the age related lower NCVs in children. Needle EMG findings are similar to those in ALS: decreased recruitment with fast firing units, increased amplitude, duration and complexity of MUAPs, and fibrillation potentials—all in a widespread distribution. Fasciculations are not as prominent in hereditary SMA as in acquired motor neuron disease.

SMA II, also known as the chronic or intermediate form of Werdnig-Hoffman disease, is similar to SMA I both clinically and electrodiagnostically, but is less malignant. Weakness is noted later, after the age of about 3 months and usually between 6 and 24 months, and survival is longer, sometimes into adulthood. SMA III, or Kugelberg-Welander disease classically presents in adolescence with lower extremity weakness which is proximal, asymmetric, and sometimes accompanied by calf hypertrophy. The electrodiagnostic picture is similar to SMA I, except the distribution of abnormalities may be more localized. Due to extreme chronicity and efficient reinnervation, fibrillations may be difficult to demonstrate. Some patients have a characteristic finger tremor due to spontaneous and contraction fasciculations (40).

Other hereditary motor neuronopathies related to SMA include neurogenic arthrogryposis multiplex congenita and a progressive, malignant, childhood bulbar form (Fazio-Londe disease). SMA sometimes occurs in association with microcephaly, mental retardation, deafness, retinitis pigmentosa, optic atrophy or spinocerebellar ataxia.

OTHER MOTOR NEURONOPATHIES

Rarely, disease of the motor neuron may present in a scapuloperoneal distribution, in a facioscapulohumeral distribution or as a distal form of SMA which clinically resembles CMT disease but with preserved sensation and reflexes. Kennedy's syndrome (bulbospinal atrophy) is an X-linked disorder which usually presents with bulbar dysfunction in young adulthood, has no significant UMN component, and frequently permits long survival. Gynecomastia and characteristic facial fasciculations may provide diagnostic clues (41).

Disorders deserving consideration when a patient presents with an unusual form of motor neuronopathy include: poliomyelitis (unvaccinated, postvaccination or due to a nonpolio enterovirus), spinal cord tumor or syrinx, diffuse gliomatosis, hexosaminidase A deficiency, hyperthyroidism, hyperparathyroidism, previous electric shock injury, previous spinal radiotherapy, toxin exposure, retroviral infection, paraproteinemia and occult neoplasm (especially lymphoma) (42). Motor neuronopathy may occur as a component of a more extensive neurologic disorder, such as multisystem atrophy, Jakob-Creutzfeldt, Machado-Joseph or polyglucosan (Lafora) body disease.

Sensory Neuronopathy (Dorsal Root Ganglionopathy)

The clinical and electrodiagnostic resemblance between sensory neuronopathy and sensory neuropathy is close. In sensory neuronopathies, the brunt of the pathology falls on the sensory neurons in the dorsal root ganglion. The disorder was first described by Denny-Brown, and has since gone by a variety of names, most referring to the condition as a sensory neuropathy (Table 13.4). The dorsal root ganglion cells degenerate and there may be inflammation. Clinically, patients have the subacute onset of pain, paresthesias and sensory loss which affects large more than small fibers. Strength is preserved, but reflexes disappear. There is often a disabling sensory ataxia which

TABLE 13.4
Common Synonyms for Sensory Neuronopathy

Subacute sensory neuropathy
Carcinomatous/lymphomatous sensory neuropathy
Malignant sensory neuropathy
Denny-Brown neuropathy
Primary sensory neuropathy
Ganglioradiculitis
Acute sensory neuronopathy
Chronic idiopathic ataxic neuropathy
Idiopathic sensory neuronopathy

may be accompanied by pseudoathetosis. CSF protein is frequently increased. When the disorder occurs as a paraneoplastic effect, the anti-Hu antibody may be present (43).

Although classically a remote effect of small cell carcinoma of the lung, sensory neuronopathy is associated with a number of other conditions, including pyridoxine intoxication, Sjögren's syndrome, and lymphoma (44). It can occur as a fairly acute, presumably immunologically mediated syndrome which requires urgent immunosuppressive treatment to prevent a disabling outcome.

Electrodiagnostically, involvement is typically diffuse, with globally low amplitude or absent sensory responses in the face of normal motor conduction studies, a normal needle exam, and absent H reflexes but intact F waves.

Key Points

- Neuronopathies are acquired or hereditary disorders that affect the motor or sensory nerve cell body.

- Amyotrophic lateral sclerosis (ALS) and the hereditary spinal muscular atrophy (SMA) syndromes account for the vast majority of neuronopathies. Various combinations of involvement of upper and lower motor neurons produce different clinical patterns of involvement, from pure upper to pure lower motor neuron.

- Before making a diagnosis of a motor neuron disease, the electrodiagnostic medicine consultant should demonstrate the presence of diffuse neuropathic abnormalities without other explanation. Sensory conduction studies are generally normal. Motor NCV may be slowed in proportion to axon loss. Needle examination changes reflect chronic denervation with reinnervation. Large amplitude, long duration, polyphasic MUPs, fibrillations and fasciculations are usually demonstrable in a multinerve/multiroot distribution involving at least three extremities. The head and the thoracic paraspinals count as extremities. The more typical the EMG abnormalities the greater the diagnostic confidence. Patients with very early, rapidly progressive or very chronic disease may not display all the expected features.

- The etiology of sporadic ALS is probably multifactorial. Glutamate driven excitotoxicity seems to play a major role. About 20% of familial cases have a mutation of the superoxide dismutase gene.

- A significant proportion of ALS patients are initially misdiagnosed.

- The electrodiagnostic medicine consultant is confronted with several regularly recurrent differential diagnostic exercises. Patients with benign fasciculations have no other clinical or electrodiagnostic abnormalities and a very favorable long term prognosis. Ulnar and peroneal neuropathies usually produce sensory abnormalities and the distribution of motor abnormalities is limited to the ulnar or peroneal nerve. Deep palmar branch ulnar lesions are more difficult to distinguish from motor neuron disease. Cervical spine disease causes frequent confusion. Cervical spondylosis is common and can closely simulate ALS. Cervical and lumbar radiculopathies can usually be distinguished by the restricted distribution and the presence of pain and segmental reflex depression. Multifocal motor neuropathy is distinguished by conduction blocks. Myasthenia gravis and early bulbar ALS are often difficult to distinguish. Monomelic motor neuron disease may only be distinguishable from ALS by its behavior over time. ALS and inflammatory myopathies may both cause generalized weakness, diffuse fibrillations and an elevated CK. Postpolio syndrome is probably not related to ALS. Rare ALS patients present in the ICU as failure to wean from the ventilator.

- The common hereditary SMA syndromes are all variants of the same basic genetic defect that causes the mechanisms of normal preprogrammed cell death (apoptosis) to go awry. They are clinically divided into different types primarily by age at onset and long term prognosis. The electrodiagnostic picture is essentially the same as for ALS, with some variations.

- Sensory neuronopathies are much rarer than the motor syndromes. Patients usually present with severe ataxia and have globally abnormal sensory action potentials without any other electrodiagnostic abnormality.

References

1. Ringel SP, Murphy JR, Alderson MK, et al. The natural history of amyotrophic lateral sclerosis. Neurology 1993;43:1316–1322.
   Using 42 strength and functional assessments recorded monthly, the natural history of ALS is described in 167 patients. Mean age at onset was 57.4 years, and symptoms were present for 2.64 years before study entry. There was a highly variable rate of decline within the group of patients, but no differences in rate of decline. The median survival was 4.0 years for the study cohort but 2.1 years for newly diagnosed cases. Decline in pulmonary function most closely correlated with death. See also: Brooks, B.R. Natural history of ALS: symptoms, strength, pulmonary function, and disability. Neurology 1996;47: S71–81.

2. Tucker T, Layzer RB, Miller RG, et al. Subacute, reversible motor neuron disease. Neurology 1991;41:1541–1544.
   Four patients with a clinical syndrome closely resembling amyotrophic lateral sclerosis recovered completely, without treatment, 5 to 12 months after onset. Electrodiagnostic tests revealed acute and chronic denervation, with normal motor and sensory nerve conduction studies. Although such cases are rare, the possibility of spontaneous recovery should always be considered when counseling patients with suspected ALS.

3. Tsai CP, Ho HH, Yen DJ, et al. Reversible motor neuron disease. Eur Neurol 1993;33:387–389.
   A 69-year-old male with a clinical syndrome resembling ALS recovered almost completely in approximately 1.5 years.

4. Lambert EH. Electromyography in amyotrophic lateral sclerosis. In: Norris FH, Kurland LT, eds. Motor neuron diseases: research on amyotrophic lateral sclerosis and related disorders. New York: Grune & Stratton, 1969.
   The often quoted first detailed description of the EMG findings in ALS. Source of the Lambert criteria. Numerous pertinent observations: mean increase in MUAP amplitude 4X and up to 10X normal; mean increase in MUAP duration 35%, up to 2X normal; occurrence of complex potentials with parasites; pseudomyopathic units; abnormalities of neuromuscular transmission; benign vs. malignant fasciculations; and slowing of NCV.

5. Eisen A. Amyotrophic lateral sclerosis. Intern Med 1995;34:824–832.
   The final cascade of amyotrophic lateral sclerosis (ALS) coincides with the onset of clinical neurological deficits and involves multifactorial interactive mechanisms, including excitotoxicity, free radical accumulation and possibly immunological disturbances. They are probably predated by months or years by thus far unidentified triggers. Selective vulnerability of the corticomotoneuronal system in ALS is likely due to degradation of several gene products essential to transmitter, receptor and nerve growth factor maintenance specific to this functional system.

6. Gutmann L, Mitsumoto H. Advances in ALS. Neurology 1996;47:S17–8, 1996.
   A concise review of current concepts regarding the pathogenesis of ALS. See also: Rothstein JD. Excitotoxicity hypothesis. Neurology 1996;47:S19–25; Siddique T, Nijhawan D, and Hentati A. Molecular genetic basis of familial ALS. Neurology 1996;47:S27–34; Smith RG, Siklos L, Alexianu ME, Engelhardt JI, et al. Autoimmunity and ALS. Neurology 1996;47:S40–5.

7. Miller RG, Bouchard JP, Duquette P, et al. Clinical trials of riluzole in patients with ALS. ALS/Riluzole Study Group-II. Neurology 1996;47:S86–90.
   Two double-blinded, placebo-controlled clinical trials of riluzole have now been carried out in more than 1,100 patients with ALS. The results of both studies show a modest benefit in prolonging survival that is statistically significant. These results led to the availability of this drug by the Food and Drug Administration for use in the United States beginning in early 1996. This is the first drug that has been available for ALS. It begins a new era in both basic and clinical research in an

attempt to find a cure for this disease. See also:Mitsumoto H, Olney RK. Drug combination treatment in patients with ALS: current status and future directions. Neurology 1996;47: S103–7; Sufit R, Newman D. The impact of the approval of riluzole. Neurology 1996;47:S117.

8. Denys EH. AAEM case report #5: Amyotrophic lateral sclerosis. Muscle Nerve 1994;17:263–268.

40-year-old man presented with a gradual onset of gait unsteadiness and weakness in the arms. The stretch reflexes were normal in the upper extremities but hyperactive in the lower extremities with bilateral Babinski signs. A myelogram revealed a partial obstruction at C-5–6. Two prior electromyograms, 7 and 5 months prior to admission, reportedly showed positive waves only in two peroneal supplied muscles. Repeat electromyographic testing demonstrated normal nerve conduction velocities and needle electrode abnormalities in upper and lower extremities as well as thoracic paraspinal muscles allowing a diagnosis of amyotrophic lateral sclerosis (ALS). The importance of electromyographic testing in clinically nonaffected areas is stressed as well as its role in patients presenting with upper motor neuron signs. It is the task of the clinical electromyographer to consider other entities in the differential diagnosis, such as a multifocal motor neuropathy with conduction blocks and design the tests accordingly. The role of electromyography in the prediction of the course of ALS by assessing the degree of reinnervation is discussed. This will become increasingly important in the design of treatment trials.

9. Tahmoush AJ, Gillespie JA, Hulihan JF, et al. Clinical and electrophysiological assessments in ALS patients. Electromyogr Clin Neurophysiol 1991;31:491–496.

Three clinical and four electrophysiological assessments were performed in a cross-sectional study of 87 ALS patients. The association between Norris ALS and mean muscle strength scores is significant, and these scores are significantly correlated with mean interference pattern, mean denervation potential and mean compound muscle action potential scores respectively. Scatterplots of the data and regression lines suggest linear relationships between each of these assessments. See also: Kelly JJ, Jr., Thibodeau L, Andres PL, Finison LJ. Use of electrophysiologic tests to measure disease progression in ALS therapeutic trials. Muscle Nerve 1990;13:471–479.

10. Layzer RB. The origin of muscle fasciculations and cramps. Muscle Nerve 1994;17:1243–1249.

See Chapter 8 for abstract.

11. Kuncl RW, Cornblath DR, Griffin JW. Assessment of thoracic paraspinal muscles in the diagnosis of ALS. Muscle Nerve 1988;11:484–492.

In ALS patients, distal limb muscles and thoracic paraspinal muscles were affected more frequently than proximal limb and cranial muscles. These patterns suggest selective vulnerability of specific neuronal populations. The vulnerability of truncal muscles, illustrated by thoracic paraspinal wasting or head and shoulder drooping, was a helpful differential sign in diagnosing ALS. Thoracic paraspinal electromyography was especially valuable in distinguishing ALS from other disorders, such as combined cervical and lumbar spondylotic amyotrophy or polymyositis, which may masquerade as ALS. The finding of denervation atrophy on biopsy of thoracic paraspinal muscles was diagnostic in difficult cases. Because the thoracic paraspinal muscles are frequently affected in ALS and spared in spondylotic amyotrophy, their assessment provides a practical strategy in differentiating ALS from other motor syndromes.

12. Behnia M, Kelly JJ. Role of electromyography in amyotrophic lateral sclerosis. Muscle Nerve 1991;14:1236–1241.

A review of the role of electrodiagnostic testing in ALS in a large ALS clinic. Over 31 months, 133 patients with a clinical diagnosis of ALS were tested. In most, nerve conduction studies were normal, and needle electrode examination showed active denervation in the upper and lower limbs or the limbs and bulbar muscles (Lambert's criteria). However, 50 of 133 patients did not fulfill Lambert's criteria at presentation. This study reveals that a large proportion of patients with a clinical diagnosis of ALS fail to have classical findings on initial electrodiagnostic studies, and reveals several caveats of electrodiagnostic testing in these patients.

13. Cornblath DR, Kuncl RW, Mellits ED, et al. Nerve conduction studies in amyotrophic lateral sclerosis. Muscle Nerve 1992;15:1111–1115.

The question often arises whether in the presence of severe atrophy and reduction of the CMAP amplitude abnormal CV exceeds what can be expected from ALS alone. To determine the limits of abnormality in classic ALS, this study prospectively evaluated NCS data from 61 patients who met a strict clinical definition of ALS. In nerves with reduced AMP, CV rarely fell to less than 80% of the lower limit of normal, and DL and F rarely exceeded 1.25 times the upper limit of normal. Utilizing the entire data set and regression analyses, 95% confidence limits for expected values for CV, F, and DL as a function of AMP were calculated. These limits thus derived suggest criteria for NCS abnormalities in ALS and may be useful in differentiating ALS from other illnesses.

14. Ross MA. Electrodiagnostic assessment of amyotrophic lateral sclerosis. In: 1996 AAEM Course E: update on motor neuron disorders. 1996:

This course handout reviews the electrodiagnosis of ALS, including information on advanced techniques such as single fiber, scanning and macro EMG. Suggested electrodiagnostic criteria for the diagnosis, based on the criteria used for the CNTF study, are included.

15. Bernstein LP, Antel JP. Motor neuron disease: decremental responses to repetitive nerve stimulation. Neurology 1981;31:202–204.

To 2 Hz repetitive stimulation, six patients with rapidly progressive ALS had a decrement of 7.6 ± 1.3% at baseline which repaired immediately after exercise and increased to 13.6 ± 1.2% two minutes after exercise. Only one of eight patients with slowly progressive disease had any decrement. The decrement correlated better with disease progression than with CMAP amplitude. Decrements up to 10% are generally considered normal.

16. Belsh JM, Schiffman PL. Misdiagnosis in patients with amyotrophic lateral sclerosis. Arch Intern Med 1990; 150:2301–2305.

A review of records of 33 patients with a definitive diagnosis of ALS showed that 43% were initially misdiagnosed. Mean time to correct diagnosis was 16.0 ± 9.3 months for the misdiagnosed group, and 7.6 ± 4.1 months for the rest of the patients. Two of three patients with an initial symptom of dyspnea were misdiagnosed. Three patients underwent laminectomies because of misdiagnosis. Age, stage of disease, and unusual presenting symptoms were not identified as causes of misdiagnosis. Most likely causes were physicians' failure to consider the diagnosis and lack of familiarity with the common clinical presentations of amyotrophic lateral sclerosis.

17. Brooks BR. El Escorial World Federation of Neurology criteria for the diagnosis of amyotrophic lateral sclerosis. Subcommittee on Motor Neuron Diseases/Amyotrophic Lateral Sclerosis of the World Federation of Neurology Research Group on Neuromuscular Diseases and the El Escorial "Clinical limits of amyotrophic lateral sclerosis" workshop contributors. J Neurol Sci 1994; 124 Suppl:96–107.

18. Chaudhuri KR, Crump S, al-Sarraj S, et al. The validation of El Escorial criteria for the diagnosis of amyotrophic lateral sclerosis: a clinicopathological study. J Neurol Sci 1995;129 Suppl:11–12.

19. Oba H, Araki T, Ohtomo K, et al. Amyotrophic lateral sclerosis: T2 shortening in motor cortex at MR imaging. Radiology 1993;189:843–846.

The MR images of 14 of 15 ALS patients showed T2 shortening in precentral cortices, while the images of all but one of the control patients showed no such finding. In three of eight brains at autopsy, sections from the precentral cortex showed sparsely distributed, intensely stained astrocytes and macrophages. Abnormal iron deposition associated with the degenerative process could be the source of T2 shortening, which is a useful MR imaging finding in the diagnosis of ALS.

20. Yagishita A, Nakano I, Oda M, et al. Location of the corticospinal tract in the internal capsule at MR imaging. Radiology 1994;191:455–460.

This study reviewed MR images of 100 control subjects and 35 patients with ALS and brain specimens from seven control subjects and five ALS patients. In the posterior IC, the brain specimens from control subjects demonstrated a pale area with large axons and thick myelin sheaths. In five ALS patients, the brain specimens showed degeneration of the CST in the same region. MR images demonstrated abnormal hyperintensity that represented degeneration of the CST in five of 35 ALS patients. In the same region, hyperintense foci were found in the control subjects.

21. Blexrud MD, Windebank AJ, Daube JR. Long-term follow-up of 121 patients with benign fasciculations. Ann Neurol 1993;34:622–625.

121 patients with a diagnosis of benign fasciculations were identified. All had a normal neurological examination and normal electrophysiological studies, except for fasciculation potentials. None of the patients developed symptomatic motor neuron disease on follow up 2 to 32 years after diagnosis.

22. Eisen A, Stewart H. Not-so-benign fasciculation. Ann Neurol 1994;35:375–376.

A letter in comment to reference 21, stating that 6.7% of a series of ALS patients had fasciculations as the initial and only symptom.

23. Parry GJ. AAEM case report #30: multifocal motor neuropathy. Muscle Nerve 1996;19:269–276.

A 73-year-old man with a 16-year history of fasciculations and 15 years of weakness in his right arm was diagnosed with focal motor neuron disease. After 10 years of purely motor symptoms, he developed mild paresthesias although his sensory examination remained normal. Reflexes were reduced or absent in the weak muscles but were normal elsewhere. Nerve conduction was studied in nerves innervating weak muscles and showed severe motor conduction block. Sensory nerve conduction studies were minimally abnormal, showing reduced amplitudes with normal velocities. Based on the clinical picture and the presence of severe motor conduction block, the patient was diagnosed with multifocal motor neuropathy. Treatment with high-dose intravenous immunoglobulin was given with significant improvement in strength and partial resolution of the conduction block. As this case demonstrates, this treatable disorder may occasionally be mistaken for motor neuron disease although the resemblance is only superficial, and it should never be mistaken for amyotrophic lateral sclerosis.

24. Donofrio PD. AAEM case report#28: monomelic amyotrophy. Muscle Nerve 1994;17:1129–1134.

Monomelic amyotrophy is a rare form of motor neuron disease usually presenting as painless asymmetric weakness and atrophy in the distal upper extremities of young adults. Only rarely are the legs involved and pyramidal findings are uncommon. Monomelic amyotrophy is most often observed in people of Japanese and Indian heritage and affects men almost exclusively. Most cases are sporadic. Laboratory testing is frequently normal or nonspecific except for electrophysiologic studies which typically demonstrate reduced compound muscle action potential amplitudes, fasciculations, and features consistent with acute and chronic denervation in distal upper extremity muscles. Necropsy in 1 patient identified anterior horn cell shrinkage, necrosis, and gliosis in appropriate spinal cord segments. Symptoms and signs often progress for several years before spontaneously arresting. The differential diagnosis for monomelic amyotrophy is broad, including processes which affect the cervical cord, roots, brachial plexus, and individual or multiple nerves in the upper extremity.

25. Harrington TM, Cohen MD, Bartleson JD, et al. Elevation of creatine kinase in amyotrophic lateral sclerosis: potential confusion with polymyositis. Arth Rheum 1983;26:201–205.

CK levels were elevated in 43% of a group of 100 ALS patients. Mean level was 240 units, range 59–1,327 (normal male <95, normal female <59). Seven patients were initially misdiagnosed as having polymyositis and given high dose steroids. CK elevations up to approximately 20X normal occur regularly in ALS patients.

26. Eisen A, Berry K, Gibson G. Inclusion body myositis (IBM): myopathy or neuropathy? Neurology 1983;33:1109–14.

Muscle biopsies from 6 elderly sporadic and 1 familial cases of IBM showed characteristic vacuoles and filamentous inclusions. Routine EMG studies, near nerve sensory recordings and single fiber EMG were done. Distal weakness, asymmetry, loss of reflexes, normal or only mild CK elevation, decreased MUAP recruitment, grouped atrophy, angular fibers and markedly increased fiber density all suggest a neurogenic component in some patients.

27. Achari AN, Anderson MS. Myopathic changes in amyotrophic lateral sclerosis: pathologic analysis of muscle biopsy changes in 111 cases. Neurology 1974;24:477–481.

67% of muscle biopsies from a group of 111 ALS patients had myopathic along with neurogenic changes. 25% of biopsies showed neurogenic changes only and 7% were normal. Patients with myopathic changes on biopsy had higher CKs. Myopathic changes included central nuclei, fiber rounding, basophilic degeneration, vacuolar changes, and (in 11 patients) an interstitial focal mononuclear cell infiltrate. Two cases were indistinguishable from primary myositis. The cases were "clinically classical" motor neuron disease whose EMGs showed "unequivocal evidence of diffuse anterior horn cell involvement."

28. Windebank AJ, Litchy WJ, Daube JR, et al. Late effects

of paralytic poliomyelitis in Olmsted County, Minnesota. Neurology 1991;41:501–507.

Sixty-four percent of 50 survivors of previous paralytic polio complained of new symptoms of muscle pain, fatigue, and weakness after a period of prolonged stability. This led to changes in lifestyle or activity in only 18%. The likelihood of expressing new complaints was not related to present age or interval since polio, and electrophysiologic testing did not distinguish between those with or without new problems. The development of new difficulties in a limb was most strongly predicted by significant paralysis of that limb at the time of the acute illness. Patients with leg weakness were twice as likely to complain of new problems compared to those with arm weakness. Elevated creatine kinase levels were present only in those with new complaints.

29. Armon C, Daube JR, Windebank AJ, et al. How frequently does classic amyotrophic lateral sclerosis develop in survivors of poliomyelitis? Neurology 1990; 40:172–174.

There is a paucity of reports of classic ALS developing in survivors of paralytic poliomyelitis. A report of a patient with classic ALS and an antecedent paralytic disease thought to have been poliomyelitis from which she recovered completely. If the paucity of ALS preceded by true poliomyelitis is not merely a matter of underreporting, antecedent paralytic poliomyelitis may have a protective role against the development of ALS.

30. Windebank AJ, Litchy WJ, Daube JR, et al. Lack of progression of neurologic deficit in survivors of paralytic polio: a 5-year prospective population-based study. Neurology 1996;46:80–84.

A prospective, population-based cohort study of polio survivors in Olmsted County, Minnesota, between 1986 and 1993. Fifty individuals who had had past paralytic polio underwent completed detailed quantitative clinical and electrophysiologic studies at entry and after 5 years. These studies demonstrated stable neuromuscular function within the cohort, although 60% of the individuals were symptomatic. In two-thirds of the symptomatic patients, the causes of their symptoms were unrelated to earlier polio. For the 20% of patients who had unexplained muscle pain, perception of weakness, and fatigue, a mechanical disorder most likely underlies their symptoms.

31. Bolton CF. Neuromuscular complications of sepsis. Intensive Care Med 1993;19 Suppl 2:S58-S63.

Sepsis and multiple organ failure are major problems in medical and surgical intensive care units. Critical illness polyneuropathy occurs in 70% of these patients. Difficulty in weaning from the ventilator is an early sign. Electrophysiological studies are necessary to establish the diagnosis; these studies show an axonal degeneration of peripheral nerve fibres. Recovery occurs in weeks or months, depending upon severity. Muscle biopsy reveals denervation atrophy. Sepsis itself does not induce a neuromuscular transmission defect, but neuromuscular blocking agents may increase the severity of critical illness polyneuropathy. If steroids are used in addition to neuromuscular blocking agents, a severe myopathy may result. Other effects on muscle are cachectic myopathy and panfascicular muscle fibre necrosis. A variety of combinations of these conditions may affect the same patient. Only well-designed prospective studies will determine the true effect of these medications on the neuromuscular system in septic patients.

32. Bolton CF. Sepsis and the systemic inflammatory response syndrome: neuromuscular manifestations. Crit Care Med 1996;24:1408–1416.

The systemic inflammatory response syndrome is a new concept in which infection and trauma induce a systemic inflammatory response affecting the microcirculation to organs throughout the body. The nervous system is commonly affected in the forms of septic encephalopathy and critical illness polyneuropathy. Neuromuscular blocking agents and corticosteroids may have additional toxic effects on the neuromuscular system that are manifest as transient neuromuscular blockade, an axonal motor neuropathy, or a thick filament myopathy. Clinical examination in the critical care unit is often unreliable and electrophysiologic studies, at times accompanied by magnetic resonance imaging of the spinal cord, measurement of the CK concentration, and muscle biopsy, are often necessary to establish the diagnosis.

33. Kuisma MJ, Saarinen KV, Teirmaa HT. Undiagnosed amyotrophic lateral sclerosis and respiratory failure. Acta Anaesthesiol Scand 1993;37:628–630.

Two patients suffering from exacerbation of chronic respiratory insufficiency due to previously undiagnosed amyotrophic lateral sclerosis are reported. Both patients had a false diagnosis of asthma. A central etiology was suspected when weaning from mechanical ventilation proved unsuccessful during respiratory failure, necessitating intensive care. A neurologic examination and a typical electroneuromyography recording confirmed the diagnosis of amyotrophic lateral sclerosis.

34. Bolton CF, Doyle JJ, Gooch JL, et al. 1996 AAEM Course A: Critical Care Electrodiagnosis. Rochester: Am Assoc of Electrodiag Med, 1996:

This course handout covers several topics relevant to electrodiagnostic medicine in the intensive care unit.

35. Russman BS, Iannacone ST, Buncher CR, et al. Spinal muscular atrophy: new thoughts on the pathogenesis and classification schema. J Child Neurol 1992;7:347–353.

One hundred and forty-one SMA patients were evaluated on at least four occasions over a 3-year period. The patients have been grouped by age of onset, as well as by function at the time of initial evaluation. The muscle strength of 96 patients aged 5 years or older was evaluated at 6-month intervals. The new observations made are: (1) The present classification schema is not valid; for example, 49 patients with onset of weakness before 6 months of age (type I or Werdnig-Hoffmann disease), whose life span is said to be only 2 to 4 years, participated in the study and are 4 months to 31 years of age. (2) Thirty-seven patients were evaluated over an 18-month period. None lost strength during this time but four lost function. Although the period of observation was short, the results suggest that the loss of function in patients with spinal muscular atrophy might be explained by a process other than cell death that allows patient strength to be maintained and simultaneously prevents the motor unit from achieving its normal adult potential.

36. McDonald CM. Autosomal recessive predominantly proximal spinal muscular atrophy. In: 1996: AAEM Course F: update on motor neuron disorders. Rochester: Am Assoc of Electrodiag Med, 1996.

A course handout with a concise review of the SMA syndromes, including the genetics, natural history, physical examination findings, electrodiagnosis and management.

37. Zerres K, Rudnik-Schoneborn S. Natural history in proximal spinal muscular atrophy. Clinical analysis of 445 patients and suggestions for a modification of existing classifications. Arch Neurol 1995;52:518–523.

A group of 445 patients was subdivided into SMA types I, II, III, and IV on the basis of achieved motor development and age at onset. Survival probabilities at 2, 4, 10, and 20 years of age were 32%, 18%, 8%, and 0%, respectively, in patients with SMA type I (those who were never able to sit) and 100%, 100%, 98%, and 77%, respectively, in patients with SMA type II (those who were able to sit but were unable to walk). Patients with SMA type III (those who were able to walk, and had age at onset younger than 30 years) were subdivided into those with an age at onset before (SMA type IIIa) and after (SMA type IIIb) 3 years. The probabilities of being ambulatory at 10, 20, and 40 years after onset were 73%, 44%, and 34%, respectively, in patients with SMA type IIIa, and they were 97%, 89%, and 67%, respectively, in patients with SMA type IIIb.

38. Jones HR, Jr. EMG evaluation of the floppy infant: differential diagnosis and technical aspects. Muscle Nerve 1990;13:338–347.
The usual reason for EMG studies in the newborn and young infant is to evaluate a floppy baby. The electromyographer must not only be aware of important differences in normal physiologic parameters but must also be familiar with a spectrum of diseases that are not typically encountered in the adult. The most common disorders affecting the peripheral motor unit are infantile motor neuron disease and the congenital myopathies, but a large number of other diseases warrant consideration.

39. David WS, Jones HR, Jr. Electromyography and biopsy correlation with suggested protocol for evaluation of the floppy infant. Muscle Nerve 1994;17:424–430.
EMG data were correlated with results of muscle and nerve biopsies in 41 of 80 infants with nonarthrogrypotic floppy infant syndrome who had concomitant biopsies (38) or other diagnostic analyses (3). A diagnosis was made of Werdnig-Hoffmann disease (WHD) in 15, a congenital infantile polyneuropathy (IPN) in 3, neuromuscular transmission defect (NMTD) in 2, myopathy in 12, and presumed "central" hypotonia in 9. A very positive correlation rate between nerve conduction studies with electromyography and biopsy results was found in 93% with WHD and 100% in IPN. Only 40% with biopsy-proven myopathy had an abnormal EMG. Only once did the results of electromyography and biopsy conflict.

40. Hausmanowa-Petrusewicz I, Karwanska A. Electromyographic findings in different forms of infantile and juvenile proximal spinal muscular atrophy. Muscle Nerve 1986;9:37–46.
Quantitative EMG was performed in 223 infantile and juvenile cases of SMA, which were classified into 3 groups: (A) form Ia, Werdnig-Hoffmann disease; (B) forms Ib and II, intermediate forms; and (C) form III, Kugelberg-Welander disease. The groups differed in the occurrence of spontaneous activity; only groups A and B showed spontaneous rhythmic firing of motor units, whereas in long-standing cases, pseudomyotonic volleys appeared. The parameters of individual MUAPs differed in the different forms of the disease. Group A showed, in addition to long potentials of high amplitude, some short and low amplitude potentials, and the histograms of amplitudes and durations were bimodal. In the long-standing cases, the values of these parameters were shifted to longer durations and higher amplitudes of motor unit potentials. However, in long-standing cases of the benign group C, the short, low potentials appeared as well as so-called linked potentials. In the very early stage of the disease, the children who were found to be suffering from chronic forms of SMA—both malignant and benign—had an EMG record that was slightly different from that of acute form Ia. Their EMG record shows more so-called "spinal" signs, particularly in the benign group C (Kugelberg-Welander disease). These increasing features of chronic anterior horn cell involvement followed a pattern of reinnervation and hypertrophy of muscle fibers. These phenomena were particularly seen in the benign group C. These findings indicate that in the early stage of SMA, the EMG not only has diagnostic, but also prognostic, value.

41. Ferrante MA, Wilbourn AJ. The characteristic electrodiagnostic features of Kennedy's disease. Muscle Nerve 1997;20:323–329.
A study of the clinical and electrodiagnostic (EDX) features of 19 patients with Kennedy's disease to define the EDX features, their distribution, their clinical correlation, and to determine whether they are unique to this disorder. Findings included: (1) the percentage with SNAP abnormalities is high (95%); (2) M wave abnormalities are less frequent (37%) and less pronounced; (3) the needle electrode examination is always abnormal (100%), revealing acute and chronic motor axon loss, with the latter predominating; (4) the clinical onset is heterogeneous for both the site of onset (bulbar, upper extremity, lower extremity, combination) and the symptomatology (sensory, motor, sensorimotor); (5) focal onsets were reported in the majority (79%); and (6) there is a strong correlation between the clinical onset (both site and symptomatology) and the maximal EDX abnormalities. Thus, the EDX features of Kennedy's disease are consistent with a slowly progressive and very chronic degeneration of the anterior horn cells and dorsal root ganglia. Although the clinical onsets are heterogenous, the EDX features are homogenous and unique, consisting of a diffuse, very slowly progressive anterior horn cell disorder coupled with a sensory neuropathy/neuronopathy that mimics an acquired process. See also: Trojaborg W, Wulff CH. X-linked recessive bulbospinal neuronopathy (Kennedy's syndrome): a neurophysiological study. Acta Neurol Scand 1994;89: 214–219.

42. So YT, Olney RK. AAEM case report #23: acute paralytic poliomyelitis. Muscle Nerve 1991;14:1159–1164.
A 56-year-old man with acute paralytic poliomyelitis is described. The illness started with fever and diarrhea after an overseas trip, and an enterovirus other than poliovirus was isolated from the patient's stool. The onset of weakness was rapid and asymmetric, with primary involvement of the lower extremities. Nerve conduction studies revealed low amplitude motor responses after the first week, with normal results for sensory studies. Serial electromyographic studies were performed, documenting acute denervation followed later by reinnervation in the distribution of multiple segments. The clinical and electrodiagnostic features of acute poliomyelitis are reviewed. See also: Younger DS, Rowland LP, Latov N, et al. Lymphoma, motor neuron diseases, and amyotrophic lateral sclerosis. Ann Neurol 1991;29:78–86. Fisher M, Mateer JE, Ullrich I, et al. Pyramidal tract deficits and polyneuropathy in hyperthyroidism, Combination clinically mimicking amyotrophic lateral sclerosis. Am J Med 1985;78:1041–1044. Gericke CA, Zschenderlein R, Ludolph AC. Amyotrophic lateral sclerosis associated with multiple myeloma, endocrinopathy and skin changes suggestive of a POEMS syndrome variant. J Neurol Sci 1995;129 Suppl:58–60. Specola N, Vanier MT, Goutieres F, et al. The juvenile and chronic forms of GM2 gangliosidosis: clinical and enzymatic heterogeneity. Neurology 1990;40:145–150. Matsushima K, Kocha H, Watanabe R, et al. Diffuse cere-

brospinal gliomatosis mimicking amyotrophic lateral sclerosis. Intern Med 1993;32:476–479.

43. Pourmand R, Maybury BG. AAEM case report #31: paraneoplastic sensory neuronopathy. Muscle Nerve 1996; 19:1517–1522.

Sensory neuronopathy presents with sensory ataxia and no weakness. The site of pathology is in the dorsal root ganglia. Electrodiagnostic studies show absence of sensory nerve action potentials and preservation of motor nerve function. Elderly individuals with sensory ataxia and typical electrodiagnostic findings of sensory neuronopathy should be evaluated for underlying carcinoma.

44. Griffin JW, Cornblath DR, Alexander E, et al. Ataxic sensory neuropathy and dorsal root ganglionitis associated with Sjogren's syndrome. Ann Neurol 1990;27: 304–315.

Eleven women and two men developed sensory and autonomic neuronopathies in association with features of primary Sjögren's syndrome. Sjögren's syndrome had not been previously diagnosed at the time of neurological presentation in 11 of the 13. All had prominent loss of kinesthesia and proprioception. The course ranged from an abrupt, devastating onset to indolent progression over years. Sensory NCSs and nerve biopsy demonstrated a wide spectrum in the severity of loss of large myelinated fibers. The cutaneous nerves of 6 patients had perivascular mononuclear infiltrates without necrotizing arteritis. Examination of biopsy specimens of dorsal root ganglia in 3 patients revealed lymphocytic (T-cell) infiltration in the dorsal roots and ganglia, with focal clusters around neurons. The possibility of Sjögren's syndrome should be considered in patients, especially women, who develop acute, subacute, or chronic sensory and autonomic neuropathies, with ataxia and kinesthetic loss.

14

Radiculopathies

The neck, an organ most complex,
Has little use in either sex;
Its function's little more, at best,
Than tying to the head, the chest.

Edwin D. Kilbourne, M.D.

It seems humans barely achieve full maturity before their tissues begin an accelerating phase of degeneration. Nowhere is this more evident than in the spine. The intervertebral disc is the largest avascular structure in the body, depending for sustenance on the diffusion of nutrients across the endplate. Another avascular structure, the lens of the eye, offers interesting parallels. Both begin to desiccate and lose elasticity in the 5th-6th decade; individuals in this age group develop presbyopia and are prone to intervertebral disc rupture. In the 7th-9th decade, the tendency is to hardening and calcification resulting in cataracts and spinal stenosis. Unfortunately, the clinical success in dealing with degenerative spine disease is far less than in dealing with degenerative lens disease.

Clinical Pathoanatomy

Knowledge of the anatomical details of the spine, the spinal nerves, and the paravertebral muscles is integral to performing electrodiagnostic medicine consultations in patients with suspected radiculopathy. The following discussion covers the static and dynamic anatomy and pathoanatomy of the spine; the intervertebral disc; the spinal ligaments; the spinal roots, nerves and ganglia; and the paravertebral muscles.

THE SPINE

The vertebrae are separated by intervertebral discs, which are composed of an outer fibrous ring, the annulus fibrosus, and an inner gelatinous core, the nucleus pulposus (NP). The "posterior elements" of the vertebral bodies spread out to encircle the spinal cord and form the spinal canal. Extending backwards from the vertebral body, with varying degrees of slant, are the pedicles. The pedicles end in a bony mass, which has smooth upper and lower surfaces, the superior and inferior articulating facets, which are separated by the pars interarticularis. The facets allow a gliding action between adjacent vertebrae. From the facet masses, the transverse processes jut laterally and the laminae extend backwards to join in the midline and complete the circle. From the junction point of the laminae, the spinous process extends backward a bit further (Fig. 14.1). The lateral recess is the corner formed by the pedicle, vertebral body, and superior articular facet (Fig. 14.2). Hypertrophy of the facet can cause lateral recess stenosis. The neural foramen has an entrance, a middle zone, and an exit. The lateral recess of the spinal canal merges into the entry zone of the foramen. The dorsal root ganglion (DRG) occupies the midzone.

The spinal nerve passes outward from the spinal canal through the intervertebral foramen, a passageway formed by the vertebral body anteriorly, pedicles above and below, and the facet mass and its articulation, the zygapophyseal joint, posteriorly. The uncovertebral joints (of Luschka), which are not true joints, are the points where the posterolateral surface of a cervical vertebra comes into apposition with a neighboring vertebra. Degenerative osteophytes projecting into the intervertebral foramen from the uncovertebral "joints" may narrow it and cause radiculopathy (Fig. 14.1). The uncovertebral joints are not present in the lumbosacral spine.

The tough anterior longitudinal ligament (ALL) extends lengthwise along the anterior aspect of the vertebral column providing anterior reinforcement for the annulus. The posterior longitudinal ligament (PLL) extends along the posterior aspect of the vertebral

FIGURE 14.1. Lateral view of the cervical spine, showing the vertebral bodies separated by intervertebral discs, the pedicles merging into the facet joint with its superior and inferior facets and intervening pars interarticularis. The facets are oblique in the cervical region, more vertical in the lumbosacral spine. The uncovertebral joints are not true joints, but just the opposing surfaces of the vertebral bodies. The uncovertebral processes may form osteophytes, or "spurs," which then project into the foramen.

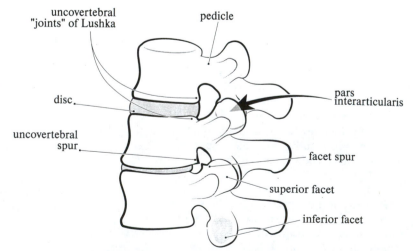

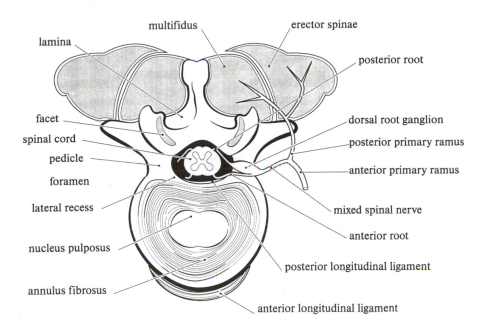

labels on figure:
lamina
multifidus
erector spinae
facet
posterior root
spinal cord
dorsal root ganglion
pedicle
posterior primary ramus
foramen
anterior primary ramus
lateral recess
mixed spinal nerve
nucleus pulposus
anterior root
annulus fibrosus
posterior longitudinal ligament
anterior longitudinal ligament

FIGURE 14.2. Cross section of a vertebral body with one pedicle cut away to show the contents of the intervertebral foramen, with the dorsal root ganglion lying in the midzone. Note the location of the multifidus muscle compartment and the innervation of the paraspinal muscles by the posterior primary ramus. The posterior longitudinal ligament is incomplete laterally, and disc ruptures tend to occur in a posterolateral direction. When a facet joint becomes enlarged due to osteoarthritis it may encroach on the lateral recess, where the nerve root is entering the foramen.

bodies and reinforces the discs posteriorly. Compared with the ALL, the PLL is weak and flimsy and narrows as it descends. Disc herniations tend to occur posterolaterally, especially in the lumbosacral region, in part because of the lateral incompleteness of the PLL (Fig. 14.3). In the cervical region, the PLL may ossify and contribute to spondylotic narrowing. The ligamentum flavum extends along the posterior aspect of the spinal canal. It buckles and folds during neck extension and may also contribute to canal narrowing.

The static anatomy of the spine provides only a partial understanding of the changes that occur on motion. Direct measurements have shown that the pressure within the disc varies markedly with different postures and activities. It is lowest when lying supine, increases by fourfold on standing and increases a further 50% when leaning forward. The pressure is 40% higher when sitting than standing. The higher pressure when sitting is clinically relevant, as patients with lumbosacral disc ruptures characteristically have more pain sitting than standing. Eating meals from the mantelpiece is virtually pathognomonic. The intradiscal pressure during a situp is astronomical.

The size of the intervertebral foramina decrease with extension and with ipsilateral bending. In extension, the facet joints draw closer together and the posterior quadrants of the spinal canal narrow. The longitudinal and flavum ligaments alternately stretch and buckle during flexion and extension. The spinal cord stretches during extension. Tethering by the dentate ligaments accentuates the mechanical stresses laterally. Cervical roots stretch with flexion and may an-

gulate at the entrance to the foramen. The intraspinal subarachnoid pressure varies with respiration and increases markedly with Valsalva or restriction of venous outflow. Like veins everywhere, the epidural and radicular veins change in size with posture and respiration. All these dynamic changes, which are especially relevant in the presence of pathology, form the basis for clinical tests and historical questions useful for distinguishing the various causes for back and neck pain.

THE INTERVERTEBRAL DISC

The annulus provides circumferential reinforcement for the disc; the spherical NP allows the vertebral bodies above and below to glide and slip across it, like a ball bearing. The NP is eccentrically placed, closer to the posterior aspect of the disc (Fig. 14.2). The relative thinness of the annulus posteriorly is another factor contributing to the tendency of disc herniations to occur in that direction.

The great majority of the weight bearing function of a normal disc is borne by the NP, which contains proteoglycans, macromolecules which heartily imbibe fluid. Early in life, the NP is 90% water, but undergoes progressive desiccation over time. With desiccation of the nucleus and loss of compressibility, the annulus must assume more of the weight burden. This increased load, in the face of its own degenerative weakening, then makes the annulus prone to tears. Intradiscal proteoglycans are innocuous, but spilled

FIGURE 14.3. Posterior view of the cauda equina with exiting nerve roots. The nerve roots move laterally en route to their exit foramina. A posterolateral HNP has compressed the S1 root as it passes by the L5-S1 interspace. The dorsal root ganglion lies well lateral and below, out of harm's way, so that the peripherally recorded sensory nerve action potential would not be affected. A central HNP at any interspace could affect multiple roots.

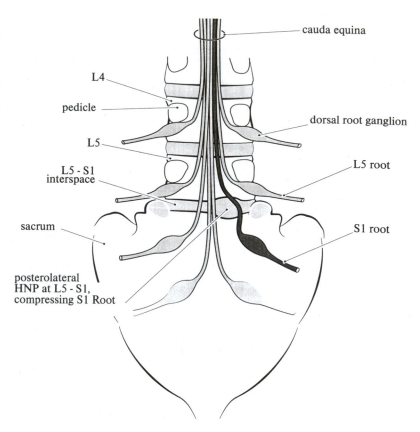

into the epidural space in the course of disc rupture they can incite an inflammatory response.

THE SPINAL ROOTS

The anterior and posterior roots arise from the spinal cord and arc laterally toward the exit foramen. The DRG lies on the posterior root at the midzone of the foramen, and just beyond this point the two roots join to form the mixed spinal nerve. The location of the DRG is of immense clinical and electrodiagnostic importance (vide infra). Just after its exit from the foramen the spinal nerve divides into anterior and posterior primary rami. The anterior ramus innervates the limb muscles, the posterior the paravertebral muscles. Most limb muscles receive innervation from more than one root.

In the cervical spine, the nerve root exits over the vertebral body of like number, i.e., the C6 root exits at C5-6. The C8 root exits beneath C7 and all subsequent roots exit beneath the vertebral body of like number, i.e., the L5 root exits at L5-S1. The roots exit more or less horizontally in the cervical spine, although there is a slight downward slant. The downward slant increases through the thoracic region. When the cord

terminates at the level of L1-2, the remaining roots drop vertically downward in the cauda equina to their exit foramina (Fig. 14.3). In the cervical region, there is about a one segment discrepancy between the cord level and the spinous process, in the thoracic region about two segments, in the lumbosacral region three to four segments. Therefore, the L5 nerve root exiting at the L5-S1 interspace has arisen as a discrete structure at L1-L2 and had to traverse the interspaces at L2-3, L3-4 and L4-5 before exiting at L5-S1, sliding laterally all the while. So, the L5 root could be injured by a central disc at L2-3 or L3-4, a posterolateral disc at L4-5, or a far lateral disc or lateral recess stenosis at L5-S1. A posterolateral disc at L4-5 is the most likely culprit, but not the sole suspect. The clinician must correlate the EMG localization of a given root with the radiographic and clinical information to deduce the vertebral level involved and the proper course of action.

Clinical and EMG localization of radiculopathies depends heavily on detailed knowledge of dermatomal and myotomal anatomy (see Chapter 3). Unfortunately, available charts always vary in some detail. Our knowledge of segmental anatomy began with detailed anatomical dissections, and has been supplemented in the modern era with clinical and EMG information. Wolf's small monograph contains an eloquent discussion of dermatomes and myotomes, their origins and their variability, in addition to a wealth of information on the clinical assessment of the peripheral nervous system (1). EMG-derived myotomal data is of the greatest utility for EMG assessment of suspected radiculopathy (2).

THE PARASPINAL MUSCLES

The anatomical details of the structure and innervation of the paravertebral muscles are highly relevant to the electrodiagnostic evaluation of radiculopathies (3). Paraspinal abnormalities are the earliest and sometimes only changes to develop. The anatomy of the paravertebral muscle mass is complex, but for electrodiagnostic purposes, it can practically be divided into the multifidus compartment versus everything else. Most of the paraspinal muscles arise from one common embryologic precursor, and there is extensive longitudinal overlap of innervation. This creates two problems for the EMGer: 1) the redundant innervation provides a mechanism for efficient reinnervation after a solitary root lesion, minimizing detectable abnormalities, and 2) the level at which paraspinal abnormalities appear may not correspond with the level of the lesion. In contrast, the deep multifidus innervation arises from a single root. Multifidus abnormalities in radiculopathy are therefore both more likely to be present and are more localizing. They are not localizing enough, however, to reliably indicate the vertebral level of the injury, but other factors come into play in this limitation, as discussed.

Pathology of Degenerative Spine Disease

With aging and recurrent micro and macro trauma, degenerative spine disease develops. This involves both the disc (degenerative disc disease, or DDD) and the bony structures and joints (degenerative joint disease, or DJD). These processes are separate but related. Together DDD and DJD are referred to as spondylosis.

Small tears in the annulus may cause nonspecific, nonradiating low back pain (LBP). More extensive tears lead to disc bulging or protrusion, in which the disc herniates but remains beneath the PLL. Frank ruptures breach the PLL and allow a full blown herniation of the nucleus pulposus (HNP) into the epidural space. Most HNPs in the lumbosacral spine occur in a posterolateral direction; occasionally they are directly lateral or central (Fig. 14.3). Which nerve roots are damaged depends largely on the direction of the herniation. In the face of disc herniation, the root may be damaged not only by direct compression but also by an inflammatory process induced by discal proteoglycans, ischemia due to pressure and by adhesions and fibrosis.

The anterior elements, vertebral body and pedicles, normally bear 80–90% of the weight. As degenerative changes advance with desiccation and loss of disc height, the posterior elements (facets, pars and laminae) may come to carry up to 50% of the weight bearing function. This increases the work of the posterior elements and accelerates their degenerative changes. They react to the increased weight bearing role by becoming hypertrophic and elaborating osteophytes.

Osteoarthritis and synovitis of the facet joints is another source of problems. In response to the increased loading attendant on loss of disc height and shift of weight bearing posteriorly, the facet joints develop degenerative changes: laxity of the capsule, instability, subluxation and bony hypertrophy with osteophyte formation. The friction induced by minor instability and microtrauma leads to the formation of osteophytes. In the cervical spine, there is the added element of hypertrophy of the uncinate processes and the development of uncovertebral spurs. Degenerative osteophytes arising simultaneously from the uncus and from the vertebral body end plate region may become confluent and create a spondylotic bar or ridge which stretches across the entire extent of the spinal canal. Like any arthritic joint, the facet may enlarge, impinging on the intervertebral foramen or the spinal canal, especially in the lateral recess. Loss of disc height causes the PLL and the ligamentum flavum to buckle and bulge into the canal. The degenerative changes in the discs and bony elements eventually produce cervical or lumbar spondylosis and may culminate in the syndrome of spinal stenosis.

All these degenerative changes leave less room for the neural elements. In the sagittal plane, the average cervical spinal cord is about 8 mm and the average cervical spinal canal about 14 mm. A sagittal canal diameter less than 10 mm may put the spinal cord at risk. The epidural space is normally occupied primarily by epidural fat and veins. When disc herniations and osteophytes intrude into the space, the resultant clinical manifestations depend in large part on how much room there is to accommodate them. Patients blessed by nature with capacious spinal canals can asymptomatically harbor a surprising amount of pathology. Patients with congenitally narrow canals and those who have undergone past spinal fusion procedures are at increased risk for developing spinal stenosis. Compression of vascular structures may introduce an additional complication of cord and/or root ischemia.

Several different clinical syndromes may ensue from degenerative spine disease, including: simple, single level radiculopathy; multilevel radiculopathy; cauda equina syndrome; cervical myelopathy; cervical radiculomyelopathy; neurogenic claudication; lateral recess syndrome; and occasionally a central cord or Brown-Sequard syndrome. Electrodiagnostic medicine is most helpful in evaluating the radiculopathy component, and the remainder of the discussion will focus on nerve root syndromes. Rarely, radiculopathy results from other processes, such as tumor (e.g., neurofibroma, meningioma, metastasis), infection (e.g., Lyme disease, zoster, CMV), infiltration (e.g., meningeal neoplasia, sarcoidosis), or ischemia (e.g., diabetes) (4).

Because of the varied pathology involved, different types of radiculopathy occur in disc disease and spondylosis. The process is frequently multifactorial, involving some combination of disc herniation and spondylosis. The most straightforward clinical syndrome is unilateral "soft disc" rupture. A similar clinical picture can result from a foraminal osteophyte, a "hard disc." Some patients have soft disc superimposed on hard disc. It is clinically, radiologically and sometimes surgically, difficult to distinguish between soft disc and hard disc. Osteophytes, spurs, and foraminal stenosis are more common than simple soft disc in the etiology of cervical radiculopathy. In the Radhakrishnan et al series, soft disc, i.e., not present in association with significant spondylosis, was responsible in only 22%, the remainder had hard disc or a combination (5). A central HNP may compress the spinal cord or cauda equina.

Modern imaging techniques have become a mixed blessing. MRI shows abnormalities of the spine (disc bulges and protrusions) in patients who have no symptoms (6). With the high false positive rate of imaging studies, it is increasingly necessary to identify the dysfunctional root by other means, such as clinical evaluation and EMG. Low back pain is extremely common. Given the high incidence of MRI abnormalities in the population, how many of the innumerable episodes of acute, self limited back and neck pain suffered by humankind, usually attributed to musculoskeletal problems, are in reality discogenic?

Pathophysiology of Radiculopathy

The pathophysiology of radiculopathy is essentially the same regardless of etiology. Root compression due to HNP or spur tends to be concentrated on the distal portion of the root, proximal to the DRG. As with any nerve compression syndrome, the large myelinated fibers bear the brunt of the damage, and the degree of injury depends on the intensity and duration of the compressive force (2,7). Demyelination is the primary change with mild compression; more severe insults produce axon loss. Even with large lesions the damage is usually only partial. With recovery, remyelination and axon regrowth occur. In the muscle, collaterals sprout from undamaged axons and these provide another mechanism for reinnervation.

After root compression a number of events occur. If severe enough to produce conduction block or immediate axonal disruption, there is decreased recruitment in the affected muscle. The degree depends on the cross innervation by other roots and the number of roots involved. With a moderate injury the remaining motor units increase their firing rate to compensate for the lost contribution of the involved axons to contractile power. This change is detectable immediately after injury. With a purely demyelinating root lesion there is no further change. If there is loss of axons, denervation develops in the target muscles, and spontaneous and increased insertional activity in the form of spike and positive sharp fibrillations gradually materialize. It requires days to weeks for fibrillations to appear after any nerve injury, and root lesions are no exception.

Fibrillations appear and disappear on a schedule determined by the severity of injury, the distance from the injury, the extent of collateral innervation, and the efficiency of reinnervation. Not all muscles of a myotome are affected equally. Abnormalities evolve in a proximal to distal gradient, appearing first in the paraspinals, then in proximal limb muscles and last in distal limb muscles. The denervated muscle fibers are then slowly reinnervated over months by either collateral sprouts from uninvolved axons or by regrowth from the site of injury. Due to healing and reinnervation, the fibrillations disappear in the same sequence in which they emerged. The paraspinals reinnervate first, with resolution of spontaneous activity, and this pattern evolves centrifugally down the extremity. Fibrillations disappear last from the distal muscles. So the fibrillations may appear first in the paraspinals, but also disappear first from the paraspinals.

Reinnervation also changes the architecture of the motor unit. As the motor unit territory of axons that have provided reinnervation increases, they oversee more muscle fibers. Initially, the reinnervating sprouts are immature and conduct erratically and slowly due to incomplete myelination. Sometimes they do not produce a muscle fiber discharge at all, either because of conduction failure in the sprout or failure of the new, immature, unstable neuromuscular junction to function properly. This produces fragmentation, polyphasicity, and instability of the MUAP as each terminal fiber makes its contribution to the MUAP spike erratically. Rather than one smooth spike resembling a QRS complex, the MUAP is composed of multiple, independent spikes. The ultimate example is the "nascent" MUAP of early reinnervation: small amplitude, highly polyphasic (often 10 or more components), and firing at an extremely high rate in a futile attempt to generate power. Sometimes the sprout conducts so slowly that the action potential generated by its subject muscle fibers is detached from the main body of the MUAP and becomes a late component, trailing far behind. These are also referred to as parasites or satellite potentials and can only be truly appreciated with delay line analysis. As the reinnervating sprouts mature and myelinate more uniformly, their variability in conduction velocity diminishes. The discharge of the motor unit becomes more coordinated and the number of phases or turns decreases. The unit simplifies. However, because of the increased number of muscle fibers now firing in synchrony, the amplitude increases. Muscle fibers far from the electrode now make a contribution, which is seen by the electrode as an increase in MUAP duration.

When reinnervation is complete, the resultant picture is one of a decreased number of MUAPs. The remaining MUAPs have increased amplitude, duration and complexity, sometimes with late components, and they discharge rapidly. On delay line analysis the units are stable, with no variability in configuration; any late components present do not jitter or block. Chronic repetitive discharges (CRDs) may appear after 4–6 months and remain indefinitely, but fibrillations are absent (7). This is the picture of static, healed, stable radiculopathy.

When radiculopathies affect multiple levels, as often occurs in advanced cervical or lumbar spondylosis, these changes are more profound and long lasting. Reinnervation is inefficient because there are few healthy roots remaining. There is often a mixture of chronic neurogenic MUAP changes mixed with active fibrillations, indicating a dynamic and ongoing process.

General Principles of Electrodiagnosis in Radiculopathy

The electrodiagnostic procedures of use in evaluation of radiculopathy include motor and sensory nerve conduction studies (NCS), late responses, needle electrode examination (NEE) and evoked potentials. The general picture is one of normal motor and sensory NCS, with abnormalities in a myotomal distribution, including paraspinals, on NEE. Some general rules help avoid error. The sensory potentials should be normal, as discussed further below. Motor studies are abnormal only in proportion to axon loss. The NEE abnormalities should be in a myotomal distribution, involving at least two muscles, preferably several, having the same myotomal but different peripheral nerve innervation. Always surround abnormality with normality to avoid missing a diffuse process, such as polymyositis, nonspecific diffuse increased insertional activity, or motor neuron disease (2,7). Normal paraspinals do not exclude radiculopathy. Fibrillation potentials isolated to a paraspinal focus are consistent with but not diagnostic of radiculopathy. Diffuse paraspinal fibrillations can occur in a number of conditions (2). The vertebral level location of fibrillations does not reliably indicate the root involved. And lastly, a normal study does not exclude radiculopathy.

The mainstay of diagnosis is the NEE. Most electrodiagnostic medicine consultants (EMCs) are reluctant to diagnose radiculopathy unless fibrillation potentials are present. Relying on MUAP abnormalities in isolation invites overdiagnosis. Normal muscles may contain 5–15% polyphasic MUAPs (7). Unless the MUAP changes are pronounced and unequivocal (clearly decreased recruitment, increased size, markedly polyphasic) and clearly in a myotomal distribution, the examiner should remain conservative, err on the side of undercalling, and make some noncommittal statement. EMG has clear limitations in the evaluation of radiculopathy. One of its strengths is that a normal individual virtually never has an abnormal EMG. A low incidence of false positives should be good reason to rely on the study when it is abnormal. Soft call diagnosis of radiculopathy based on equivocal MUAP changes alone does everyone a disservice.

The timing of the electrodiagnostic medicine consultation in radiculopathy is crucial. Although there is some disagreement, most EMGers use a general rule that it requires about 7–10 days after onset to detect fibrillations in the paraspinal muscles and 2–3 weeks in the limb muscles. With rare exception, patients are in full electrical flower at about 3 weeks (7). The findings on needle examination are thus heavily dependent on timing. A study done too early may be normal, a study done too late may also be normal or show only chronic neurogenic MUAP changes but no fibrillations. A study could show fibrillations in the paraspinals only, because limb muscles have not had time for them to develop, or in the limb muscles only because the paraspinals have reinnervated.

Motor NCS are typically normal in radiculopathies. The damage to the root is usually only partial. In the face of a severe radiculopathy with marked motor loss, there may be loss of M wave amplitude due to neurogenic atrophy, and mild to moderate slowing of motor nerve conduction velocity due to involvement of the fastest conducting fibers. The situation is the same as for motor neuron disease and axonal polyneuropathies, i.e., conduction slowing and loss of M wave amplitude in proportion to the degree of axon loss. Peripheral motor conduction slowing occurs most commonly when a severe L5 radiculopathy producing foot drop causes diffuse slowing of the peroneal nerve, which can be mistaken for peroneal neuropathy. The lack of focal changes across the fibular head and the normality of the superficial peroneal sensory nerve action potential (SNAP) should help identify the radicular nature of the process.

Like the motor NCS, the SNAPs are also normal in radiculopathies. The sensory neuron in the dorsal root ganglion, residing in relative safety in the midzone of the intervertebral foramen, is not often compressed by either HNP or osteophytic spur. The intact and uninvolved cell body is able to maintain its peripheral process in continued health, although the central process may be lost or damaged. The peripherally recorded SNAP thus remains normal, even in the face of radicular sensory loss or abnormalities of the relevant SEP (8).

There are some exceptions to the otherwise reliable rule of normal SNAPs in radiculopathy. Recent anatomical studies have shown that although the majority of DRGs lie directly beneath the pedicle, in about one third of specimens the center of the ganglion in the lumbar region may overlay the lateral portion of the disc (9). Occasionally, a free disc fragment from a far lateral HNP may migrate out into the foramen and impinge on the DRG. Similarly, severe lateral recess stenosis due to hypertrophy of the superior facet may compromise the DRG (10). Sometimes, the DRG may lie in an ectopic intraspinal location, well proximal to its usual position, making it vulnerable to involvement by HNP or spur (11). Such ectopic DRGs have been mistaken for tumors, with unfortunate results.

For the reasons discussed, the status of the paraspinal muscles is critical in the assessment of radiculopathies. To ensure an adequate paraspinal survey, it is imperative to maximize the chances of examining the multifidus compartment (vide supra). Haig et al. developed a technique for localizing the multifidus based on the injection of latex dye and subsequent dissection of cadavers (3). The needle should be inserted 2.5 cm lateral to the midline at an angle of 45° and driven to the periosteum, then withdrawn slightly.

The progress and final position of the needle is monitored by the insertional activity produced. In obese subjects, the angle should be changed to 60° if insertional activity is not obtained. Unfortunately, no multifidus muscle arises from the spinous process of S1.

Limitations of EMG in the Diagnosis of Radiculopathy

As discussed, the root level of injury bears an inconstant relationship to the vertebral level of injury. Referring physicians, especially surgeons, usually think in terms of a vertebral interspace. The EMC should think in terms of roots and not be seduced into thinking that electrodiagnosis can identify the vertebral level, especially in the lumbosacral spine. For instance, the electrodiagnostic medicine diagnosis should be "L5 radiculopathy," not "L5-S1 radiculopathy."

Most limb muscles are innervated by at least two roots. This minimizes both the degree of weakness and the electrical changes which occur in radiculopathy. The uninvolved root provides a source of collateral sprouts for reinnervation. In addition, most root lesions are only partial, and the uninvolved axons at the affected level also provide reinnervation. The motor unit in a typical limb muscle contains a few hundred muscle fibers. Fortunately, dysfunction of only a few axons will set hundreds of muscle fibers to fibrillating, and this amount of denervation is usually readily detected by NEE, if done in the proper time frame. When multiple roots are involved, reinnervation rescue is less effective and the abnormalities are even more pronounced. When the root lesion is mild and produces only demyelination, no fibrillations appear and the only abnormality may be changes in MUAP recruitment, the detection of which is often subjective and equivocal. Demyelinating lesions severe enough to cause marked recruitment changes also generally damage enough axons to produce fibrillations. With mild radiculopathies, the EMG may eventually revert to normal, even in the face of continued symptoms (2).

Although the F wave assesses the proximal structures, including the roots, most EMCs have found the F of more theoretical than practical value in the evaluation and management of radiculopathy. Only a few uninvolved axons and multiple root innervation suffice to preserve the minimal F latency. Even when root demyelination occurs, the involved segment is so short it has little detectable effect on the overall latency of the very long F wave loop. When F abnormalities are unequivocal, other more definitive changes are usually detectable. The same arguments can be applied to the H-reflex, with the additional problems that it only assesses the S1 segment (the FCR H-reflex is seldom used), and that any H-reflex abnormality is heralded by clinically detectable changes in the ankle reflex. There is disagreement about whether the amplitude or the latency is the more important parameter. The late responses can sometimes serve as useful confirmation of pathology in the face of equivocal abnormalities on the NEE. The hypothetical utility of SEPs in radiculopathy has also not been realized (7).

Cervical Radiculopathy

A recent population based study of cervical radiculopathy provided a wealth of interesting information (5). The incidence is highest at ages 50–54, with a mean age of 47 and a male predominance. Other series have also found a similar mean age and male predominance (12,13). In the population based study, there was a decline in incidence after age 60 (the patients are developing spondylosis and spinal stenosis). There was a history of physical injury or exertion in only 15%; the most common precipitants were shoveling snow or playing golf. The onset was acute in half, subacute in a quarter and insidious in a quarter, with the majority of patients symptomatic for about 2 weeks before diagnosis. Surgery was done in 26%. The disease tends to recur: 31% of patients had a previous history of cervical radiculopathy and 32% had a recurrence during follow-up. At last follow-up, 90% of the patients had minimal to no symptoms. Others have noted this favorable long-term prognosis.

There are a number of clinical conditions that may be confused with cervical radiculopathy. These primarily include brachial plexopathies, entrapment neuropathies, and non-neuropathic mimickers. The more common musculoskeletal conditions causing confusion include shoulder pathology (bursitis, tendinitis, impingement syndrome), lateral epicondylitis, and DeQuervain's tenosynovitis. Cervical myofascial pain, facet joint disease and cervical vertebral body pathology can cause neck pain with referred pain to the arm. (Patients with cervical strain due to whiplash rarely have radiculopathy. There were zero cases of HNP due to whiplash in the Radhakrishnan et al series [5]). Lyme disease can cause meningitis and radiculitis, producing neck and arm pain. A rare patient with subarachnoid hemorrhage may present with neck pain without headache. Cervical epidural abscess or hematoma may present with neck pain and various neurologic signs. Pain can be referred to the neck, arm, or shoulder from the heart, lungs, esophagus, or upper abdomen.

CLINICAL SIGNS AND SYMPTOMS IN CERVICAL RADICULOPATHY

Because EMG has its greatest yield when focused on weak muscles and on the region of likely pathology, familiarity with the clinical details is useful in planning the examination. The electrodiagnostic medicine consultation should include an appropriate history and physical examination to direct and guide the study. Two classic articles detail the history and examination findings in cervical radiculopathy (12,14). The annotated bibliography provides a summary, but both are worth detailed perusal.

Yoss et al. evaluated 100 patients with surgically confirmed single level cervical radiculopathies (12). They were confident enough after this experience to recommend dispensing with myelography to guide future surgery! Their findings are useful in guiding an EMG. The highly and suggestively localizing findings from these 100 patients are summarized in Table 14.1. Murphey et al. reviewed 648 cases of surgically treated single level cervical radiculopathies (14). Findings in terms of pain radiation and neurological deficits were similar to Yoss et al. The Memphis series did emphasize the occurrence of pain in the pectoral region in 20% of their cases; they opined that neck, periscapular and pectoral region pain was referred from the disc itself, and that arm pain was the result of nerve root compression.

In the Radhakrishnan et al. series, cervicobrachial pain was present at the onset in 98% and was radicular in 65% (5). Paresthesias were reported by 90%, almost identical to the Yoss series. Pain on neck movement was present in 98%, paraspinal muscle spasm in 88%, decreased reflexes in 84% (triceps 50%, biceps or brachioradialis 34%), weakness in 65%, and sensory loss in 33%. The diagnostic criteria used by Radhakrishnan et al. are summarized in Table 14.2. Using these criteria, 45% of the patients were judged to have definite cervical radiculopathy, 30% probable, and 25% possible. In the Cleveland clinic series, 70% had motor and sensory symptoms, 12% had motor symptoms only, and 18% had sensory symptoms only (13).

The clinical evaluation preceding the EMG should screen for the presence of nonradicular pathology, and determine which cervical root(s) is most likely involved. Patients with bicipital tendinitis, deQuervain's, a hemiparesis and the like should be sent away if politically possible. Those with findings suggesting a

TABLE 14.1
Clinical Findings in 100 Cervical Radiculopathy Patients (12)

Clinical Finding	Highly Localizing To	Suggestively Localizing To
Pain only in neck and shoulder		C5
Presence of scapular/interscapular pain		C7 or C8
No pain below elbow		C5
Pain involving the posterior upper arm		C7
Pain involving the medial upper arm		C7 or C8
Paresthesias limited to the thumb	C6	
Paresthesias limited to index and middle	C7	
Paresthesias limited to ring and small	C8	
Whole hand paresthesias		C7
Depressed triceps reflex	C7 or C8	
Depressed biceps and brachioradialis reflexes	C5 or C6	
Weakness of spinati	C5	
Weakness of deltoid	C5 or C6	
Weakness of triceps	C7	
Weakness of hand intrinsics	C8	
Sensory loss over thumb only		C6 or C7
Sensory loss involving middle finger	C7	
Sensory loss involving small finger	C8	

specific root level should receive an electrodiagnostic assessment directed at that level. Those who may have cervical radiculopathy but no clues to a given level should receive a generic root screen of six limb muscles plus the paraspinals (15). The specifics of the electrodiagnostic examination are discussed further below.

Localizing information in suspected cervical radiculopathy is obtainable from the history—especially from patterns of pain radiation and paresthesias. Radiating pain on coughing, sneezing or straining at stool is significant but seldom elicited. Increased pain on shoulder motion suggests nonradicular pathology. Relief of pain by resting the hand atop the head is reportedly characteristic of cervical radiculopathy, but I have seen this phenomenon with a Pancoast tumor. Hand paresthesias at night suggest carpal tunnel syndrome, but CTS can occur in association with cervical radiculopathy ("double crush syndrome"), so nocturnal acroparesthesias do not exclude radiculopathy.

Physical examination in patients with suspected cervical radiculopathy should include an assessment of the range of motion of the neck and arm, a search for root compression signs, detailed examination of strength and reflexes, a screening sensory examina-

TABLE 14.2
Summary of Diagnostic Criteria for Cervical Radiculopathy from 1994 Population Based Study (5)

Symptoms

Neck pain, arm pain or combined neck and arm pain

Paresthesia, hyperesthesia, or dysesthesia in a nerve root distribution

Muscle weakness

Signs

Sensory changes in a dermatomal distribution

Weakness, atrophy or fasciculation, in a myotomal distribution

Unilateral diminished deep tendon reflexes

Diagnostic tests/surgical verification

Electromyographic evidence of acute denervation in cervical paraspinal muscles and/or in a myotome

Demonstrable abnormality on myelography, computer-assisted myelography, or MRI correlating with cervical radiculopathy

Identification of an affected cervical root at surgery

tion and probing for areas of muscle spasm or trigger points. The cervical spine range of motion is highly informative. Patients should be asked to put chin to chest and to either shoulder, each ear to shoulder and to hold the head in full extension; these maneuvers all affect the size of the intervertebral foramen. Pain produced by movements that close the foramen suggest cervical radiculopathy. Pain on the symptomatic side on putting the ipsilateral ear to the shoulder suggests radiculopathy, but increased pain on leaning or turning away from the symptomatic side suggests a myofascial origin. Radiating pain with the head in extension and tilted slightly to the symptomatic side is highly suggestive of cervical radiculopathy; brief breath holding in this position will sometimes elicit the pain. The addition of axial compression (Spurling's maneuver) does not seem to add much. Light digital compression of the jugular veins until the face is flushed and the patient is uncomfortable will sometimes elicit radicular symptoms: unilateral shoulder, arm, pectoral or scapular pain, or radiating paresthesias into the arm or hand (Naffziger sign). This is a highly specific but insensitive finding. An occasional patient has relief of pain with manual upward neck traction. Patients with a globally restricted cervical spine range of motion often have extensive degenerative disease.

Pain or limitation of motion of any upper extremity joint should signal the possibility of nonradicular pathology. The patient should be asked to put the shoulder through a full active range of motion, touching the hand to the opposite shoulder and the opposite ear, then reaching behind as high between the scapulae as possible. Any pain or limitation of motion on the symptomatic side suggests bursitis, capsulitis, tendinitis or impingement syndrome rather than cervical radiculopathy as the etiology of the patient's pain.

A focused but detailed strength exam should at least assess the power in the deltoids, spinati, biceps, triceps, pronators, wrist extensors, EIP, APB and interossei. The sensory exam should concentrate on the hand, and particularly assess touch, since the large, myelinated fibers conveying light touch are more vulnerable to pressure injury than the smaller fibers carrying pain and temperature. Reflex exam should include not only the standard upper extremity reflexes, but the knee and ankle jerks and plantar reflexes as well. Increased lower extremity reflexes and extensor plantar responses suggest myelopathy complicating the radiculopathy.

Based on the foregoing, Table 14.3 outlines the clinical data that favor the diagnosis of cervical radiculopathy.

TABLE 14.3

Clinical Signs and Symptoms That Favor a Diagnosis of Cervical Radiculopathy

- Age 35–60
- Acute/subacute onset
- History of cervical or lumbosacral radiculopathy
- Cervicobrachial pain radiating to shoulder, periscapular region, pectoral region, or arm
- Paresthesias in arm or hand
- Pain on neck movement—especially extension or ipsilateral bending
- Positive root compression signs
- Radiating pain with cough, sneeze, or bowel movement
- Myotomal weakness
- Decreased reflex(es)
- Dermatomal sensory loss
- Pain relief with hand on head
- Pain relief with manual upward traction

ELECTRODIAGNOSIS IN CERVICAL RADICULOPATHY

The Quality Assurance committee of the American Association of Electrodiagnostic Medicine has recently reviewed the utility of EMG in the evaluation of patients with cervical radiculopathy and formulated a practice parameter addressing this problem (16). A meticulous, stringent review of the literature identified 10 high quality articles addressing the issue. The sensitivity of EMG for detecting abnormalities was in the range of 60–70%. The sensitivity is significantly higher in patients with motor involvement than in those with only pain or sensory abnormalities, and the yield increases with increasing severity of disease. Because EMGs are rarely abnormal in normal subjects, the test is highly specific. There is a 65–85% correlation of EMG abnormalities with imaging and surgical findings (16). C7 root lesions are the most common (±60%), C6 next most common (±20%), with C5 and C8 lesions making up about equal proportions of the remainder (2,5,12–14).

The examiner should tailor the EMG to probe the muscles most likely to be involved. In the absence of clear clinical direction, one must resort to a generic root screen. Choosing which muscles to study, and how many, has heretofore been a matter of personal opinion and preference. Recent investigations have provided some guidance. Lauder and Dillingham concluded that a screen of six limb muscles plus the paraspinals had a yield of 93–98%, and that examining more muscles made no significant additional contri-

TABLE 14.4
High Yield Muscles for Cervical Radiculopathy Screens (13)*

C5	C6	C7	C8
IS 83%	ANC 100%	Triceps 93%	EIP 100%
Deltoid 83%	FCR 80%	FCR 93%	FDI 83%
BR 83%	PRT 78%	ANC 78%	ADM 83%
BB 71%	BR 71%	PRT 61%	FPL 67%
PS 71%	PS 63%	PS 31%	PS 80%

* Defined by the presence of fibrillation potentials.
Overall, the paraspinal muscles were abnormal in 48%.
ADM, abductor digiti minimi; ANC, anconeus; BB, biceps brachii; BR, brachioradialis; EIP, extensor indicis proprius; FCR, flexor carpi radialis; FDI, first dorsal interosseous; IS, infraspinatus; PRT, pronator teres; PS, paraspinal muscles.

bution (15). Levin, et al studied 50 patients with surgically proven single level cervical radiculopathies (13). They found stereotyped patterns with C5, C7 and C8 lesions, but a variable pattern with C6 lesions which could resemble C5 or C7. The muscles of highest yield for each level are shown in Table 14.4. Based on the information from these two studies, the following six limb muscle survey seems reasonable as a generic root screen: deltoid or infraspinatus; brachioradialis; triceps or anconeus; flexor carpi radialis; extensor indicis proprius and first dorsal interosseous. This would provide at least two reasonably high yield muscles for each root. The brachioradialis, anconeus, and flexor carpi radialis are particularly useful since they are high yield for more than a single root. If the clinical history and examination suggest a particular root, modification of the screen to include more high yield muscles from the suspected level should be productive.

Lumbosacral Radiculopathy

It goes without saying that low back pain (LBP) is a major cause of misery in humans; about 70% suffer from at least an occasional episode (17). And although many patients suffer with sciatica at some time, clinically significant radiculopathy occurs in only 4% to 6% of the population. Estimates of the direct and indirect costs of back pain and related disorders range as high as $100 billion per year. The 5% of patients who become temporarily or permanently disabled from back pain account for 75% or more of these costs (18,19). The first step down the road to disability is usually an

episode of LBP of suspected discogenic origin, often with radicular symptoms. Lumbar spine surgery does not always meet with success, and a failed back patient gradually evolves from what may or may not have been a true radicular syndrome. Abnormalities on imaging studies are common in asymptomatic subjects and only loosely associated with symptoms and neurologic examination (6,18). Specialized evaluation, including electrodiagnostic medicine consultation, can help avoid subjecting patients with back pain to unnecessary surgical procedures.

There are numerous potential origins for LBP. Most benign self limited episodes of LBP presumably arise from musculoligamentous structures, and discomfort is localized to the low back region. But there are numerous pain sensitive structures which can underlie a clinical episode of back pain: the intervertebral disc, especially the outer fibers of the annulus; the facet joints; other bony structures; and spinal nerve roots. In addition, pain can be referred to the lower back from visceral structures in the abdomen and pelvis. The back may also be involved in systemic diseases, such as spondyloarthropathies.

Involvement of some of these pain sensitive structures can produce referred pain that radiates to the extremity (buttock, hip, thigh) and can simulate the radiating pain of nerve root origin. A study of 1293 cases of LBP concluded that referred pain to the lower limb most often originated from sacroiliac and facet joints. Referred pain to the extremity occurred nearly twice as often as true radicular pain, and frequently mimicked the clinical presentation of radiculopathies (20). Investigations have demonstrated that considerable pain can be referred to the buttock and thigh with disease limited to the disc, the facet joint or the sacroiliac joint (21–23). A study of 92 patients with chronic LBP concluded that 39% had annular tears or other forms of internal disc disruption as the etiology of their pain. No available clinical test differentiated between patients with internal disc disruptions and those with compressive radiculopathy (24). A similar situation seems to exist with facet join pain (25).

The first suggestion that a patient may have nerve root compression usually comes because of radiating pain into one or both lower extremities. Conservative therapy still usually suffices, even in patients with HNPs, and only 5–10% of patients ultimately warrant surgery (17). Operative intervention is generally appropriate only when there is a combination of definite disk herniation shown by imaging studies, a corresponding syndrome of radicular pain, a corresponding neurologic deficit, and a failure to respond to conservative therapy (17). At some point in the clinical course of such patients, an EMG is often requested to help elucidate the presence and degree of radicular dysfunction. The role of the EMC is to help identify patients who have radicular syndromes, and separate them from those with other etiologies of LBP. But distinguishing radiating referred pain from radiating radicular pain can be difficult.

The clinical and electrodiagnostic evaluation should be organized and planned to accomplish at least the following aims: 1) assist in identifying patients whose pain is of nonneurologic origin; 2) help separate patients who have true radicular pain from those who have radiating referred pain from a more proximal source, such as a diseased facet joint or a diseased, but not ruptured, disc; 3) in the case of true radicular pain, focus the EMG on the muscles most likely to be involved; and 4) exclude conditions that can mimic radiculopathy, such as peroneal neuropathy at the fibular head.

CLINICAL SIGNS AND SYMPTOMS IN LUMBOSACRAL RADICULOPATHY

Deyo et al. reviewed the information which could be obtained from the history and physical examination in patients with LBP (26). They suggest trying to answer three basic questions: is there a serious, underlying systemic disease present, is there neurologic compromise that might require further evaluation, and are there psychological factors leading to pain amplification. Signs that suggest the possibility of underlying systemic disease include: a history of cancer, unexplained weight loss, pain lasting longer than one month, pain unrelieved by bed rest, fever, focal spine tenderness, morning stiffness, improvement in pain with exercise, and failure of conservative treatment.

The utility, or lack thereof, of various physical examination findings has been studied. The straight leg raising (SLR) test remains the mainstay in detecting radicular compression. The test is performed by slowly raising the symptomatic leg with the knee extended. Tension is transmitted to the nerve roots between about 30° and 70° and pain increases. Pain at less than 30° raises the question of nonorganicity, and some discomfort and tightness beyond 70° is routine and insignificant. There are various degrees or levels of positivity. Ipsilateral leg tightness is the lowest level, pain in the back more significant and radiating pain in the leg highly significant. When raising the good leg produces pain in the symptomatic leg (crossed straight leg raising sign), the likelihood of a root lesion is very high.

The positivity of the SLR should be the same with the patient supine or seated. If a patient with a positive supine SLR does not complain or lean backwards when the extended leg is brought up while in the seated position (e.g., under the guise of doing the plantar response), it is suggestive of nonorganicity. The SLR can be enhanced by passively dorsiflexing the patient's foot just at the elevation angle at which the increased root tension begins to produce pain. A quick snap to the sciatic nerve in the popliteal fossa just as stretch begins to cause pain (bowstring sign, or popliteal compression test) accomplishes the same end. Patients with hip disease have pain on raising the leg whether the knee is bent or straight; those with root stretch signs only have pain when the knee is extended. Pain from hip disease is maximal when the hip is flexed, abducted and externally rotated by putting the patient's foot on the contralateral knee and pressing down slightly on the symptomatic knee (FABERE test). There are other procedures for checking the SI joints.

The neurologic examination should include assessment of power in the major lower extremity muscle groups, but especially the dorsiflexors of the foot and toes, and the evertors and invertors of the foot. Plantar flexion of the foot is so powerful that manual testing rarely suffices. Having the patient do ten toe raises with either foot is a better test. Sensation should be tested in the signature zones of the major roots (1). The status of knee and ankle reflexes is informative about the integrity of the L3–4 and S1 roots. There is no good reflex for the L5 root, but the hamstring reflexes are occasionally useful. The medial and lateral hamstrings are both innervated by both L5 and S1, but the medial hamstring tends to be more L5 and the lateral more S1. An occasional L5 radiculopathy produces a clear selective diminution of the medial hamstring reflex. In a patient with absent ankle jerks and a question of neuropathy, loss of the lateral hamstring with preservation of the medial helps confirm radicular pathology. Preservation of the lateral hamstring jerk with an absent ankle jerk suggests a length dependent process, i.e., peripheral neuropathy.

Studies have found that only 8 of 27 physical tests investigated successfully discriminated between patients with chronic LBP and normal controls. The eight useful tests were: pelvic flexion, total flexion, total extension, lateral flexion, straight leg raising, spinal tenderness, bilateral active straight leg raising, and sit-up (26). Tests for nonorganicity are very useful. Pain during simulated spinal rotation, pinning the patients hands to the sides while rotating the hips (no spine rotation occurs as shoulders and hips remain in a constant relationship) suggests nonorganicity. Likewise, a discrepancy between the positivity of the SLR between the supine and seated position, pain in the back on pressing down on top of the head,

TABLE 14.5
Differential Diagnostic Points in Patients with Low Back Pain Syndromes

Disorder	Site of Involvement	Local Pain	Referred Radiating Pain	Radicular Radiating Pain	Pain Increased By	Pain Decreased By	Positive SLR	Weakest Muscles	Decreased Reflex	High Yield EMG Muscles	Other
L5 radiculopathy—HNP	L5 root-postero-lateral HNP @ L4-5	Back	Buttock, posterior thigh	Buttock, post. thigh, lower leg, dorsum of foot, big toe	Sitting > standing, cough, sneeze, spinal flexion	Standing, lying	Yes	TA, EHL, TP, EDL/EDB PL, TFL, GMD	MHS (±)	TA, TP, PL, EHL, GMX MHS	
L5 radiculopathy—lateral recess syndrome	L5 root—lateral recess stenosis	Back	Buttock, posterior thigh	Buttock, post. thigh, lower leg, dorsum of foot, big toe	Standing, extension	Spinal flexion	No				Age 30–55 for HNP, older for lateral recess stenosis; generally leg pain > back pain
S1 radiculopathy—HNP	S1 root-postero-lateral HNP @ L5-S1	Back	Buttock, posterior thigh	Buttock, post. thigh, lower leg, heel, lateral foot/toes	Sitting > standing, cough, sneeze, spinal flexion	Standing, lying	Yes	Gastroc, FDL, short toe flexors, decreased	Ankle, LHS (±)	GMX gastroc., AH, EDB	
S1 radiculopathy—lateral recess syndrome	S1 root—lateral recess stenosis	Back	Buttock, posterior thigh	Buttock, post. thigh, lower leg, heel, lateral foot/toes	Standing, extension	Spinal flexion	No	# toe raises			
Discogenic pain	Intervertebral disc-torn annulus; internal disruption	Back	Buttock, posterior thigh	None	Sitting, spinal flexion	Lying	No	No weak muscles, possible splinting due to pain	None	None	
Facet pain	Facet joint	Back	Buttock, posterior thigh	None	Lying supine, extension, rotation	Walking, flexion	No	No weak muscles	None	None	Pain may decrease with facet block
Musculoligamentous pain	Musculo-ligamentous structures of low back	Back	Buttock, posterior thigh	None	Walking, bending, stooping, minor movements	Sitting or lying	Negative or equivocal, not radiating	No weak muscles	None	None	Frequently follows unaccustomed exertion of the back; trigger points

Condition	Structure	Pain	Referred pain		Aggravated by	Relieved by					Other
Spinal stenosis	Cauda equina, multi-level radiculopathy	Back	Buttock, posterior thigh	Depends on root and level	Walking, standing	Sitting, leaning forward	Variable	Depends on root	Depends on root	Depends on root	No signs of peripheral vascular insufficiency
High lumbar disc	L2,3,4, usually HNP	Back	Buttock	Anterior thigh	Sitting	Lying	No	Quads, adductors	Knee	RF, IP, add. long	+ Reverse SLR
Hip disease	Hip joint, trochanteric bursa	Hip, buttock	Groin, anterior thigh, lateral thigh, knee	None	Standing, walking, hip rotation	Sitting or lying supine	No	None	None	None	+ FABERE (see text)
SI joint disease	SI joint	Back, buttock	Posterior thigh	None	Resting	Repetitive movement, exercise, activity	No	None	None	None	Age <30, male, history of pain > 3 months, morning stiffness, + SI joint maneuvers
Bony spine pain, e.g., metastatic disease, osteomyelitis	Vertebral body	Back	Buttocks, thighs	None	Nothing specific	Nothing specific	No	None	None	None	Boring, relentless pain, worse at night, history of cancer, history of unexplained weight loss, age > 50
Viscerogenic pain	Viscera, e.g., colon, rectum, prostate, uterus & adnexa, aortoiliac vessels	Variable, sometimes none	Back	None	Nothing specific	Nothing specific	No	None	None	None	Evidence of visceral disease; pain unrelated to activity or posture
Nonorganic		Back and any other; often back + neck	None	None	No consistent pattern	No consistent pattern	Variable and non-organic	None	None	None	Nonorganic physical signs, depression, disability, litigation

The table outlines what is generally true, it is not a statement of absolutes.
AH, abductor hallucis; EDB, extensor digitorum brevis; EDL, extensor digitorum longus; EHL, extensor hallucis longus; FDL, flexor digitorum longus; GMD, gluteus medius; GMX, gluteus maximus; HNP, herniated nucleus pulposus; IP, iliopsoas; LHS, lateral hamstrings; MHS, medial hamstrings; PL, peroneus longus; RF, rectus femoris; TA, tibialis anterior; TFL, tensor fascia lata; TP, tibialis posterior; SLR, straight leg raising.

widespread and excessive "tenderness," general over-reaction during testing, and nondermatomal/nonmyotomal neurologic signs. The presence of three of these signs suggests, if not nonorganicity, at least embellishment (26).

The major radicular syndromes include HNP, lateral recess stenosis, and spinal stenosis with cauda equina compression. Virtually all patients with radiculopathy have sciatica. The odds of a patient without sciatica having radiculopathy have been estimated at 1 : 1,000 (26). The details of the sciatica are noteworthy, including the exact pattern of radiation, influence of body position and movement, and presence or absence of neurologic symptoms.

With HNP or lateral recess stenosis, leg pain usually predominates over back pain. With HNP, the pain is typically worse when sitting, better when standing, better still when lying down, and generally worse in flexed than extended postures—all reflecting the known changes in intradiscal pressure that occur in these positions. With lateral recess stenosis, the pain is worse with standing or walking, relieved by sitting with the torso flexed or by lying down. Patients with HNP tend to have a positive SLR; those with recess stenosis do not. The essence of the recess stenosis picture then is pain on standing, lack of pain on sitting and a negative SLR. The essence of the HNP picture is pain worse on sitting, lessened with standing and a positive SLR. Patients with HNP are usually in the 30–55 age range, those with lateral recess stenosis a bit older. As with cervical radiculopathy, pain may exacerbate with cough, sneeze or Valsalva.

As patients mature into the seventh decade and beyond, the liability to disc rupture decreases, but degenerative spine disease attacks in a different form. Osteophytic spurs and bars; bulging discs; thickened laminae and pedicles; arthritic, hypertrophied facets; and thickened spinal ligaments all combine to narrow the spinal canal and produce the syndrome of spinal stenosis. An extension posture contributes to spinal stenosis by causing narrowing of the foramina and dorsal quadrants, and buckling of the ligamentum flavum. Narrowing of the canal compresses neural and possibly vascular structures. Flexing the spine, as by leaning forward, stooping over or sitting down opens the canal and decreases the symptomatology.

Patients with spinal stenosis and neurogenic claudication experience pain, weakness, numbness and paresthesias/dysesthesias when standing or walking. Symptoms decrease with sitting or bending forward. An occasional patient will have a bizarre symptom, such as spontaneous erections or fecal incontinence brought on by walking. Differentiation from vascular claudication is made by the wide distribution of symptoms, the neurologic accompaniments, and the necessity to sit down for relief. Vascular claudication tends to produce focal, intense, crampy pain in one or both calves and the pain subsides if the patients just stops and stands. Patients with vascular claudication have even more symptoms walking uphill, because of the increased leg work. Neurogenic claudication may decrease when walking uphill because of the increased spinal flexion in forward leaning. Patients with vascular claudication have as much trouble riding a bicycle as walking because of the leg work involved, whereas forward flexion on the bicycle opens up the spinal canal, allowing patients with neurogenic claudication to ride a bike with greater ease than they can walk.

An investigation of 68 patients with lumbar spinal stenosis found that pseudoclaudication, or neurogenic claudication, was the most common symptom, producing pain, numbness, or weakness on walking, frequently bilaterally and usually relieved by flexing the spine. Mild neurologic abnormalities occurred in a minority of patients. EMG showed one or more involved roots in 90% of patients (27).

The vast majority of lumbosacral radiculopathies are due to degenerative spine disease. The EMC must remain mindful that other disease processes can occur and may require exclusion. Patients with AIDS may develop an acute lumbosacral polyradiculopathy with a rapidly progressive flaccid paraparesis and areflexia, frequently associated with sphincter disturbances, which is due to cytomegalovirus infection and responds to ganciclovir. Patients may develop back pain and radiculopathy with epidural abscess or hematoma, diffuse meningeal neoplasia, diabetes, and other conditions (4).

Helpful points in the differential diagnosis of back and leg pain are summarized in Table 14.5.

Electrodiagnosis

If the history and examination prior to EMG suggest a particular root, then the needle examination should focus on that level. In the absence of clear localizing information a generic root screen is reasonable. Because more than 95% of lumbar HNPs occur posterolaterally at L4–5 or L5-S1, a generic root search is appropriately focused on the L5 and S1 nerve levels (17).

Lauder et al. retrospectively studied 247 electrodiagnostically confirmed lumbosacral radiculopathies, combining the most frequently abnormal individual muscles into different screens (28). They concluded that five muscle screens, including paraspinal muscles, identified 94–98% of the lesions, and that adding additional muscles resulted in an insignificantly increased yield. The paraspinal muscles alone identified 88%, but of course provided no localization. A screen of four limb muscles plus the paraspinals may be adequate, especially if employing Haig's paraspinal mapping technique (28,29). However, all the high yield L5 or S1 muscles in the best four limb muscle screen are in the sciatic distribution, and in the absence of paraspinal fibrillations the diagnosis of radiculopathy is not secure under such circumstances. The five-muscle group of tibialis anterior, EHL, gastrocnemius, tensor fascia lata, and adductor longus, plus the paraspinals, detected 98.4% of the radiculopathies. Other five-muscle combinations had yields ranging from 96.4% to 98.0%. The highest yield muscles found in this study are shown in Table 14.6.

Wilbourn and Aminoff proposed a general lower extremity survey of seven limb muscles, plus the paraspinals (7). However, two of these are intrinsic foot muscles, which are a tradeoff between a potentially higher yield because of distal position versus a recognized tendency to show abnormalities even in asymptomatic, normal controls. However, Lauder et al. found for S1 radiculopathies that the medial gastrocnemius had a slightly higher yield than the abductor hallucis and a much higher yield than the EDB. Therefore, the following five limb muscles seem reasonable for a generic screen: rectus femoris or adductor longus; tibialis anterior; gastrocnemius; gluteus maximus; tibialis posterior or peroneus longus or EHL.

There is general agreement that examination of the paraspinal muscles is very useful in the evaluation of suspected cervical or lumbosacral radiculopathy (30). There are other important issues that merit discussion. Paraspinal abnormalities should be interpreted with extreme caution in patients who have undergone laminectomy. Fibrillations can persist for years after surgery even in patients who have no evidence of recurrent radiculopathy (31). Though it has not been specifically studied, there is no reason to suspect that this limitation would apply to patients who have undergone anterior cervical discectomy.

Some asymptomatic patients may have minor degrees of spontaneous and increased insertional activity isolated to the paraspinals, and abnormalities limited to the paraspinals may not necessarily indicate the presence of radiculopathy, especially in older patients (32). Fibrillations isolated to the paraspinal muscles may occur in a number of conditions, and in such cases are not restricted to the symptomatic region—again the need to surround abnormality with normality. Paraspinal fibrillations may occur in patients with diabetes, occult carcinoma, and other conditions, as well as transiently after myelography (33).

Key Points

- The vertebrae are separated by discs, composed of an annulus fibrosus and a nucleus pulposus (NP). Posterior elements form the spinal canal. The lateral recess merges into the entry zone of the intervertebral foramen, and the dorsal root ganglion (DRG) lies in the midzone of the foramen. The location of the DRG is of immense clinical importance.
- Spinal nerves pass outward through the foramen. Degenerative osteophytes projecting into the foramen from the uncovertebral joints may cause radiculopathy.
- The anterior and posterior spinal ligaments reinforce the vertebral column. HNPs most often occur posterolaterally because of lateral incompleteness of the posterior ligament and the eccentrically posterior position of the NP.
- Clinically important changes occur on spinal motion.
- After exiting from the foramen, the spinal nerve divides into anterior and posterior primary rami, which innervate the limb muscles and paravertebral muscles respectively. The anatomical details of the structure and innervation of the paravertebral muscles are highly relevant to the electrodiagnostic evaluation of radiculopathies.
- Degenerative spine disease involves both the disc and the bony structures and joints. These processes are separate but related. Because of the varied pathology involved, different types of radiculopathy may occur in disc disease and spondylosis.
- The pathophysiology of radiculopathy is essentially the same regardless of etiology. Demyelination is the primary change with mild compression; more severe insults pro-

TABLE 14.6
High Yield Muscles for Lumbosacral Radiculopathy Screens (28)*

Muscle	Yield
Rectus femoris	83% for L3 or L4
Adductor longus	80% for L3 or L4
Tibialis anterior	78% for L5, 64% for L5 or S1, 92% for L4 or L5
Tibialis posterior	81% for L5
Peroneus longus	84% for L5
Extensor hallucis longus	87% for L5
Gluteus maximus	61% for L5 or S1
Extensor digitorum brevis	67% for S1, 33% for L5
Medial hamstring	60% for L5
Gastrocnemius group	96% for S1
Abductor hallucis	90% for S1

* Defined by the presence of fibrillation potentials.

duce axon loss. With recovery, remyelination and axon regrowth occur. Collateral sprouts from undamaged axons also provide reinnervation. After an axon loss injury, fibrillations appear and disappear on a schedule determined by the severity of injury, the distance from the injury, the extent of collateral innervation, and the efficiency of reinnervation. Abnormalities evolve in a proximal to distal gradient, appearing first in the paraspinals and last in distal limb muscles. Reinnervation follows the same centrifugal pattern. Fibrillations appear first in the paraspinals, but also disappear first from the paraspinals.

- For greatest information, the multifidus compartment of the paraspinals must be examined.

- The electrodiagnostic procedures of use in evaluation of radiculopathy include motor and sensory conduction studies, late responses, and needle electrode examination (NEE). The general picture is one of normal motor and sensory conduction studies, with abnormalities in a myotomal distribution, including paraspinals, on NEE.

- The mainstay of diagnosis is the NEE. As a general rule, it requires about 7–10 days after onset to detect fibrillations in the paraspinal muscles and 2–3 weeks in the limb muscles. A study done too early may be normal, a study done too late may also be normal or show only chronic neurogenic MUAP changes but no fibrillations. A study could show fibrillations in the paraspinals only, because limb muscles have not had time for them to develop, or in the limb muscles only because the paraspinals have reinnervated.

- Preservation of the SNAP helps exclude pathology involving the plexus or peripheral nerve.

- EMG has its greatest yield when focused on weak muscles and on the region of likely pathology, so familiarity with the typical clinical picture of cervical and lumbosacral radiculopathy is useful in planning the examination.

- The electrodiagnostic medicine consultation should always include an appropriate history and physical examination to direct and guide the study. The clinical evaluation preceding the EMG should screen for nonradicular pathology, and determine which root(s) is most likely involved.

- Localizing information can be obtained from the history, especially from patterns of pain radiation and paresthesias, and from the physical examination.

- The electrodiagnostic medicine consultant should tailor the EMG to probe the weakest muscles. In the absence of clear clinical direction, one must resort to a generic root screen. Choosing which muscles, and how many, has heretofore been a matter of personal opinion and preference. Recent investigations have provided some guidance. A screen of six limb muscles plus the paraspinals for cervical radiculopathy, and five limb muscles plus paraspinals for lumbosacral radioculopathy has a high yield if radiculopathy is present.

References

1. Wolf JK. Segmental neurology: a guide to the examination and interpretation of sensory and motor function. Baltimore:University Park Press, 1981.
   See Chapter 3 for abstract.

2. Wilbourn AJ, Aminoff MJ. AAEE minimonograph #32: the electrophysiologic examination in patients with radiculopathies. Muscle Nerve 1988;11:1099–1114.
   A brief history of the evolution of radiculopathy as a clinical entity, and the use of electrodiagnostic studies to diagnose it, are provided. Root anatomy and the concept of myotomes and dermatomes are reviewed, as is the pathophysiology of radiculopathy. The value and limitations of the various electrophysiologic procedures used in the diagnosis of radiculopathies are discussed, including motor and sensory nerve conduction studies, late responses, somatosensory evoked potentials, nerve root stimulation, and the needle electrode examination. The specific muscles are enumerated which most often appear abnormal on needle electromyography with lesions of the various roots. The electrodiagnostic differentiation of root lesions from plexus lesions is described, and the various electrodiagnostic findings with lumbar canal stenosis are discussed. Finally, the value and limitations of the electrodiagnostic assessment in the evaluation of patients with suspected radiculopathies are reviewed.

3. Haig AJ, Moffroid M, Henry S, et al. A technique for needle localization in paraspinal muscles with cadaveric confirmation. Muscle Nerve 1991;14:521–526.
   Description of a technique for localization of the EMG needle electrode into the multifidus which relies on palpation of bony structures and needle insertion at certain angles and depths. The technique was evaluated by injecting latex dye in 199 locations in 13 cadavers. Dissection demonstrated that the technique was accurate in 97%, 93%, and 82% of injections into the multifidus, longissimus, and iliocostalis. See also: Stein J, Baker E, Pine ZM. Medial paraspinal muscle electromyography: techniques of examination. Arch Phys Med Rehabil 1993;74:497–500.

4. Naftulin S, Fast A, Thomas M. Diabetic lumbar radiculopathy: sciatica without disc herniation. Spine 1993; 18:2419–2422.
   Diabetic radiculopathy commonly presents with severe unilateral pain of sudden onset that is usually located in the lower extremity, frequently in the proximal segments. Occasionally, bilateral asymmetric pain may be observed. Weakness of hip or thigh muscles, decreased sensation and hypo- or areflexia are commonly observed. The clinical picture can resemble that of high lumbar disc herniation. Electrodiagnostic and radiological studies may help differentiate between the two conditions.

5. Radhakrishnan K, Litchy WJ, O'Fallon WM, et al. Epidemiology of cervical radiculopathy. A population-based study from Rochester, Minnesota, 1976 through 1990. Brain 1994;117:325–335.
   An epidemiological survey of cervical radiculopathy in Rochester, Minnesota, 1976–90, through the records-linkage system of the Mayo Clinic ascertained 561 patients (332 males and 229 females). Ages ranged from 13 to 91 years; the mean age +/− SD was 47.6 +/− 13.1 years for males and 48.2 +/− 13.8 years for females. A history of physical exertion or trauma preceding the onset of symptoms occurred in only 14.8% of cases. A past history of lumbar radiculopathy was present in 41%. The median duration of symptoms prior to diagnosis was 15 days. A monoradiculopathy involving C7 nerve root was the most frequent, followed by C6. A confirmed disc protrusion was responsible for cervical radiculopathy in 21.9% of patients; 68.4% were related to spondylosis, disc or both. During the median duration of follow- up of 4.9 years, recurrence of the

condition occurred in 31.7%, and 26% underwent surgery for cervical radiculopathy. A combination of radicular pain and sensory deficit, and objective muscle weakness were predictors of a decision to operate. At last follow-up 90% of our population-based patients were asymptomatic or only mildly incapacitated due to cervical radiculopathy. The average annual age-adjusted incidence rates per 100,000 population for cervical radiculopathy in Rochester were 83.2 for the total, 107.3 for males and 63.5 for females. The age-specific annual incidence rate per 100,000 population reached a peak of 202.9 for the age group 50–54 years.

6. Jensen MC, Brant-Zawadzki MN, Obuchowski N, et al. Magnetic resonance imaging of the lumbar spine in people without back pain. N Engl J Med 1994;331: 69–73.

The relation between abnormalities in the lumbar spine and low back pain is controversial. This study examined the prevalence of abnormal findings on MRI of the lumbar spine in 98 asymptomatic people, without back pain. Scans were read independently by two neuroradiologists who did not know the clinical status of the subjects. Abnormal MRI scans from 27 people with back pain were mixed randomly with the scans from the asymptomatic people. The following standardized terms were used to classify the five intervertebral disks in the lumbosacral spine: normal, bulge (circumferential symmetric extension of the disk beyond the interspace), protrusion (focal or asymmetric extension of the disk beyond the interspace), and extrusion (more extreme extension of the disk beyond the interspace). Nonintervertebral disk abnormalities, such as facet arthropathy, were also documented. Thirty-six percent of the 98 asymptomatic subjects had normal disks at all levels. With the results of the two readings averaged, 52 percent of the subjects had a bulge at least one level, 27 percent had a protrusion, and 1 percent had an extrusion. Thirty-eight percent had an abnormality of more than one intervertebral disk. The prevalence of bulges, but not of protrusions, increased with age. The most common nonintervertebral disk abnormalities were Schmorl's nodes (herniation of the disk into the vertebral-body end plate), found in 19 percent of the subjects; annular defects (disruption of the outer fibrous ring of the disk), in 14 percent; and facet arthropathy (degenerative disease of the posterior articular processes of the vertebrae), in 8 percent. The findings were similar in men and women. On MRI examination of the lumbar spine, many people without back pain have disk bulges or protrusions but not extrusions. Given the high prevalence of these findings and of back pain, the discovery by MRI of bulges or protrusions in people with low back pain may frequently be coincidental.

7. Wilbourn AJ, Aminoff MJ. Radiculopathies. In: Brown WF, Bolton CF, eds. Clinical electromyography. 2nd ed. Boston: Butterworth-Heinemann, 1993:177–209.

A superb and comprehensive discussion of the details of the electrodiagnosis of radiculopathies. An update and expansion of the AAEM minimonograph on radiculopathies by the same authors (reference 2). The chapter ends with a very useful set of conclusions and recommendations.

8. Benecke R, Conrad B. The distal sensory nerve action potential as a diagnostic tool for the differentiation of lesions in dorsal roots and peripheral nerves. J Neurol 1996;223:231–239.

See Chapter 7 for abstract.

9. Cohen MS, Wall EJ, Brown RA, et al. 1990 AcroMed Award in basic science. Cauda equina anatomy. II: Extrathecal nerve roots and dorsal root ganglia. Spine 1990;15:1248–1251.

Inconsistent data exist regarding the anatomy of the spinal nerve roots lateral to the thecal sac. A newly developed in situ technique was used to precisely define anatomic parameters on 20 fresh human cadavers. The take-off angle of the nerve roots from the thecal sac decreases from a mean of approximately 40 degrees from L1-L5 to 22 degrees at S1. The motor bundles are directly ventral to the sensory fibers within individual roots extrathecally. Dorsal root ganglia size varies with vertebral level. The majority of ganglia lie directly beneath the vertebral pedicles and one third overlie a portion of the lateral intervertebral disc. These previously undescribed relationships may aid in the understanding of lumbosacral neurocompressive disorders and are important to note during pedicle screw insertion, posterolateral decompression for spinal trauma, and paravertebral approaches for lateral disc herniations.

10. Sasaki K. Magnetic resonance imaging findings of the lumbar root pathway in patients over 50 years old. Eur Spine J 1995;4:71–76.

In patients with degenerative disease of the lumbar spine, stenosis not only in the entrance zone but also in the mid- and exit zones of the nerve root pathway can occur. With the development of MRI, it has become easier to assess stenosis of the root pathway, especially in the mid- and exit zones. This study looked at the incidence of severe exit-zone stenosis of L3–5 roots in 45 patients aged over 50 years. The incidence of severe exit-zone stenosis at the L3 root was < 20% at all ages. On the other hand, L4 and L5 nerve root stenosis increased with age and severe stenosis affected 70% of L4 roots and 80% of L5 roots in patients in their seventies. The incidence of deformation or disappearance of the dorsal root ganglion (DRG) was 10% or less at L3 and L5 roots, while it was 10% at L4 root.

11. Kikuchi S, Sato K, Konno S, et al. Anatomic and radiographic study of dorsal root ganglia. Spine 1994;19: 6–11.

Anatomic and radiographic studies investigated normal variation of dorsal root ganglia in lumbosacral roots. The positions of dorsal root ganglia were classified into three types: intraspinal, intraforaminal, and extraforaminal. At L4 and L5 nerve roots, they were mostly intraforaminal, whereas at S1, they were mostly intraspinal. Proximally placed ganglia had a high frequency of ganglionic indentation. The incidence of intraspinal dorsal root ganglia was much higher clinically than in anatomic studies. Variations in connecting patterns or positions of dorsal root ganglia may be related to the occurrence and variety of radicular symptoms. The dorsal root ganglia is clinically important, and its location may correspond to clinical symptoms.

12. Yoss RE, Corbin KB, MacCarty Collin S, et al. Significance of symptoms and signs in localization of involved root in cervical disc protrusion. Neurology 1957;7:673–683.

An investigation of 100 Mayo Clinic patients with a surgically and radiologically verified single level cervical radiculopathy whose symptoms were relieved after decompression. The history and physical examination were able to localize the correct level in 87 patients, and to 1 of 2 levels in 10; in only 3 patients was the clinical information seriously misleading. Roots involved were: C7–69, C6–19, C8–10 and C5–2. Only 56% of the patients had neck or shoulder pain, and it was more common in C5 or C6 lesions (71%) than in C7 or C8 lesions (52%). In contrast, 99% of patients had pain in the upper arm, but is was poorly localized in most. Pain in the medial upper arm was always due to a C7 or C8 lesion. Pain in the forearm was seen in 88%, but again was usually poorly localized. Neither patient (only 2) with C5 lesions had pain below the elbow. Hand paresthesias occurred in 91%. The most common pattern involved thumb and index finger and was most often but not always due to C6. The second most common pattern involved the index and middle fingers and was always due to C7. In 6 of 7 patients with paresthesias limited to the ring and little fingers, the lesion involved C8. Reflexes were diminished in 72%. A decreased triceps jerk was always due to C7 or C8. In 7 or 8 patients where biceps and brachioradialis jerks were decreased together, the lesion was at C5 or C6. Unequivocal muscle weakness was seen in 75% of the patients, spread among all levels: 100% of the C5 patients had weakness, 68% of C6, 65% of C7 and 80% of C8. Weakness of the spinati was always due to a C5 lesion, of deltoid or brachioradialis always C5 or C6, of triceps always C6 or C7, of hand intrinsics always C8. In contrast to the frequency of paresthesias, only 24 patients had detectable sensory loss and in 23 of these it was limited to the hand. There were few specific patterns. Involvement of thumb and index was usually C6 but could be C7, involvement of the middle finger was always C7, and involvement of the ring and small fingers was always C8.

13. Levin KH, Maggiano HJ, Wilbourn AJ. Cervical radiculopathies: comparison of surgical and EMG localization of single root lesions. Neurology 1996;46:1022–1025.

A study of 50 cases of surgically proven solitary root lesions studied preoperatively with EMG. Studies classified as abnormal only by the demonstration of fibrillation potentials on needle examination. Lesions occurred at: C7—56%, C6—18%, C5—14%, and C8—12%. With C5,7,&8 radiculopathies, changes were relatively stereotyped. The root lesion with the most variable presentation was C6: in half the patients the pattern resembled C5 and in the other half the findings resembled C8. Contains a very useful tabulation of the yield of different muscles in lesions of the various roots.

14. Murphey F, Simmons JCH, Brunson B. Surgical treatment of laterally ruptured cervical disc: review of 648 cases, 1939–1972. J Neurosurg 1973;38:679–683.

An analysis of 648 surgically treated patients with single level cervical radiculopathy, with follow up on 380. The authors concluded that hard disc alone rarely caused radiculopathy, most had soft disc superimposed; 90% of patients awoke one morning with pain in the neck and rhomboid region, very few had a history of trauma. Referred pain to the anterior chest occurred in 20%. Although the documentation is not as detailed as in Yost, et al (Neurology 1957), the essence of the clinical syndromes is similar.

15. Lauder TD, Dillingham TR. The cervical radiculopathy screen: optimizing the number of muscles studied. Muscle Nerve 1996;19:662–665.

A follow up to the previous study of lumbosacral radiculopathy by the same investigators (reference 28) In studying 175 patients with EMG proven cervical radiculopathy and assessing the yield of various muscle screens, the authors concluded that examination of 6 limb muscles plus the paraspinals detected 93–98%, and that examination of more muscles did not increase the diagnostic accuracy. The most productive screen (98.3%) included deltoid, triceps, APB, ECRL, FCU, ADM and paraspinals. Not as rich in detail as the lumbosacral study, but highly useful, especially in combination with the Cleveland clinic study (reference 13).

16. So YT, et al. Literature review on the utility of electromyography in evaluating patients with cervical radiculopathy. Muscle Nerve, in press.

An extensive review of the available literature, choosing only articles that met rigorous, predetermined criteria. Ultimately, 10 studies were included in a final tabulation of the sensitivity of EMG compared with clinical, radiological and surgical findings. The sensitivity of EMG varied, but most estimates were in the 50–70% range. EMG abnormalities were highly correlated with motor weakness. Correlation with imaging studies was 65–85%. The review concludes that EMG confirms a clinical diagnosis of cervical radiculopathy with a moderate degree of sensitivity and a high degree of specificity.

17. Deyo RA, Loeser JD, Bigos SJ. Herniated lumbar intervertebral disk. Ann Intern Med 1990;112:598–603.

Low back pain is common, but a herniated intervertebral disk is the cause in only a small percentage of cases. Most symptomatic disk herniations result in clinical manifestations (pain, reflex loss, muscle weakness) that resolve with conservative therapy, and only 5% to 10% of patients require surgery. Sciatica is usually the first clue to disk herniation, but sciatica may be mimicked by other disorders that cause radiating pain. Because more than 95% of lumbar disk herniations occur at the L4–5 or L5-S1 levels, the physical examination should focus on abnormalities of the L5 and S1 nerve roots. Plain radiography is not useful in diagnosing disk herniation, but more sophisticated imaging (myelography, CT or MRI) should generally be delayed until a patient is clearly a surgical candidate.

18. Wipf JE, Deyo RA. Low back pain. Med Clin North Am 1995;79:231–246.

Radiographic abnormalities of the lumbar spine, including disk protrusion, are common in asymptomatic subjects and only loosely associated with symptoms and neurologic examination. prognosis of low back pain is an important component of therapy. Most patients with simple back pain recover with symptomatic treatment. Plain radiographs are indicated for evaluation of patients with radiculopathy and those with risk factors for underlying medical conditions. The majority of patients with back pain, even those with radiculopathy, improve with conservative management and surgery is unnecessary. Surgical consultation, imaging studies, (and EMG!) are indicated for patients with persistent or progressive neurologic deficits or persistent sciatica with nerve root tension signs. Acute radiculopathy with bilateral neurologic deficits, saddle anesthesia, or urinary symptoms is suggestive of cord compression or cauda equina syndrome and requires urgent surgical referral.

19. Frymoyer JW, Cats-Baril WL. An overview of the incidences and costs of low back pain. Orthop Clin North Am 1991;22:263–271.

Although a precise estimate is impossible, it is plausible that the direct medical and indirect costs of these conditions are in the range of more than $50 billion per annum, and could be as high as $100 billion at the extreme. Of these costs, 75% or more can be attributed to the 5% of people who become disabled temporarily or permanently from back pain—a phenomenon that seems more rooted in psychosocial rather than disease determinants. Within this overall equation, spinal surgery plays a relatively small role, although the contribution to disability probably has more than passing significance. The future challenge, if costs are to be controlled, appears to lie squarely with prevention and optimum management of disability, rather than perpetrating a myth that low back pain is a serious health disorder.

20. Bernard TN, Jr., Kirkaldy-Willis WH. Recognizing specific characteristics of nonspecific low back pain. Clin Orthop 1987;266–280.

A retrospective review of 1293 cases of low back pain treated over a 12-year period revealed that sacroiliac joint syndrome and posterior joint syndromes were the most common referred-pain syndromes, whereas herniated nucleus pulposus and lateral spinal stenosis were the most common nerve root compression lesions. Referred pain syndromes occur nearly twice as often and frequently mimic the clinical presentation of nerve root compression syndromes. Combined lesions occurred in 33.5% of cases. Lateral spinal stenosis and herniated nucleus pulposus coexisted in 17.7%. Distinguishing radicular from referred pain, recognition of coexisting lesions, and correlation of diagnostic imaging with the overall clinical presentation facilitates formulation of a rational plan of therapy.

21. Milette PC, Fontaine S, Lepanto L, et al. Radiating pain to the lower extremities caused by lumbar disk rupture without spinal nerve root involvement. Am J Neuroradiol 1995;16:1605–13.

Lumbar diskography was performed in 235 consecutive patients. In 17 patients, severe and persistent low back pain, with unilateral or bilateral radiation to the lower extremities, was provoked by contrast injection into only one disk. One milliliter of 1% lidocaine was then slowly injected in the center of these disks. A 75% to 100% reduction of the low back pain was experienced by 13 patients, and a 75% to 100% reduction of the radiating pain was experienced by 16 patients within 60 seconds after the intradiskal injection of lidocaine. Radiographs demonstrated radial tears through the entire annulus thickness in 16 of 17 disks. Results suggest that, in some patients with low back pain and unilateral or bilateral radiation to the lower extremities, the pain arises from within the disk. In these cases, pain radiating to the lower limb seems to be a referred type and seems unrelated to direct nerve root compression or irritation by a disk fragment in the epidural space.

22. Schwarzer AC, Aprill CN, Derby R, et al. The relative contributions of the disc and zygapophyseal joint in chronic low back pain. Spine 1994;19:801–806.

This study sought to determine the relative contribution of the disc and the zygapophyseal joint as a pain source in patients with chronic low back pain. Ninety-two consecutive patients with chronic LBP were studied with discography and zygapophyseal joints blocks; 39% had at least one positive discogram. Eight patients responded to both a screening zygapophyseal joint block and a confirmatory block. Only three patients had both a positive discogram and a symptomatic zygapophyseal joint. In patients with chronic LBP, the combination of discogenic pain and zygapophyseal joint pain is uncommon.

23. Schwarzer AC, Aprill CN, Bogduk N. The sacroiliac joint in chronic low back pain. Spine 1995;20:31–37.

The true prevalence of SI joint pain is unknown and despite a plethora of clinical tests, none has been validated against an established criterion standard. This study sought to establish 1) its prevalence, 2) the validity of pain provocation, 3) whether any arthrographic abnormalities predict a response to joint block, and 4) whether certain pain patterns discriminate patients with this diagnosis. Forty-three consecutive patients with chronic LBP, maximal below L5-S1, were investigated with sacroiliac joint blocks. 30% obtained relief of pain. Groin pain was the only pain referral pattern found to be associated with response to sacroiliac joint block. The sacroiliac joint is a significant source of pain in patients with chronic LBP.

24. Schwarzer AC, Aprill CN, Derby R, et al. The prevalence and clinical features of internal disc disruption in patients with chronic low back pain. Spine 1995;20:1878–1883.

Internal disc disruption has been postulated as an important cause of LBP. Ninety-two consecutive patients with chronic LBP and no history of previous lumbar surgery underwent a standard physical examination and CT discography at a minimum of two levels. Diagnostic criteria for internal disc disruption were fully satisfied in 39% of patients, most commonly at L5-S1 and L4-L5. None of the clinical tests used could differentiate between those patients with internal disc disruption and other patients.

25. Schwarzer AC, Aprill CN, Derby R, et al. Clinical features of patients with pain stemming from the lumbar zygapophysial joints. Is the lumbar facet syndrome a clinical entity? Spine 1994;19:1132–1137.

Previous studies have demonstrated a wide range of prevalence for zygapophysial joint pain and conflicting results with regard to clinical signs. 176 consecutive patients with chronic LBP were investigated with zygapophysial joint blocks. 47% had a definite or greater response to a screening injection at one or more levels but only 15% had a 50% or greater response to a confirmatory block. Response to zygapophysial joint injection was not associated with any single clinical feature or set of clinical features. The zygapophysial joint is an important source of pain but the existence of a "facet syndrome" must be questioned.

26. Deyo RA, Rainville J, Kent DL. What can the history and physical examination tell us about low back pain? JAMA 1992;268:760–765.

A highly clinical, pithy and practical discussion of what can be learned from the clinical encounter with a LBP patient. Includes a brief review of the anatomic and physiologic origins of LBP syndromes, the prevalence of diseases that cause LBP, and clues on how to recognize underlying systemic disease, detect neurologic compromise and find evidence of psychogenic overlay. Concludes with a useful summary and recommendations. Keys to recognizing systemic disease are the presence of systemic symptoms and failure of bed rest to relieve the pain. Neurologic involvement is suggested by sciatica or pseudoclaudication. Pain radiating below the knee is more likely of true radicular origin than pain radiating only to the posterior thigh. Problematic items in the psychosocial history include depression, failure of previous treatments, substance abuse and disability issues. Frankly reviews what is useful and not useful in the physical examination. Very helpful is a discussion of findings on physical examination which might suggest nonorganicity.

27. Hall S, Bartleson JD, Onofrio BM, et al. Lumbar spinal stenosis. Clinical features, diagnostic procedures, and results of surgical treatment in 68 patients. Ann Intern Med 1985;103:271–275.

A review of 68 patients with strictly defined, myelographically proven, surgically confirmed lumbar spinal stenosis. Pseudoclaudication was the commonest symptom (94%) and was described by patients as pain (93%), numbness (63%), or weakness (43%). Symptoms were frequently bilateral (68%) and generally relieved by flexing the lumbosacral spine. Neurologic abnormalities were found in a minority of patients and were usually mild. Electromyography showed one or more lumbosacral radiculopathies in 34 of 37 patients examined. Radiographic evidence of degenerative disk or joint disease was found in 63 patients. All patients had stenosis on myelography, with narrowing at L2, L3, and L4 being the commonest; 30% had multi-level stenosis. Two of ten CTs were normal. Surgery was extensive; 72% of patients had three or more laminae removed. At a mean of 4 years after surgery, 84% of patients reported that surgery had yielded good to excellent results.

28. Lauder TD, Dillingham TR, Huston CW, et al. Lumbosacral radiculopathy screen. Optimizing the number of muscles studies. Am J Phys Med Rehabil 1994;73:394–402.

The literature is unclear as to which muscles and how many are required for a sensitive lumbosacral radiculopathy (LSR) screen. A retrospective study of 247 electrodiagnostically confirmed LSRs in 201 patients over a 3-yr period was conducted to determine how many muscles are required to identify a LSR. All LSRs showed abnormal spontaneous activity (positive waves or fibrillation potentials) in two or more muscles innervated by the same nerve root level but different peripheral nerves. All cases were categorized by radiculopathy level, and the most frequently abnormal individual muscles were combined into different muscle screens. The frequency with which each muscle screen identified a radiculopathy was the frequency with which one or more muscles in the screen displayed abnormal spontaneous activity divided by the total number of radiculopathies. The paraspinal muscles (PM) alone identified 88% of LSRs. Without PM, two muscle screens identified only 14–68%, three muscle screens identified 37–89% and four muscle screens identified 45–92%. Including PM, three muscle screens identified 86–94% of LSRs, four muscle screens identified 91–97% and five muscle screens yielded 94–98% identification. Seven to ten muscle screens resulted in minimal improvements in identifying a LSR with 98–99% identification. The authors conclude that five muscle LSR screens, including PM, are sufficient to identify LSRs while minimizing patient discomfort and examiner time.

29. Haig AJ, Talley C, Grobler LJ, et al. Paraspinal mapping: quantified needle electromyography in lumbar radiculopathy. Muscle Nerve 1993;16:477–484.

In the diagnosis of LBP, the presence of a high percentage of false positive findings on radiologic imaging studies has lead to a more definitive role for electrodiagnosis as a confirmatory test. The paraspinal muscles are a crucial part of the electrodiagnostic examination for radiculopathy. To date, no technique for paraspinal evaluation has been validated. Based on previously documented anatomical techniques, the authors have designed a method of paraspinal examination termed "paraspinal mapping" (PM). EMG needles are placed in five carefully chosen locations and inserted in multiple directions. Individual scores for these insertions are added to determine a total PM sensitivity score. The first 50 studies using PM were compared to peripheral EMG, imaging studies, and pain drawings. Results indicate that the technique is easy to perform. Sensitivity scores relate well with these tests. In this limited and uncontrolled population, PM had higher sensitivity for abnormalities than either peripheral EMG or imaging studies. Because of the anatomical validity of PM, future studies may show it to be useful in localizing the level of radiculopathy independently from peripheral EMG, and to support clinical findings and imaging studies.

30. Czyrny JJ, Lawrence J. The importance of paraspinal muscle EMG in cervical and lumbosacral radiculopathy: review of 100 cases. Electromyogr Clin Neurophysiol 1996;36:503–508.

A random retrospective chart review was performed on 49 patients with cervical and 51 with lumbosacral radiculopathy to determine the frequency of EMG abnormalities in the paraspinal and limb muscles. Criteria for abnormality was the pres-

ence of spontaneous activity in two muscles in a myotomal pattern in the limb, or in the paraspinal muscles. 20/49 (40.8%) of the cervical radiculopathy patients and 10/ 51 (19.6%) of the lumbosacral radiculopathy patients had abnormalities only in the paraspinal muscles. These results indicate that especially in the cervical spine, a significant percentage of patients with radiculopathy will be missed if examination of the paraspinal muscles is not part of the evaluation. Examination of the paraspinal muscles is an important part of the electrodiagnostic evaluation of a patient with suspected radiculopathy.

31. See DH, Kraft GH. Electromyography in paraspinal muscles following surgery for root compression. Arch Phys Med Rehabil 1975;56:80–83.

To help determine if paraspinal muscle EMG following laminectomy is useful in patients with a suspected recurrence, the paraspinal muscles were examined in 20 patients who had undergone laminectomy for lumbosacral root compression and had no evidence of recurrent radiculopathy. EMG was done 1 cm and 3 cm lateral from the midline from L3 through S2. The interval between surgery and EMG ranged from 3–1/2 to 41 months. Seventeen of the 20 cases showed fibrillation potentials and positive sharp waves; of these, 15 were abnormal at three or more levels and 13 at both 1 cm and 3 cm from the midline. The study concluded that patients who have undergone laminectomy for root compression may demonstrate EMG abnormalities in the paraspinal muscles for periods of up to 41 months postoperatively even without recurrent radiculopathy, even up to 3 cm lateral to the midline and at multiple vertebral levels. See also: Johnson EW, Burkhart JA, Earl WC. Electromyography in postlaminectomy patients. Arch Phys Med Rehabil 1972;53:407–409.

32. Date ES, Mar EY, Bugola MR, et al. The prevalence of lumbar paraspinal spontaneous activity in asymptomatic subjects. Muscle Nerve 1996;19:350–354.

Fibrillations and positive sharp waves in the lumbosacral paraspinals in patients without previous back surgery has been generally considered abnormal, consistent with posterior rami denervation. In some cases, it is the only abnormality on the electromyographic examination. This study was undertaken to determine the prevalence of abnormal spontaneous activity in lumbosacral paraspinals in asymptomatic individuals. Nine (14.5%) of 62 subjects studied had positive sharp waves or fibrillations noted on the needle examination of bilateral lumbosacral paraspinal muscles. There was a significant increase in the prevalence of abnormal activity with increasing age. This suggests that caution should be taken in attributing radiculopathy as the etiology of low back pain when electromyographic lumbosacral paraspinal abnormalities are the only positive findings in the middle-aged or older individual. See also: Haig AJ. The prevalence of lumbar paraspinal spontaneous activity in asymptomatic subjects. Muscle Nerve 1996;19:1503–1504; Campbell WW, Jensen ME, Motgi G, et al. Electrodiagnostic-radiographic correlation in patients with suspected radiculopathy and fibrillations confined to paraspinal muscles. Muscle Nerve 1991;14:888–889.

33. Watson R, Waylonis GW. Paraspinal electromyographic abnormalities as a predictor of occult metastatic carcinoma. Arch Phys Med Rehab 1975;56:216–218.

A retrospective review was conducted to determine whether membrane irritability localized primarily to the paraspinal muscles could predict the presence and localization of spinal metastatic disease. In 1800 EMGs, 91 met the following criteria: (1) three or more paraspinal segments involved, (2) little or no membrane irritability in the anterior rami, and (3) no previous surgery on the paraspinal area. The proven discharge diagnoses were carcinoma in 24%, herniated nucleus pulposus in 28%, degenerative disc disease in 16%, diabetes mellitus in 9% and miscellaneous in 8%; in 15% no diagnosis could be made. See also: LaBan MM, Tamler MS, Wang AM, Meerschaert JR. Electromyographic detection of paraspinal muscle metastasis. Correlation with magnetic resonance imaging. Spine 1992;17:1144–1147; Weber RJ, Weingarden SI. Electromyographic abnormalities following myelography. Arch Neurol 1979;36:588–589.

15

Plexopathies

The brachial and lumbosacral plexi are anatomically complex. Attempts to retain the details are a constant reminder of the fallibility of human memory for most physicians. Clinical disorders reflect the anatomical intricacies. Electrodiagnostic techniques are potentially very helpful (1–3). Needle electrode examination (NEE) can help localize the lesion and judge its completeness and its evolution. Limitations of the clinical examination due to pain, weakness or contractures can sometimes be overcome. Sensory potential abnormalities help exclude radiculopathy (see Chapter 14) (4). Late responses, proximal stimulation and SEPs can help assess the integrity of proximal structures. The following discussion will focus on the most common plexus disorders with an emphasis on the electrodiagnostic aspects.

Clinical Pathoanatomy

The brachial plexus (BP) arises from the anterior primary rami of C5-T1. The phrenic nerve, the long thoracic nerve to the serratus anterior, and the dorsal scapular nerve to the rhomboids come off at root level and can sometimes aid in localization. The posterior primary rami leave the spinal nerve just after its exit and innervate the paraspinal muscles. The status of the paraspinals is integral to localizing a process to the brachial or lumbosacral plexus. The anterior primary rami form the plexus. C5 and C6 join to form the upper trunk. The suprascapular nerve to the supraspinatus and infraspinatus comes off the upper trunk and is of occasional use in localization. The spinati are the most proximal muscles innervated by the plexus. The C7 anterior primary ramus continues as the middle trunk. The C8 and T1 rami combine to form the lower trunk. The trunks are named for their relationship to one another.

The three trunks then bifurcate into anterior and posterior divisions. All the posterior divisions come together to form the posterior cord, which then divides into its two major terminal branches, the radial and axillary nerves. The anterior divisions form the medial and lateral cords. The cords are named for their anatomical relationships to the axillary artery. The lateral cord terminates in two major branches: the musculocutaneous nerve and the lateral head of the median nerve. The lateral component of the median carries all median sensory functions and the motor innervation to the pronator teres and flexor carpi radialis. The medial cord also terminates in two major branches: the medial head of the median nerve and the ulnar nerve. The medial head of the median nerve carries all the other median motor functions, but has no sensory component. After giving off the medial head to the median nerve, the medial cord continues as the ulnar nerve.

The foregoing is the bulk of what the electrodiagnostic medicine consultant (EMC) needs to know about brachial plexus anatomy. Some additional details are occasionally useful. The medial antebrachial cutaneous nerve (MABC), which supplies sensation to the medial forearm, arises from the medial cord via the lower trunk. The MABC sensory potential is easily obtainable and can help distinguish C8 radiculopathy from plexopathy. It is primarily useful in the evaluation of suspected thoracic outlet syndrome (TOS). The lateral antebrachial cutaneous (LABC) nerve is the distal continuation of the musculocutaneous, which arises from the lateral cord. It is frequently helpful in evaluating suspected pathology of the upper plexus. Figure 15.1 is an electrodiagnostically oriented plexus diagram.

The roots and trunks of the plexus lie in the posterior triangle of the neck, the cords lie in the axilla, and the divisions span the gap and lie approximately beneath the clavicle. The plexus is sometimes divided into a supraclavicular portion, roots and trunks, and an infraclavicular portion, divisions, cords and terminal branches. The plexus is also broadly divided into upper (upper trunk, lateral cord) and lower (lower trunk and medial cord) parts. Some pathologic processes have a predilection for different parts of the plexus.

The lumbosacral plexus (LSP) is in fact two plexi, even three if one counts the coccygeal plexus as a component. The lumbar portion of the plexus originates from the anterior primary rami of L1-L4. It lies

in or just posterior to the psoas muscle, where it is at risk for damage due to retroperitoneal hematoma. L4 and L5 give rise to the lumbosacral trunk, which joins the lumbar plexus to the sacral plexus. Roots from S1-S3 join the lumbosacral trunk to complete the sacral plexus, which lies along the posterolateral wall of the pelvis, between the piriformis muscle and the major vessels. The lumbosacral plexus ends as a plethora of branches, but many are sensory nerves of no significant electrodiagnostic import.

The major motor branches of the lumbosacral plexus are the femoral nerve (L2-4), which supplies the iliopsoas, sartorious and quadriceps, the obturator (L2-4), which supplies the adductors and gracilis, and the sciatic (L4-S3), which supplies all muscles distal to the knee. The sciatic has two components, the common peroneal and the tibial, which are two separate nerves lying in a common sheath. The superior gluteal (L4-S1) innervates the gluteus medius and tensor fascia lata. The inferior gluteal (L5-S2) innervates the gluteus maximus. The status of the gluteal muscles is important in differentiating between radiculopathy, plexopathy and sciatic mononeuropathy. The pudendal branches of the plexus supply the genitalia and the anal spincter.

The most important sensory branches are the saphenous, which is a continuation of the femoral nerve, and the lateral femoral cutaneous (LFC) nerve, which arises from the lumbar plexus, courses around the pelvic brim and exits beneath the inguinal ligament adjacent to the anterior superior iliac spine. There are standard techniques for recording sensory potentials from both the saphenous and the LFC, but they are often difficult to obtain even in normal subjects.

Pathophysiology of Plexopathy

Many pathologic processes may affect either the brachial or lumbosacral plexus. Whereas the vast majority of radiculopathies are due to compression, the plexus may fall victim to a number of different pathologic processes. Some of these include: external compression (e.g., backpack or rucksack palsy), compression from an internal process (e.g., encroachment on the lower plexus from a Pancoast tumor, or on the lumbar plexus from a retroperitoneal hematoma), inflammatory and dysimmune disorders (e.g., brachial "plexitis"), radiation injury, ischemia, and acute trauma due to traction, laceration, missile wounds and so forth. The plexus may be involved in systemic processes such as systemic lupus or sarcoid. Some of

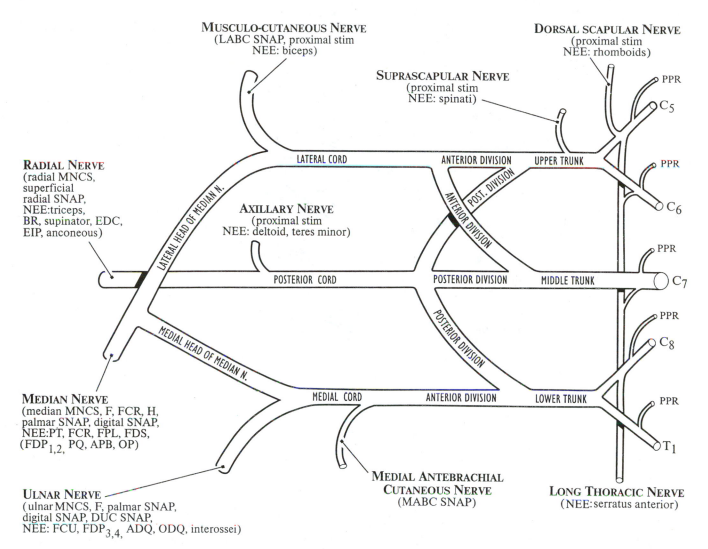

MUSCULO-CUTANEOUS NERVE
(LABC SNAP, proximal stim
NEE: biceps)

DORSAL SCAPULAR NERVE
(proximal stim
NEE: rhomboids)

SUPRASCAPULAR NERVE
(proximal stim
NEE: spinati)

PPR

C5

PPR

RADIAL NERVE
(radial MNCS,
superficial
radial SNAP,
NEE:triceps,
BR, supinator, EDC,
EIP, anconeous)

LATERAL CORD

ANTERIOR DIVISION

UPPER TRUNK

C6

PPR

AXILLARY NERVE
(proximal stim
NEE: deltoid, teres minor)

LATERAL HEAD OF MEDIAN N.

POST. DIVISION

ANTERIOR DIVISION

POSTERIOR CORD

POSTERIOR DIVISION

MIDDLE TRUNK

C7

PPR

POSTERIOR DIVISION

MEDIAL HEAD OF MEDIAN N.

C8

PPR

MEDIAN NERVE
(median MNCS, F, FCR, H,
palmar SNAP, digital SNAP,
NEE:PT, FCR, FPL, FDS,
(FDP$_{1,2}$, PQ, APB, OP)

MEDIAL CORD

ANTERIOR DIVISION

LOWER TRUNK

PPR

T1

**MEDIAL ANTEBRACHIAL
CUTANEOUS NERVE**
(MABC SNAP)

LONG THORACIC NERVE
(NEE: serratus anterior)

ULNAR NERVE
(ulnar MNCS, F, palmar SNAP,
digital SNAP, DUC SNAP,
NEE: FCU, FDP$_{3,4}$, ADQ, ODQ, interossei)

FIGURE 15.1. Electrodiagnostically oriented diagram of the brachial plexus. The plexus is stripped of all but the major branches of electrodiagnostic importance. The primary electrodiagnostic procedures for evaluating a particular branch are indicated.

these processes are by nature progressive. All these mechanisms of injury make the pathophysiology of plexopathies complex and the electrodiagnostic evaluation challenging.

With pressure injuries, the same general rules apply as for other nerves. Mild lesions produce primarily demyelination and can cause severe clinical deficits, but have an excellent prognosis. Conduction studies distal to a demyelinating injury are normal. If stimulation is carried out proximal to the lesion (difficult in plexus cases), there is conduction slowing, conduction block, or temporal dispersion. The needle electrode examination (NEE) shows a decreased number of MUAPs that discharge rapidly in an attempt to recoup through firing rate the lost contribution to power of

normal numbers of units. No fibrillations appear and the motor unit architecture does not change.

With more severe injuries there is axon loss. The peripherally recorded sensory potential disappears early. After 1–3 weeks, fibrillations emerge; their intensity and distribution depend on the extent of axon loss. The M wave amplitude of denervated muscle decreases, and the conduction velocity (CV) of the relevant nerve may show slowing in proportion to the axon loss. Reinnervation occurs slowly—the fibrillations disappear and the motor unit architecture changes with the appearance of complex and polyphasic units, initially unstable, small and very complex, maturing into large amplitude, long duration, less complex, stable units.

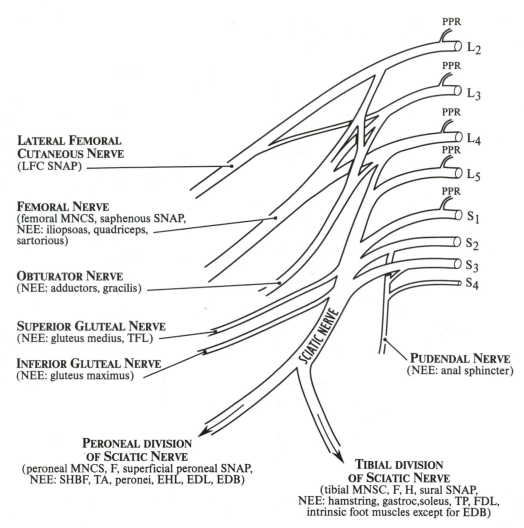

PPR

L$_2$

PPR

L$_3$

PPR

L$_4$

PPR

L$_5$

PPR

S$_1$

S$_2$

S$_3$

S$_4$

**LATERAL FEMORAL
CUTANEOUS NERVE**
(LFC SNAP)

FEMORAL NERVE
(femoral MNCS, saphenous SNAP,
NEE: iliopsoas, quadriceps,
sartorious)

OBTURATOR NERVE
(NEE: adductors, gracilis)

SUPERIOR GLUTEAL NERVE
(NEE: gluteus medius, TFL)

INFERIOR GLUTEAL NERVE
(NEE: gluteus maximus)

SCIATIC NERVE

PUDENDAL NERVE
(NEE: anal sphincter)

**PERONEAL DIVISION
OF SCIATIC NERVE**
(peroneal MNCS, F, superficial peroneal SNAP,
NEE: SHBF, TA, peronei, EHL, EDL, EDB)

**TIBIAL DIVISION
OF SCIATIC NERVE**
(tibial MNSC, F, H, sural SNAP,
NEE: hamstring, gastroc,soleus, TP, FDL,
intrinsic foot muscles except for EDB)

FIGURE 15.2. Electrodiagnostically oriented diagram of the lumbosacral plexus. The plexus is stripped of all but the major branches of electrodiagnostic importance. The primary electrodiagnostic procedures for evaluating a particular branch are indicated.

With plexus lesions there may be the additional complication of disease progression. Many of the conditions that affect the plexus are not static. Pancoast tumors continue to grow, radiation damage tends to progress, and systemic diseases such as lupus continue their activity. This can lead to a complex picture of extreme chronicity, with mixed chronic neurogenic MUAP changes and fibrillations. The MUAPs may be both large amplitude/long duration and unstable, reflecting a dynamic, ongoing process. Fibrillations do not completely disappear, but may decrease in numbers and become low amplitude. Chronic repetitive discharges may emerge. With radiation injury, myokymic discharges frequently develop.

Electrodiagnosis of Plexopathies

Procedures useful in the evaluation and management of plexopathies include motor and sensory conduction studies, late responses, NEE, root stimulation, and SEPs (1). The sensory potential is especially relevant. Diseases of any severity affecting the plexus attenuate or abolish the sensory nerve action potential (SNAP) in the distribution of the involved nerve(s). With axon loss, the SNAP decreases in amplitude and may show CV slowing or latency prolongation in proportion to the decreased number of conducting fibers and random involvement of the largest, fastest conducting axons. With severe lesions the SNAP disappears early. In contrast, radiculopathies do not affect the SNAP, as discussed in Chapter 14. In some plexopathies, the SNAP may not demonstrate abnormalities; the yield is increased by doing multiple SNAPs, including the symptomatic segments, and making side to side comparisons (4).

Motor conduction studies, including CV, distal latency, and M wave amplitude distal to the lesion remain normal in purely demyelinating, neuropraxic lesions. Conduction across the lesion may reveal conduction slowing or a decrease in amplitude of the M wave, which may be accompanied by temporal dispersion. With remyelination, slowing or temporal dispersion when conducting across the lesion may be the only residual.

Following lesions with extensive axon loss, peripheral conduction studies may remain normal for several days. Conduction across the lesion may show slowing or dispersion. With severe lesions, conduction block may be complete. As the process matures, the peripheral conduction parameters become abnormal, with CV slowing and a decline in M wave amplitude in proportion to the axon loss. Late responses become abnormal immediately. With significant conduction block the F and H waves usually disappear. Early on, abnormal late responses and decreased recruitment may be the only detectable abnormalities. With the full electrodiagnostic picture has developed, the late responses tend to be abnormal in proportion to the rest of the examination. Supraclavicular or root stimulation may help demonstrate conduction block or slowing across the lesion.

The NEE typically shows abnormalities in proportion to the extent of the lesion and the time since onset, as discussed in the pathophysiology section. The key to diagnosis in plexopathies is demonstrating abnormalities on NEE that are in the distribution of a plexus component, trunk(s) or cord(s). Additionally, the paraspinal muscles should be normal in a process restricted to the plexus. However, some "plexus" lesions are in fact radiculoplexopathies, with pathologic changes not only in the plexus but also involving the roots. Diabetic lumbosacral plexopathy is the most obvious example. As always, the electrodiagnostic information must be correlated with the rest of the clinical data to reach a final diagnosis. Occasionally, examination of the root innervated rhomboids, serratus anterior, or diaphragm may help to localize a lesion to the brachial plexus. Examination of the gluteal muscles and tensor fascia lata is integral to the localization of a lesion to the lumbosacral plexus. Respiratory synkinesias sometimes appear in brachial plexopathies when there is aberrant regeneration during healing and diaphragm motor axons reinnvervate the biceps. MUAPs in the biceps fire synchronously with respiration—the "breathing arm."

Plexopathies

The most common and clinically important conditions affecting the brachial plexus include: acute brachial plexopathy (neuralgic amyotrophy, or brachial plexitis), trauma, neoplasms, postradiation plexopathy, obstretrical palsies, postsurgical plexopathy, the "stinger" or "burner" phenomenon in football players, and thoracic outlet syndrome. It may rarely be involved in a number of other conditions, including lupus, lymphoma, Ehler-Danlos syndrome and infectious or parainfectious disorders (Table 15.1).

The LSP has a somewhat less eclectic but still intimidating repertoire. The most common conditions include diabetes (diabetic amyotrophy), neoplasms, postradiation plexopathy, and an idiopathic form that may be analogous to acute brachial plexopathy. The LSP may rarely be involved in systemic disorders such

TABLE 15.1
Causes of Brachial Plexopathy

Infectious/parainfectious/injections

Immunizations	Herpes zoster
Serum sickness	HIV
Botulinum toxin	EBV
Interleukin-2	CMV
Interferon	Parvovirus
Heroin	Yersiniosis
Lyme disease	

Hereditary

Hereditary neuralgic amyotrophy
HNPP
Ehlers-Danlos syndrome

Physical injury

Radiation therapy	Stretch
Cardiac surgery	External pressure (e.g.,
Birth injury	backpack palsy, seat belts,
Shoulder dislocation	Posey palsy)
Penetrating wounds	

Other

Neuralgic amyotrophy	Post liver transplant
SLE	Lymphoma
Pregnancy	Metastatic disease
Systemic vasculitis	Pancoast tumor

as retroperitoneal hemorrhage, aortic aneurysm, amyloidosis, sarcoid, and infectious or parainfectious disorders (see Table 15.4).

Disorders of the Brachial Plexus

NEURALGIC AMYOTROPHY

This condition has gone by a number of names, most frequently brachial plexitis, Parsonage-Turner syndrome, and acute brachial plexus neuropathy. Neuralgic amyotrophy (NA) is the currently preferred nosology because it does not imply unpossessed knowledge of precise location or pathophysiology.

NA is a fairly stereotyped clinical syndrome characterized by the acute onset of pain in the shoulder and upper arm, followed by weakness of variable severity, primarily affecting upper arm and shoulder muscles (5). It runs a protracted course of slow, sometimes incomplete recovery, and sometimes as one arm is recovering the other is stricken. Recurrence is not rare. As in Guillain-Barre syndrome many patients have some antecedent event, such as viral infection, immunization or surgery.

The pain in NA is a defining feature. It tends to begin abruptly and is very intense, often more severe at night. After a variable interval, usually 3–10 days, weakness begins in the shoulder and upper arm. Occasionally, the weakness begins in, is limited to, or is maximal in a specific peripheral nerve distribution, classically the anterior interosseous or long thoracic. Sensory loss is minimal or absent. The primary differential diagnostic consideration is cervical radiculopathy (Table 15.2).

The typical electrodiagnostic picture is one of a spotty axon loss process involving either the plexus or multiple nerves arising from the plexus, sparing the paraspinals (6). Motor conduction studies are usually normal. Sensory potentials are sometimes, not invariably, of low amplitude. Late responses may be prolonged or absent. NEE typically reveals fibrillations and MUAP changes, maximal in the most affected muscles, but frequently present in uninvolved muscles on the affected or the unaffected side. The abnormalities are sometimes spotty and not in a well-defined plexus distribution.

Some cases of NA are familial. Patients with a syndrome resembling NA can have hereditary neuropathy with liability to pressure palsies (HNPP), which is due to a mutation or deletion in the PMP22 gene on chromosome 17. Both familial NA and HNPP are autosomal dominant. Although there was early speculation that HNPP might be the mechanism for familial NA, further genetic studies have shown that these are separate and unrelated entities (7). The plexopathy in HNPP is often painless and may follow minor trauma.

RADIATION AND NEOPLASTIC PLEXOPATHIES

Like radiation damage to other parts of the neuraxis, radiation plexopathy appears after a delay of months to years. This is also the time frame in which the radiation therapy (RT) may have kept a tumor at bay. The problem is to distinguish recurrent tumor from radiation brachial plexopathy (RBP), a difficult and important differential (Table 15.3). Pain can occur with either condition, but is more likely to be an early

TABLE 15.2
Differential Diagnosis—Neuralgic Amyotrophy vs. Cervical Radiculopathy

Neuralgic Amyotrophy	*Cervical Radiculopathy*
Increased pain on arm/shoulder movement	Increased pain on neck movement
Severe pain	Moderate pain
Weakness follows pain	Weakness coincides with pain
Minimal sensory dysfunction	Major sensory dysfunction
Abnormal SNAP	Normal SNAP
No paraspinal denervation	Paraspinal denervation
Abnormal needle exam in a plexus distribution	Abnormal needle exam in a myotome distribution
Shoulder/upper arm pain	Radiating radicular pain
Younger (12–47)	Older (13–91)
	Positive root compression signs

TABLE 15.3
Differential Diagnostic Points in Neoplastic vs. Radiation Induced Brachial Plexopathy

Neoplastic Plexopathy	*Radiation Plexopathy*
Horner's syndrome common	Horner's syndrome rare
Presents with pain	Presents with paresthesias
Pain is predominant symptom	Paresthesias and sensory loss are the predominant symptoms
More lower plexus (equivocal)	More upper plexus (equivocal)
Imaging study shows discrete mass	Imaging study is normal or shows only loss of tissue planes
Diffuse motor and sensory conduction abnormalities	Abnormal SNAPS/normal MNCVs
	Conduction block across plexus
	Myokymia
	Fasciculation potentials
	Paraspinal fibrillations

and dominant symptom in neoplastic brachial plexopathy (NBP). Sensory dysfunction with numbness and paresthesias is more likely to be the predominant symptom with RBP, but some patients have significant pain. Weakness and reflex changes occur in either condition. Early studies suggested that RBP had an upper plexus and NBP a lower plexus distribution, but this was not substantiated in subsequent investigations as a reliable differentiator because of the amount of overlap between the two groups. Most patients in both groups have involvement of the lower trunk or the entire plexus (8).

Motor nerve conduction studies tend to be abnormal in proportion to axon loss, with loss of M wave amplitude and normal or mildly slowed NCVs. A decrease in amplitude or loss of sensory potentials is common. Conduction block across the plexus on Erb's point stimulation is more common in RBP, but complicated by technical limitations, such as the frequent induration and edema of the supraclavicular fossa in these patients (8). As a generalization, patients with RBP tend to have abnormal sensory and relatively normal motor conduction studies and those with NBP have both motor and sensory abnormalities, but the conduction features do not reliably distinguish between the two groups. NEE is usually very abnormal in either condition, with chronic neurogenic MUAP changes and fibrillations. Patients with RBP are much more likely to have prominent fasciculations. The presence of myokymia is highly suggestive of RBP, and is clearly the most useful electrodiagnostic discriminating feature. Even patients who ultimately

prove to have NBP have usually had plexus RT as well, and the incidence of myokymia in pure NBP not complicated by past RT is unknown.

Harper et al. found that the presence or absence of pain as the presenting symptom, the temporal profile of the illness, a discrete mass on CT, and myokymic discharges on EMG most reliably predicted the underlying cause of the plexopathy. Distribution of weakness and nerve conduction studies were not useful in discriminating between the two groups (8). A study of RBP in 79 breast cancer patients from an oncologic rather than a neurologic viewpoint revealed that 35% developed RBP. In 50% the process was panplexus, but of those with more focality, 18% had involvement of the upper trunk only, and only 4% the lower trunk. RBP was more common after RT plus cytotoxic therapy than after RT alone. Most patients had no significant latency between RT and the onset of symptoms, raising the possibility of chemotherapy enhancement of radiation effects (9). A painful, short latency brachial plexopathy may also occur during or after RT for Hodgkin's disease.

POSTOPERATIVE BRACHIAL PLEXOPATHY

The brachial plexus can sustain injury in a number of ways: missile and stab wounds, motor vehicle (especially motorcycle) accidents, football, and iatrogenic misadventures. The iatrogenic plexopathies primarily occur during cardiac surgery. The stinger or burner that frequently affects football players is likely a mild form of plexus injury.

Postoperative brachial plexopathies were noted to increase dramatically following the advent of modern open heart and coronary bypass surgical procedures. Postoperative plexopathies can occur as a presumably immunologically mediated event after procedures on parts of the body remote from the plexus. But the most common situation by far is for plexopathy to follow coronary artery bypass graft (CABG) procedures. A number of injury mechanisms have been postulated, including hyperabduction of the arm, displacement of the clavicle, first rib fracture with plexus laceration, overzealous sternal spreading causing stretch or compression of the plexus between the clavicle and first rib, and laceration of the plexus during attempted internal jugular (IJ) vein cannulation. Injuries continued to occur when the arms were routinely adducted at the patient's sides.

In a series of 421 CABG patients studied at the Cleveland Clinic, there was a 13% incidence of peripheral nervous system complications, and the majority were plexopathies. The study analyzed 451 different variables. In 74% of the plexopathy patients, there was a correlation between the site of jugular cannulation and the side of the injury, suggesting inadvertent laceration or compression by hematoma. In four of the remaining six patients, an internal mammary graft was used. These grafts require greater sternal retraction, and seem more likely to stretch the plexus. So, either jugular cannulation or internal mammary grafting seemed to explain 21 of the 23 cases in this series (10). Blaming IJ cannulation has not gone unchallenged in the surgical literature.

In a large prospective study, 27 of 1000 CABG patients developed postoperative brachial plexus injuries. Patients who underwent grafting of the internal mammary artery had a 10-fold increased incidence of plexus injury (10.6%) as compared with those who did not (<1%) (11). Optimal positioning and the use of minimal retraction may lessen but not eliminate these injuries.

In most cases of post-CABG plexopathy, the damage is primarily to the lower trunk or medial cord. Horner's syndrome may accompany the variable pain, numbness and weakness. EMG changes closely correlate with the clinical severity of the injury. The majority of deficits resolve within several weeks, suggesting that the predominant pathophysiology is demyelination. Induced hypothermia may somehow play a role by increasing the susceptibility to nerve injury.

Peripheral nerve compression injuries may also occur in this setting. In the Cleveland Clinic series, there were 5 ulnar neuropathies in the 421 patients (10). In a prospective study of 20 patients undergoing CABG, conduction slowing across the elbow was present in

one-third *preoperatively*, and conduction abnormalities developed in an additional 27% of the ulnar nerves postoperatively, all of which were *asymptomatic* and most of which resolved electrically on followup (12). So, in addition to plexopathies, there appears to be a high incidence of mild, asymptomatic and undetected ulnar neuropathies following CABG.

TRAUMATIC PLEXOPATHIES

Traumatic plexopathies are primarily due to stretch, or to blunt or penetrating trauma. Motorcyclists are particularly prone to upper plexus stretch when falling so that the shoulder and head are forced in opposite directions. The classic lower plexus stretch results from a fall through the ceiling in which the patient breaks the fall by grabbing the overhead rafters, abruptly jerking the arms overhead. Most traumatic plexopathies affect the supraclavicular portion or are diffuse. A frequent confounding injury is root avulsion, in which the stretch is severe enough to wrench one or more spinal roots from the cord. The plexus may also suffer external compression, as in backpack palsy or seat belt trauma, or be damaged in the course of shoulder dislocation or fracture of the clavicle. External compression palsies can be severe in susceptible individuals. In one case, the initial manifestation of HNPP was an acute, severe backpack palsy in a young paratrooper. He stood, wearing an 80-lb rucksack, in preparation to jump, but the jump was delayed for 30–45 min because of wind conditions in the drop zone. In that span of time, he developed an acute, panplexus deficit and the left arm became flail. He jumped anyway! Recovery was prolonged and incomplete.

Stretch injuries of the plexus occur during childbirth. These most often involve the upper plexus (Erb's palsy), much less often the lower plexus (Klumpke's palsy) or the entire plexus. High birth weight and complicated deliveries are predisposing factors. Prognosis is usually good (13). Some neonates have had fibrillation potentials detected in the first few days of life, suggesting an intrauterine mechanism of injury, such as compression by an amniotic band.

The "stinger" or "burner" phenomenon is common in American football. After a block or tackle, a player may develop sudden, intense, dysesthetic pain in the shoulder and arm. The injury is now thought to involve the upper trunk of the plexus rather than the cervical roots, and the mechanism is uncertain. Traction when the head and shoulder are forcibly separated is one possibility, as in a mild form of the often devastating upper plexus injury that occurs in motocyclists. A study at West Point showed that it is more likely that the symptoms result from the shoulder pad being forcefully pushed into Erb's point (14). Some players have persistent symptoms, the "prolonged burner" syndrome.

Electrodiagnostic assessment in traumatic plexopathies seeks to ascertain the distribution of the damage, the completeness of the lesion, the predominant pathophysiology and whether or not there is an associated root avulsion. The findings vary with the severity and location of the lesion. A mild to moderate lesion would likely show normal motor conductions, low amplitude SNAPs, delayed or absent late responses, and recruitment abnormalities on NEE in a distribution of a trunk or cord of the plexus, sparing the paraspinals. More severe lesions would typically show absent SNAPs and late responses, low M wave amplitude in affected muscles, possibly with MNCV slowing in proportion to axon loss, with more severe MUAP abnormalities and fibrillations on NEE. Nerve root or Erb's point stimulation can help in some instances, as can SEPs (1).

If there is root avulsion, the DRG and the peripheral processes remain intact and the peripherally recorded sensory potentials remain normal in the face of clinical anesthesia and marked motor abnormalities in the same distribution. However, it is difficult to avulse a root without some associated plexus stretch. Myelography may show a traumatic meningocele in root avulsion, but both false positive and false negative studies occur. The correlation between the myelographic and the neurophysiologic data was only 50% in a recent study (15).

THORACIC OUTLET SYNDROME (TOS)

TOS has a long and controversial history. It was firmly established in the minds of physicians as a cause of acroparesthesias and arm pain for 40 odd years before the medical community discovered the far more common entities of carpal tunnel syndrome (CTS) and cervical radiculopathy. In evaluating a patient with acroparesthesias, TOS is one of the first possibilities to come to mind for many nonneurologists, and nearly the last thing to come to mind for neurologists, especially electrodiagnostic medicine consultants. First rib resections for TOS are commonly performed in the USA, occasionally with disastrous results (16). The likelihood of undergoing surgery may be related to the potential for reimbursement; first rib resections are very rare among Colorado Medicaid patients (17).

Surgeons are still struggling to clearly define TOS as a clinical entity nearly 100 years after its original description (18). The surgical literature is inconsistent and often contradictory. In one center where TOS is

felt to be common, 409 patients underwent TOS surgery in a 19-year span (19). In contrast, a peripheral nerve surgeon believes surgery for TOS should be a rare event (20). And where Jamieson et al. find a TOS patient to operate on about every 2 weeks, most EMCs, who see patients with acroparesthesias and arm pain with high frequency, count themselves fortunate to encounter one convincing case of TOS every 2 years. Perceptions about the prevalence of TOS between surgeons and neurologists are at variance on the order of 100:1. References 18 and 21 are polemics which illustrate the differences between the medical and surgical viewpoints (18, 21).

We should probably recognize five types of TOS: arterial, venous, true neurogenic, disputed neurogenic and the droopy shoulder syndrome. Everything about disputed neurogenic TOS is arguable: its mechanism, its symptoms, its electrodiagnosis, even its existence. Terms such as scalenus anticus, costoclavicular, and hyperabduction syndrome are outdated and falling into disuse. Various structures have been incriminated in causing compression of the neurovascular structures at the thoracic outlet, including cervical ribs or bands, elongated C7 transverse process, scalenus anterior muscle, the pectoralis minor tendon and the humeral head.

Vascular TOS is most common in young athletes, especially competitive throwing athletes (pitchers, quarterbacks) and swimmers. Arterial or venous insufficiency, with occlusion, stenosis, poststenotic dilatation, or aneurysm/pseudoaneurysm formation of the subclavian or axillary artery, or occlusion of the subclavian vein is sometimes demonstrable radiographically (22). The humeral head may compress the axillary artery in hyperabduction and external rotation, i.e., the throwing position. In one case, a young competitive swimmer developed a cool, blue, swollen arm only when doing the butterfly stroke. Vascular TOS may develop without a cervical rib or band and respond to simple anterior scalene resection.

There is substantial agreement about the entity of true neurogenic TOS (TNTOS): it is rare, most often due to compression of the lower trunk of the plexus by a cervical rib or band, and typically presents with medial arm pain, ulnar/C8 distribution sensory dysfunction and thenar muscle wasting in a young woman. The electrodiagnostic picture is characteristic. Patients have a low amplitude or absent ulnar SNAP, a low amplitude median M wave recorded from the thenar muscles, generally normal conduction velocities except for slowing in proportion to axon loss, delayed or absent median and ulnar F waves responses, and chronic neurogenic MUAP changes in the distribution of the lower trunk, sparing the paraspinals. The MABC SNAP is abnormal more frequently than the ulnar SNAP. The reason for the paradoxical involvement of ulnar sensory and median motor fibers is unclear, but may be related to the internal fascicular anatomy and selective fascicular vulnerability of the lower trunk. A recent report convincingly documents the occurrence of TNTOS in a competitive swimmer due to compression by a thickened, fibrous band within a hypertrophied anterior scalene muscle (22). TNTOS is readily confused with ulnar or median neuropathy or C8 radiculopathy.

Ulnar conduction slowing across the plexus with stimulation at Erb's point was touted for many years, after the 1972 NEJM publication of Urschel and Razzuk, as the best method of electrically demonstrating the pathology in TOS. The technique failed utterly in the hands of most EMGers. Wilbourn and Lederman later exposed the illustration purporting to demonstrate conduction delay as having been fabricated, prompting an editorial reprimand with a lecture regarding authorship responsibilities (23). To this day, there is still no convincing evidence that such across plexus conduction studies have any utility. Other techniques, especially SEPs, have been advocated but also proved disappointing, likely due largely to the rarity of compression of neural structures in suspected TOS.

The major problem arises with the entity now called disputed neurogenic TOS (DNTOS). Roos, a leading surgical proponent of TOS and its surgical management, contends that 97% of the cases of TOS are of the neurologic type. Because TNTOS is rare, DNTOS accounts for the vast majority of cases" (21). Surgeons divide TOS into upper plexus and lower plexus types, and the description of symptoms sounds suspiciously like cervical radiculopathy to the neurological ear (21). TOS partisans disagree about many aspects of this syndrome. As Wilbourn pointed out, "No other alleged neurologic disorder has so many of its fundamental concepts in dispute, with so many of the disputes being between its proponents" (21). The profusion of symptoms attributed to DNTOS, not only arm pain and numbness but also migraine headaches and a host of other complaints, challenges credulity. The symptoms are in essence a resurrection of the concepts of the scalenus anticus syndrome, which were largely discredited with the appreciation of the symptomatology of CTS and cervical radiculopathy (21). Surgeons, renowned for cursory exams, through "detailed history and thorough physical examination" detect deficits that elude neurologists (13, 21).

One of the main criteria for the diagnosis, a positive Adson's maneuver, was shown 50 years ago to be positive in 80% of normal asymptomatic individuals (13). The elevated arm stress test (EAST maneuver), touted

for TOS, is frequently positive in patients with CTS and in normal controls (13). No confirmatory tests can reliably substantiate the diagnosis of DNTOS, which eludes all but clinical surgical evaluation and can only be proven by surgical exploration, a self-fulfilling prophecy (21). The surgical treatment is not without risk; in one laboratory, about as many patients were seen with postoperative brachial plexopathies as with TNTOS (16, 21).

In this context, it is interesting to compare two 1995 papers. One reports unequivocal TNTOS in a patient with no cervical band (22). The other reports 14 patients with symptoms which clearly fall into the DNTOS category; 13 had cervical bands and all had "abnormally attached or enlarged" scalene muscles (24).

The droopy shoulder syndrome shares many similarities with DNTOS (25). Some believe it accounts for most cases of TOS. Almost all droopy shoulder syndrome patients are slender young women with long graceful necks and horizontal or downsloping, rather than the normal slightly upsloping, clavicles. The T2 vertebra may be visible on lateral cervical spine films because of the low lying shoulders. Symptoms have been attributed to chronic brachial plexus stretch due to the low hanging shoulders. Pain in the shoulder, arm, hand, and sometimes neck and head, and paresthesias are the usual symptoms. Supraclavicular percussion and downward traction on the arms exacerbates, and passive elevation decreases, the symptoms. Treatment is with shoulder strengthening exercises. The prudence of separating droopy shoulder syndrome from other instances of DNTOS is debatable (13).

Disorders of the Lumbosacral Plexus

Processes that affect the lumbosacral plexus primarily include diabetes, cancer, and radiation. There is a syndrome of idiopathic lumbosacral plexopathy (LSP) that may be analogous to neuralgic amyotrophy involving the brachial plexus, but with some important differences. Table 15.4 lists some causes of LSP.

DIABETIC AMYOTROPHY

Diabetes can affect the peripheral nervous system in many different ways. One classification lists nine different varieties of diabetic "neuropathy." Like neuralgic amyotrophy, diabetic amyotrophy has a stereotyped clinical presentation. The typical patient is older, with Type II diabetes, usually mild and occasionally not previously diagnosed. Symptoms begin

TABLE 15.4
Causes of Lumbosacral Plexopathy

Infections/parainfectious/injections

Lyme disease	EBV
Immunizations	HIV
Heroin	CMV

Physical injury

Trauma
Radiation therapy
Obstetrical injury

Other

Diabetes mellitus	Lymphoma
Cancer	Aortic aneurysm
Bradley's syndrome	Sarcoid
Retroperitoneal hematoma or abscess	Amyloid
	Vasculitis
Idiopathic	Collagen vascular disease

subacutely with pain in one hip or thigh which becomes severe. Weakness of the hip flexors, gluteal muscles and quadriceps ensues and the patient begins to lose weight, often 20 lb or more. Pain continues, the quadriceps atrophies, and the knee jerk disappears. Similar but milder pain, weakness and atrophy occur on the opposite side. At its zenith, the patient has painful, bilateral but asymmetric, weakness and wasting of the thighs along with substantial weight loss. The process eventually stabilizes and a slow and occasionally incomplete recovery follows over months to a couple of years (26).

The clinical deficit most often involves the lumbar plexus diffusely. The sacral plexus is minimally involved or spared, though patients sometimes develop a mild foot drop. Examination shows bilateral but asymmetric weakness and wasting of the hip flexors, adductors, gluteal muscles, hamstrings and quadriceps. The knee jerk is usually absent, often with preservation of the ankle reflexes. Sensory loss is minimal or absent. The differential diagnosis primarily includes high lumbar HNP, involving L2, L3, or L4 (Table 15.5).

The electrodiagnostic picture is one of axon loss in a lumbar plexus distribution. Femoral conduction studies may show a decreased M wave amplitude and increased latency in proportion to axon loss. If there is coexistent diabetic distal axonopathy, other conduction abnormalities may be present but are not due to

the amyotrophy. Paraspinal fibrillations are frequently present and do not necessarily indicate structural radiculopathy; diabetic amyotrophy may in fact be a radiculoplexopathy. The paraspinal fibrillations are often diffuse in the lumbosacral region and may even extend into the thoracic paraspinals; they are not limited to the symptomatic level. Patients with diabetic amyotrophy are in the age group where imaging studies commonly show disc disease, but high lumbar HNPs account for only a tiny fraction of disc ruptures. Statistically, odds are much higher that a patient with this syndrome will have diabetic amyotrophy than an HNP. But, the patient *must* have diabetes. In one memorable, preMRI case a patient with a consistent clincal picture, but no diabetes, eventually was found to have a Schwannoma on the L3 root.

RADIATION AND NEOPLASTIC PLEXOPATHIES

Neoplasms may metastasize to the LSP, or directly invade it. The most common tumors are colorectal, breast, and cervical carcinomas, sarcomas and lymphomas. As with the brachial plexus, radiation therapy (RT) given as treatment for the tumor may itself damage the plexus. One is then presented with the conundrum of distinguishing neoplastic lumbosacral plexopathy (NLSP) from radiation lumbosacral plexopathy (RLSP). The distinction of NLSP from neoplastic involvement of the spinal cord, cauda equina or meninges can be difficult. RT can sometimes damage the anterior horn cells in the lumbosacral enlargement, especially when given for lymphoma.

Patients with LSP due to tumor typically present with insidious pelvic or lumbosacral pain with variable radiation into the leg, followed by paresthesias,

TABLE 15.5
Differential Diagnosis of Diabetic Amyotrophy vs. High Lumbar HNP

Diabetic Amyotrophy	*HNP*
Diabetes mellitus	
Bilateral asymmetrical weakness	Unilateral weakness
Constant pain	Increased pain with cough, sneeze, sitting or flexion; decreased pain with extension
Multi-root fibrillation potentials	Single root fibrillation potentials
Diffuse paraspinal fibs	Focal paraspinal fibs
Weight loss	Positive reverse SLR

sensory loss and weakness with variable involvement of bowel and bladder function. Examination usually shows weakness in a unilateral, multiroot distribution, accompanied by sensory loss and reflex asymmetry. Leg edema and a palpable mass are occasionally present. The process may affect the upper, lower or entire plexus (27). Sarcomas, colorectal tumors, and lymphomas tend to involve the lower plexus. EMG abnormalies are often more extensive than the clinical exam would predict. Many cancer patients also have clotting abnormalities that may predispose them to develop retroperitoneal hemorrhage with a resultant LSP, but the onset is more acute.

Radiation plexopathy usually presents after a long latency period, mean 6.5 years, with progressive asymmetric leg weakness (28). Most have had more than 4,000 rads but some patients suffer RLSP at doses as low as 3,000 rads. Pain is present at onset in only 10% and occurs at some time in the course in only 50%. Weakness is bilateral in most. Helpful EMG findings in RLSP include paraspinal fibrillations (50%), fasciculations (35%) and myokymia. In a study of 20 patients with RLSP, myokymia was present in 60% vs. none of 21 patients with NLSP. Paraspinal fibrillations probably result from RT damage to roots, and this condition has also been called a radiculoplexopathy. Prognosis is poor in either condition. RLSP causes major disability and NLSP predicts poor survival (28). Table 15.6 lists some points in the differential between NLSP and RLSP.

IDIOPATHIC LUMOSACRAL PLEXOPATHY

Whether there is a primary, spontaneous "plexitis" affecting the LSP analogous to the entity of neuralgic amyotrophy of the brachial plexus has been a matter of conjecture. If so, it occurs at only a fraction of the incidence of the upper extremity condition. Bradley et al. described six patients with a painful lumbosacral plexopathy associated with a high sedimentation rate and which responded to immunosuppression. All had bilateral but asymmetric lower extremity weakness. Sural nerve biopsies in each case showed axonal degeneration and perivascular inflammatory infiltrates, but there was no evidence of systemic vasculitis. Although half the patients were diabetic, the plexopathies were not thought to be on the basis of diabetes. An immunologically mediated process with an ischemic mechanism was suspected (29).

In a recent report of five patients with idiopathic, unilateral, lumbosacral plexopathy, the age range was from 37–75, four were female, only one had an antecedent viral infection, and all had pain primarily in the leg (only one patient had back pain and that was slight). Weakness was diffuse in three, distal in one and proximal in one; four had sensory loss (30). None had evidence of radiculopathy on imaging studies. The ESR was mildly elevated in two. Motor conduction studies were normal in three, showed low M wave ampitudes in one, and a low tibial M wave with absent peroneal response in the other; 8 of the 13 sensory potentials studied were normal. With minimal exception, needle examination showed denervation in clinically weak muscles; two had paraspinal fibrillations. The leg pain was a prominent and persistent symptom in all.

Other causes of LSP include aortic aneurysm, amyloidosis, sarcoidosis and obstetrical injury (31–34). An ischemic plexopathy can be mistaken for an incomplete spinal cord injury (35). Additional etiologies for LSP are listed in Table 15.4.

Common Clinical Scenarios

1. Neuralgic amyotrophy (NA) vs. cervical radiculopathy (CR).

Table 15.2 outlines some features useful in the differential diagnosis. Patients with NA tend to be somewhat younger than those with CR, although there is much overlap. A patient in the 2nd or 3rd decade is much more likely to have NA. Patients with CR have other signs of radiculopathy such as pain on neck motion and root compression signs. CR usually causes prominent paresthesias, but sensory involvement in NA is inconspicuous. In CR, the NEE abnormalities are in a myotomal distribution and involve the paraspinals, and the SNAP is normal. In NA, the NEE abnormalities are spotty,

TABLE 15.6
Differential Diagnosis of Neoplastic vs. Radiation Lumbosacral Plexopathy

Neoplastic	*Radiation Therapy*
Presents with pain	Presents with indolent leg weakness
Uilateral weakness	Bilateral weakness
Short latency	Long latency
Unilaterally decreased reflexes	Bilaterally decreased reflexes
Discrete mass on imaging study	Normal or nondescript imaging study
Palpable mass	Myokymia on EMG
Leg edema	Paraspinal fibrillations
Hydronephrosis	Radiation dose >4,000 rads

may be present in the asymptomatic limb, do not involve the paraspinals, and the SNAP is usually (not always, particularly with mild cases) abnormal.

2. Neoplastic vs. radiation induced plexopathy.

The archetypical patient with RBP underwent RT for breast cancer several years ago, has had paresthesias with minimal pain in the affected extremity for several months, has no Horner's syndrome, no abnormality of motor conduction, fasciculations and myokymia on NEE, paraspinal fibrillations, and an imaging study showing only ill defined loss of tissue planes. In contrast, the classic patient with NBP has a history of lung cancer discovered several months ago, and presents with severe pain in the affected extremity of several weeks' duration, has a Horner's syndrome, abnormal motor as well as sensory conduction studies, fibrillations in the limb but none in the paraspinals, no fasciculations or myokymia, and an imaging study showing a discrete mass in the plexus (Table 15.3).

Similar logic applies to the LSP. The usual patient with NLSP presents early in the course with painful, unilateral leg weakness, accompanied by leg edema and a pelvic or rectal mass. In a study of 85 patients with LSP due to tumor, the combination of leg pain and edema, weakness, a palpable mass and hydronephrosis strongly predicted tumor (27). The typical patient with RLSP presents several years after RT with painless, bilateral, asymmetric weakness and has myokymia on EMG (28). Table 15.6 outlines some features in the differential diagnosis.

3. Post-CABG plexopathy vs. ulnar neuropathy at the elbow.

Clinical findings which favor a brachial plexus localization include weakness in nonulnar lower trunk or medial cord muscles (e.g., APB, FPL, EIP), sensory dysfunction involving the medial arm or forearm, sensory loss over the entire ring finger, and a depressed triceps reflex. Findings which favor ulnar neuropathy include weakness limited to ulnar innervated muscles, sensory loss which splits the ring finger and does not extend more than 2–4 cm proximal to the wrist crease and a positive Tinel's sign in the ulnar groove. Helpful electrodiagnostic findings in ulnar neuropathy include focal slowing, conduction block or temporal dispersion across the elbow, F wave abnormalities limited to the ulnar nerve, and needle exam abnormalities limited to ulnar muscles. Findings that would indicate lower brachial plexopathy include

an abnormal median as well as ulnar F wave, abnormal MABC SNAP, and needle exam changes outside the ulnar distribution.

4. Diabetic amyotrophy vs. high lumbar radiculopathy

Differential diagnostic features are summarized in Table 15.5. In diabetic amyotrophy the pain is primarily on one side, but usually involves the other side to at least some degree, at least when the syndrome is fully developed. The pain is constant, not affected by movement or other factors, and involves the hip and thigh primarily. In radiculopathy, the pain also involves the back, varies with position, and is strictly unilateral. The patient with diabetic amyotrophy has almost always lost weight, sometimes a great deal. Abnormalities on NEE are usually diffuse, involving the hip, gluteal, quadriceps, adductor and hamstring muscles. In radiculopathy, the NEE changes are more restricted.

Key Points

- Plexopathies are complicated both because of the intricacies of the anatomy and because of the variety of disease processes involved. Electrodiagnosis plays an integral part in the clinical evaluation and management of patients with plexopathies.

- The brachial plexus arises from the anterior primary rami of C5-T1; the posterior primary rami innervate the paraspinal muscles, the status of which is vital in localization. The plexus is composed of trunks, divisions, cords and terminal branches. Many of the twigs and branches shown in traditional anatomical diagrams add confusing complexity but are of scant or no clinical relevance.

- The lumbosacral plexus is in reality a lumbar plexus and a sacral plexus joined by the lumbosacral trunk.

- Many different pathologic processes can affect the brachial and lumbosacral plexi. The electrodiagnostic procedures useful for evaluation of plexopathies include motor and sensory conduction studies, late response studies, needle electrode examination (NEE) and SEPs. Of these, the NEE is the mainstay of diagnosis and localization.

- The key to diagnosis is demonstrating abnormalities in the distribution of some plexus component, sparing the paraspinals.

- The status of the sensory potentials is critical for distinguishing plexopathy from radiculopathy.

- Neuralgic amyotrophy (NA), aka brachial plexitis, Parsonage-Turner syndrome, is a stereotyped clinical syndrome with acute pain in the shoulder and upper arm, followed by weakness in an upper plexus distribution with minimal sensory involvement, a slow recovery and a spotty axon loss pattern on EMG. The features that help to separate NA from cervical radiculopathy are summarized.

- It can be very difficult to separate brachial plexopathy due to tumor invasion from that due to radiation therapy. Myokymia, paraspinal fibrillations, no pain, and slow evolution suggest radiation plexopathy.

- Lower trunk plexopathies occur in 5–10% of patients undergoing CABG, for unclear reasons. Trauma from internal jugular cannulation is the major suspected etiology.

- Traumatic plexopathies can also result from stretch, external pressure, and penetrating wounds. Electrodiagnostic evaluation is primarily oriented toward determining the distribution, completeness and pathophysiology and ascertaining whether there is an associated root avulsion.

- Thoracic outlet syndrome (TOS) is a very controversial entity which is either very common or very rare depending on outlook and definition. True neurogenic TOS has a characteristic clinical and electrodiagnostic picture. A plethora of symptoms has been attributed to the so-called disputed neurogenic form of TOS, which largely defies attempts at electrodiagnosis.

- Diabetic amyotrophy is the most common disorder affecting the lumbosacral plexus (LSP). It has a characteristic and stereotyped clinical presentation. The primary differential is with high lumbar disc.

- Separating radiation induced from neoplastic lumbosacral plexopathy is similar to the differential for the brachial plexus.

- A form of idiopathic or spontaneous lumbosacral plexopathy, analogous to neuralgic amyotrophy of the brachial plexus probably exists, but is much less common and much less well defined.

References

1. Aminoff MJ, Olney RK, Parry GJ, et al. Relative utility of different electrophysiologic techniques in the evaluation of brachial plexopathies. Neurology 1988;38:546–550.
   Results of detailed electrophysiologic studies in 23 patients with suspected brachial plexopathies. In 5 with neurogenic TOS, needle EMG and the size of ulnar SNAPs and thenar M waves were important in localizing the lesion; F-response and SEP studies were of more limited utility. All electrodiagnostic studies were normal in 10 patients with nonneurogenic TOS. In traumatic (3) or idiopathic brachial plexopathy (5), needle EMG was especially helpful but, in the former, SEP studies helped to guide management and, in the latter, to confirm the proximal site of the lesion when peripheral SNAPs were normal. The presence of preserved but small SNAPs but absent M waves in patients with traumatic plexopathies suggested a combined pre- and postganglionic lesion.

2. Goldstein B. Applied anatomy and electrodiagnosis of brachial plexopathies. Phys Med Rehab Clin North Am 1994;5:477–493.
   A review of the anatomic and electrodiagnostic fundamentals important in evaluating brachial plexopathies, organized along a practical pathophysiologic principle and regional anatomic approach. See also Mukerji SK, Castillo M, Wagle AG. The brachial plexus. Sem Ultrasound, CT, MRI 1996;17:519–538.

3. Wilbourn AJ. Electrodiagnosis of plexopathies. Neurol Clin North Am 1985;3:511–259.
   A review of the electrodiagnostic features of axon loss and segment demyelinating types of plexopathy and the EMG differentiation of plexopathies from other neurogenic lesions.

4. Rubin M, Lange DJ. Sensory nerve abnormalities in brachial plexopathy. Eur Neurol 1992;32:245–247.
   SNAP amplitude should be abnormal in brachial plexopathies (BP) which cause axonal degeneration in distal segments. 56 patients with BP were identified. In diffuse BP, 88% showed low amplitude or absent median or ulnar SNAP. Three of 5 patients with upper trunk BP had low amplitude or absent SNAP (1 median, 1 radial, 1 lateral antebrachial cutaneous). 75% of patients with lower trunk/medial cord BP had low amplitude or absent SNAP. Overall, 82.5% of patients had low amplitude or absent SNAP when a sensory nerve in the distribution of signs was studied. Testing multiple sensory nerves to include symptomatic regions enhances the diagnostic yield of SNAP in BP. See also Benecke R, Conrad B. The distal sensory nerve action potential as a diagnostic tool for the differentiation of lesions in dorsal roots and peripheral nerves. J Neurol 1980;223:231–239.

5. Subramony SH. AAEE case report #14: neuralgic amyotrophy (acute brachial neuropathy). Muscle Nerve 1988;11:39–44.
   Neuralgic amyotrophy is characterized by acute onset of arm pain, followed by a variable interval of flaccid paralysis in the distribution of the brachial plexus on one or sometimes both sides. Electromyography reveals findings suggestive of an axonal degeneration process affecting various portions of the brachial plexus or individual nerves emanating from it, sometimes difficult to localize to discrete cords, trunks, or nerves. Diagnosis is established by excluding other causes, including compression and vasculitides. Prognosis for recovery is excellent.

6. England JD, Sumner AJ. Neuralgic amyotrophy: an increasingly diverse entity. Muscle Nerve 1987;10:60–68.
   In 9 cases of neuralgic amyotrophy, clinical and EMG findings suggested lesions of individual peripheral nerves or peripheral nerves branches occurring singly (mononeuropathy) or in various combinations (mononeuropathy multiplex). There were 4 occurrences of isolated denervation of the pronator teres muscle; 4 occurrences of anterior interosseous nerve lesions; 3 occurrences of lateral antebrachial cutaneous nerve lesions; 2 occurrences of long thoracic nerve lesions; and one occurrence each of a median nerve trunk lesion, a median palmar cutaneous branch lesion, a suprascapular nerve lesion, and an axillary nerve lesion. "Neuralgic" pain was a prominent feature in all cases, and the location of the pain correlated with the location of the nerve lesion. This entity is considerably more diverse than generally appreciated.

7. Chance PF, Lensch MW, Lipe H, et al. Hereditary neuralgic amyotrophy and hereditary neuropathy with liability to pressure palsies: two distinct genetic disorders. Neurology 1994;44:2253–2257.
   Hereditary neuralgic amyotrophy with predilection for the brachial plexus (HNA) and hereditary neuropathy with liability to pressure palsies (HNPP) are autosomal dominant disorders associated with episodic, recurrent brachial neuropathies.

HNPP is associated with a deletion or abnormal structure of the PMP22 gene on chromosome 17p11.2-12. The genetic locus for HNA is unknown. To address the possibility that HNPP and HNA might be identical disorders or allelic variations at the same locus, the authors investigated three HNA pedigrees with markers from the HNPP region. They did not find the 17p11.2-12 deletion associated with HNPP, nor an abnormality in PMP22 structure with HNA. This analysis provides genetic evidence, in addition to that suggested by the clinical, electrophysiologic, and pathologic differences, that HNA and HNPP are distinct disorders. See also Gouider R, et al. HNA and HNPP: two distinct clinical, electrophysiologic and genetic entities. Neurology 1991;44:2250–2252.

8. Harper CM Jr., Thomas JE, Cascino TL, et al. Distinction between neoplastic and radiation-induced brachial plexopathy, with emphasis on the role of EMG. Neurology 1989;39:502–506.
Clinical, radiologic, and electrophysiologic studies are retrospectively reviewed for 55 patients with neoplastic and 35 patients with radiation-induced brachial plexopathy. Breast and lung cancer accounted for 78% of the patients, and the final diagnosis was neoplastic plexopathy in 52% of the breast cancer patients and 94% of the lung cancer patients. Neoplastic plexopathy (NP) patients had a shorter course. The median interval between the diagnosis of cancer and the onset of plexopathy was 18 months (0-276) in neoplastic plexopathy, as compared with 60 months (4-408) for the radiation plexopathy (RP) patients. Moderate to severe pain occurred in 80% of neoplastic vs. 26% of radiation plexopathies. Horner's was present in 33% or neoplastic vs. 6% of radiation plexopathies. Some abnormality of median motor conduction was present in 55% of neoplastic vs. 34% of radiation plexopathy motor nerves studied, but abnormalities of ulnar and musculocutaneous motor conduction was the same in both groups. The incidence of sensory conduction abnormalities was the same in both groups. Paraspinal fibrillations were present in 23% of the RP group but only 2% of the NP group. Myokymic discharges occurred in 63% of RP vs. 4% of NP and fasciculations in 31% vs. 15%. The pronator teres and APB were the muscles most commonly having myokymia. The presence or absence of pain as the presenting symptom, temporal profile of the illness, presence of a discrete mass on CT of the plexus, and presence of myokymic discharges on EMG contributed significantly to the prediction of the underlying cause of the brachial plexopathy. The distribution of weakness and the results of nerve conduction studies were of no help in distinguishing neoplastic from radiation-induced brachial plexopathy.

9. Olsen NK, Pfeiffer P, Mondrup K, et al. Radiation-induced brachial plexus neuropathy in breast cancer patients. Acta Oncol 1990;29:885–890.
The incidence and latency period of radiation-induced brachial plexopathy (RBP) were assessed in 79 breast cancer patients. Clinically, 35% of the patients had RBP; 19% had definite RBP, i.e., were physically disabled, and 16% had probable RBP. Fifty percent had affection of the entire plexus, 18% of the upper trunk only, and 4% of the lower trunk. In 28% of cases assessment of a definite level was not possible. RBP was more common after radiotherapy and chemotherapy (42%) than after radiotherapy alone (26%) but the difference was not statistically significant (p = 0.10). In most patients with RBP the symptoms began during or immediately after radiotherapy, and were thus without significant latency. Chemotherapy might enhance the radiation-induced effect on nerve tissue, thus diminishing the latency period.

10. Lederman RJ, Breuer AC, Hanson MR, et al. Peripheral nervous system complications of coronary artery bypass graft surgery. Ann Neurol 1982;12:297–301.
Among 421 patients undergoing CABG, 13% developed PNS complications. Most common was a brachial radiculoplexopathy, the majority of which (21 of 23) affected the lower trunk or medial cord. In 17 cases there was a correlation between the site of jugular vein canulation and the side affected, suggesting that needle trauma played a role. Most PNS deficits were transient, and lasting disability was rare. See also Hanson, et al. Mechanism and frequency of brachial plexus injury in open-heart surgery. Ann Thor Surg 1983; 36:675–679.

11. Vahl CF, Carl I, Muller-Vahl H, Struck E. Brachial plexus injury after cardiac surgery. The role of internal mammary artery preparation: a prospective study on 1000 consecutive patients. J Thorac Cardiovasc Surg 1991;102:724–729.
Brachial plexus injury is a typical complication after median sternotomy. A prospective study was performed on 1000 consecutive patients to determine whether preventive actions, including lower position and least possible opening of the sternal retractor, help to reduce the complication rate. 27 patients suffered postoperative brachial plexus injury. Patients without preparation of the internal mammary artery had a complication rate of less than 1%, whereas the complication rate of those patients with preparation of the internal mammary artery was as high as 10.6%. The main symptoms were continuous pain and motor and sensory disturbances. Most frequent were lesions corresponding to the roots C8-T1. 6 patients had Horner's syndrome; 3 had ptosis only with no other signs of Horner's syndrome. Symptoms persisted in 8 patients more than 3 months after the operation, and 1 patient still had intractable pain. Increasing use of internal mammary artery grafts in coronary bypass demands measures to protect the brachial plexus.

12. Watson BV, Merchant RN, Brown WF. Early postoperative ulnar neuropathies following coronary artery bypass surgery. Muscle Nerve 1992;15:701–705.
Ulnar neuropathies following surgery are common. However, they often go undetected during the early postoperative period, because the patient may be unaware of symptoms related to the neuropathy. Nerve conduction studies are useful in localizing the lesion, but are usually employed only in cases developing signs and symptoms. This study examined the incidence, time of onset, and outcome of clinical and subclinical ulnar neuropathies. Electrophysiological studies were carried out preoperatively, immediately following surgery, and 4 to 6 weeks postoperatively in 20 coronary artery bypass patients. Conduction velocity across the elbow was reduced in 3 limbs (8%) postoperatively, all of which were detected immediately following surgery. One patient developed conduction block and weakness in ulnar supplied intrinsic hand muscles. Denervation was seen in 2 cases and, in 1 case (5%), a right brachial plexus injury was clinically evident 5 days following surgery. All newly developing ulnar neuropathies were asymptomatic, with most recovering to their preoperative electrophysiological status at follow-up.

13. Stewart JD. Focal peripheral neuropathies. 2nd ed. New York: Raven Press, 1993:
A succinct review of the anatomy and disorders affecting the brachial and lumbosacral plexi. The emphasis is on clinical evaluation and management.

14. Markey KL, Di Benedetto M, Curl WW. Upper trunk brachial plexopathy. The stinger syndrome. Am J Sports Med 1993;21:650–665.

    A study of the cause of upper trunk brachial plexopathy in football players, a "stinger" or a "burner." This injury has been thought to result from traction from lateral flexion of the neck. At the United States Military Academy, a 4-phase study of 261 tackle football players investigated this injury. Electromyography and nerve root stimulation studies were used to delineate the lesion, which was found in a total of 32 players. The study demonstrated that a much more common mechanism of injury resulting in the stinger syndrome is probably compression of the fixed brachial plexus between the shoulder pad and the superior medial scapula when the pad is pushed into the area of Erb's point, where the brachial plexus is most superficial.

15. Trojaborg W. Clinical, electrophysiological, and myelographic studies of 9 patients with cervical spinal root avulsions: discrepancies between EMG and X-ray findings. Muscle Nerve 1994;17:913–922.

    In traumatic brachial plexus injuries, the most important diagnostic question concerns the presence or absence of a preganglionic nerve root lesion. EMG and motor and sensory NCSs were performed in 17 patients with traumatic plexus injuries who had myelographic evidence of nerve root avulsion; in 8 of these clinical and electrophysiological features confirmed the X-ray findings. However, in 9 cases there was a discrepancy between myelographic and neurophysiological data regarding the actual number and sites of roots avulsed. Thus, in 2 cases myelography showed avulsion of one more root than did conduction studies and EMG; in 2 others, there was discordance as to the specific roots avulsed; in 4 cases fewer nerve roots seemed to be avulsed radiologically than predicted clinically, and in 1, none at all, although clinical and electrophysiological data were compatible with avulsion of four roots. In 6 cases recovery showed that avulsions indicated by clinical and electrophysiological considerations could not have occurred.

16. Wilbourn AJ. Thoracic outlet syndrome surgery causing severe brachial plexopathy. Muscle Nerve 1988;11:66–74.

    Hundreds of first rib resections are performed yearly in the United States to treat a controversial type of neurogenic thoracic outlet syndrome (NTOS). This surgery was thought to be devoid of serious neurological complications until 1982. However, that year Dale unearthed the rather astounding fact that the members of a single surgical society were aware of nearly 300 brachial plexus injuries resulting in motor deficits that had occurred during such operations, although almost none had been reported in the literature. In this report the features of the two main types of NTOS ("true" and "disputed") are discussed. The history of brachial plexus injury occurring during TOS surgery is traced back to the late nineteenth century. The clinical and electrophysiological features of eight patients who sustained such injuries are described in detail, the literature on this topic is reviewed, and the location and causes for these injuries are discussed. See also Cherington M, et al. Surgery for thoracic outlet syndrome may be hazardous to your health. Muscle Nerve 1986;9:632–634.

17. Cherington M, Cherington C. Thoracic outlet syndrome: reimbursement patterns and patient profiles. Neurology 1992;42:943–945.

    TOS is one of the most controversial subjects in clinical medicine. In spite of the increasing skepticism voiced in the medical literature, many patients continue to be diagnosed as having TOS and treated surgically. Colorado is one of the leading states where TOS surgery is performed. We have examined the 1989 data as collected by the Colorado Hospital Association and have defined a patient profile and reimbursement pattern. Of the 174 patients who underwent surgery, women outnumbered men by three to one (132 to 47), even when worker's compensation was the payer. The data show that patients who do not have private insurance or worker's compensation are rarely diagnosed as having TOS. Medicaid patients almost never undergo surgery.

18. Luoma A, Nelems B, Campbell JN, Naff NJ, Dellon AL, Wilbourn AJ. Thoracic outlet syndrome: thoracic surgery perspective, neurosurgical perspective and a plea for conservatism. Neurosurg Clin North Am 1991; 2:187–245.

    This trilogy is in debate format, written by thoracic surgeons, neurosurgeons, and a neurologist. It focuses on the controversial subtype of TOS, which presents with primarily sensory symptoms, normal neurologic examination, normal electrodiagnostic study results, and normal neck x-ray films. At present, this entity is so variable in its "typical" presentation that it has no characteristic profile. Although some physicians now are attempting to narrow its boundaries, the goal of fashioning a syndrome that has general acceptance remains to be achieved; consequently, the surgeons are urged by the neurologist to review the literature critically, and to err toward conservatism.

19. Jamieson WG, Chinnick B. Thoracic outlet syndrome: fact or fancy? A review of 409 consecutive patients who underwent operation. Can J Surg 1996;39:321–326.

    409 patients operated on for TOS were studied to determine what findings are helpful in substantiating this diagnosis and what are the results of decompressive thoracic outlet surgery in the management of TOS. The average age was 36 years, and 83% were women. Patients presented with neurologic type (368 ⟨90%⟩), arterial impingement (29 ⟨7%⟩) and venous obstructive symptoms (12 ⟨3%⟩). The series included 44 patients with bilateral symptoms and 26 patients with cervical ribs. Some form of litigation or compensation was associated with 177 patients. Transaxially first rib resection was done in 93% and supraclavicular thoracic outlet decompression in 7% of the patients. Preoperatively, in the 368 patients who had neurologic TOS, 99% displayed supraclavicular brachial plexus tenderness and 98% exacerbation of symptoms with arms in the abduction external rotated position. There were eight complications of surgical intervention (1.9%). In the follow-up group, there were no details, no subclavian/axillary artery or view damage and no brachial plexus injury. Seventy-eight percent of the patients with neurologic TOS in this group improved postoperatively; 21% had complete relief, 32% had good relief and 25% had fair relief. Twenty-two percent showed no improvement. The authors conclude that signs and symptoms helpful in making the diagnosis of neurologic TOS are supraclavicular tenderness on palpation and exacerbation of symptoms with the arms in the abducted external rotated position. The surgical procedures are safe. Patients with TOS refractory to medical management can benefit from thoracic outlet decompression. (Author's note: this is the surgical line, along with the hook and the sinker.)

20. Mackinnon SE, Patterson GA, Novak CB. Thoracic outlet syndrome: a current overview. Semin Thorac Cardiovasc Surg 1996;8:176–182.

    TOS and the surgery associated with this diagnosis have a controversial reputation. The majority of patients with TOS seen in the context of the work place will have a multiplicity of components to their symptomatology, including multilevel nerve compression and muscle imbalance of the neck, shoulder, and back. Identification and conservative management of these problems make the necessity for surgery for thoracic outlet syndrome a rare event. Decompression of the brachial plexus, with or without first rib resection, is a technically demanding surgical procedure requiring expertise in peripheral nerve, vascular and thoracic surgery.

21. Roos DB, Wilbourn AJ, Hachinski V. The thoracic outlet syndrome is underrated/overdiagnosed. Arch Neurol 1990;47:327–330.

From the controversies in neurology section. Roos, a surgeon, and Wilbourn, a neurologist, debate TOS from their respective points of view, with a comment by Hachinski. Roos contends that neurologic TOS accounts for 97% of all cases, can be divided into upper and lower plexus forms, does not respond well to conservative therapy and that the diagnosis is clinical. In many cases, the most gratifying results are the remarkable relief of severe headaches and return to normal sleep patterns. Wilbourn reviews the history, clinical signs and symptoms and therapy, focusing on the disputed TOS syndrome, and concludes convincingly that it is highly overdiagnosed.

22. Katirji B, Hardy RW, Jr. Classic neurogenic thoracic outlet syndrome in a competitive swimmer: a true scalenus anticus syndrome. Muscle Nerve 1995;18:229–233.

Neurogenic TOS is caused by compression of the lower brachial plexus, usually by a cervical rib or a fibrous band. A 16-year-old girl had progressive weakness and wasting of her right hand. She had been a competitive long distance freestyle and butterfly swimmer since age 8 years. A neurological exam at age 20 revealed severe atrophy and weakness of all intrinsic right hand muscles, more so of the thenar muscles, and hypesthesia along the ulnar aspect of the hand and forearm. EMG, which showed a severe chronic axon loss lower trunk brachial plexopathy with minimal fibrillations, was typical for classic neurogenic TOS. Chest and cervical spine X-rays and MRI of the cervical spine were normal. A supraclavicular exploration confirmed the absence of a cervical rib or band. The lower trunk was thickened under the scalenus anticus which was sectioned. Clinical and EMG follow-up 2.5 years later showed no significant changes. This is the first case of true neurogenic TOS caused by scalenus anticus compression occurring in a competitive swimmer.

23. Urschel HC, Jr, Razzuk MA. Management of the thoracic-outlet syndrome. N Engl J Med 1972;286:1140–1143.

The original article purporting to demonstrate conduction delay across the thoracic outlet. The figure showing the abnormality consists of two sets of four sweeps, one from a normal control and the other from a patient with TOS. The fourth tracing from the patient is merely the third tracing repeated on a slower sweep speed. When challenged 12 years later, the authors had a specious explanation for the subterfuge. See also Wilbourn AJ, Lederman RJ. Evidence for conduction delay in thoracic-outlet syndrome is challenged. N Engl J Med 1984;310:1052–1053.

24. Liu JE, Tahmoush AJ, Roos DB, et al. Shoulder-arm pain from cervical bands and scalene muscle anomalies. J Neurol Sci 1995;128:175–180.

14 patients were identified with (1) pain and sensory changes in a brachial plexus distribution, (2) aggravation of pain with use of the affected extremity, and (3) pain on palpation over the brachial plexus. All patients had minimal or no intrinsic hand muscle atrophy. Only one patient had cervical ribs. Nerve conduction studies were normal, and EMG showed mild chronic neuropathic changes in 2 patients. None of the patients responded to conservative therapy over a prolonged period (7–12 months). A compressive brachial plexopathy from abnormally attached or enlarged scalene muscles that affected both upper and lower trunks of the brachial plexus was found at surgery in all patients. In 13 patients, at least one fibrous band compressed the lower trunk of the brachial plexus. Therefore, neurogenic thoracic outlet syndrome can occur from cervical bands and scalene muscle anomalies without intrinsic hand muscle atrophy, cervical ribs, enlarged C7 transverse processes, or EMG abnormalities.

25. Swift TR, Nichols FT. The droopy shoulder syndrome. Neurology 1984;34:212–215.

A report that patients with thoracic outlet syndrome have: (1) low-set, "droopy" shoulders and long swan neck; (2) pain in the neck, shoulder, chest, arms, or hands; (3) aggravation of symptoms by downward traction and relief by propping up the arms; (4) occurrence in women; (5) absence of abnormal vascular, neurologic, and electrical findings; (6) a Tinel's sign over the brachial plexus; and (7) T-2 vertebra visible above the shoulders on lateral cervical spine films. The authors contend droopy shoulder syndrome accounts for most cases of thoracic outlet syndrome but is largely unrecognized by physicians. See also Clein LJ. The droopy shoulder syndrome. Can Med Assoc J 1976;114:343–344.

26. Chokroverty S, Sander HW. AAEM case report #13: diabetic amyotrophy. Muscle Nerve 1996;19:939–945.

Report of a case fulfilling the criteria for the diagnosis of diabetic amyotrophy. Based on the clinical and EMG features, diabetic amyotrophy is a recognizable clinical entity that can be differentiated from other diabetic neuropathies. The site of the lesion and the pathogenesis remain controversial. The course of the illness is variable with gradual, but often incomplete, improvement.

27. Jaeckle KA, Young DF, Foley KM. The natural history of lumbosacral plexopathy in cancer. Neurology 1985;35:8–15.

A study of 85 cancer patients with lumbosacral plexopathy and documented pelvic tumor by CT or biopsy. Three clinical syndromes were delineated: lower (L4–S1), 51%; upper (L1–L4), 31%; and pan-plexopathy (L1–S3), 18%. Seventy percent of patients had the insidious onset of pelvic or radicular leg pain, followed weeks to months later by sensory symptoms and weakness. The quintet of leg pain, weakness, edema, rectal mass, and hydronephrosis suggests plexopathy due to cancer. CT showed pelvic tumor in 96%. On myelography, epidural extension, usually below the conus medullaris, was seen in 45%.

28. Thomas JE, Cascino TL, Earle JD. Differential diagnosis between radiation and tumor plexopathy of the pelvis. Neurology 1985;35:1–7.

A study of 20 patients with lumbosacral radiculoplexopathy from RT and 30 patients with plexus damage from pelvic malignancy. Indolent leg weakness occurred early in radiation disease, whereas pain marked the onset of tumor plexopathy. Eventually, all radiation cases had weakness, which was bilateral in most of them and painless in one-half of them. Tumor patients typically had unilateral weakness, which was painful in all of them. Radiation disease often resulted in serious neurologic disability. Of the tumor patients, 86% were dead within 3 1/2 years after onset of neurologic symptoms.

29. Bradley WG, Chad D, Verghese JP, et al. Painful lumbosacral plexopathy with elevated erythrocyte sedimentation rate: a treatable inflammatory syndrome. Ann Neurol 1984;15:457–464.
   6 patients had a painful lumbosacral plexopathy, elevated ESR and sural nerve biopsy showing axonal degeneration and perivascular inflammation. None of the patients had cancer or an underlying systemic vasculitis. 5 were treated with immunosuppressants and in 4 the plexopathy improved or was arrested. The pathogenesis is unclear.

30. Hinchey JA, Preston DC, Logigian EL. Idiopathic lumbosacral neuropathy: a cause of persistent leg pain. Muscle Nerve 1996;19:1484–1486.
   A report of 5 cases of idiopathic lumbosacral plexopathy. See text for details.

31. Plecha EJ, Seabrook GR, Freischlag JA, et al. Neurologic complications of reoperative and emergent abdominal aortic reconstruction. Ann Vasc Surg 1995;9:95–101.
   Patients undergoing abdominal aortic reconstructions are at increased risk for ischemic neurologic complications. Between 1986 and 1992, 5 patients sustained ischemic injuries to the spinal cord, nerve roots, or lumbosacral plexus. Physical exam and EMG localized the injury to the level of the cauda equina or lumbosacral plexus. The incidence of neurologic deficits during this study period was 18% (3/17) in patients requiring aortofemoral graft excision for infection. Neurologic deficits after reoperative and emergent abdominal aortic reconstructions are uncommon but devastating complications. Of particular concern is the incidence of neurologic deficits after removal of aortofemoral grafts with disruption of collateral flow to the spinal cord and nerve roots.

32. Antoine JC, Baril A, Guettier C, et al. Unusual amyloid polyneuropathy with predominant lumbosacral nerve roots and plexus involvement. Neurology 1991;41:206–208.
   Report of a 25-year-old patient with a progressive asymmetric peripheral neuropathy of the distal lower limbs. Imaging studies showed enlargement of lumbosacral roots, plexus, and proximal sciatic nerve. Sacral plexus biopsy revealed amyloidosis.

33. Zuniga G, Ropper AH, Frank J. Sarcoid peripheral neuropathy. Neurology 1991;41:1558–1561.
   A study of 10 patients with sarcoidosis and peripheral neuropathy. Six had a subacute or chronic axonal sensorimotor neuropathy without cranial neuropathy, beginning months to years after established systemic sarcoidosis. Four patients had atypical neuropathies: acute Guillain-Barre syndrome, mononeuritis multiplex, unilateral lumbosacral plexopathy, and a purely sensory neuropathy, all before systemic sarcoidosis became evident, and all except one had cranial nerve abnormalities. Autopsy in one patient with sensorimotor neuropathy showed only scattered foci of lymphocytes in spinal roots and ganglia with nerve fiber loss.

34. Feasby TE, Burton SR, Hahn AF. Obstetrical lumbosacral plexus injury. Muscle Neve 1992;15:937–940.
   Injuries to the lumbosacral plexus during labor and delivery have been reported in the literature for years, but have lacked electrophysiologic testing to substantiate the location of the nerve injury. A report of 2 cases with comprehensive electrophysiologic testing which localized the site of this obstetrical paralysis to the lumbosacral trunk (L4-5) and S–1 root where they join and pass over the pelvic rim. The paralysis may be mild or severe. Small maternal size, a large fetus, midforceps rotation, and fetal malposition may place the mother at risk for this nerve injury.

35. Cifu DX, Irani KD. Ischaemic lumbosacral plexopathy in acute vascular compromise: case report. Paraplegia 1991;29:70–75.
   Report of a patient with marked lower extremity weakness, hypotonia, hyporeflexia, and a functioning bowel and bladder 3 months following a stab wound to the left ventricle, thought to represent an incomplete spinal cord injury due to ischemia. NCSs showed slowed velocities, prolonged distal latencies and decreased amplitudes of all lower extremity nerves. EMG revealed denervation of all proximal and distal lower extremity musculature, with normal paraspinalis. 3 other cases of ischaemic lumbosacral plexopathy, mimicking an incomplete spinal cord injury, have been reported.

C H A P T E R

16

Generalized Peripheral Neuropathies

OUTLINE

Peripheral neuropathies are conditions that affect peripheral nerve axons, their myelin sheaths, or both, producing a variety of signs and symptoms. As in arthritis or anemia, a diagnosis of peripheral neuropathy is relatively meaningless, as dozens of conditions could be responsible. Greater precision is required to have any clinical usefulness. Table 16.1 lists some of the major and most common etiologies of peripheral nerve disease, but is far from exhaustive. A recent major textbook lists more than 100 neuropathies of electrodiagnostic interest (1).

The electrodiagnostic characterization is integral to the evaluation of patients with neuropathy, permitting a greater accuracy of diagnosis and helping to define the distribution, the pathophysiology, the severity and sometimes the prognosis. The electrodiagnostic profile of a neuropathy can help focus the differential diagnosis and guide subsequent investigations and management.

The ultimate goal in neuropathy evaluations is to establish a precise etiologic diagnosis to guide treatment, if any is available. Arriving at a final diagnosis can be either simple, as in diabetes or alcoholism, or exasperatingly difficult. Except in specialized centers, the exact cause is identified only about half the time, and many of those are diabetics or alcoholics. Thus,

TABLE 16.1
Selected Causes of Peripheral Neuropathy

Inflammatory demyelinating neuropathy
  AIDP (Guillain-Barre syndrome)
  CIDP

Infectious and granulomatous neuropathy
  Leprosy
  Sarcoid
  HIV related
  Lyme disease

Neuropathy associated with systemic disease
  Diabetes
  Chronic renal disease
  Alcoholism
  Paraproteinemia
  Dysimmune neuropathies
  Hypothyroidism
  Vitamin deficiency
  Paraneoplastic neuropathy
  Amyloidosis
  Connective tissue disease
  Critical illness polyneuropathy

Ischemic neuropathy
  Peripheral vascular disease
  Vasculitis

Metabolic neuropathy
  Porphyria
  Leukodystrophy
  Lipidosis
  Bassen-Kornzweig disease
  Tangier disease
  Refsum's disease
  Fabry's disease

Hereditary neuropathy
  HMSN type I (hypertrophic form of Charcot-Marie-
    Tooth disease)
  HMSN type II (neuronal form of Charcot-Marie-Tooth
    disease)
  HMSN type III (Dejerine-Sottas disease)
  Other forms of HMSN
  HSAN type I
  HSAN type II
  HSAN type III (Riley-Day syndrome)
  Hereditary neuropathy with liability to pressure palsies
    (tomaculous neuropathy)
  Giant axonal neuropathy

Toxins
  Pharmaceuticals
  Environmental toxins

a great deal of time and energy is expended to help only a few patients. However, effective therapy is often available, ranging from aggressive immunosuppression, to discontinuing a medication, to control of an underlying systemic disease. Even patients for whom

no specific therapy is available can benefit from symptomatic treatment.

To establish an etiologic diagnosis, the neuropathy must be characterized and classified as precisely as possible. To separate the cause of a particular neuropathy from the protean possibilities, an attempt should be made to construct a profile of characteristics to narrow the differential diagnosis. From the long list of causes of neuropathy, only a short list emerges of conditions that cause a chronic, predominantly sensory, large fiber axonopathy, or an acute, predominantly motor, multifocal demyelinating neuropathy with secondary axonal damage. Using clinical, electrodiagnostic, pathologic and laboratory data, neuropathies can be classified according to their anatomical site of involvement, time course, distribution, pattern of deficit, type of functional fiber involved, and whether the process is primarily axonal, primarily demyelinating or mixed (Tables 16.2–16.10). It is helpful to classify a neuropathy in as many ways as possible, in hopes of uncovering a characteristic signature. Knowledge of the relevant anatomical, physiological and pathological concepts helps greatly in this exercise.

The onset of a neuropathy may be relatively acute or subacute, evolving over several days to several weeks, or more chronic, evolving over several months to many years. There is some unavoidable overlap in the middle, between what might be called subacute and what might be called chronic. In Tables 16.2–16.5, common, interesting or otherwise relevant neuropa-

TABLE 16.2
Acute/Subacute Myelinopathies

Uniform Diffuse Demyelination	*Segmental, Multifocal Demyelination*
Toxins	GBS†
Hexacarbons	Acute arsenic intoxication
N-hexane	Lymphoma
Methyl butyl ketone	HIV infection (early)
Na+ channel blockers	Diphtheria
tetrodotoxin	Drugs
saxitoxin	Amiodarone*
Drugs	Perhexiline*
Amiodarone*	Cytosine arabinoside*
Perhexilene*	
Doxorubicin	
Cytosine arabinoside*	

* Both patterns have been reported.
† GBS is a syndrome, not a disease, and can occur as part of several conditions.

TABLE 16.3
Subacute/Chronic Demyelinating Neuropathies

Uniform, Diffuse Demyelination	Segmental, Multifocal Demyelination
HMSN I, III, IV	CIDP and variants*
Metachromatic leukodys-trophy	Hypothyroidism
	Leprosy
Adrenoleukodystrophy	Hereditary neuropathy with liability to pressure palsies
Adrenomyeloneuropathy	
Krabbe's disease	Lyme disease
Cockayne's syndrome	HIV infection (early)
Tangier disease	Paraproteinemic neuropathy
	Cryoglobulinemia
	Lymphoma
	SLE

* Includes CIDP-MGUS, POEMS syndrome, multifocal motor neuropathy and anti-MAG neuropathy.

thies are classified into demyelinating vs. axonal, and whether the onset is acute/subacute vs. subacute/chronic. Tables 16.7–16.10 outline some of the differences in functional fiber type.

The anatomical site of involvement may range from the nerve cell body (neuronopathy, e.g., acute ataxic sensory neuronpathy), to the nerve roots (acute inflammatory demyelinating polyradiculoneuropathy), to the nerve proper, to the axon terminals (twig neuropathy, e.g., hyperparathyroidism). There are two primary patterns of involvement: generalized/symmetric vs. focal/multifocal. The time course may vary from acute, evolving over days to weeks, to chronic, evolving over months to years, to very chronic, life-long, to relapsing and remitting. Neuropathies may be predominantly motor (e.g., Guillain-Barre) or predominantly sensory (e.g., amyloidosis).

Most neuropathies produce symmetric distal involvement, but some may cause primarily proximal weakness (e.g., porphyria) or proximal sensory loss (e.g., Tangier disease) or acral sensory loss over the coolest body parts (e.g., leprosy). Sensory neuropathies may preferentially affect large fibers (e.g., vitamin B12 deficiency) or small fibers (e.g., hereditary sensory neuropathy). Particular neuropathies may or may not have associated autonomic dysfunction. As defined by the clinical, electrodiagnostic and occasionally pathologic examinations, a neuropathy may be primarily axonal (e.g., HMSN II), primarily demyelinating (e.g., CIDP), mixed but mainly axonal (e.g., chronic renal disease), or mixed but with significant demyelination (e.g., diabetes).

The following discussion will cover the relevant anatomy, physiology and pathology of peripheral nerve, the clinical evaluation of the neuropathy patient, and the clinical and electrodiagnostic differential diagnosis, concluding with a discussion of the more common neuropathic syndromes.

Anatomy of the Peripheral Nerve

Peripheral nerves are composed of myriad axons, ensheathed by myelin of varying thickness and supported by Schwann cells, all embedded in a matrix of connective tissue. Nerves are divided into discrete internal fascicular compartments by perineurium. The blood nerve barrier (BNB) is a physiologic partition, created by the perineurium and the endothelium of intrafascicular capillaries, which regulates the nerve microenvironment and acts as a diffusion barrier (2). The extreme terminal ends of nerve fibers are not protected by perineurium and have no effective BNB. Within each fascicle endoneurium separates individual axons and their Schwann cells (Fig. 16.1). Fascicles are bound together into nerve trunks by the epineurium, loose areolar connective tissue which also contains blood vessels, lymphatics and the nervi nervorum. The epineurium also serves an important cushioning role. The interfascicular epineurium lies between fascicles, the epifascicular epineurium circumferentially envelopes the entire nerve (2).

TABLE 16.4
Acute/Subacute Axonopathy

Primarily motor
Acute motor axonal neuropathy (axonal GBS)
Porphyria
Lead intoxication
Dapsone
Tick paralysis
Critical illness polyneuropathy

Primarily sensory
Paclitaxel/docetaxel (high dose)
Cisplatinum
Acute sensory neuronopathy
Pyridoxine intoxication (high dose)
Ciguatera intoxication
Miller-Fisher syndrome
Metronidazole

Mixed
Critical illness polyneuropathy

TABLE 16.5
Subacute/Chronic Axonopathy

Primarily Motor	Primarily Sensory
HMSN II and V	Distal sensory neuropathy in AIDS
Paraneoplastic motor neuropathy	Diabetes mellitus
	Chronic arsenic intoxication
Vincristine	Paclitaxel/docetaxel (usually)
	Cisplatinum
	Pyridoxine intoxication (low dose)
	Paraneoplastic neuropathy
	Chronic ataxic neuropathy
	Sjogren's syndrome
	Primary biliary cirrhosis
	Amyloidosis
	Lyme disease
	Vitamin E deficiency
	Tabes dorsalis
	Anti-sulfatide neuropathy
	Friedreich's ataxia
	Abetalipoproteinemia
	Nonsystemic vasculitic neuropathy

Mixed Sensorimotor

Amyloidosis	Paraneoplastic neuropathy
Alcoholism	Hypothyroidism
Vitamin B12 deficiency	Lyme disease
	HIV
Sarcoidosis	Connective tissue diseases
Most toxins	Vasculitic neuropathy
Most drugs	Multiple myeloma
HIV infection	Cryoglobulinemia
Diabetes mellitus	AIDS
Chronic arsenic intoxication	
Lead intoxication	

TABLE 16.6
Mixed Axonopathy/Myelinopathy

Diabetes mellitus
ESRD
GBS (cases with axon loss)
CIDP (cases with axon loss)

TABLE 16.7
Primarily Motor Polyneuropathies

GBS
CIDP
Porphyria
Dapsone
Lead
CMT disease

TABLE 16.8
Large Fiber Sensory Neuropathies

Uremia
Diabetes mellitus (pseuotabes)
Paraneoplastic neuropathy
Sjogren's syndrome
Vitamin B12 deficiency
Friedreich's ataxia
Certain toxins
    Pyridoxine
    Cisplatinum
    Metronidazole
Acute idiopathic sensory neuronopathy
CIDP

TABLE 16.9
Small Fiber Sensory Neuropathies

Diabetes mellitus (pseudosyringomyelia)
Amyloidosis
Hereditary sensory autonomic neuropathies
Leprosy

TABLE 16.10
Neuropathies with Major Autonomic Dysfunction (56)

Diabetes
Alcoholism
Amyloidosis
HSAN III (Riley-Day syndrome)
Guillain-Barre syndrome
Porphyria
Vincristine
Idiopathic pandysautonomia

Normal Nerve

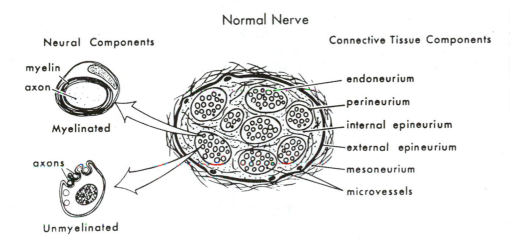

Neural Components

myelin
axon

Myelinated

axons

Unmyelinated

Connective Tissue Components

endoneurium
perineurium
internal epineurium
external epineurium
mesoneurium
microvessels

FIGURE 16.1. The normal peripheral nerve is composed of connective tissue and neural tissue components. The nerve fibers may be myelinated or unmyelinated. Reprinted with permission from Mackinnon SE, Dellon AL. Surgery of the peripheral nerve. New York: Thieme, 1988:3.

Fascicles bifurcate, join with adjacent fascicles, re-divide and recombine to create a complex internal fascicular network (Fig. 16.2). Nerves can be classified into monofascicular, oligofascicular and polyfascicular types. A polyfascicular pattern is common in regions subject to mechanical stress and where there is heavy fiber exchange, such as the brachial plexus. Plexiform fascicular exchange is most prominent proximally, and a constant fascicular pattern is present for only a short distance in proximal regions of a nerve. Fascicles innervating a particular muscle or sensory zone become more discrete and constant in position as they approach the target organ. This complex intraneural topography has important clinical and electrophysiologic implications (2).

Axons are divided into three major size groups: large myelinated, small myelinated and unmyelinated. Large myelinated axons have diameters in the 6–12 μm range, small myelinated axons 2–6 μm and unmyelinated axons 0.2–2.0 μm. Small myelinated fibers are about three times more numerous than large myelinated axons. The myelin sheath adds additional thickness. Conduction is most efficient when the ratio of the axon diameter to total fiber diameter is 0.5–0.7 (3).

Ultrastructurally, axons contain cytoskeletal elements, neurofilaments and neurotubules, which are synthesized in the cell body and move slowly down the axon at a rate of 3 mm/day. Neurotubules consist of polymerized dimers of tubulin protein forming longitudinally oriented hollow tubes about 20 nm in diameter and 1 mm long, linked by cross bridges to the neurofilaments. Neurofilaments are smaller organelles that maintain axonal structure. Neurotubules are responsible for fast antegrade and retrograde axonal transport (see below).

In myelinated axons, a single Schwann cell wraps a single internodal segment in concentric layers of

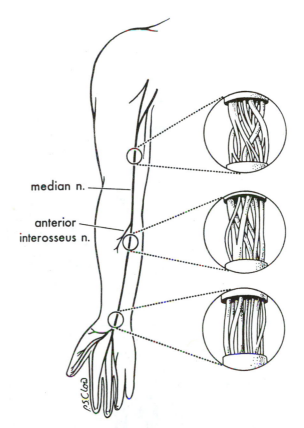

median n.

anterior
interosseus n.

FIGURE 16.2. Internal topography of the median nerve at different levels. The complexity of the internal fascicular anatomy is apparent. The degree of plexus formation between fascicles decreases in the distal portion of the nerve as the bundles approach their target muscles. Reprinted with permission from Mackinnon SE, Dellon AL. Surgery of the peripheral nerve. New York: Thieme, 1988:6.

myelin (Fig. 16.3). Schmidt-Lanterman incisures are bits of Schwann cell cytoplasm sequestered between layers of myelin. The external plasma membrane of the Schwann cell is continuous with the outermost layer of myelin, the inner membrane of the Schwann cell is immediately adjacent to the outer surface of the axolemma. The external lamina is a condensation of extracellular matrix surrounding the entire external surface of the Schwann cell. For "unmyelinated" axons, a single Schwann cell, sometimes referred to as a Remak cell, sends out processes to support several adjacent axons, lending to each primarily a cytoplasmic coat and only a minimal investment of myelin. A complex of several unmyelinated axons and their supporting Remak cell is encased by an external lamina (3). The nodes of Ranvier are gaps in the myelin coverage between the territories of adjacent

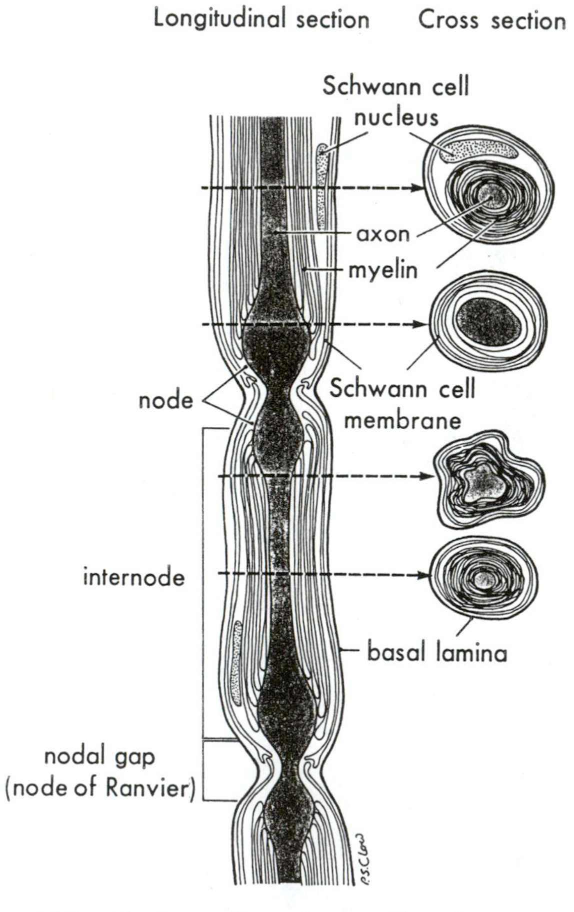

FIGURE 16.3. Single myelinated nerve fiber demonstrating the relationships between the axon, the Schwann cell and the myelin sheath at different points. Reprinted with permission from Mackinnon SE, Dellon AL. Surgery of the peripheral nerve. New York: Thieme, 1988:4.

Schwann cells. Internodal length varies with fiber size and is about 1 mm for large diameter fibers.

Peripheral nerves receive blood supply from penetrating segmental arteries usually derived from adjacent vessels. Penetrating arterioles then form an extensive longitudinal anastomotic network than runs within the nerve. Watershed zones of precarious perfusion within the nerve may explain some of the clinical manifestations seen in ischemic neuropathies, especially in vasculitis.

Physiology of Peripheral Nerve

Peripheral nerve fibers are classified according to two schemes, the ABC and the I/II/III/IV systems, both ranging from largest (A, I) to smallest (C, IV). The conduction velocity (CV) of a fiber depends on its diameter and degree of myelination, and ranges from < 1 m/sec for small, unmyelinated fibers to > 100 m/sec for large, myelinated fibers. The compound nerve action potential (NAP) recorded in vitro from mixed peripheral nerve separates fibers into groups based on their CV. A-alpha and A-gamma fibers are efferent fibers from alpha and gamma motoneurons respectively. A-beta and A-delta fibers are primarily cutaneous afferents. Group B fibers are preganglionic autonomics. Group C fibers are postganglionic autonomics, visceral afferents, and pain and temperature fibers. The Roman numeral system applies only to afferent fibers. Ia fibers arise from nuclear bag muscle spindle fibers and joint receptors, Ib fibers from Golgi tendon organs and II fibers from nuclear chain muscle spindle fibers. Class III fibers are cutaneous axons which correspond more or less to A-delta pain fibers, and type IV fibers correspond to C fibers.

Some neuropathies have a predilection for certain types and sizes of fibers. Large fiber neuropathies affect strength, reflexes and proprioception with relative sparing of pain and temperature sensation, whereas small fiber neuropathies primarily affect pain, temperature and autonomic function. Differential involvement of large vs. small sensory fibers can sometimes be discerned clinically. Standard nerve conduction studies evaluate only the conduction characteristics of the large, myelinated fibers. Autonomic studies (Chapter 9) can evaluate the autonomic system. Evaluation of nonautonomic small fibers is currently a research undertaking. The immunological and biochemical differences between fibers that might explain differential involvement are just beginning to be understood. For example, the L2 membrane protein is expressed only on motor axon Schwann cells, and the nerves to the extraocular muscles are especially rich in ganglioside GQ1b, which may relate to their involvement in Miller Fisher syndrome (3).

The axoplasm is in constant flux, containing elements which flow to and fro along its length between the cell body and the periphery. Antegrade axoplasmic flow moves from the cell body distally, retrograde flow moves centripetally. Antegrade flow has multiple components. Slow axonal transport, 1–3 mm/day, conveys cytoskeletal proteins to the periphery for maintenance and renewal of axoplasm, along with neurotransmitters, enzymes and other components. Fast axonal transport, 400 mm/day, largely transports membrane-bound vesicles that are propelled by kinesin, a microtubule associated ATPase. Abnormalities of axonal transport are likely important in the mechanism of dying back or length dependent neuropathies. Several substances produce neuropathy by disrupting the cytoskeletal elements: vinca alkaloids, taxoids, and hexacarbons for example (4). Retrograde flow moves materials from the periphery back to the cell body and is the mechanism through which some neurotrophic viruses reach the CNS.

Pathology of Peripheral Nerve

Nerve fibers react to injury through two primary mechanisms, axonal degeneration, and demyelination (3). In axonal degeneration, the cytoplasm disintegrates. Cytoskeletal elements disappear and are replaced by amorphous granular material. Eventually the axolemma becomes discontinuous and the myelin sheath, but not the Schwann cell, secondarily disintegrates. Fragments of axolemma and myelin form linear arrays of myelin ovoids. Macrophages phagocytose and eventually remove the debris. With complete axon transection, the interval from injury to total axonal fragmentation is usually less than 2 weeks. If the injury is proximal, the nerve cell body may undergo central chromatolysis. Wallerian degeneration specifically refers to the axonal degeneration distal to a traumatic nerve injury.

In demyelinating neuropathies, the primary insult is to the myelin sheath or the Schwann cell, producing varying degrees of interference with myelin maintenance. In the earliest stages, demyelination is paranodal. With progression, the rest of the internodal segment becomes involved. Segmental demyelination refers to involvement of several internodes over a segment of nerve. In some conditions the Schwann cells are involved diffusely and the demyelination is uniform along the length of the nerve, e.g., Charcot-Marie-Tooth disease. In most acquired myelinopathies, the involvement is multifocal, e.g., Guillain-Barre syndrome. In compression neuropathies, the demyelination is focal and involves only a discrete segment, e.g., carpal tunnel syndrome.

With severe demyelination, there may be secondary axon loss. In compression neuropathies, the myelin is more susceptible to injury and axon loss reflects chronicity and severity. In dysimmune inflammatory neuropathies the axon may be an accidental victim of the attack, the bystander effect. The secondary axon loss in myelinopathies and the secondary demyelination in axonopathies add another measure of clinical and electrodiagnostic complexity to the evaluation of neuropathies. Clinically and electrophysiologically these secondary changes may create a mixed picture of axonopathy and myelinopathy. For example, uremia characteristically produces an axonopathy with secondary demyelination, and severe Guillain-Barre syndrome, a primarily demyelinating and inflammatory neuropathy, is often associated with significant secondary axon loss due to the bystander effect.

Treatment implications mandate the separation of demyelinating and axonal neuropathies. The two primary techniques available for this purpose are nerve conduction studies (NCSs) and nerve biopsy, and both unfortunately have limitations. The morphologic and electrophysiologic criteria for differentiating between the two are imperfect, and subject to operator variability. Long standing peripheral nerve disease, regardless of cause, may lead to indistinguishable pathological changes (3). Studies have shown that slowing of sural nerve conduction velocity (NCV) is significantly related to loss of large fibers or demyelination on biopsy. CV is inversely proportional to the fraction of fibers with segmental or paranodal demyelination or remyelination but unrelated to the proportion of degenerating axons. In a recent study, there was significant discordance between biopsy and conduction study findings in only 23% of patients (5).

Clinical Signs and Symptoms of Peripheral Neuropathy

The cardinal manifestations of peripheral neuropathy are weakness, alterations in sensation and reflex changes. The patterns of abnormality are important in differential diagnosis, and detailed clinical examination exploring the details and specifics is often rewarded. Is the neuropathy predominantly motor or sensory? If weakness is present, is it proximal, distal or diffuse? Is there atrophy? Are the reflex changes length dependent or global? Do the sensory changes demonstrate a predilection for large or small fibers?

Is there autonomic dysfunction? Are the findings symmetric?

The age at onset, pace of evolution, presence of associated medical or neurologic conditions, and medication history are very important. The family history is crucial but often tricky, as many individuals with hereditary neuropathies do not recognize their own condition. Other family members having funny looking feet or difficult to fit shoes may be the only clue to a condition that is rampant but unrecognized in a kindred.

Quantitation of the degree of deficit is useful for longitudinal follow up. Sophisticated instrumentation is available for this purpose, but is expensive and not in wide use outside academic centers. Simple bedside testing can provide a great deal of useful information. Strength is most often described using the MRC scale. The power in small hand muscles can be nicely described using techniques that compare the patient's strength to the same muscles of the examiner (6). Two point discrimination is quantitative and easily performed. Inexpensive hand held esthesiometers can quantitate touch sensibility. Vibratory sensation is a sensitive parameter of peripheral nerve function, and can be simply quantitated by noting where the patient can perceive it and for how long, e.g., "vibration absent at the great toes and metatarsal heads, can perceive a maximally vibrating 128 Hz fork for 5 seconds over the medial malleoli." If the patient returns having lost vibration over the malleoli, the condition is progressing. If on follow up, vibration is present for 12 seconds over the malleoli and can now be perceived for 3 seconds over the metatarsal heads, the patient is improving. Functional testing is invaluable. The time required to walk a set distance or to get up from the floor, the arm and leg outstretch time, the ability to support the entire body weight on one tiptoe and similar functions are objective and quantifiable.

Electrophysiology of Peripheral Neuropathies

Demyelinating neuropathies and axonopathies produce different electrophysiologic pictures. In brief, primary myelinopathies produce marked slowing of conduction velocities with preservation of distal amplitudes, while axonopathies produce marked loss of distal amplitudes, with relative preservation of conduction velocities. When the disease process affects only the myelin, conduction is impaired because of loss of saltatory conduction. If the process is uniform and diffuse, affecting all the myelin, as in a hereditary myelinopathy, then the conduction abnormalities involve all nerves and all segments of nerves to an approximately equal degree. If the process is focal then only the involved nerve is affected. If the process is multi-focal the abnormalities may be wide-spread, but different in different nerves and in different segments of the same nerve. In either case, with a myelinopathy, the axon is intact and there is no loss of trophic influences on the target motor and sensory organs. Muscle atrophy does not occur, and denervation potentials, fibrillations and positive sharp waves do not appear in the affected muscles.

In contrast, a disease process that primarily affects the axons causes loss of the axon mediated trophic influences on target organs. The muscle becomes atrophic, with a resultant decline in M wave amplitude. Axon loss produces a diminution of sensory or compound nerve action potential amplitude. Involvement of all the axons in a nerve may render the nerve inexcitable, and no motor or sensory potentials can be elicited. However, any surviving axons will conduct at their normal velocity. If a disease process produces dropout of 50% of the axons in a nerve, the electrodiagnostic picture would be a 50% ($\pm$) loss of M wave amplitude, but a relatively normal CV. Clinical and electrophysiologic characteristics helpful in distinguishing axonopathy from myelinopathy are summarized in Table 16.11.

Unfortunately, as is often the case, things do not always follow the classical or typical pattern. Some neuropathies are truly mixed, having electrophysiologic features of both demyelination and axon loss. In addition, axonopathies can produce some degree of slowing of CV. Random involvement of axons will inevitably affect some of the largest and fastest conducting fibers, whose dropout then will lower the maximal CV. If the largest and fastest conducting axons are preferentially affected, as has been postulated for motor neuron disease, then significant slowing could occur due to an axonopathy. The severity of an axonopathy is reflected by the degree of muscle fiber atrophy and its attendant loss of M wave amplitude. A severe axonopathy can be expected to involve more of the fastest conducting fibers and will therefore produce more slowing of CV than a mild axonopathy. For this reason, if the M wave amplitude is decreased, more severe conduction slowing must be present before one can be confident of the existence of demyelination. Because of these complicating factors, criteria for demyelination have been developed. Although there is not universal consensus on criteria, the use of some criteria set is coming into increasingly wide acceptance; debate continues regarding precise details. The criteria for primary demyelination used by the

TABLE 16.11
Clinical and Electrodiagnostic Features That Help Distinguish Axonopathy from Myelinopathy

Axonopathy

Clinical	*Electrodiagnostic*
• Insidious onset • Slow progression • Slow recovery • Evidence of length dependency • Loss of ankle jerks with presence of other reflexes • Stocking distribution sensory loss • Weakness limited to distal muscles • Symmetry • Normal CSF protein	• Normal or mildly slowed nerve conduction velocities, i.e., do not meet criteria for demyelination • Decreased M wave amplitude • Decreased sensory or compound NAP amplitude • Increased DML/late response latencies proportional to CV slowing • Proximal to distal gradient of increasing abnormality on needle examination

Myelinopathy

Clinical	*Electrodiagnostic*
• More rapid onset • More rapid recovery • Mild asymmetry • Global loss of reflexes • Proximal, or diffuse weakness • Cranial nerve involvement • Motor > sensory dysfunction • Increased CSF protein	• Marked conduction velocity slowing, i.e., meets criteria for demyelination • Normal M wave amplitude • Spotty or multifocal involvement • Normal sural, abnormal median SNAP • Conduction block or temporal dispersion on proximal stimulation • Prolongation of DML or late response latencies disproportional to CV slowing • Paucity of denervation on needle examination with no proximal/distal gradient

Dutch Guillain-Barré study group are summarized in Table 16.12, and the research criteria for the diagnosis of CIDP, including the electrophysiologic criteria for demyelination are covered in Tables 16.13 and 16.14.

Although CV and amplitude are the primary parameters, other electrodiagnostic variables may be useful as well. Disproportionate prolongation of distal motor

TABLE 16.12
Criteria for Primary Demyelination Employed by the Dutch GBS Study Group

Distal motor latency > 150% of ULN

F wave latency > 150% of ULN

Motor NCV <70% of LLN

Abnormal M wave amplitude decay

Abnormal temporal dispersion

ULN, upper limit of normal; LLN, lower limit of normal; NCV, nerve conduction velocity.
Modified from Muelstee J, et al. Electrodiagnostic criteria for polyneuropathy and demyelination: application in 135 patients with Guillain-Barre syndrome (26).

TABLE 16.13
Clinical and Laboratory Criteria for the Diagnosis of CIDP

Clinical
  Mandatory
    Progressive or relapsing dysfunction of a peripheral nerve nature involving more than one limb and evolving over at least two months
    Hypo- or areflexia
  Supportive
    Large fiber sensory loss pattern
  Exclusion
    Acral mutilation, retinitis pigmentosa, ichthyosis, drug or toxin exposure, family history suggestive of a genetic neuropathy
  Sensory level
  Unequivocal sphincter disturbance
Pathologic
  Mandatory
    Nerve biopsy showing unequivocal demyelination and remyelination
  Supportive
    Nerve biopsy showing abnormalities nonspecific but consistent with CIDP
  Exclusionary
    Nerve biopsy excludes vasculitis, amyloidosis or other specific pathology
CSF
  Mandatory
    Cell count <10 if HIV negative, <50 if HIV positive
    VDRL negative
  Supportive
    Elevated protein

Modified from AAN AIDS task force. Research criteria for diagnosis of CIDP. Neurology 1991;41:617–618 (31).

TABLE **16.14**
Electrophysiologic Criteria for the Diagnosis of CIDP

Mandatory—must have three of the following four abnormalities
  Reduction in conduction velocity in two or more nerves:
    To <80% of the lower limit of normal (LLN) if amplitude is >80% of LLN
    To <70% of LLN if amplitude <80% of LLN
  Partial conduction block or abnormal temporal dispersion in one or more motor nerves, not at sites commonly prone to compression
  Prolongation of distal latency in two or more nerves:
    To >125% of the upper limit of normal (ULN) if amplitude is >80% of the LLN
    To >150% of ULN if amplitude is <80% of LLN
  Absent F waves, or prolongation of F wave latency in two or more motor nerves:
    To >120% of ULN if amplitude is >80% of LLN
    To >150% of ULN if amplitude is <80% of LLN
Supportive
  Reduction in sensory CV <80% of LLN
Absent H reflexes

Modified from AAN AIDS task force. Research criteria for diagnosis of CIDP. Neurology 1991;41:617–618 (31).

latency or late response latency, beyond that explicable on the basis of axon loss, may also indicate demyelination. Axonopathies are length dependant, due to a "dying back" process that affects the most distal nerve terminals first and involves more proximal nerve segments with progression. Disproportionate conduction abnormalities in the most distal nerves can thus indicate axonopathy. A gradient of abnormality on needle examination, with greatest involvement of the most distal muscles and progressively less involvement of more proximal muscles suggests a length dependent process.

Another major indicator of demyelination is conduction block or temporal dispersion. This is a change in amplitude or configuration of M wave waveform on stimulation proximal to a given point (Fig. 16.4). In temporal dispersion, focal demyelination of axons produces conduction slowing that involves some fibers to a greater degree than other fibers, producing a loss of synchrony. The M wave conducted through the demyelinated region is dispersed and spread out, with an increased duration and a loss of amplitude (Fig. 16.5). However, all fibers successfully conduct through the affected region, so the total area under the M wave curve remains the same with both proximal and distal stimulation. In conduction block, some

fibers are so severely demyelinated that they do not conduct at all. There is not only a diminution in M wave amplitude but also a diminution in the total area under the curve, indicating that fewer muscle fibers have been successfully depolarized with proximal stimulation as compared with distal stimulation.

Clinical weakness seems to correlate with conduction block, not with CV slowing or temporal dispersion. A great deal has been made of distinguishing between conduction block and temporal dispersion, but the distinction is of questionable utility, as both these phenomena indicate a focal demyelinating le-

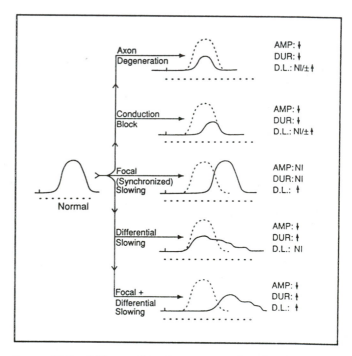

FIGURE 16.4. Effects of various types of pathophysiology on the M wave recorded proximal to a nerve lesion, comparing the normal (broken line) and the abnormal (solid line) response. Patterns include from above down: 1) axon loss, producing amplitude loss but little change in CV; 2) conduction block involving all blocked fibers to an equal degree producing loss of amplitude and slowing of CV but no change in waveform morphology; 3) synchronized focal slowing without conduction block producing slowing of CV without loss of amplitude or change in waveform morphology; 4) differential slowing with loss of amplitude and temporal dispersion due to unequal fiber involvement; there is no true conduction block and the fastest fibers are unaffected; 5) a combination of 3 and 4 with conduction slowing and temporal dispersion. Amp, amplitude; dur, duration; DL, distal latency. Reprinted with permission from Wilbourn AJ. Electrodiagnosis with entrapment neuropathies. In: 1992 AAEM plenary session I: entrapment neuropathies. Rochester: AAEM, 1992:23.

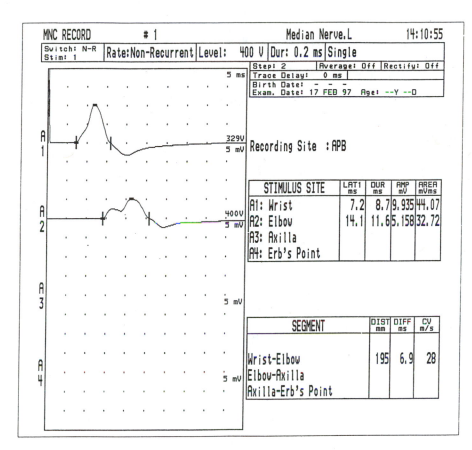

```
MNC RECORD        # 1              Median Nerve.L      14:10:55
Switch: N-R  Rate:Non-Recurrent Level:   400 V Dur: 0.2 ms Single
Stim: 1
                                        5 ms  Average: Off  Rectify: Off
                                              Trace Delay:      0 ms
                                              Birth Date:  - - -
                                              Exam. Date: 17 FEB 97  Age: --Y --D
A
1                                  329V  Recording Site : APB
                                   5 mV

A                                  400V
2                                  5 mV
```

STIMULUS SITE	LAT1 ms	DUR ms	AMP mV	AREA mVms
A1: Wrist	7.2	8.7	9.935	44.07
A2: Elbow	14.1	11.6	5.158	32.72
A3: Axilla				
A4: Erb's Point				

SEGMENT	DIST mm	DIFF ms	CV m/s
Wrist-Elbow	195	6.9	28
Elbow-Axilla			
Axilla-Erb's Point			

FIGURE 16.5. A median nerve conduction study in a patient with CIDP. The CV was 28 m/s. On proximal stimulation the M wave amplitude has decreased by 47%, but the duration has increased by 33% so that the area of the negative spike has decreased by only 25%; the double hump indicates desynchronization. Although visually impressive, this abnormality would not meet strict criteria for conduction block. However, it is still strong evidence of a demyelinating process.

sion in the subjacent nerve (7). As a result, the fairly simple criteria of a significant loss of negative spike or peak to peak amplitude with proximal stimulation as compared with distal stimulation may suffice to indicate demyelination, and whether the loss of amplitude is due to conduction block, temporal dispersion, or a combination of the two is relatively immaterial.

Care must be taken not to confuse M wave amplitude loss due to length-dependent phase cancellation with loss of amplitude due to conduction block or temporal dispersion (8). Length-dependent phase cancellation is always problematic with proximally recorded sensory or compound nerve action potentials (9). It is not usually an issue with motor conduction studies so long as the CV is fairly normal. With severe slowing, however, length-dependent phase cancellation may become an issue even in motor studies. In addition, proximal amplitude loss due to anomalous innervation should not be confused with conduction block. Submaximal stimulation may lend the appearance of conduction block, particularly in chronic de-

myelinating neuropathies, in which the electrical threshold for activation may be abnormally increased.

Demyelination may occur in two major patterns. Disorders that affect the myelin diffusely due to a genetic defect, biochemical abnormality or the effect of certain drugs or toxins produce global, uniform demyelination. There is little variation from nerve to nerve or from segment to segment of any given nerve (10,11). In the majority of patients with familial demyelinating neuropathy, distal motor latencies are prolonged in proportion to CV, the median and ulnar forearm CV does not vary by > 5 m/sec, and there is no evidence of conduction block or temporal dispersion. Such uniform conduction slowing suggests a generalized dysfunction of myelin or Schwann cells. Of course, conduction block, temporal dispersion or disproportionate segmental slowing could occur due to a superimposed compression neuropathy, so abnormalities of the median nerve at the wrist, ulnar at the elbow or peroneal at the fibular head should be interpreted cautiously. In addition, with very slow CVs phase cancellation may come into play and produce an appearance resembling conduction block over long nerve segments.

In acquired demyelinating neuropathies, the distal motor latency and the CV vary more randomly, differences between median and ulnar CV of > 5 m/sec or even > 10 m/sec are common, and conduction block or temporal dispersion may occur. Such a pattern of conduction abnormality suggests a multifocal attack on the peripheral nervous system, which may become widespread but does not affect the myelin diffusely.

Common Neuropathies

The following sections discuss some of the clinical and electrodiagnostic aspects of the more common or interesting neuropathic syndromes seen in electrodiagnostic medicine practice. Space limitations do not permit discussion of every syndrome. Detailed elaboration is available elsewhere (1,12,13).

DIABETIC NEUROPATHY

Approximately 50% of patients with diabetes have peripheral nerve involvement after 25 years of the disease. Several schemes have been used to classify the numerous different forms of diabetic neuropathy (Table 16.15). Most common is a chronic, generalized, symmetric polyneuropathy, usually predominantly sensory but sometimes sensorimotor, with variable autonomic dysfunction and variable, sometimes oppressive, pain. The sensory involvement may be diffuse, predominantly small fiber, or predominantly large fiber. There are several types of asymmetric diabetic neuropathy. Almost any peripheral nerve can develop ischemia due to diabetic small vessel disease, but the third cranial nerve and the femoral nerve seem most susceptible. Diabetic amyotrophy is the most common of the asymmetric neuropathies and is better described as a radiculoplexopathy; it is discussed in detail in the chapter on plexopathies. Symmetrical proximal neuropathies also occur.

Several possible mechanisms are possibly operative in the various diabetic neuropathies. Reversible metabolic changes may account for some of the conduction abnormalities. Aldose reductase converts glucose into sorbitol, which accumulates in the nerve, decreasing myoinositol levels and impairing the action of the Na/K pump. CV begins to improve within hours of reversing hyperglycemia (13,14). Diabetic microangiopathy and intraneural hypoxia likely play a significant role as well. Enzymatic reactions between glucose and

TABLE 16.15
Some Forms of Diabetic Neuropathy

Generalized symmetric polyneuropathies
    Rapidly reversible neuropathies
        Hyperglycemic neuropathy
        Treatment induced neuropathy
    Distal sensory ± motor ± autonomic polyneuropathies
        Large fiber neuropathy (pseudotabetic)
        Small fiber neuropathy (pseudosyringomyelic)
        Acute painful neuropathy
        Ataxic neuropathy
        Acrodystrophic neuropathy
        Autonomic neuropathy
    Symmetric motor neuropathy
        Proximal symmetrical motor neuropathy
        Distal motor neuropathy
Focal and multifocal neuropathies
    Cranial mononeuropathies
    Asymmetric proximal motor neuropathy (diabetic amyotrophy)
    Truncal neuropathy (thoracoabdominal neuropathy)
    Compression and entrapment neuropathies

proteins produce advanced glycosylation end products that may contribute to neuropathy by damaging the extracellular matrix, and by enhancing basement membrane thickening and reduplication (3). Some patients, especially those with asymmetric or proximal neuropathies, may have a treatable inflammatory vasculopathy, and some diabetics have a disorder indistinguishable from CIDP (15).

Diabetic generalized sensorimotor polyneuropathy commonly shows evidence of both chronic axonal degeneration as well as significant demyelination. NCVs may be markedly reduced, but temporal dispersion and conduction block are unusual. The combination of axonal degeneration and marked conduction slowing is characteristic of diabetic neuropathy. The demyelination is beyond that expected for most axonal neuropathies, and the axon loss is in excess of that seen in most myelinopathies (13). Good diabetic control can improve the long-term outlook for patients with most forms of diabetic neuropathy (16).

NEUROPATHY OF CHRONIC RENAL FAILURE

The typical neuropathy of end stage renal disease (ESRD) is a distal, symmetric, subacute, slowly progressive sensorimotor axonopathy. Approximately 60–80% of patients with ESRD have neuropathy at the onset of dialysis. Although primarily an axonopathy, the neuropathy of ESRD may be associated with significant secondary demyelination, and there may be preferential large fiber involvement clinically and pathologically (3,17,18). Although the neuropathy may stabilize with dialysis, significant improvement occurs only after transplantation. A rapidly progressive neuropathy can occur (18). Diabetes is a common cause of ESRD, and some patients have coexistent diabetic and uremic polyneuropathy. Repeated routine nerve conduction studies have no clinical role to play in the management of ESRD neuropathy and the timing of dialysis (19).

ALCOHOLIC NEUROPATHY

The pathogenesis of the neuropathy in chronic alcoholics remains in debate. Most alcoholics suffer from malnutrition, but no specific nutritional deficiencies seem to explain the neuropathy. Alcohol has direct toxic effects on the central nervous system, and possibly on the peripheral nervous system. A recent study of 107 alcoholics showed that 32% had peripheral neuropathy by EMG, and 24% had dysautonomia. The neuropathies correlated directly with the level of alcohol intake and bore no relationship to nutritional status (20). Clinically and electrodiagnostically, the neuropathy is a nondescript, distal, symmetric, generalized sensorimotor axonopathy with variable pain, variable weakness and variable dysautonomia. Sensory dysfunction is more prominent than motor; mild weakness is common but severe weakness is rare.

VITAMIN B12 DEFICIENCY

Inhibition of the vitamin B12-dependent enzyme, methionine synthase, creates disturbed methylation reactions, leading to impaired DNA synthesis and a host of attendant complications. Neurologic manifestations include neuropathy, myelopathy and dementia. The neuropathy is said to be an axonopathy, but demyelination is prominent pathologically in the CNS and there is little electropathologic correlation information regarding the neuropathy. The electrodiagnostic evaluation in some patients with vitamin B12 deficiency reveals a significant demyelinating component, and both pathologic processes are probably at work. Clinically, the neuropathy is predominantly sensory with a predilection for large fibers. An important clue is evidence of an associated myelopathy. The combination of absent ankle jerks and upgoing toes is highly suggestive. Significant neurologic involvement can occur in the absence of hematologic abnormalities. In my experience, neither the vitamin B12 level nor the methylmalonate or homocysteine levels are reliable in excluding neurologically significant B12 deficiency.

DYSIMMUNE NEUROPATHIES

Dysimmune neuropathies are those in which peripheral nerve damage results from some aberration of the immune system. Most involve abnormalities of both cellular and humeral immunity, and most are associated with inflammation and demyelination. The two most common disorders are acute inflammatory demyelinating polyradiculoneuropathy (AIDP, Guillain-Barre syndrome [GBS]) and chronic inflammatory demyelinating polyradiculoneuropathy (CIDP) (21). A number of other less common disorders may fall under this rubric, including the demyelinating neuropathy associated with paraproteinemia, POEMS syndrome, the syndrome of multifocal motor neuropathy (MMN), the anti-MAG neuropathy, anti-sulfatide neuropathy, and GALOP syndrome (22). Acute motor axonal neuropathy (AMAN) is a variant of GBS in which the immune attack is directed at the axolemma at the nodes of Ranvier of large motor fibers. Most AMAN cases follow *Campylobacter jejuni* infection, in which antibodies directed against some epitope(s) on the organism attack GM1-reactive epitopes on the nodal axolemma (23). The possibility has been raised that some more chronic axonal neuropathies may have a dysimmune pathogenesis (22).

The resemblance of AIDP and CIDP to experimental allergic neuritis (EAN) strongly suggests that disordered cellular immunity is involved in pathogenesis. In addition, antibody and complement have been implicated in several syndromes (21). Impairment of the BNB is another important factor. The IDP syndromes may well involve a combined "land-air attack" in which sensitized cells breach the BNB, paving the way for antibodies, which then induce demyelination.

A number of antinerve antibodies have been described in association with various syndromes, but their exact pathogenetic role remains enigmatic. The antibodies described are primarily directed against glycolipid and glycoprotein components of peripheral nerve myelin. Sialic acid bearing glycolipids (gangliosides), including GM1, GD1b, and GQ1b, as well as the asialo form of GM1, are frequent targets. The majority of patients with CIDP have autoantibodies against beta tubulin. Antibodies to GM1 are particularly associated with the syndrome of MMN. Antibodies against myelin associated glycoprotein (MAG) and an associated sulfoglucoronyl paragloboside (SGPG) appear to produce a slightly different syndrome. Whether the various syndromes are distinct disease entities or variants of CIDP remains a matter of debate between lumpers and splitters (21).

Most of the dysimmune neuropathies are potentially treatable, but the best treatment may vary with the syndrome. Steroids, immunosuppressants, plasma exchange (PE), and intravenous immunoglobulin (IVIG) have all been used.

Guillain-Barre Syndrome (GBS)

GBS has an annual incidence in the U.S. of 1–2/100,000. In about 60% of cases, some antecedent event has seemingly primed and activated the immune system—preceding infection (especially CMV, EBV, or *C. jejuni*), surgery, pregnancy or immunizations. GBS is a subacutely progressive, largely reversible neuropathy producing symmetric weakness and areflexia or hyporeflexia, sparing sphincter function, and occasionally producing respiratory failure. It is primarily a motor disorder and may appear purely motor. The distribution of weakness varies, and proximal weakness is not uncommon. The weakness occasionally descends rather than ascends. Facial weakness occurs in 50%, and other cranial nerves are involved now and then. Weakness typically progresses over 1–3 weeks. About 25–30% of patients develop respiratory failure requiring a ventilator. Initial symptoms are sensory in about 70% of patients, including paresthesias and vague numbness, but there is typically minimal or no objective sensory loss. Autonomic dysfunction occurs commonly: hypotension, paroxysmal hypertension, arrhythmias, ileus, or sphincter dysfunction when the disease is severe. There is good recovery in the majority of cases; about 15% have significant residua, 5% are left with severe disability, and there is still a 5% mortality rate.

CSF protein is usually normal for the first several days, then rises, sometimes reaching extraordinary levels, and remains high for several months. Pleocytosis can occur, but more than 50 cells suggests an alternate diagnosis. Increased cells are especially common in HIV associated cases.

The 1976 swine flu/GBS epidemic prompted a set of diagnostic criteria, which were reviewed and updated in 1990 (24). Essential features for the diagnosis include progressive weakness of more than one limb, plus attenuation or loss of reflexes. Features that strongly support the diagnosis include: progression, relative symmetry, mild sensory symptoms or signs, cranial nerve involvement, autonomic dysfunction, absence of fever at the onset of the neuropathic symptoms and eventual recovery. GBS can occasionally deviate from its usual clinical picture, primarily by quirks in distribution (25).

The usual differential diagnostic exercise in GBS is to rule other processes masquerading as peripheral nerve disease. Possibilities include acute myelopathy due to spinal cord compression or transverse myelitis, acute anterior horn cell disease due to poliomyelitis or other viral infection, myopathies (especially in light of the tendency of GBS to sometimes cause weakness greater proximally, simulating the pattern commonly seen in myopathies), acute neuromuscular junction disorder, tick paralysis, poisoning due to marine toxins, or hysterical paralysis.

Electrodiagnosis of GBS

With the advent of effective treatment, early electrodiagnostic confirmation of suspected GBS has become more critical (26). There are several problems, primarily related to the nature of the pathological process. The inflammation and demyelination are characteristically spotty, some nerves may be clearly involved while others escape entirely, so as a general rule, the more nerve conduction studies performed, the more likely an abnormality will be found. The earliest pathological changes often involve the roots and proximal nerves, which are relatively inaccessible to routine conduction studies. Late response studies, F waves and H reflexes, may therefore detect abnormality when standard peripheral studies are still normal. In some patients, early involvement of distal nerve terminals, likely because of the lack of an effective BNB along the preterminal, intramuscular axon, may produce a low amplitude M wave even on distal stimulation, making it more difficult to demonstrate demyelination level slowing and conduction block. The main trunks of the major nerves are often the last segments to be involved.

In addition, clinical weakness is related to conduction block rather than to the severity of conduction slowing, so there is an imprecise correlation between the clinical deficit and the electrodiagnostic abnormalities, especially if conduction block is proximal. Patients may be improving clinically at a time when the electrodiagnostic picture is worsening or may have severe deficits when the electrical studies are not very impressive. Depending on the criteria used, most patients demonstrate characteristic electrical abnormalities at some time in the course of the illness, but 10–20% may have normal studies early in the course when there is a premium on accurate diagnosis. SEP studies appear to add little additional diagnostic sensitivity.

Several different sets of electrophysiologic criteria have been proposed for the diagnosis of GBS (24,26–28). All involve balancing early accurate confirmation of a demyelinating neuropathy against the risk of false positives. Some of the criteria for diagnosis of GBS have been adapted from those proposed for CIDP. In the latter condition, the chronicity usually leads to more impressive and widespread abnormalities, and these criteria may be too restrictive for use in the acute situation.

The Dutch GBS Study Group recently examined the sensitivity and specificity of several different sets of criteria for the early electrodiagnosis of GBS (26). Using previously published guidelines, a demyelinating neuropathy could be established in 3–36% of the patients on the initial study. Criteria developed for CIDP proved particularly disappointing. The best criteria set developed by the study group documented polyneuropathy in 85%, and specifically a demyelinating polyneuropathy in 60%, of the patients on the initial study; which was done within 2–15 days (median 6 days) of disease onset. These guidelines required the presence of at least two abnormal nerves to document the diffuse nature of the process. A nerve was considered sufficiently tested when at least five variables were examined. Neuropathy was diagnosed when three variables were abnormal, and demyelination was considered documented if at least one of six possible indicators of primary demyelination was present (Table 16.12). The requirement for three abnormal variables per nerve dropped the false positive rate to zero in the control population. The criteria developed and the reference values obtained result in conduction parameter abnormalities considerably "softer" than employed by most centers.

All studies agree that abnormalities are more common with increasing duration of illness. The incidence of demyelination increases by 10–20% on follow-up examinations done several weeks into the course (26,29). This evolution of abnormalities also has diagnostic value.

GBS is notoriously variable, both in its clinical presentation and its electrodiagnostic picture. The axonal form (AMAN) is increasingly accepted as a disease entity. Patients with AMAN have a higher incidence of associated *C. jejuni* infection and antibodies against GM1 ganglioside and a worse long-term prognosis (23). Even in ordinary demyelinating GBS, there is often clinical and electrical sparing of sensory fibers. In both GBS and CIDP, the sural SNAP may be paradoxically spared while the median digital SNAP is affected (30). This abnormal median-normal sural (AMNS) pattern occurs most commonly in demyelinating neuropathies. The extreme pattern of absent median/present sural seems relatively specific for GBS and CIDP. Some patients with GBS develop severe distal nerve segment dysfunction early in the disease, producing very low amplitude or absent M waves on distal stimulation. This pattern could result from either axonal degeneration or distal nerve twig conduction block due to preferential attack through the distally deficient BNB (25). It is not inconceivable that some instances of apparent AMAN in fact reflect severe distal demyelination. Such distal involvement could also potentially explain the AMNS sensory pattern.

As discussed later, the investigational electrodiagnostic criteria for CIDP are strict (Table 16.14). They may be too rigid to use for the diagnosis of GBS. A reasonable modification, as shown by the Dutch group, would be to assess at least five variables for each nerve (e.g., DML, MNCV, F latency, distal M wave amplitude, and evidence of temporal dispersion or conduction block) and to insist on at least three abnormal variables before diagnosing neuropathy. At least two, and preferably more, nerves should display a neuropathic pattern before diagnosing polyneuropathy. At least two, and preferably more, nerves should have at least one of the criteria for primary demyelination before diagnosing a demyelinating polyneuropathy.

In the final analysis, almost any pattern of electrodiagnostic abnormality, including the absence of any abnormality, could be consistent with early GBS. The diagnosis should depend on the total clinical picture, with the electrophysiologic features as one of the pillars of support.

The electrodiagnostic picture can also provide useful prognostic information (25). The best indicator of prognosis is M wave amplitude. Patients having a M wave amplitude less than 10–20% of the lower limit of normal have a poor prognosis, and those with normal M wave amplitude have an excellent prognosis. There is no significant correlation between long term outcome and conduction block or conduction velocity. There is disagreement about whether fibrillation potential intensity has prognostic implications.

Chronic Inflammatory Demyelinating Polyradiculoneuropathy (CIDP) and Variants

GBS and CIDP are probably variants of the same disease process that develop over different time courses (21,28). CIDP likely represents as many as 10–20% of all initially undiagnosed neuropathies, and is important to recognize because of the likelihood it may respond to treatment. The clinical and electrophysiologic criteria for the diagnosis are summarized in Tables 16.13 and 16.14 (31). To distinguish CIDP from GBS, which is fully developed in 90% of patients by 4 weeks, the condition must evolve over a period of at least 8 weeks. Obtaining pathologic confirmation of the diagnosis is sometimes difficult, and the need for nerve biopsy is debatable (25). If clinical, EMG, and CSF criteria are met, nerve biopsy serves mostly to exclude other conditions.

There are several variants of the CIDP syndrome in which a demyelinating polyneuropathy occurs in association with other clinical and electrodiagnostic features (22) (Table 16.16). CIDP sometimes occurs in association with a monoclonal gammopathy of undetermined significance (MGUS). The CIDP-MGUS patients tend to be slightly older, have a more chronic course, more sensory involvement, and more predominantly lower extremity involvement. POEMS syndrome is essentially CIDP associated with osteosclerotic myeloma. The clinical picture of the neuropathy is essentially the same as for CIDP, but patients have other abnormalities on clinical and laboratory evaluation. The electrodiagnostic features of CIDP-MGUS and POEMS syndrome are basically the same as for CIDP. The neuropathy associated with antibody to myelin associated glycolipid (MAG) tends to be symmetric, with predominantly lower extremity involvement and more striking sensory alterations. Electrophysiologically, the anti-MAG neuropathy is a primarily demyelinating syndrome. The hallmark and most consistent feature of the disorder is striking prolongation of distal motor latencies. Conduction block is not characteristic. A purely sensory variant of CIDP has been reported, which may develop motor involvement late in the course (22).

A major conceptual problem has developed in understanding so-called multifocal motor neuropathy (MMN), particularly its relationship to motor neuron disease and its potential to present as a treatable mimicker of ALS (32). The original report described patients with very chronic, asymmetric weakness involving the upper extremities more than the lowers, associated with impressive conduction block. The authors speculated that the condition was probably a variant of CIDP and most current evidence supports

this conclusion (33). Parry and Clark later reported patients with weakness, atrophy, cramps, fasciculations and preserved reflexes with minimal sensory complaints or findings, all initially thought to have ALS (34). Further experience has shown that with careful evaluation some degree of clinical sensory involvement is the rule rather than the exception in MMN (22,25,33). SNAPs tend to be normal, suggesting there may be sensory conduction disturbance in some segment of nerve not usually tested. There is an association between this syndrome and antibodies against GM1 and other gangliosides. Patients with ALS, and other neurologic conditions, may also have antiganglioside antibodies, albeit usually at lower titers than those with MMN.

Many patients with MMN respond to IVIG, which is also of benefit in AIDP, and probably in CIDP (35). It appears more and more likely that so-called MMN is probably not a separate entity but a variant of CIDP characterized by asymmetry and prominent conduction block (25). Many patients, perhaps most patients, do have sensory complaints and findings. No great effort is usually required to demonstrate conduction block and patients typically have major conduction abnormalities in addition to conduction block (33).

The dysimmune neuropathies are primarily demyelinating syndromes, with the single exception of the anti-sulfatide neuropathy. These patients develop a painful, predominantly sensory, predominantly axonal clinical syndrome associated with antibody reactivity to peripheral nerve sulfatide components and a generalized axonopathy electrophysiologically (22).

Electrodiagnosis of CIDP and Variants

The electrodiagnostic approach in CIDP differs somewhat from that in GBS. In the acute condition, the clinical and electrodiagnostic exercise is to exclude other pathology masquerading as an acute neuropathy. If the weakness is due to a neuropathy, GBS is the overwhelming diagnostic possibility. In contrast, a plethora of conditions can produce a chronic neuropathy, and the differential diagnostic exercise is usually between CIDP and other neuropathies, rather than between CIDP and nonneuropathic mimickers. As a result, the electrophysiologic criteria employed for diagnosis are more stringent (31) (Table 16.14). Bromberg found no significant difference in diagnostic sensitivity comparing three different sets of electrodiagnostic criteria for primary demyelination in chronic polyneuropathy and estimated a sensitivity of approximately 66% as the practical limit for the electrodiagnosis of CIDP (36).

TABLE 16.16
Variants of CIDP

CIDP-MGUS
POEMS syndrome
Anti-MAG neuropathy
GALOP syndrome
Sensory CIDP
Multifocal motor neuropathy?

INFECTION RELATED NEUROPATHIES

The peripheral nervous system disorders complicating HIV infection are heterogeneous and highly prevalent (37). Inflammatory demyelinating neuropathy occurs early in the course of the disease, frequently at the time of seroconversion, which is clinically and electrophysiologically indistinguishable from AIDP and CIDP. In the late stages of the disease, usually when the CD4 count is < 50, the most common neuropathy is a painful, distal, sensory axonopathy. Less commonly, HIV patients may develop lymphomatous or vasculitic neuropathy. Neuropathies may also occur due to antiretroviral therapy, other drugs, malnutrition, and vitamin B12 deficiency. H zoster frequently causes radiculopathy and CMV may produce a severe polyradiculoneuropathy or diffuse mononeuritis multiplex.

Lyme disease can produce several different peripheral neurologic complications in up to one third of the patients with late disease. Vasculitis is likely an important pathophysiologic mechanism. Most common are a mild, chronic, axonal sensorimotor polyradiculoneuropathy, and facial nerve palsy (38). Electrodiagnostic evaluation frequently shows mild motor and sensory conduction slowing, and both proximal and distal axonal involvement. Chronic neurologic manifestations usually improve, but may not resolve, even with appropriate treatment.

CRITICAL ILLNESS POLYNEUROPATHY

Sepsis and multiorgan failure may trigger critical illness polyneuropathy, a common cause of severe generalized weakness and weaning failure in critically ill patients (39). Critical illness polyneuropathy may occur in some form in as many as 50% of critically ill patients who have been septic for more than two weeks. The origin is likely multifactorial and related to the systemic inflammatory response syndrome. The pattern of weaning failure gradually changes from that of the underlying disease to one of neuromuscular ventilatory failure. Proximal, including facial and paraspinal, muscles are often involved, and tendon reflexes may be preserved. Critical illness polyneuropathy is most often a distal, sensorimotor axonopathy, but a purely motor form may represent a variant. Differentiation from early AIDP with minimal electrodiagnostic abnormalities may be problematic. Recovery is usually rapid and clinically complete, although electrodiagnostic evaluation may disclose residua.

PARANEOPLASTIC NEUROPATHIES

Neuromuscular complications of cancer can result from direct effects of the tumor, from side effects of therapy, or from paraneoplastic syndromes (40). Through remote effects, tumors can produce a paraneoplastic subacute sensory axonopathy or sensory neuronopathy, or, more commonly, a nondescript distal sensorimotor axonopathy. Paraproteinemic disorders and lymphomas may cause a demyelinating neuropathy resembling AIDP or CIDP. Tumors may also produce vasculitis with an attendant neuropathy. In most instances, the paraneoplastic effect is immunologically mediated. The anti-Hu antibody (type 1 antineuronal nuclear autoantibody [ANNA-1]) is a polyclonal IgG directed against neurons throughout the central and peripheral systems, and associated primarily with the subacute sensory neuropathy/neuronopathy syndrome and chiefly with underlying small cell lung carcinoma, which is sometimes otherwise silent. The tumor expresses neuronal antigens or antigenically indistinguishable epitopes, and induces cross reaction with various tissues in the nervous system. An immune response intended to limit the growth and spread of a neoplasm is then misdirected and causes autoimmunologically-mediated neurologic injury. The anti-Hu antibody likely enters the dorsal root ganglion through an incomplete BNB to cross react with dorsal root ganglion neurons, inciting inflammation and cell loss.

VASCULITIC NEUROPATHIES

Polyarteritis nodosa (PAN), Churg-Strauss syndrome, and hypersensitivity angiitis account for most instances of vasculitic neuropathy (3). Other causes include rheumatoid arthritis, SLE, undifferentiated connective tissue disease, Wegener's granulomatosis, primary Sjogren's syndrome, lymphoid granulomatosis, and cryoglobulinemia. Vasculitis may also complicate cancer, HIV infection and Lyme disease. Peripheral neuropathy is often an early and dominant feature of systemic necrotizing vasculitis, and may be the only manifestation of the underlying process (41). PAN and Churg-Strauss syndrome are characterized by inflammation of medium and small arteries, and hypersensitivity angiitis with inflammation of capillaries and venules. A painful, multiple mononeuropathy syndrome is the most common clinical presentation, but as more nerves are involved the neuropathy may become confluent and appear as a generalized but asymmetrical polyneuropathy. A distal symmetrical polyneuropathy also occurs. Nerve conduction abnormalities are variable. Sensorimotor axonopathy is the most common picture, but conduction block and severe slowing of motor CV may be seen. Electrodiagnostic studies may reveal abnormalities in patients with no symptoms of neuropathy. Electrical abnormalities of the sural nerve correlate well with the subsequent yield on biopsy. Some patients have vasculitis isolated to the peripheral nervous system, the syndrome of nonsystemic vasculitic neuropathy. The clinical and electrodiagnostic features and pathology are similar to PAN, but the peripheral nervous system is affected in isolation and other systems are spared. It may be an organ-specific variant of PAN.

HEREDITARY NEUROPATHIES

There are numerous forms of hereditary neuropathy (Table 16.17). The widely used Dyck classification scheme divides the hereditary neuropathies into motor-sensory (HMSN) and sensory-autonomic forms (HSAN), numbering the subtypes. The many other forms of hereditary neuropathy are not included under this scheme. The HMSN syndromes are still often referred to as Charcot-Marie-Tooth (CMT) disease.

HMSN I, aka peroneal muscular atrophy, or the hypertrophic form of CMT disease, or CMT 1, is a uniform, diffuse demyelinating neuropathy with marked slowing of NCV which does not vary significantly from nerve to nerve or from segment to segment, with no evidence of conduction block or temporal dispersion (10). NCVs are frequently as slow as 50% of normal and there is often secondary axon loss. Clinically, CMT 1 is a slowly progressive, symmetric distal sensorimotor neuropathy with associated muscle wasting most evident distal to the knee (stork leg, or inverted champagne bottle deformity), palpably enlarged nerves, and frequently accompanied by skeletal deformities such as pes cavus or scoliosis. Sensory dysfunction is less prominent than motor dysfunction. Nerve pathology demonstrates demyelination, remyelination and onion bulb formation. CMT disease may increase the susceptibility to chemotherapy induced neuropathy (42). CMT 1 is most often transmitted as an autosomal dominant, but may be X-linked. The dominant form is divided into CMT 1A, located on chromosome 17, and CMT 1B, located on chromosome 1. CMT 1A is much more common, and usually involves duplication of the region of 17p which codes for peripheral myelin protein (PMP-22). The abnormal genes in the other forms also involve Schwann

TABLE 16.17
Hereditary Neuropathies

Syndrome	Dyck Classification	Synonyms
CMT 1	HMSN I	Hypertrophic form of CMT
CMT 2	HMSN II	Neuronal form of CMT
Dejerine-Sottas disease	HMSN III	Infantile hypertrophic neuropathy
Refsum's disease	HMSN IV	Phytanic acid storage disease
Acrodystrophic neuropathy	HSAN I	Multiple
Morvan's disease	HSAN II	Multiple
Riley-Day syndrome	HSAN III	Familial dysautonomia
HNPP		Tomaculous neuropathy
Giant axonal neuropathy		
Seitelberger's disease		Neuroaxonal dystrophy
Hereditary amyloidosis		Numerous types
Porphyrias		
MLD		
ALD/AMN		
Krabbe's disease		Globoid cell leukodystrophy
Fabry's disease		Angiokeratoma corporis diffusum
Bassen-Kornzweig disease		Abetalipoproteinemia
Tangier disease		Analphalipoproteinemia

ALD, adrenoleukodystrophy; AMN, adrenomyeloneuropathy; CMT, Charcot-Marie-Tooth; HMSN, hereditary motor sensory neuropathy; HNPP, hereditary neuropathy with liability to pressure palsies; HSAN, hereditary sensory autonomic neuropathy; MLD, metachromatic leukodystrophy.

cell and myelin proteins—P_0 (an important myelin structural protein) in CMT 1B and connexin-32 (which localizes to nodes of Ranvier and Schmidt-Lanterman incisurae) in CMT 1X (43).

HMSN II, aka the neuronal form of CMT disease, or CMT 2, makes up about one-third of the cases of autosomal dominant CMT. It is associated with selective degeneration of lower motor neurons and dorsal root ganglion cells. There is considerable overlap between CMT 1 and CMT 2. The clinical picture is identical except for the presence of nerve hypertrophy in CMT 1, and both are autosomal dominant. CMT 2 will also likely prove to result from more than one type of genetic abnormality. Electrophysiologically, conduction slowing is less severe and may be absent. Distal sensory potentials are abnormal in about half the cases.

Hereditary neuropathy with liability to pressure palsies (HNPP) is the genetic mirror image of CMT 1A (44). In CMT 1A, the PMP-22 gene on chromosome 17 is duplicated (70% of cases) or sustains a point mutation, whereas the same region shows large deletions in HNPP. Clinically, patients with HNPP present in the second or third decade with a mononeuropathy, multiple mononeuropathy or brachial plexopathy, often precipitated by trivial trauma. Conduction studies may show a mild underlying neuropathy, but the prominent abnormality is a focal or multifocal picture of demyelinating lesions at common pressure sites. Nerve biopsy shows characteristic focal hypermyelination involving many internodes, causing segments of thickened myelin resembling links of sausage (tomaculi), hence tomaculous neuropathy (3). Recall the optimal ratio of axon diameter to fiber diameter is 0.5–0.7 for most efficient conduction. The hypermyelination of HNPP alters this ratio; too much of a good thing?

The rare hereditary sensory autonomic neuropathies (HSAN) are divided into three groups according to the degree of involvement of the modalities and the age of onset. All are primarily sensory axonopathies by EMG. HSAN I is dominantly inherited, and features small fiber sensory loss and painless foot ulcers, with onset in the second decade. HSAN II presents in infancy with anesthesia and mutilation of the extremities. HSAN III (Riley-Day syndrome, familial dysautonomia) causes small fiber sensory loss with prominent autonomic dysfunction.

AMYLOIDOSIS

Amyloidosis develops in a variety of circumstances. It may occur as a primary process, or complicate paraproteinemias or any chronic systemic disease, espe-cially chronic renal failure and dialysis. Many cases are familial. The disease causes intercellular deposition of insoluble, beta pleated fibrillary protein. Presentations are highly variable, and the disease should be suspected in the presence of unexplained proteinuria, cardiomyopathy, congestive heart failure, hepatosplenomegaly or cranial neuropathy. Peripheral neuropathy occurs in approximately 10% of cases, and the most severe neuropathies tend to occur in the familial forms. The mechanism whereby amyloid deposition causes neuropathy remains obscure, but mechanical compression, ischemia and metabolic abnormality have been invoked as explanations. Amyloid deposition in the transverse carpal ligament produces carpal tunnel syndrome. The utility of sural nerve biopsy in diagnosis has been questioned (45).

Hereditary amyloidosis with neuropathy has many forms that have had colorful designations, e.g., Portugese, van Allen, Indiana, Finnish, German, but are now referred to as familial amyloid polyneuropathy (FAP) types I-IV. Most are due to mutations in the gene coding for the protein transthyretin (prealbumin), the primary component of amyloid protein. FAP type I produces a sensory dominant neuropathy characterized by dissociated sensory loss in a small fiber pattern, autonomic dysfunction, pain and trophic changes, with amyloid deposition in the endoneurium of peripheral nerve, dorsal root ganglia and sympathetic ganglia. Type II often presents with CTS. Type III is associated with a painful, distal axonopathy. Type IV FAP is characterized by progressive cranial neuropathy, corneal dystrophy, and distal sensorimotor neuropathy. The abnormal amyloid subunit protein in type IV is derived from a variant molecule of gelsolin, an actin modulating cytoskeletal protein. The electrophysiological findings in type IV are distinctive.

Nonhereditary amyloidosis is divided into primary and dysproteinemic types, which are clinically and electrophysiologically indistinguishable. The progressive neuropathy is primarily sensory, small fiber and accompanied by dysautonomia. Electrodiagnostically the neuropathy is a distal, symmetric sensorimotor axonopathy.

TOXIC NEUROPATHIES

Although an important consideration in the differential diagnosis of peripheral nerve disease, toxic neuropathies are either rare conditions or fairly obvious, as in the chemotherapy patient. Potential toxins include heavy metals, environmental toxins and pharmaceutical agents. There are numerous potential offenders, and this discussion must of necessity focus on only a few agents.

Intoxication with several heavy metals may cause neuropathy, but the agents of greatest practical importance are lead and arsenic. There is a correlation between cumulative exposure to lead and electrophysiologic abnormalities (46). Classically, lead produces a predominantly motor neuropathy with a predilection for the radial nerve and presents with wrist drop. Demyelination is impressive experimentally, but human lead neuropathy is an axonopathy (12). The neuropathy of arsenic intoxication is usually a sensory > motor axonopathy, but in acute cases the electrodiagnostic picture may resemble AIDP (47,48).

Hexacarbon neuropathies are due to exposure to either n-hexane or methyl butyl ketone (MBK); the neurotoxic effect from both agents is primarily mediated by their common metabolite 2,5-hexanedione (49,50). These agents produce giant axonal swellings that contain accumulations of neurofilaments resembling those in hereditary giant axonal neuropathy. Exposure may occur occupationally or recreationally (glue sniffing, huffer's neuropathy). The neuropathy is primarily a distal, sensorimotor axonopathy with secondary demyelination, and severity correlates with duration of exposure. Worsening may continue after cessation of exposure (coasting), but the long-term prognosis is good.

CHEMOTHERAPY RELATED NEUROPATHIES

The majority of toxic neuropathies are iatrogenic and related to drugs used to treat a variety of conditions ranging from cancer and AIDS to gout. Unfortunately, the antimitotic effects of several important chemotherapeutic agents is accompanied by incidental damage to the peripheral nervous system. The newest class of agents, the taxoids, paclitaxel and docetaxel, bind to tubulin and promote microtubule polymerization, leading to the accumulation of bundles of disordered microtubules which interrupt normal mitotic operations, and possibly interfere with axonal transport (51). The vinca alkaloids, vincristine and vinblastine, in contrast produce microtubule dissembly, which impairs neurotubule function and axonal transport. Cisplatin is a heavy metal complex which cross links DNA in a manner similar to alkylating agents. Several agents show promise in partially negating the neurotoxic side effects of chemotherapeutic agents, especially amifostine blocking the effects of taxoids.

The neuropathy of vincristine is a sensorimotor axonopathy with variable dysautonomia. The neuropathies of both cisplatin and paclitaxel/docetaxel are predominantly sensory and dose dependent (51,52). The cisplatin neuropathy is predominantly large fiber with loss of proprioception and sensory ataxia. Chemotherapy may unmask a previously unrecognized neuropathy (42).

OTHER DRUG RELATED NEUROPATHIES

Among the numerous medications that may cause neuropathy, colchicine and pyridoxine merit particular mention because of the prevalence of their use. Like some chemotherapeutic agents, colchicine interferes with microtubule growth and impairs microtubule dependent functions; it may cause a generalized, sensorimotor axonopathy, frequently associated with a myopathy (14). Pyridoxine, commonly used for such conditions as premenstrual syndrome and carpal tunnel syndrome, has significant neurotoxic potential, primarily for dorsal root ganglion neurons. It is also frequently prescribed, in potentially toxic doses, for the empiric treatment of neuropathies which are seldom if ever due to pyridoxine deficiency. Initial reports described a profound, often permanent, ataxic neuropathy with massive doses. Lower doses, in the 100–200 mg/day range, taken over a long period can also produce neuropathy; 500–1,000 mg tablets are available over the counter (53). The daily requirement is in the range of 2 mg/day.

Most pharmaceuticals cause a chronic, generalized, sensorimotor axonopathy. Notable exceptions are the sensory neuropathy/neuronopathy due to pyridoxine, cisplatin and the taxoids, and the motor neuropathy of dapsone. Amiodarone, perhexiline, and ara-C may cause a myelinopathy (12).

MONONEUROPATHY MULTIPLEX

A mononeuropathy affects only one peripheral or cranial nerve, and the most common etiology is trauma. The term mononeuropathy multiplex, or multiple mononeuropathy, refers to a condition producing two or more nontraumatic mononeuropathies. A patient with more than one mononeuropathy at common entrapment sites likely has multiple compression syndromes rather than mononeuropathy multiplex in the true sense of the term. Occasionally, features suggesting both generalized polyneuropathy and mononeuropathy multiplex may be present simultaneously. Late in the course of mononeuropathy multiplex, when many nerves have become involved, the pattern may begin to resemble a generalized polyneuropathy. Subtle asymmetry on clinical or electrodiagnostic testing is an important clue to the possibility of such a confluent or summated mononeuropathy multiplex syndrome. Any generalized neuropathy may render nerves more susceptible to injury, producing a focal accentuation of the diffuse process due to the vulnera-

TABLE 16.18
Some Etiologies of Mononeuropathy Multiplex

Vasculitis
- Churg-Strauss
- Polyarteritis nodosa
- Wegener's granulomatosis
- Non-systemic vasculitic neuropathy

Connective tissue disorders
- SLE
- Rheumatoid arthritis
- Sjogren's syndrome
- Cryoglobulinemia
- Hypereosinophilic syndrome

Infection
- Leprosy
- HIV, especially with CMV infection
- Lyme disease
- Malaria
- Infective endocarditis

Paraneoplastic
- Lymphoma, angiotropic large cell
- Leukemia

Other
- Sarcoid
- Burns
- Neurofibromatosis 2
- Focal perineuritis

ble nerve syndrome. For instance, a patient with a mild, generalized neuropathy due to diabetes may present with CTS, and the underlying polyneuropathy only becomes apparent with electrodiagnostic testing of apparently unaffected nerves.

Usually, the primary diagnostic concern in a patient with mononeuropathy multiplex is vasculitis causing multiple nerve infarctions (54,55). In underdeveloped countries, leprosy is an important consideration. Some etiologies of mononeuropathy multiplex are listed in Table 16.18.

Key Points

- Electrodiagnostic characterization is integral to the clinical attempt to define a specific etiology for a peripheral neuropathy from the myriad possibilities. Neuropathies may be classified in several different ways in hopes of defining a characteristic signature.

- Important anatomical considerations include the relationships between axons and their supporting elements, the blood nerve barrier, the blood supply and the complex intraneural fascicular topography.

- Physiologists classify peripheral nerves according to the A-C and the I-IV schemes that relate fiber size to conduction velocity (CV) and to function.

- Some neuropathies have a predilection for certain types and sizes of fibers. The immunological and biochemical substrate underlying this differential involvement remain poorly understood.

- Axoplasmic flow moves cytoskeletal elements and other constituents to and from the axon. Abnormalities of axoplasmic flow are likely important in the mechanism of length dependent neuropathies. Several substances produce neuropathy by interfering with axoplasmic flow.

- Pathologically, nerve fibers react to injury by axonal degeneration or demyelination, or some combination of the two.

- Treatment implications mandate the separation of demyelinating and axonal neuropathies. Some clinical and electrodiagnostic features helpful in differentiation are reviewed in Table 16.11.

- The cardinal manifestations of peripheral neuropathy are weakness, alterations in sensation, and reflex changes. The patterns of abnormality are important in differential diagnosis.

- Axonopathies and myelinopathies produce quite different electrodiagnostic profiles. Primary myelinopathies can produce marked slowing of CV with preservation of distal amplitudes, while axonopathies can produce marked loss of distal amplitudes with relative preservation of CV.

- Demyelinating neuropathies are divided into those which cause uniform, diffuse demyelination and those which cause segmental, multifocal demyelination; the likely etiologies of these two patterns are different.

- Conduction block and temporal dispersion on stimulation of a proximal nerve site which is not present on distal stimulation is a hallmark of acquired demyelination.

- Common neuropathies can be divided into those which evolve acutely to subacutely over several days to several weeks, and those which evolve subacutely to chronically over several months to several years. Tables 16.2–16.6 classify axonopathies and myelinopathies by these differing time courses.

- Diabetic neuropathy is very common; approximately 50% of patients have neuropathy after 25 years of the disease.

- Diabetic neuropathy is divided into a number of subtypes; the most common is a generalized, sensorimotor axonopathy. Diabetic and uremic neuropathies can be associated with a significant degree of demyelination.

- The neuropathy of alcoholism may be due to nutritional deficiency or the toxic effects of ethanol, or to a combination of effects.

- The dysimmune neuropathies are important to recognize because they are often either treatable primary conditions or they signal the presence of a major systemic disease process.

- The electrodiagnosis of acquired demyelinating neuropathies is complex. The use of some set of criteria for demyelination is increasingly accepted, but the details remain unsettled. Criteria used for CIDP may not be well suited to the evaluation of acute Guillain-Barre syndrome.

- Critical illness, infection related, paraneoplastic, vasculitic, hereditary, amyloidotic, and toxic neuropathies are reviewed. The differential diagnosis of mononeuropathy multiplex is reviewed in Table 16.18.

References

1. Dumitru D. Electrodiagnostic medicine. Philadelphia: Hanley & Belfus, 1995.

2. Wertsch JJ, Oswald TA, Roberts MM. Role of intraneural topography in diagnosis and localization in electrodiagnostic medicine. PMR Clin North Am 1994;5:465–475.
   Focal nerve lesions may not reflect isolated involvement of only the apparently affected branch but instead may indicate a more proximal lesion involving certain discrete individual fascicles. For precise anatomic localization of peripheral nerve lesions, one should include consideration of the internal topography of peripheral nerves. See also Matloub HS, Yousif NJ. Peripheral nerve anatomy and innervation pattern. Hand Clin 1992;8:201–214; Myers RR. Anatomy and microanatomy of peripheral nerve. Neurosurg Clin North Am 1991;2:1–20; Jabaley ME, Wallace WH, Heckler FR. Internal topography of major nerves of the forearm and hand: a current view. J Hand Surg (Am) 1980;5:1–18.

3. Anthony DC, Vogel FS. Peripheral nervous system. In: Damjanov I, Linder J, eds. Anderson's pathology. 10th ed. St. Louis: Mosby, 1996.2799–2831.
   An excellent review of both clinical and pathological aspects of peripheral nerve disease. Covers normal anatomy and physiology, reactions to injury, pathological techniques, indications for nerve biopsy and the pathological findings in common neuropathies.

4. Graham DG, Amarnath V, Valentine WM, et al. Pathogenetic studies of hexane and carbon disulfide neurotoxicity. Crit Rev Toxicol 1995;25:91–112.
   The toxic effects of n-hexane result in neurofilament-filled swellings of the distal axon in both central and peripheral nervous systems. Hexane requires metabolism to 2,5-hexanedione. Progressive cross-linking of the stable neurofilament during its anterograde transport in the longest axons may result in the accumulation of neurofilaments within axonal swellings.

5. Logigian EL, Kelly JJ, Jr., Adelman LS. Nerve conduction and biopsy correlation in over 100 consecutive patients with suspected polyneuropathy. Muscle Nerve 1994;17:1010–1020.
   Since the observation that CIDP was steroid responsive, it has become important to differentiate it from axonal neuropathy. This study examined the correlation between routine NCSs and sural nerve biopsy (SNB) in 100 patients. Neuropathy was classified physiologically and histologically as normal, axonal, demyelinative, or indeterminate using specific NCS and SNB criteria. Physiological and histological diagnoses were concordant in 63%, and minimally discordant in 14% of patients. The authors concluded that: (1) except for sensory neuropathy, routine motor NC studies generally suffice in identifying demyelinative neuropathy; (2) NC slowing in axonal neuropathy is usually slight but may result in significantly prolonged distal motor latencies when M wave amplitude is very low, and prolonged F wave latency when motor CV is slightly low; and (3) the physiologic criteria employed in this study rarely misclassifies neuropathy as demyelinative in patients with predominant axon loss on biopsy.

6. Wolf JK. Segmental neurology: a guide to the examination and interpretation of sensory and motor function. Baltimore: University Park Press, 1981.
   See Chapter 3 for abstract.

7. Cornblath DR, Sumner AJ, Daube J, et al. Conduction block in clinical practice. Muscle Nerve 1991;14:869–871.
   A consensus article drafted by 9 authorities. The loss of M wave amplitude and/or area on proximal stimulation necessary to call conduction block has been put at 20–60% in different published guidelines. Problems related to determining conduction block in the face of slow CV, high excitation threshold and temporal dispersion are reviewed. Computer modeling has shown phase cancellation due to desynchronization can lead to loss of both amplitude and area. For these reasons, a discrepancy in amplitude or area between proximal and distal stimulation sites should only suggest the presence of conduction block. Three methods for further investigation are discussed.

8. Rhee EK, England JD, Sumner AJ. A computer simulation of conduction block: effects produced by actual block versus interphase cancellation. Ann Neurol 1990;28:146–156.
   A reduction in M wave amplitude and area following proximal versus distal stimulation is the accepted hallmark of conduction block; however, quantitative criteria for determining conduction block remain ambiguous. In this study, digitized records of individual MUAPs elicited by incremental stimulation in vivo were arithmetically combined in a computer simulation of M wave generation. Through simulation of possible phase interaction patterns of individual MUAPs, we have shown that abnormal temporal dispersion alone can produce reductions in M wave area of up to 50%, values that are commonly thought to represent conduction block. Measurements of M wave amplitude and area in determining conduction block may be misleading if there is significant abnormal temporal dispersion. See also Olney RK. Consensus criteria for the diagnosis of partial conduction block. Muscle Nerve, in press.

9. Wilbourn AJ. Sensory nerve conduction studies. J Clin Neurophysiol 1994;11:584–601.
   See Chapter 7 for abstract.

10. Lewis RA, Sumner AJ. The electrodiagnostic distinctions between chronic familial and acquired demyelinative neuropathies. Neurology 1982;32:592–596.
    A comparison of the electrodiagnostic studies of 40 patients with chronic acquired demyelinative neuropathy and 18 patients with familial demyelinative neuropathy. Patients with acquired neuropathy had differential slowing of CV when distal segments were compared to more proximal conduction velocities in the same nerve, when equivalent segments of different nerve were compared, and when dispersion of M waves was examined. Conduction block was noted in some patients. Patients with familial disease had uniform conduction slowing of all nerve segments and conduction block was not seen. Chronic acquired demyelinative neuropathy is characterized by

multifocal slowing of nerve conduction, whereas familial demyelinative neuropathy is characterized by uniform conduction slowing. Disproportionate changes between DML and CV, differences in ulnar and median forearm CV > 5 m/sec or the presence of conduction block or temporal dispersion suggest an acquired process. However, see also Inaba A, Yokota T, Shiojiri T, Yamada M. Two siblings with nerve conduction abnormalities indicating an acquired type of demyelinating neuropathy. Muscle Nerve 1997;20:608–610.

11. Miller RG, Gutmann L, Lewis RA, et al. Acquired versus familial demyelinative neuropathies in children. Muscle Nerve 1985;8:205–210.
This study extends the observations on the electrophysiologic differences between chronic acquired demyelinative neuropathy and the demyelinative form of CMT disease to include the genetically determined demyelinating neuropathies seen in metachromatic leukodystrophy, Krabbe's leukodystrophy, and Cockayne's syndrome. The electrophysiologic features of metachromatic leukodystrophy (five patients), Krabbe's (four patients), and Cockayne's syndrome (three patients) were all similar. There was uniform slowing of conduction (both in different nerves and in different nerve segments), and conduction block was not seen. These findings are consistent with a uniform degree of demyelination in multiple nerves and throughout the entire length of individual axons. Thus, uniform slowing of nerve conduction constitutes strong evidence for a familial demyelinative neuropathy, as opposed to the multifocal slowing seen in acute and chronic acquired demyelinative neuropathy.

12. Donofrio PD, Albers JW. AAEM minimonograph #34: polyneuropathy: classification by nerve conduction studies and electromyography. Muscle Nerve 1990;13:889–903.
This superb paper thoroughly reviews the reported electrodiagnostic features of various peripheral neuropathies. The authors reviewed 252 reports, and classified neuropathies into uniform demyelinating, segmental demyelinating, motor > sensory axon loss, axon loss sensory, sensorimotor axon loss and mixed axon loss, demyelinating categories. All the information is presented in tables. Accurate electrodiagnostic classification leads to a more focused and expedient identification of the etiology of polyneuropathy in clinical situations.

13. Albers JW. Clinical neurophysiology of generalized polyneuropathy. J Clin Neurophysiol 1993;10:149–166.
Clinical electrophysiologic measures derive from sound neurophysiologic principles and provide sensitive, objective information useful in the evaluation of generalized polyneuropathy. Clinicians use electrodiagnostic information to confirm clinical findings, localize specific abnormalities to a degree not clinically possible, and identify the underlying pathophysiology. Although the primary role of clinical electromyography is diagnostic, test results are sufficiently sensitive to identify subclinical findings and to monitor small changes related to disease progression or treatment response. In some peripheral disorders, electrodiagnostic information provides the most sensitive indicator of prognosis. Classification of generalized polyneuropathy using electrophysiologic information focuses the differential diagnosis, directs the subsequent evaluation, and often suggests a specific diagnosis or class of disorders. Awareness of these disorders relates to increased utilization of clinical electrophysiology and identification of characteristic electrodiagnostic features that result in their recognition.

14. Schaumburg HH, Berger AR, Thomas PK. Disorders of peripheral nerves. 2nd ed. Philadelphia: F.A. Davis, Co. 1992.

15. Krendel DA, Costigan DA, Hopkins LC. Successful treatment of neuropathies in patients with diabetes mellitus. Arch Neurol 1995;52:1053–1061.
Twenty-one patients with diabetes mellitus were given anti-inflammatory and/or anti-immune treatment for progressive peripheral neuropathy, using IVIG, prednisone, cyclophosphamide, plasma exchange, and azathioprine alone or in combination. Fifteen patients had evidence of axonal neuropathy by electrophysiologic studies (group A). All 15 patients had non-insulin-dependent diabetes mellitus, 10 patients had weight loss, and 13 patients had prominent involvement of thighs and/or thoracic bands consistent with diabetic amyotrophy or mononeuropathy multiplex. Small vessel disease was seen in all 10 patients who underwent biopsy, with perivascular or vascular inflammation seen in seven patients. Six patients had demyelinating neuropathy by electrophysiologic criteria (group B). All these patients had insulin-dependent diabetes mellitus, and no one had weight loss. The process was asymmetric in three patients and involved thoracic or abdominal regions in two patients. Onion bulbs were seen in all four patients who underwent biopsy, but no vascular inflammation or occlusion was seen. In all patients in both groups, worsening of their conditions stopped and improvement started after beginning treatment. Neuropathies responsive to anti-inflammatory and/or anti-immune therapy in patients with diabetes mellitus include (1) multifocal axonal neuropathy caused by inflammatory vasculopathy, predominantly in patients with non-insulin-dependent diabetes mellitus indistinguishable from diabetic proximal neuropathy or mononeuropathy multiplex, and (2) demyelinating neuropathy indistinguishable from chronic inflammatory demyelinating polyneuropathy, predominantly in patients with insulin-dependent diabetes mellitus. See also Younger DS, Rosoklija G, Hays AP, et al. Diabetic peripheral neuropathy: a clinicopathologic and immunohistochemical analysis of sural nerve biopsies. Muscle Nerve 1996;19:722–727.

16. The Diabetes Control and Complications Trial Research Group. The effect of intensive diabetes therapy on the development and progression of neuropathy. Ann Intern Med 1995;122:561–568.
A multicenter, randomized, controlled clinical trial which followed 1441 diabetic patients, comparing intensive therapy with three or more daily insulin injections or continuous subcutaneous insulin infusion guided by four or more glucose tests per day compared with conventional therapy with one or two daily insulin injections. Intensive therapy reduced the development of confirmed clinical neuropathy by 64%. Nerve conduction velocities generally remained stable with intensive therapy but decreased significantly with conventional therapy. The study concluded that intensive therapy markedly delays or prevents the development of polyneuropathy.

17. Angus-Leppan H, Burke D. The function of large and small nerve fibers in renal failure. Muscle Nerve 1992;15:288–294.
Thermal thresholds were measured in 20 patients with ESRD to determine the extent of small afferent fiber involvement and to compare this with the clinical and electrophysiological evidence of large fiber involvement. Abnormalities of standard NCSs were found in 16 patients, but abnormal thermal thresholds were found in only 6. In the NCSs, the amplitudes of nerve potentials were reduced more than their CVs consistent with

an axonopathy. This study found little evidence of significant dysfunction of small afferent fibers in ESRD and, when such changes occurred, they did not correlate with the clinical evidence of polyneuropathy. The functional sparing of axons of small diameter is consistent with the relative sparing of these axons in pathological studies.

18. Ropper AH. Accelerated neuropathy of renal failure. Arch Neurol 1993;50:536–539.
A report of four patients with ESRD on peritoneal dialysis who developed a partly reversible acute uremic neuropathy which simulated GBS or CIDP.

19. Phillips LH, Williams FH. Are nerve conduction studies useful for monitoring the adequacy of renal dialysis? Muscle Nerve 1993;16:970–974.
This report addresses the question of whether there is evidence to indicate that routine use of NCS is helpful to monitor the adequacy of present-day dialysis, and concludes that there is insufficient evidence to allow one to answer the question.

20. Monforte R, Estruch R, Valls-Sole J, et al. Autonomic and peripheral neuropathies in patients with chronic alcoholism. A dose-related toxic effect of alcohol. Arch Neurol 1995;52:45–51.
This cross-sectional study of 107 alcoholic patients and 61 controls found that autonomic and peripheral neuropathies were common among alcoholics and were not related to age, nutritional status, or other alcohol-related diseases. Alcohol appears to be toxic to autonomic and peripheral nerves in a dose-dependent manner.

21. van der Meche FGA, van Doorn PA. Guillain-Barre syndrome and chronic inflammatory demyelinating polyneuropathy: immune mechanisms and update on current therapies. Ann Neurol 1995;37:S14-S31.
GBS and CIDP most likely represent parts of a continuum, arbitrarily separated by their time course. The pathogenesis of inflammatory demyelinating polyneuropathies has not been elucidated yet, but involvement of the immune system has been firmly established. Preceding infections, especially with C. jejuni, and the analysis of antiganglioside antibodies lend new support to the hypothesis of molecular mimicry between epitopes on infectious agents and peripheral nerve constituents as one of the mechanisms in GBS. In GBS, the efficacy of IVIG was established after earlier positive findings with plasma exchange. Even with these treatments it should be anticipated that one fourth of patients after IVIG and one third of patients after plasma exchange will show further deterioration in the first 2 weeks after onset of treatment. Despite this, just one treatment course usually is indicated in the individual patients and no valid arguments were found to switch to the other treatment modality. In CIDP, prednisone, plasma exchange and IVIG are effective in a proportion of patients. The last two are equally effective. Patients may respond to one of these if a previous treatment failed, and here switching therapy may be effective due to the chronic course of the disease. The mechanism of IVIG in inflammatory neuropathies is discussed. There is evidence that idiotypic-antiidiotypic interaction may play a role, but several other mechanisms also may be involved.

22. Campbell WW. Chronic dysimmune neuropathies. In press.
A review of chronic dysimmune neuropathies, including CIDP and its variants. There are several different forms of chronic dysimmune peripheral neuropathy, which are associated with several different types of antinerve antibody and with several different patterns of abnormality on electrodiagnostic testing.

CIDP is far and away the most common chronic dysimmune syndrome. A clinical and electrodiagnostic picture resembling CIDP can occur in patients with monoclonal gammopathies of undetermined significance. Patients with CIDP should be screened to exclude osteosclerotic myeloma associated with the POEMS syndrome. The syndrome of multifocal motor neuropathy is often not purely motor, and is probably a variant or subtype of CIDP. The neuropathy associated with antibody to MAG produces a predominantly lower extremity, sensory > motor demyelinating syndrome with marked prolongation of distal motor latencies. Elderly patients with a striking and disproportionate gait disturbance may be suffering from the GALOP syndrome, possibly another variant of CIDP. Patients with a painful, predominantly sensory axonopathy may harbor antibodies to peripheral nerve sulfatides. See also Uncini A, Sabatelli M, Mignogna T, et al. Chronic progressive steroid responsive axonal polyneuropathy: a CIDP variant or a primary axonal disorder? Muscle Nerve 1996;19:365–371.

23. Hafer-Macko C, Hsieh S, Li CY, et al. Acute motor axonal neuropathy: an antibody-mediated attack on axolemma. Ann Neurol 1996;40:635–644.
The acute motor axonal neuropathy (AMAN) form of GBS is a paralytic disorder characterized by variable degeneration of motor fibers and by sparing of sensory fibers, with little demyelination or inflammation. Most cases have antecedent infection with C. jejuni, and many have antibodies directed toward GM1. In 7 fatal cases of AMAN, immunocytochemistry demonstrated IgG and complement bound to the axolemma of motor fibers, most frequently at the nodal axolemma. The results suggest that AMAN is due to an antibody and complement mediated attack on the axolemma of motor fibers.

24. Asbury AK, Cornblath DR. Assessment of current diagnostic criteria for Guillain-Barre syndrome. Ann Neurol 1990;27 Suppl:S21-S24.
Elaboration on the diagnostic criteria for GBS first published in 1978. Reviews the clinical features required for the diagnosis, features strongly supportive of the diagnosis, features that cast doubt on the diagnosis, and features that rule out the diagnosis. The electrodiagnostic criteria are expanded and specific detail added.

25. Parry GJ. Guillain-Barre Syndrome. New York: Thieme, 1993.
A monograph which reviews the history, epidemiology, pathology, clinical features, diagnosis and treatment of GBS. The electrodiagnostic evaluation section includes a discussion of the morphological basis for nerve conduction abnormalities, review of conduction block and the mechanisms of conduction slowing and temporal dispersion. Nerve conduction and needle EMG characteristics in GBS are discussed at length, with a concluding section on designing an electrophysiologic study for suspected GBS. Includes a brief chapter on CIDP.

26. Meulstee J, van der Meche FG. Electrodiagnostic criteria for polyneuropathy and demyelination: application in 135 patients with Guillain-Barre syndrome. Dutch Guillain-Barre Study Group. J Neurol Neurosurg Psychiatry 1995;59:482–486.
Since the development of effective but expensive therapeutic strategies for the treatment of GBS, early confirmation of the diagnosis has become very important. Electrodiagnostic criteria were developed for the discrimination of polyneuropathy and in particular for demyelination. The sensitivity and specificity of these criteria were determined in 135 patients with GBS in an early stage of the disease, along with 45 healthy

volunteers. The algorithms used to develop the criteria consisted of sets of selected electrodiagnostic variables, each of them relevant to the detection of polyneuropathy. Each set was applied on all of three consecutive electrodiagnostic examinations within one month of disease onset. Application of the best set resulted in 85% of patients with GBS fulfilling the criteria for polyneuropathy at the first examination (mean time interval six days of disease onset), whereas none of the healthy volunteers fulfilled the criteria (sensitivity 85%, specificity 100%). The set of criteria for the detection of demyelination was fulfilled by 60% during the first examination (by 66% and 72% during the second and third examination). Application of criteria for demyelinating polyneuropathy as defined by others resulted in substantially lowered incidence (3%-46%). The authors conclude that these criteria for the electrodiagnostic delineation of polyneuropathy are the most sensitive to date, with respect to the early confirmation of the diagnosis of GBS.

27. Albers JW. AAEE case report #4: Guillain-Barre syndrome. Muscle Nerve 1989;12:705–711.

A case report of a 33-year-old woman who awoke with distal paresthesias, mild incoordination, and progressive weakness. Examination 3 days later demonstrated weakness of the extremities, greater in distal muscles than in proximal ones, mild facial weakness, distal vibratory loss, and areflexia. Electrodiagnostic studies provided evidence of an acquired demyelinating polyradiculoneuropathy of recent onset. Motor conduction studies revealed abnormal temporal dispersion and partial conduction block. Preserved sural responses with abnormal median sensory conduction studies supported the diagnosis of GBS, as did subsequent cerebrospinal fluid examinations documenting increasing total protein, identification of preceding cytomegalovirus injection with increasing serum convalescent titer, and progressive clinical improvement after a brief plateau. The role of electrodiagnosis in establishing the diagnosis and prognosis in Guillain-Barre syndrome is reviewed.

28. Albers JW, Kelly JJ, Jr. Acquired inflammatory demyelinating polyneuropathies: clinical and electrodiagnostic features. Muscle Nerve 1989;12:435–451.

The acquired demyelinating polyneuropathies include acute (AIDP, Guillain-Barre syndrome, GBS) and chronic (CIDP, dysproteinemic) forms which differ primarily in their temporal profile. They are inflammatory-demyelinating diseases of the peripheral nervous system and likely have an immunologic pathogenesis. Although these neuropathies usually have a characteristic presentation, the electromyographer plays a central role in their recognition, since the demyelinating component of the neuropathy, which greatly reduces the differential diagnosis, is often first identified in the electromyography laboratory. In AIDP, the electromyographer, in addition to establishing the diagnosis, can sometimes predict the prognosis. Recognition of the chronic and dysproteinemic forms of acquired demyelinating polyneuropathy is important since they are treatable. The dysproteinemic forms also may be associated with occult systemic disorders that also may require treatment, independent of the neuropathy.

29. Ropper AH, Wijdicks EF, Shahani BT. Electrodiagnostic abnormalities in 113 consecutive patients with Guillain-Barre syndrome. Arch Neurol 1990;47:881–887.

A study of electrodiagnostic testing on 113 consecutive patients with GBS. The most common motor conduction abnormalities were proximal conduction block alone (27%), proximal block associated with a distal lesion (27%), and generalized slowing (22%). Other combinations of abnormalities each occurred in fewer than 10% of patients. 37% of patients initially had normal

sensory nerve conduction study results, most often in association with proximal conduction block. The characteristic early electrodiagnostic changes in GBS were often present when cerebrospinal fluid concentration was still normal. Extensive early fibrillations occurred in 10 patients, 6 of whom recovered well. Patients with early generalized slowing of motor NCV combined abnormalities, or low muscle action potential amplitudes in ulnar, median, and peroneal nerves generally, but not always, had poorer outcomes than patients with conduction block in one nerve segment. There was no consistent relationship between results of electrophysiologic studies and overall clinical grade or limb power, except that none of the patients with an isolated proximal block had virtual or complete paralysis in the same limb.

30. Bromberg MB, Albers JW. Patterns of sensory nerve conduction abnormalities in demyelinating and axonal peripheral nerve disorders. Muscle Nerve 1993;16:262–266.

The pattern of an abnormal median-normal sural (AMNS) sensory response is associated with GBS and CIDP and considered unusual in other types of neuropathy, although specificity and sensitivity of this pattern have not been evaluated. This study compared sensory responses (patterns and absolute values) in patients with GBS, CIDP, diabetic polyneuropathy (DP), and motor neuron disease (MND). The AMNS pattern occurred more frequently in recent onset GBS (39%) compared with CIDP (28%), DP (14%-23%), or MND (22%) patients. This pattern was found in 3% of control subjects. The extreme pattern of an absent median-present sural response occurred only in GBS and CIDP patients and in no other groups. These findings may reflect early distal nerve involvement particularly in GBS patients which is highlighted by differences in median and sural nerve recording electrode placement. In the appropriate clinical setting, the AMNS pattern, an absent median-present sural response pattern, or a reduced median amplitude compared with the sural amplitude supports a diagnosis of a primary demyelinating polyneuropathy.

31. Ad Hoc Subcommittee AAN AIDS Task Force. Research criteria for diagnosis of chronic inflammatory demyelinating polyneuropathy (CIDP). Neurology 1991;41: 617–618.

CIDP is a pattern recognition diagnosis, based on clinical signs and symptoms, electrodiagnostic studies and CSF examination. This paper reviews the clinical, electrophysiologic, pathologic CSF and other laboratory features of the disease, classifying these into mandatory, supportive and exclusionary diagnostic criteria.

32. Pestronk, A. Invited review: motor neuropathies, motor neuron disorders, and antiglycolipid antibodies. Muscle Nerve 14:927–936, 1991.

High titers of IgM anti-GM1 antibodies are commonly found in the serum of patients with some lower motor neuron disorders and peripheral neuropathies. Enzyme-linked immunosorbent assays (ELISA) are useful for the detection and quantitation of anti-GM1 antibodies. Testing for serum anti-GM1 activity is indicated in the diagnostic evaluation of lower motor neuron syndromes. The presence of high titers of anti-GM1 antibodies mandates careful electrophysiologic testing for the motor conduction block that is found in multifocal motor neuropathy, a treatable disorder. Quantitation of anti-GM1 antibodies may also be a useful guide in the treatment of multifocal motor neuropathy. Further study of antiglycolipid antibodies in motor neuron disorders and peripheral neuropathies may provide clues to the events that stimulate these antibodies and to the pathogenesis of such syndromes.

33. Parry GJ. AAEM case report #30: multifocal motor neuropathy. Muscle Nerve 1996;19:269–276.
    A 73-year-old man with a 16-year history of fasciculations and 15 years of weakness in his right arm was diagnosed with focal motor neuron disease. After 10 years of purely motor symptoms, he developed mild parasthesias although his sensory examination remained normal. Reflexes were reduced or absent in the weak muscles but were normal elsewhere. Nerve conduction was studied in nerves innervating weak muscles and showed severe motor conduction block. Sensory nerve conduction studies were minimally abnormal, showing reduced amplitudes with normal velocities. Based on the clinical picture and the presence of severe motor conduction block, the patient was diagnosed with multifocal motor neuropathy. Treatment with high-dose intravenous immunoglobulin was given with significant improvement in strength and partial resolution of the conduction block. As this case demonstrates, this treatable disorder may occasionally be mistaken for motor neuron disease although the resemblance is only superficial, and it should never be mistaken for amyotrophic lateral sclerosis. Multifocal motor neuropathy is an inflammatory, demyelinating neuropathy which, like chronic inflammatory demyelinating polyneuropathy (CIDP), is probably immune-mediated. It differs from typical CIDP by virtue of a marked predilection for motor axons, a strikingly restricted distribution, and a protracted course. Treatment with high-dose intravenous immunoglobulin is frequently helpful, but other forms of immune manipulation are less effective.

34. Parry GJ, Clarke S. Multifocal acquired demyelinating neuropathy masquerading as motor neuron disease. Muscle Nerve 1988;11:103–107.
    A report of five patients with pure motor neuropathy characterized by multifocal weakness, muscle atrophy that was sometimes profound, cramps, and fasciculations with relatively preserved reflexes. The clinical picture led to an initial diagnosis of motor neuron disease in all cases, but nerve conduction studies revealed multifocal conduction block confined to motor axons and predominantly involving proximal nerve segments. Routine sensory nerve conduction studies, ascending compound nerve action potentials, and somatosensory evoked potentials were all normal even through nerve segments in which motor conduction was severely blocked. Onset of symptoms was insidious, and progression was indolent. In two cases, after many years of neuropathy, sensory abnormalities developed but remained clinically trivial. These unusual cases probably have the same pathogenesis as previously described patients with persistent multifocal conduction block. Distinction from motor neuron disease is critical, since chronic demyelinating neuropathy may respond to treatment.

35. van der Meche FGA, van Doorn PA. The current place of high-dose immunoglobulins in the treatment of neuromuscular disorders. Muscle Nerve 1997; 20:136–147.
    Positive effects of high-dose IVIG have been demonstrated in open studies in dermato- and polymyositis, myasthenia gravis and inflammatory neuropathies. Randomized trials have demonstrated efficacy in dermatomyositis, GBS and CIDP, and smaller ones in multifocal motor neuropathy. Trials are underway in myasthenia gravis and the Lambert-Eaton syndrome.

36. Bromberg MB. Comparison of electrodiagnostic criteria for primary demyelination in chronic polyneuropathy. Muscle Nerve 1991;14:968–976.
    Sensitivity of 3 sets of electrodiagnostic criteria for establishing primary demyelination were assessed in 70 patients with clinically established CIDP. The criteria use different abnormal values, one adjusts for the effects of axonal loss, while another relies only on CV. However, even when consideration is given to sufficient number of nerves tested, there was no significant difference (P = 0.37) in diagnostic sensitivity among them, with 48% to 64% of CIDP patients fulfilling criteria for primary demyelination. Specificity was assessed by applying the criteria to 47 patients with motor neuron disease and 63 patients with diabetic polyneuropathy. No patients met any of the criteria. Further analysis shows that as sensitivity increases specificity decreases, because of overlapping distributions of nerve conduction abnormalities in these neuropathic disorders. A sensitivity of approximately 66% is a practical limit for electrodiagnostic criteria in CIDP.

37. Dalakas MC, Cupler EJ. Neuropathies in HIV infection. Baillieres Clin Neurol 1996;5:199–218.
    Peripheral neuropathies represent the most common neurological manifestation in patients infected with HIV infection occurring either early in the infection or during the course of the illness. They present as acute or chronic demyelinating neuropathies (GBS or CIDP), mononeuritis multiplex, ganglioneuronitis, CMV related polyradiculoneuropathy, autonomic neuropathy or distal painful sensory neuropathy. They are multifactorial in etiology. Their putative cause (viral, autoimmune, toxic, nutritional, co-infections) are often dictated by the stage of the underlying HIV disease. The virus, which is not found within ganglionic neurones or Schwann cells but only within the endoneurial macrophages, may generate a tissue-specific autoimmune attack by secretion of cytokines that promote trafficking of activated T cells and macrophages within the endoneurial parenchyma. The wide use of the neurotoxic antiretroviral nucleoside analogues ddC, ddI, d4T and 3TC, exacerbate or trigger subclinical neuropathy in many of these patients. See also Lange DJ. AAEM minimonograph #41: neuromuscular diseases associated with HIV-1 infection. Muscle Nerve 1994;17:16–30.

38. Logigian EL, Steere AC. Clinical and electrophysiologic findings in chronic neuropathy of Lyme disease. Neurology 1992;42:303–311.
    A study of 25 patients with Lyme disease and chronic peripheral neuropathy. All had immunologic evidence of exposure to Borrelia burgdorferi and no other identifiable cause of neuropathy. The authors conclude that Lyme disease can be associated with a reversible, mild chronic axonal sensorimotor polyradiculoneuropathy or polyradiculopathy.

39. Hund EF, Fogel W, Krieger D, et al. Critical illness polyneuropathy: clinical findings and outcomes of a frequent cause of neuromuscular weaning failure. Crit Care Med 1996;24:1328–1333.
    A description of the clinical and electrophysiologic features and outcomes of critically ill patients with neuromuscular causes of failure to wean from mechanical ventilator support in 7 patients seen during a 3-yr period. Muscle and nerve biopsy was done in three patients, and detailed electrodiagnostic studies were done in all patients 3 to 6 wks after the onset and repeated 3 months to 3.5 yrs later in those patients who survived. All patients had moderate-to-severe limb weakness with marked muscle atrophy. Tendon reflexes were decreased in three patients, exaggerated in two patients with intracranial lesions, and absent in two patients. EMG demonstrated severe acute denervation, with striking involvement of proximal mus-

cles. Muscle and nerve biopsies showed severe neurogenic atrophy and axonal degeneration without inflammation. There was no evidence of primary myopathy. Critical illness polyneuropathy is a frequent cause of neuromuscular weaning failure in critically ill patients, regardless of the type of primary illness. Involvement of proximal (including facial and paraspinal) muscles is striking. Tendon reflexes are often preserved. Recovery is usually rapid and clinically complete, although incomplete on electrodiagnostic study. Failure to recognize the development of neuropathy in these patients may lead to erroneous conclusions about the ability to wean them from the ventilator.

40. Smitt PS, Posner JB. Paraneoplastic peripheral neuropathy. Baillieres Clin Neurol 1995;4:443–468.
Paraneoplastic peripheral neuropathies are not common, and are out-numbered by the far more common peripheral neuropathies that occur either as a direct result of the cancer (metastases) or its treatment (usually chemotherapy). Nevertheless, paraneoplastic peripheral neuropathies are important because they may be the first sign of an otherwise occult cancer and/or because they may substantially disable the patient even when the cancer itself is asymptomatic. Paraneoplastic disorders are sometimes marked by the presence of autoantibodies that react with proteins both in the underlying cancer and in the nervous system. Their discovery may lead to an early diagnosis and potential cure of the underlying cancer.

41. Said G. Vasculitic neuropathy. Baillieres Clin Neurol 1995;4:489–503.
Vasculitis is a common and treatable cause of neuropathy. In most cases, necrotizing arteritis of the type observed in polyarteritis nodosa is responsible for the lesions, but classification of vasculitis is still uncertain. The neuropathy often occurs in the context of a multisystem disorder, but in a substantial proportion of patients, especially among patients seen by neurologists, the neuropathy is the first and only manifestation of vasculitis. In such cases, the diagnosis can only be reached by performance of a nerve and muscle biopsy. Ischemic nerve lesions can also result from secondary vasculitis in a number of inflammatory, infectious and immune-mediated disorders of the peripheral nervous system.

42. Graf WD, Chance PF, Lensch MW, et al. Severe vincristine neuropathy in Charcot-Marie-Tooth disease type 1A. Cancer 1996;77:1356–1362.
A general predisposition for vincristine-related neuropathy has been observed in persons with a family history of hereditary neuropathies. This retrospective series investigated the association between the DNA rearrangement found in patients with CMT 1A and susceptibility to the neurotoxicity of vincristine in 3 families. These cases show that 17p11.2–12 duplication predisposes patients to severe neurotoxicity from vincristine and that this drug should be avoided with patients with CMT1A. Patients with other hereditary neuropathies may also be at risk for severe neurotoxic reactions.

43. Ionasescu VV. Charcot-Marie-Tooth neuropathies: from clinical description to molecular genetics. Muscle Nerve 1995;18:267–275.
Ninety-five families with CMT neuropathies were studied clinically, electrophysiologically, and by molecular genetics. Fifty-four families (56.8%) were type 1A mapped at 17p11.2-p12 and DNA duplication was present in 50 (92.6% of CMT1A families). One family with type 1B (1.1%) mapped at 1q22-q23 showed a point mutation of the myelin P0 gene. Eighteen families (18.9%) were type CMT2 based on electrophysiological studies. Molecular genetics was not yet conclusive. Twenty CMT families were with X-linked dominant inheritance (CMTX1) (21.1%) mapped at Xq13.1 and connexin 32 (CX32) point mutations were present in 15 families (75%) (five nonsense mutations, eight missense mutations, two deletions). Two CMT families (2.1%) with X-linked recessive inheritance showed no point mutations of CX32 and their mapping was different from CMTX1, respectively at Xp22.2 for CMTX2 and at Xq26 for CMTX3.

44. Vandenberghe A, Latour P, Chauplannaz G, et al. Molecular diagnosis of Charcot-Marie-Tooth 1A disease and hereditary neuropathy with liability to pressure palsies by quantifying CMT1A-REP sequences: consequences of recombinations at variant sites on chromosomes 17p11.2–12. Clin Chem 1996;42:1021–1025.
The most frequent form of Charcot-Marie-Tooth disease (CMT1A; OMIM118.220) is the result of a duplication on chromosome 17 in pll.2-p12. This region contains PMP22, a gene expressed in peripheral myelin. The mutation results from an unequal crossing-over involving repeated sequences, CMT1A-REP, located on both sides of the duplicated region. The reciprocal product of this recombination is a deletion of the same region, which is associated with hereditary neuropathy with liability to pressure palsies (HNPP; OMIM162.500).

45. Simmons Z, Blaivas M, Aguilera AJ, et al. Low diagnostic yield of sural nerve biopsy in patients with peripheral neuropathy and primary amyloidosis. J Neurol Sci 1993;120:60–63.
Sural nerve biopsy reportedly a sensitive method for diagnosing primary amyloidosis. In this study, 6 of 9 patients with peripheral neuropathy due to amyloidosis had a sural nerve biopsy which demonstrated no amyloid. Subsequent examination of other tissue or of the contralateral sural nerve eventually resulted in the correct diagnosis. Sural nerve biopsy may be less sensitive than previously believed for the diagnosis of amyloidosis in patients with peripheral neuropathy secondary to amyloid.

46. Yeh JH, Chang YC, Wang JD. Combined electroneurographic and electromyographic studies in lead workers. Occup Environ Med 1995;52:415–419.
NCS and EMG studies were performed on 31 lead workers of a battery recycling factory and 31 sex and age matched controls. A non-parametric analysis showed that there was a trend of higher index of cumulative exposure to lead with more severe electromyographic changes.

47. Oh SJ. Electrophysiological profile in arsenic neuropathy. J Neurol Neurosurg Psychiatry 1991;54:1103–1105.
Comprehensive electrophysiological studies were performed on 13 patients with arsenic neuropathy. The most prominent finding was a marked abnormality in sensory nerve conduction in the presence of moderate abnormalities in motor nerve conduction. The motor nerve conduction studies and needle EMG were typical of those seen in axonal degeneration which was confirmed by sural nerve biopsy.

48. Donofrio PD, Wilbourn AJ, Albers JW, et al. Acute arsenic intoxication presenting as Guillain-Barre-like syndrome. Muscle Nerve 1987;10:114–120.
Arsenic-induced polyneuropathy is traditionally classified as an axonal-loss type, electrodiagnostically resulting in low amplitude or absent sensory and motor responses, relatively preserved proximal and distal motor conduction rates, and distal denervation. We report four patients with a subacute onset progressive polyradiculoneuropathy following high-dose arsenic poisoning. In three patients, early electrodiagnostic testing

demonstrated findings suggestive of an acquired segmental demyelinating polyradiculoneuropathy. Serial testing confirmed evolution into features of a distal dying-back neuropathy. We hypothesize that arsenic toxicity and the resultant biochemical derangement of the peripheral nerve cell leads to subtle changes in axonal function that produce, initially, segmental demyelination and eventually distal axonal degeneration. Acute arsenic toxicity must be suspected in patients with clinical and electrodiagnostic features supporting Guillain-Barre syndrome.

49. Chang CM, Yu CW, Fong KY, et al. N-hexane neuropathy in offset printers. J Neurol Neurosurg Psychiatry 1993;56:538–542.

In printing factory workers with symptomatic peripheral neuropathy due to exposure to n-hexane the initial change in the NCS was reduced amplitude of the sensory action potentials, followed by reduced amplitude of the motor action potentials, reduction in motor CVs and increase in distal latencies. These changes indicate primary axonal degeneration with secondary demyelination. Sural nerve biopsy in a severe case showed giant axonal swellings due to accumulation of 10nm neurofilaments, myelin sheath attenuation and widening of nodal gaps.

50. Bos PM, de Mik G, Bragt PC. Critical review of the toxicity of methyl n-butyl ketone: risk from occupational exposure. Am J Ind Med 1991;20:175–194.

Methyl n-butyl ketone (MBK) was considered rather harmless until an outbreak of peripheral neuropathy occurred in 1973 among workers exposed to MBK. From the viewpoint of neurotoxicity, 2,5-hexanedione is the most important metabolite. The neurotoxicity is potentiated by several compounds, while MBK itself potentiates the toxicity of other chemicals. Peripheral neuropathy may develop in workers exposed to only a few ppm of MBK.

51. New PZ, Jackson CE, Rinaldi D, et al. Peripheral neuropathy secondary to docetaxel (Taxotere). Neurology 1996;46:108–111.

Docetaxel (Taxotere), a semisynthetic analogue of the antitumor agent paclitaxel, inhibits tubulin depolymerization. Paclitaxel produces a peripheral neuropathy. This study delineates clinically and electrophysiologically the characteristics of a peripheral neuropathy due to docetaxel. Serial neurologic exams, quantitative sensory testing and nerve conduction studies were done in 186 patients receiving docetaxel in phase I and phase II protocols. Twenty-one patients developed mild to moderate sensory neuropathy. Ten of these patients also developed weakness of varying degree in proximal and distal extremities. In summary, docetaxel produced a sensorimotor peripheral neuropathy in 11% of the patient population. See also Neurology 1996;46:2–3 & 104–107.

52. LoMonaco M, Milone M, Batocchi AP, et al. Cisplatin neuropathy: clinical course and neurophysiological findings. J Neurol 1992;239:199–204.

Sixteen patients treated with cisplatin were clinically and neurophysiologically tested before, during and up to 12 months after administration. The first symptoms of polyneuropathy occurred in 4 of 9 patients after the second course (cumulative dose 400 mg/m2). One month after treatment 1 of 9 patients was asymptomatic, 5 complained of symptoms and 3 showed clinical and neurophysiological signs of polyneuropathy. Three months after treatment all patients were affected. Clinical and neurophysiological signs of severity progression were noted up to 6 months after treatment. with CDDP

53. Dalton K, Dalton MJ. Characteristics of pyridoxine over-dose neuropathy syndrome. Acta Neurol Scand 1987; 76:8–11.

A raised serum B6 level was present in 172 women of whom 60% had neurological symptoms, which disappeared when B6 was withdrawn and reappeared in 4 cases when B6 was restarted. The mean dose of B6 in the 103 women with neurological symptoms was 117 ± 92 mgs, compared with 116.2 ± 66 mgs in the control group. There was a significant difference (p < 0.01) in the average duration of ingestion of B6 in the neurotoxic group of 2.9 ± 1.9 years compared with 1.6 ± 2.1 years in controls. The symptoms were paresthesia, hyperesthesia, bone pains, muscle weakness, numbness and fasciculation, most marked on the extremities and predominantly bilateral unless there was a history of previous trauma to the limb. These women were taking a lower dose of B6 than previously described which may account for the complete recovery within 6 months of stopping B6.

54. Hawke SH, Davies L, Pamphlett R, et al. Vasculitic neuropathy. A clinical and pathological study. Brain 1991; 114:2175–2190.

The clinical, electrophysiological and pathological features and prognosis of 34 patients with peripheral neuropathy caused by necrotizing vasculitis were evaluated. The causes included polyarteritis nodosa and its Churg-Strauss variant, rheumatoid arthritis, undifferentiated connective tissue disease, Wegener's granulomatosis, primary Sjogren's disease, and chronic lymphocytic leukemia with cryoglobulinemia; 2 patients had no evidence of systemic vasculitis. Mononeuritis multiplex was the most common clinical manifestation, followed by asymmetrical polyneuropathy and distal symmetrical polyneuropathy. Pain was a frequent symptom. Nerve conduction studies were abnormal in all cases, and in 3 patients there was conduction block or severe slowing of motor conduction. Necrotizing vasculitis was present in sural nerve biopsies of most cases, and severe active axonal degeneration was a dominant feature. Immunofluorescent staining of blood vessels for immunoglobulin, C3 and fibrinogen was positive in all cases in which it was performed, even when there was no cellular infiltration. All patients were treated with prednisone alone or in combination with other immunosuppressive agents, or with plasmapheresis. Long-term follow-up studies demonstrated that although the peripheral neuropathy usually improved and caused only mild to moderate functional disability, the long-term prognosis of the systemic disease was poor with a 5-yr survival of only 37%.

55. Olney RK. AAEM minimonograph #38: neuropathies in connective tissue disease. Muscle Nerve 1992;15:531–542.

Neuropathies are common in patients with known or suspected connective tissue disease. A vasculitic mononeuropathy multiplex is often seen in patients initially presenting with polyarteritis nodosa or developing arteritis as a complication of rheumatoid arthritis. However, vasculitic neuropathy may become confluent and present as distal symmetrical polyneuropathy or occur without systemic necrotizing vasculitis. Distal symmetrical polyneuropathies without associated vasculitis are also common in many connective tissue diseases. Compression neuropathies, especially carpal tunnel syndrome, occur with increased frequency in rheumatoid arthritis. Finally, certain neuropathies may be the major presenting feature of particular connective tissue diseases. For example, trigeminal neuropathy often heralds the onset of systemic sclerosis or mixed connective tissue disease, and sensory neuronopathy may be the initial presenting feature of Sjogren's syndrome.

56. McLeod JG. Invited review: autonomic dysfunction in peripheral nerve disease. Muscle Nerve 1992;15:3–13. The autonomic nervous system is affected in most peripheral neuropathies, but only in a small number of conditions, such as diabetes, amyloidosis, GBS, porphyria, and familial dysautonomia, is autonomic dysfunction of clinical importance. The pathological changes in the peripheral autonomic nervous system are similar to those in the peripheral somatic nerves. Autonomic disturbances are most likely to occur when there is acute demyelination or damage to small myelinated and unmyelinated fibers. Autonomic investigations should include tests of both sympathetic and parasympathetic function. Treatment consists of management of the underlying cause of peripheral neuropathy, physical and pharmacological measures.

17

Focal Neuropathies

Focal neuropathies may result from compression, entrapment, ischemia, stretch, direct trauma such as lacerations and missile wounds, involvement in fractures or dislocations, and other processes. Compression and entrapment neuropathies are among the commonest disorders seen in electrodiagnostic medicine; carpal tunnel syndrome (CTS) is the most frequent single diagnosis made in most laboratories. An understanding of the general pathology and pathophysiology of focal neuropathies, as well as the clinical and electrodiagnostic details of the individual syndromes, is integral to proper management (1–3). Both clinical and electrodiagnostic evaluation are important for management; each has a different but meaningful contribution to make (4).

The terms compression and entrapment are often used more or less interchangeably, sacrificing some accuracy. *Compression neuropathy* refers to nerve damage due to pressure applied to a nerve, whatever the source. The term *entrapment neuropathy* is appropriate when the pressure is exerted by some anatomical or pathoanatomical structure, such as the transverse carpal ligament in CTS. All entrapment neuropathies are compression neuropathies, but not all compression neuropathies are due to entrapment. Entrapment neuropathies are all chronic conditions; compression neuropathies due to externally applied pressure can develop acutely over several hours (postoperative ulnar neuropathy, tourniquet paralysis, Saturday night radial nerve palsy), subacutely over days to weeks (peroneal neuropathy at the fibular head due to prolonged bed rest or a short leg cast), or chronically over months to years (ulnar neuropathy in the retroepicondylar groove). In some instances, a nerve is injured by relatively low force applied repetitively over a long period (retroepicondylar ulnar neuropathy, ulnar neuropathy at the wrist due to bicycling, peroneal neuropathy at the fibular head due to habitual leg crossing). Almost any nerve in the body can be compressed or entrapped, and by definition involvement is limited to the distribution of a single peripheral nerve.

Pathology and Pathophysiology of Compression/Entrapment Neuropathies

At the most minimal levels of nerve compression, reversible symptoms without accompanying structural changes, the familiar "falling asleep" sensation, is the primary manifestation. Referred to as acute, or rapidly reversible, physiological block, these symptoms are due to nerve ischemia. Transient symptoms in some entrapment syndromes, such as the nocturnal paresthesias in CTS, may have an ischemic component. Although ischemic infarction of nerve clearly occurs, as in vasculitis, in most instances of compression or entrapment the clinical manifestations are primarily related to pathological changes in the myelin sheath or axon directly due to pressure; ischemia seems to play a relatively minor role in most instances. Venous engorgement at low levels of pressure has been postulated to induce a cascade of events which culminates in fiber damage, but this concept is controversial (5). In certain acute and chronic compression syndromes in which axon loss is disproportionate to the apparent level of applied pressure or to the accompanying demyelination, ischemia may be a significant factor (6).

Pathological changes involving the myelin sheath are the earliest indication of pressure applied to a nerve. Low levels of force produce selective paranodal demyelination. The integrity of the paranodal region is crucial for normal conduction, and paranodal demyelination may produce conduction abnormalities seemingly out of proportion to the severity of the myelin loss. Greater levels of force cause myelin loss along a longer section of the nerve, involving both paranodal and internodal sections, referred to as segmental demyelination. Depending on the length of the segment involved, conduction velocity may simply slow or conduction may fail entirely, producing conduction block (CB). CB may rarely involve all the fibers, in which case it is termed "complete." More commonly, CB is partial, involving some fibers while others have varying degrees of focal slowing without block. The electrodiagnostic picture is frequently a complex mixture of CB, varying degrees of focal slowing, and axon loss (see Fig. 16.4).

The pathology of acute and chronic compression neuropathy differs in some details. The best experimental model for relatively acute compression neuropathies, such as Saturday night palsy or postoperative neuropathy, is tourniquet paralysis in the baboon. The most characteristic feature of tourniquet paralysis is marked distortion of internodes with intussusception of one internode into the adjacent internode under the edges of the tourniquet, where a large pressure gradient exists between normal nerve and compressed nerve (Fig. 17.1). Distortion and intussusceptions do not occur to any degree under the body of the tourniquet, despite equally high pressures but without a gradient between adjacent segments (5). The paucity of abnormalities under the body of the cuff is further evidence against an ischemic mechanism of injury.

In contrast, in the guinea pig model of chronic compression, abnormalities of myelin are prominent throughout the length of the compressed segment, rather than just at the edges, and myelin intussusception is not seen. Instead, pressure causes displacement of myelin from the center of the internode toward the ends (rather like squeezing a tube of toothpaste in the middle), producing an appearance resembling two tadpoles swimming in opposite directions (5). Eventually the "heads" of the tadpoles break down, producing demyelination.

With more severe compression the added element of axonal damage appears. Wallerian degeneration refers to the axonal degeneration distal to a focal lesion. The typical electrodiagnostic concomitants of Wallerian degeneration are mild distal conduction slowing, low M wave amplitudes from the affected muscles even with stimulation distal to the inciting lesion, and denervation changes on needle examination.

Not all nerve fibers are equally susceptible to pressure injury. In experimental compression, large fibers are more susceptible than small, and peripheral fibers more vulnerable than central ones. In addition, different fascicles within a nerve at a given point exhibit different susceptibility to pressure injury, mostly reflecting the relationship between the fascicle's position within the nerve and the force vectors being applied (7). Such selective fascicular vulnerability is clinically important. Several problematic phenomena are probably explicable on this basis, including sparing of the forearm flexors with ulnar lesions at the elbow, different degrees of involvement of different hand muscles in ulnar neuropathy, lumbrical sparing in CTS and the varying electrophysiologic picture in

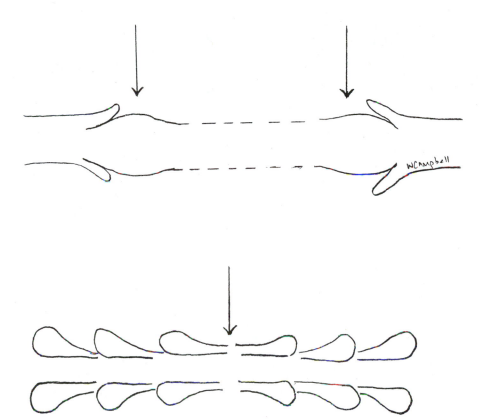

FIGURE 17.1. Arrows indicate points of compression. Acute compression causes intussusception of one internode into the adjacent internode at the margins of the compression (top). Chronic compression does not cause intussusception but a displacement of myelin toward the ends of the internode, creating bulbous distortions (bottom).

common peroneal mononeuropathy at the fibular head. Selective fascicular vulnerability creates another level of difficulty in the clinical and electrodiagnostic evaluation of focal neuropathies, and the traditional concept of focal neuropathies as transverse lesions with equal involvement of all fibers below the level of the lesion needs revision (7–10).

Peripheral nerves have significant potential for repair and recovery. After nerve compression is relieved, or proceeding pari passu with chronic repetitive trauma, nerve repair occurs. Axolemmal and partially digested myelin proteins are mitogenic for Schwann cells and induce proliferation and elaboration of myelin. Remyelination after purely demyelinating processes occurs over a period of several weeks to several months. Usually, myelin repair is complete within 12 weeks. But the new internodes replacing the damaged myelin across the repaired segment are abnormally short, and the myelin abnormally thin. Such short internodes conduct more slowly than normal. So long as no CB exists function is unimpaired, but conduction studies may reveal residual slowing. Thus, conduction abnormalities may persist after clinical resolution, despite a good outcome.

Because of continuous attempts at remyelination in chronic lesions, acute demyelinating lesions are more prone to produce CB, and chronic lesions more prone to produce focal slowing. Only a minority of nerves studied intraoperatively at the time of decompressive surgery display CB, whereas most show segmental conduction slowing (11,12). The repair of CB with slow remyelinated segments imposes a major limitation in the electrodiagnostic detection of focal neuropathies. CB is easy to detect, but demonstrating focal slowing over a short segment, especially if it is synchronous, may require special techniques (13,14).

With axonal damage, recovery is much more protracted. Reinnervation after axon loss occurs by sprouting, which has two patterns. In the periphery, intact axons adjacent to injured ones rapidly send collateral sprouts to denervated muscle fibers, and possibly to denervated sensory receptors. At the site of injury, the intact stump of the injured axon forms growth cones which attempt to span any gap present and regenerate the axon. Growth cones contain growth factors, such as growth associated protein and nerve growth factor, which promote axon regeneration. The endoneurial tubes, or Schwann cell tubes, survive for a variable period of time after injury. If the growth cones can span the gap and regenerating axons can find their way into a Schwann cell tube, reinnervation is enhanced. Axons then grow at a rate of about 1–3 mm/day from the injury site to the target. The usual estimate of axon regrowth of one mm/day or one inch/month is an average. Regeneration is faster in the young than in the old and faster in proximal segments than distal ones. Axons which grow into the wrong tube produce aberrant reinnervation, or misdirection. When intraneural fibrosis prevents axons from spanning the gap, the proliferating fibers form a chaotic mass of disorganized, contorted axons known as a traumatic neuroma. A neuroma in continuity is one formed on a nerve which remains grossly intact but is severely disrupted internally.

As attempts at repair and regeneration occur at the injury site, important changes are occurring in the target organs. Muscle fibers deprived of innervation and not promptly rescued by collateral sprouts undergo neurogenic atrophy. After some period, atrophic fibers are replaced by fat and fibrosis. As a general rule, muscle fibers that have not been reinnervated within 1 year begin to undergo irreversible changes. The nonneural elements of sensory receptors are more hardy. Even without innervation they may survive intact for long periods, and even late reinnervation may restore important sensory function. The distribution of sensory loss generally changes little after 1–2 years, but functionally appropriate sensory reinnervation by collateral sprouting has been reported as long as seven years after nerve injury. However, long-standing sensory denervation may result in reorganization of the sensory cortex and permanent changes in perception may persist even after reinnervation.

Traumatic nerve injuries can be classified by several systems. Seddon's system, the most commonly used classification scheme, divides nerve injuries into three types: neurapraxia, axonotmesis, and neurotmesis (Table 17.1). In neurapraxia, the injury involves only the myelin. Although the initial deficit may be severe, recovery is rapid and usually complete within 12 weeks. In axonotmesis there is discontinuity of axons. The nerve trunk remains intact and in continuity, and regenerating axons can find their way into surviving endoneurial tubes. Axonotmesis is almost invariably associated with at least some degree of neurapraxia. In neurotmesis, the nerve is discontinuous. Supporting elements as well as axons are disrupted, and the nerve is separated into a proximal and distal stump with an intervening gap of variable width. Regenerating axons must first span any gap present and find the distal stump before reinnervation can proceed. Sunderland added two useful subclasses of axonotmesis. In a third degree injury, there is endoneurial fibrosis which inhibits regeneration and results in variably incomplete recovery. In a fourth degree injury, nerve continuity

TABLE 17.1
Classification of Nerve Injury

Seddon	Process	Sunderland
Neurapraxia	Conduction block	First degree
Axonotmesis	Axon severed but endoneurium intact	Second degree
	Axon discontinuity, endoneurial tube discontinuity, perineurium and funicular arrangement preserved	Third degree
	Loss of countinuity of axons, endoneurial tubes, perineurium and funiculi; epineurium intact	Fourth degree
Neurotmesis	Loss of continuity of the entire nerve trunk	Fifth degree

is maintained only by scar formation and there is no effective reinnervation. The Sunderland first, second and fifth degree lesions correspond to Seddon's neurapraxia, axonotmesis and neurotmesis.

In neurapraxia, there is no axonal loss. Recovery occurs over days to weeks and there is no Tinel's sign at the site of the lesion. With a second degree injury, axonal regeneration produces a Tinel's sign at the injury site which then advances distally at the average rate of one inch/month. With a third degree injury, the Tinel's also advances, but ultimate recovery is incomplete and aberrant reinnervation may occur. With a fourth degree injury, the Tinel's sign never advances beyond the injury site and no recovery occurs. Fifth degree (neurotmetic) injuries are associated with lacerating injuries. Neither fourth or fifth degree lesions improve without surgery.

The Vulnerable Nerve Syndrome

Patients with generalized polyneuropathies, sometimes mild and previously unrecognized, are at increased risk of developing a superimposed compression neuropathy. The existence of this "vulnerable nerve syndrome" often mandates at least some clinical and electrophysiologic screening of seemingly uninvolved nerves to exclude an underlying generalized process with focal accentuation. It is frequently challenging to dissect the relative contributions of generalized neuropathy and focal neuropathy to the clinical and electrodiagnostic picture under such circumstances. A special subtype of vulnerable nerve syndrome is the controversial "double crush" phenomenon, wherein a nerve harboring one lesion develops a second lesion downstream from the first; CTS in association with cervical radiculopathy is the most common example. Whether the presence of one nerve lesion predisposes to the development of a second, or whether extraneural pathology common to multiple sites is the mechanism remains unclear (15). Patients with hereditary liability to pressure palsies suffer from the ultimate vulnerable nerve syndrome and are extremely prone to develop compression neuropathies after only trivial trauma.

Electrodiagnostic Evaluation

Nerve conduction studies and needle electromyography can contribute greatly to the diagnosis and the management of focal neuropathies. But pitfalls abound. The evaluation of diseased nerve is fraught with even more potential for technical mishap than is the case for normal nerve. The ideal situation for electrodiagnostic evaluation of focal neuropathy exists when one can stimulate or record proximal and distal to the lesion. When this is not possible, one must rely on special techniques such as F or H wave latencies, supplemented by needle examination, to localize the lesion.

Because sensory fibers are more sensitive than motor fibers to the effects of pressure, abnormalities of the nerve action potential (NAP), either sensory or compound, often precede abnormalities of motor conduction studies. While sensitive, however, changes in the NAP are often nonlocalizing. NAP abnormalities can reflect pathology in the sensory fibers anywhere at or distal to the dorsal root ganglion. With severe compression, the NAP is often simply absent, a finding of no mean significance in helping to exclude radiculopathy and gauge the severity of the neuropathy, but of no value in localization. When present, the NAP may show loss of amplitude with distalmost stimulation (indicating loss of axons), slowing, or CB (a difference in amplitude or area above vs. below the lesion). The interpretation of CB in sensory or compound NAPs is hampered by technical factors, such as the conspicuous dependency of the amplitude on the distance from the recording electrode, and biologic factors, such as phase cancellation.

Motor conduction studies, while less sensitive, are usually more localizing. Several types of abnormalities occur (see Fig 16.4). A lesion producing uniform demyelination and equal slowing of all fibers at a certain point causes synchronous focal slowing, with no change in the waveform shape or amplitude above as compared with below the lesion. A process affecting some fibers more than others, but not causing CB in any fiber, creates asynchronous or differential focal slowing with fragmentation and temporal dispersion of the waveform on stimulating above the lesion, but no loss of total area under the M wave curve. A lesion causing CB in some fibers, usually associated with focal slowing in unblocked fibers, produces a lower amplitude, often dispersed waveform on stimulating above the lesion, with some loss of total area under the curve: the picture of partial CB. With a severe lesion producing complete CB, stimulation above the lesion elicits no M wave. The most convincing localizing abnormalities in focal neuropathies are CB, partial or complete, or asynchronous focal slowing with loss of amplitude and waveform dispersion above a given point.

In the presence of CB and the ability to stimulate the nerve proximal and distal to the lesion, localization is easy. However, because the nerve's incessant efforts at repair often produce a lesion characterized predominantly by focal slowing, such simple maneuvers often do not suffice. In such cases, the probability of detecting the lesion depends on the length of nerve segment examined. Longer nerve segments produce the lowest experimental error, but including normal nerve with the pathologic segment masks the focal slowing, so the longer the segment studied the lower the likelihood of detecting the lesion. When attempting to localize a lesion not associated with CB, "inching" techniques involving the serial stimulation or recording from short nerve segments, 1 or 2 cm long, may be useful (13,14,16).

Any process producing axon loss can cause secondary slowing of CV or prolongation of distal latencies due to random drop out of the fastest conducting fibers. The presence of axon loss is signaled by a loss of M wave amplitude or area on distal stimulation. In the presence of axon loss and a low amplitude M wave, greater slowing should be present before diagnosing a focal neuropathy. These issues are addressed in more detail in Chapters 13 and 16.

Focal neuropathies are primarily demyelinating processes, but no criteria exist for the degree of slowing or latency prolongation in relation to M wave amplitude loss as for generalized neuropathies. The electrodiagnostic medicine consultant must nevertheless bear these factors in mind and make appropriate adjustments before diagnosing a focal neuropathy. For instance, median nerve entrapment at the ligament of Struthers causing axon loss may well produce mild slowing of CV distal to the point of compression, mild prolongation of distal motor and sensory latency and loss of M wave and SNAP amplitude. These are all secondary changes, and the distal latency prolongations should not lead to a diagnosis of CTS. An L5 radiculopathy can sometimes cause dramatic axon loss and secondary conduction changes in the peroneal nerve, which should not be mistaken for peroneal neuropathy.

Following acute nerve trauma, conduction in the segment distal to the injury is preserved for a period of time. There is a progressive decline in conduction velocity and loss of nerve excitability over a period of 3–10 days. Because of retained conduction in the distal stump, conduction abnormalities in the 3–10 days after onset may be misleading in terms of the underlying pathophysiology. During the acute phase, the electrodiagnostic picture may be one of "pseudo-conduction block," with no response elicitable on stimulating proximal to the lesion, no recruitable MUAPs and an absence of fibrillation potentials on needle examination, but relatively preserved distal conduction. The examiner should exercise caution about pronouncements during this interval. The greatest information would accrue from a single electrodiagnostic evaluation if done approximately 3 weeks post injury (3). Still, some valuable information can be obtained by early studies. If MUAPs under voluntary control are present, the lesion must be incomplete. If complete axon loss is destined to occur, retained conduction in the distal stump may present a transient opportunity for precise localization (17). The remainder of this discussion assumes the lesion is fully developed.

Focal Neuropathy Syndromes

While CTS, ulnar neuropathy at the elbow, peroneal neuropathy at the knee, retrohumeral radial neuropathy and facial neuropathy comprise the majority of focal neuropathies, virtually any nerve in the body can be compressed or entrapped. Many other interesting and important focal neuropathies occur, some of which are summarized in Table 17.2. Several excellent monographs and other publications discuss these less common syndromes (5,15,18–25).

CARPAL TUNNEL SYNDROME

Some of the relevant anatomy is depicted in Figure 17.2. The median nerve crosses from the distal forearm to the hand through the carpal tunnel. The walls and floor of the tunnel are formed by the carpal bones and the roof by the transverse carpal ligament (TCL). The TCL evolves from the antebrachial fascia at about the level of the wrist crease and extends 4–6 cm into

the palm. The passageway is narrowest 2.0–2.5 cm distal to its origin, which corresponds to the usual site of median nerve compression (13,26). Lying with the median nerve in the canal are the eight tendons of the flexor digitorum profundus and superficialis and the tendon of the flexor pollicis longus, surrounded by a complex synovial sheath.

The palmar cutaneous branch of the median nerve leaves the main trunk 5–8 cm proximal to the wrist crease. It travels through its own separate passageway in the TCL and provides sensation to the thenar eminence; it does not traverse the carpal tunnel. Loss of sensation over the thenar eminence is not part of CTS and suggests a lesion proximal to the wrist. After exiting the tunnel, the median nerve gives off its recurrent thenar motor branch, which curves backward and radially to innervate the thenar muscles. The nerve ends by giving off terminal motor branches to innervate the first and second lumbricals, then dividing into common digital sensory branches. More proximal median nerve anatomy is depicted in Figure 3.6.

Entrapment of the median nerve beneath the TCL is often brought on or exacerbated by excessive hand/wrist/finger movements; the combination of repetitive finger flexion with wrist motion seems to be the most hazardous ergonomic stress. Both vocational and recreational activities (e.g., gardening, metal scavenging, fly fishing, refinishing furniture, knitting/needlepoint, karate) can incite or aggravate the condition. The classical concept of repetitive motion induced chronic tenosynovitis has recently been questioned, and the relationship between carpal canal size and CTS risk remains debatable (15). Rarely CTS can result from mass lesions narrowing the passageway (e.g., ganglion, osteophyte, lipoma, aneurysm, anomalous muscle) (26). Numerous systemic conditions predispose to CTS, including rheumatoid arthritis, diabetes mellitus, chronic renal insufficiency, hypothyroidism, amyloidosis, myeloma, and pregnancy. There seems to be an autosomal dominant familial form (27).

CTS produces a characteristic clinical picture of hand pain, numbness, and paresthesias (all usually more severe at night), along with varying degrees of weakness (28,29). Proximal upper extremity pain, usually in the forearm but sometimes as far as the shoulder, is less typical but not uncommon. Many patients initially complain of "whole hand" symptoms, and rarely, for unclear reasons, a patient with CTS may present with ulnar distribution paresthesias (26). The reason for the nocturnal exacerbation of symptoms remains obscure, but the diagnosis should remain suspect in the absence of this feature.

Findings on examination vary with the severity of the condition. Patients with mild CTS may have a

TABLE 17.2
Clinical and Electrodiagnostic Features of Some Uncommon Focal Neuropathies

Syndrome	Clinical Features	Electrodiagnostic Features
Posterior interosseous neuropathy	Finger drop without wrist drop; pure motor; entrapment in the region of the supinator muscle	Motor conduction abnormalities difficult to detect; radial NAP normal; NE: denervation limited to PIN distribution
Median neuropathy due to supra-condylar spur	Median entrapment by the ligament of Struthers running from distal humeral spur to medial epicondyle	CB or FS at level of midarm; abnormal NAP; NE: denervation of pronator teres and all distal median muscles
Pronator teres syndrome	Main trunk median entrapment at the level of the pronator teres; motor and sensory dysfunction	Median slowing in the forearm; abnormal NAP; denervation of all muscles distal to pronator with variable involvement of pronator
Anterior interosseous neuropathy	Entrapment just distal to the pronator teres after AIN leaves the main trunk; motor dysfunction only	Normal routine median motor and sensory NCS; denervation limited to AIN innervated muscles
Ulnar neuropathy at the wrist	Various combinations of motor and sensory dysfunction depending on precise location of lesion, external pressure frequently a factor (e.g., bicyclist's palsy)	Normal ulnar NCS in the forearm; normal dorsal ulnar cutaneous NAP; ± prolongation of ulnar DML, ± abnormal NAPs, various patterns of denervation
Tarsal tunnel syndrome	Entrapment behind medial malleolus; pain and sensory dysfunction in sole of foot	Diagnosis rests on demonstrating motor or sensory abnormalities in distribution of medial and/or lateral plantar nerves; ± abnormalities on NE
Meralgia paresthetica	Lateral femoral cutaneous nerve entrapment near anterior superior iliac spine; pain/numbness in lateral thigh. Obesity and tight garments predispose.	No motor abnormalities; LFC NAPs technically difficult and debatably useful; diagnosis rests on excluding other pathology, e.g., L3 radiculopathy
Femoral neuropathy	May be injured at the inguinal ligament, in the pelvis or within the psoas muscle; hip/thigh weakness with decreased knee jerk and sensory loss in saphenous distribution (medial lower leg)	Sometimes CB or FS demonstrated across inguinal ligament; with more proximal lesions diagnosis rests on NE; abnormal saphenous NAP useful but nonlocalizing

AIN, anterior interosseous neuropathy; CB, conduction block; DML, distal motor latency; FS, focal slowing; LFC, lateral femoral cutaneous nerve; NAP, nerve action potential; NCS, nerve conduction study; NE, needle electromyography; PIN, posterior interosseous nerve.
SOURCE: From Campbell WW. Electromyography and conduction studies in the diagnosis and management of entrapment syndromes. AAEM course, Fundamentals of Electrodiagnostic Medicine, 1993.

normal physical exam, or trivial sensory loss over the fingertips requiring special techniques to demonstrate. The earliest sensory loss seems to occur over the volar tip of the middle finger (5). Patients with more advanced disease have more easily demonstrable sensory loss and frequently have weakness of the thenar muscles. Patients with severe involvement demonstrate thenar atrophy and dense sensory loss. Such patients with long-standing, untreated end stage CTS often have surprisingly little symptomatology. Provocative tests, such as Tinel's, Phalen's and the carpal compression maneuver, have proven disappointing, with high proportions of false positives and

false negatives (15). The "flick" sign, in which the patient flicks the wrist to demonstrate what they do to "restore the circulation" at night is more useful but still imperfect (26). The rare "reverse Tinel's sign" with paresthesias radiating retrograde up the forearm may be more specific for CTS.

The most common differential diagnostic exercise is between CTS and cervical radiculopathy, most often C6. The two conditions can coexist. Neck and shoulder pain, weakness in C6 innervated muscles, reflex changes, sensory loss restricted to the thumb, the absence of nocturnal paresthesias, and reproduction of the paresthesias with root compression maneuvers all

FIGURE 17.2. The median nerve runs beneath the transverse carpal ligament in company with the tendons of the deep and superficial finger flexors and flexor pollicis longus and a complex synovial sheath. Synovitis of this sheath may play a role in carpal tunnel syndrome. The recurrent thenar motor branch arches backward from the radial aspect to innervate the thenar muscles. The palmar cutaneous branch comes off proximal to the wrist and does not run through the carpal tunnel.

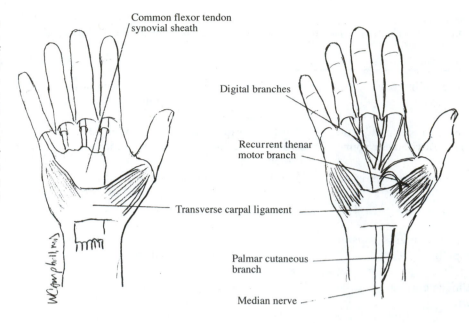

favor cervical radiculopathy. Other conditions occasionally merit consideration include proximal median neuropathy, neurogenic thoracic outlet syndrome and upper brachial plexopathy. Various musculoskeletal conditions, especially de Quervain's tendinitis, can cause hand and wrist pain suggestive of CTS. Bizarre hand paresthesias may be the presenting manifestation of vitamin B12 deficiency (30).

The earliest electrodiagnostic change is prolongation of the median NAP latency. The 8 cm palm to wrist technique is more sensitive than wrist/finger studies because of the shorter segment of unaffected nerve included (5,31). Abnormal NAP amplitude or latency, while the earliest detectable abnormality, is not localizing. With more severe involvement there is loss of NAP amplitude, prolongation of the motor distal latency, and the development of denervation in thenar muscles. For reasons not completely understood, slowing of the median CV in the forearm is not uncommon. The presence of a median to ulnar forearm anastomosis in 15–20% of the population requires constant vigilance regarding proximal and distal amplitude relationships and attention to the subtleties of the waveforms. An initial positive deflection on elbow stimulation not present on wrist stimulation, or an unrealistically fast median forearm CV, are the usual clues to CTS in association with anomalous innervation (32). Another technical hazard is spread of the stimulating current to the ulnar nerve at the wrist producing sometimes subtle changes in the waveform while spuriously lowering the distal motor latency to within the normal range (see Chapter 10).

A literature-based practice parameter on the electrodiagnosis of CTS was recently published, including an annotated bibliography of 165 references (31). The literature through 1992 was rigorously reviewed using six predetermined quality criteria, including a requirement that the diagnosis of CTS be based on clinical criteria independent of electrodiagnosis. For the use of standard surface electrodes, only eight studies of patients and six of normal subjects met all literature classification criteria. These were further culled to exclude studies in which the incidence of CTS was > 90% to avoid selection bias toward more severe cases. The median distal motor latency was prolonged in 60–74% of patients. Sensory conduction studies over a 13–14 cm distance between digit and wrist were abnormal in 49–66% of patients. Using an 8 cm distance between palm and wrist, studies were abnormal in 69–84% of patients. The difference between median and ulnar peak latency (>0.31 msec difference) had a sensitivity of 66%, but a study of controls suggests SNAP differences up to 0.5 msec may be normal (33). The difference between median and ulnar peak latency over 14 cm from wrist to ring finger (> 0.35 msec) had a sensitivity of 82%. The difference between median and radial latencies to the thumb had a sensitivity of 60–69%.

A significant minority of patients with a clinical diagnosis of CTS have normal electrodiagnostic evaluations, from 10–40% depending on the technique. Numerous special techniques have been proposed to detect the cases missed by the usual methods. But since each procedure carries its own incidence of false positives, performing multiple tests in an attempt to diagnose CTS may do more to increase the false positive rate than make any real contribution to the diagnosis in problem cases (see Chapter 5) (34).

ULNAR NEUROPATHY AT THE ELBOW

Ulnar neuropathy at the elbow (UNE) is the second most common compression neuropathy after CTS, but stands unequaled at the head of the line in complexity of clinical evaluation, electrodiagnostic picture and management. It is, in many respects, the "EMGers nightmare," the most tricky and problematic of all focal neuropathies. The pathophysiology, electrodiagnosis and management have been recently reviewed (35–38).

Anatomical details are important in understanding UNE (39,40) (Fig. 17.3, see also Fig. 3.6). After descending without branches through the upper arm, the nerve traverses the retroepicondylar groove between the medial epicondyle (ME) and olecranon process (OP). The floor of the ulnar groove is formed by the ulnar collateral ligament. The nerve then passes beneath the humeroulnar aponeurotic arcade (HUA), a dense aponeurosis joining the humeral and ulnar heads of origin of the flexor carpi ulnaris (FCU), which typically lies 1.0–2.5 cm distal to a line connecting the ME and the OP (39). After passing under the HUA, the nerve runs through the belly of the FCU, then exits through the deep flexorpronator aponeurosis lining the deep surface of the muscle 4.0–6.0 cm beyond the ME.

Important changes occur with elbow flexion. In extension, the ME and OP are juxtaposed with the HUA slack and the nerve lying loosely in the ulnar groove. With elbow flexion, the OP moves forward and separates from the ME, progressively tightening the aponeurosis across the nerve. Also, the ulnar collateral ligament bulges into the floor of the groove and the medial head of the triceps may impinge on the groove from behind. In extension the ulnar groove is smooth, round and capacious, but in flexion the nerve finds itself in inhospitable surroundings in a flattened, tortuous, and narrow canal with the HUA pulled tightly across it. With extreme flexion, the nerve may slide up to 1.4 cm distally, and it partially or completely subluxes out of its groove in many normal individuals. Anomalous muscles and fibrous bands can occasionally compress the nerve (39).

The internal fascicular organization of the nerve and varying susceptibility of different fascicles to injury may explain some of the puzzling diversity in clinical expression of ulnar neuropathies (9,10). The fibers to the first dorsal interosseous (FDI) are more susceptible to injury than those to the abductor digiti minimi (ADM). Fascicles innervating forearm flexors and the fascicles comprising the dorsal ulnar cutaneous (DUC) may paradoxically escape injury with lesions at the elbow. Different fascicles may exhibit different types of electrical pathophysiology, such as CB affecting fibers to the FDI while those to the ADM display a pure axon loss picture.

The anatomical factors account for much of the susceptibility of the ulnar nerve to injury at the elbow. The lack of protective covering over the nerve in its

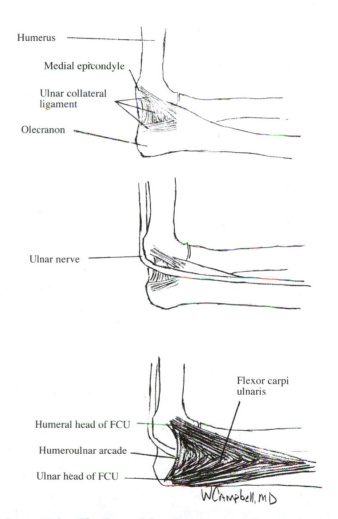

FIGURE 17.3. The floor of the ulnar groove is formed by the tripartite ulnar collateral ligament, which bulges into the groove with elbow flexion and narrows the passageway. The humeroulnar arcade (the cubital tunnel) stretches more tightly across the nerve with flexion, increasing the pressure on the nerve. After passing beneath the aponeurotic arcade, the nerve runs through the belly of the flexor carpi ulnaris and exits through the muscle's deep surface.

course through the ulnar groove accounts for its susceptibility to external pressure. Repetitive flexion and extension may predispose to UNE because of the dynamic changes in the nerve's passageway with motion. With elbow joint derangement due to trauma or arthritic changes, the nerve's vulnerability increases even further. Valgus deformities increase the stretch on the nerve with elbow flexion, and osteophytic overgrowth further narrows an often already narrow passageway. The nerve may be entrapped at the HUA or at the point of exit from the FCU (36,41,42). The role of subluxation is unclear. The proportion of UNE cases related to major elbow trauma has steadily decreased over the years, while the proportion of "idiopathic" cases has steadily increased (43).

A number of problems arise in the differential diagnosis of suspected UNE. There are at least three potential sites of ulnar compression in the region of the elbow: the ulnar groove, the HUA and the exit site from the FCU. The clinical manifestations of disease at the wrist, elbow and more proximal sites can be similar. The nerve's branching pattern limits both clinical and electrodiagnostic localization. Selective vulnerability may produce varying degrees of involvement of different fascicles (10). Forearm muscles are often spared in lesions at the elbow (9). Lesions of the brachial plexus and lower cervical roots cause signs and symptoms occasionally difficult to distinguish from UNE. Patients with anterior horn cell disease and other myelopathies may develop small hand muscle wasting resembling that seen in UNE. The sensory symptoms of UNE can mimic those of cervical radiculopathy, plexopathy and ulnar lesions at the wrist or upper arm.

A terminologic morass has grown out of imprecision in the use of terms such as tardy ulnar palsy and cubital tunnel syndrome. Tardy ulnar palsy was first used to describe UNE developing after remote elbow trauma, generally after an old fracture or dislocation. It soon degenerated into a nonspecific, generic term for any ulnar neuropathy at the elbow, on the weak presumption that remote trauma must have occurred but the patient simply couldn't recall it. Feindel and Stratford coined the term "cubital tunnel syndrome" (cubit is Latin for elbow or forearm) to refer to patients with compression of the nerve by the HUA (44). They were attempting to define a subgroup of "tardy ulnar palsy" patients who suffered from a focal entrapment at the origin of the FCU, and who could be spared a transposition procedure and managed with simple release of the aponeurotic arcade. As with tardy ulnar palsy, the term cubital tunnel syndrome soon degenerated into a useless, nonspecific, generic label for any UNE as the term increasingly grew in popularity with few bothering to read the original paper. Some clinicians use cubital tunnel syndrome to refer to ulnar groove compression and "Osborne's band" compression to refer to entrapment by the HUA. All these terms now invite confusion and miscommunication and should be stricken from the lexicon.

The physical examination of a patient with suspected UNE should include detailed assessment of strength, sensation and reflexes, and examination of the elbow for range of motion and deformity. Strength in the patient's ulnar innervated hand and forearm muscles can be semiquantitated by comparison with the examiner's like muscles. Weakness of non-ulnar C8 muscles is the usual clue to disease involving the lower brachial plexus or C8 root. This finding should in turn prompt further examination of the cervical spine and a check for Horner's syndrome. Weakness in the ulnar innervated long finger flexors and FCU may help separate UNE from a more distal lesion, though normal strength in these muscles is still entirely consistent with an elbow level lesion. Ulnar neuropathy is not the only condition that can cause hand clawing (45).

A careful sensory examination can be rewarding. The cutaneous field of the ulnar nerve does not extend more than a few centimeters proximal to the wrist crease. Involvement of the distribution of the medial antebrachial cutaneous nerve over the medial forearm excludes UNE, since this nerve runs anterior to the ME and not through the ulnar groove. Impaired sensation over the dorsum of the hand establishes the location of the lesion as proximal to the takeoff of the DUC, but sparing of the dorsal cutaneous territory does not exclude UNE because of possible selective sparing of its fascicles. Involvement of the palmar cutaneous branch distribution likewise suggests a proximal lesion. Splitting of the ring finger fairly reliably excludes plexopathy and radiculopathy.

Impaired elbow range of motion or a valgus deformity strongly suggest UNE. Reproduction of symptoms with elbow flexion and ulnar groove pressure can be informative. Examining for subluxation is seldom helpful, as this is a common phenomenon in normal individuals. Eliciting a Tinel's sign can be useful, but many normal patients "Tinel" over all their nerves; only the presence of a disproportionately active Tinel's sign over the clinically suspect ulnar nerve has any localizing value.

It is difficult to compete with British eloquence in describing the vicissitudes of the electrodiagnosis of UNE. As Payan said, "the services of an inadequate electromyographer are more dangerous than none at all"; and it is disconcertingly easy to feel inadequate when dealing with an enigmatic UNE (46).

The electrodiagnostic evaluation of ulnar neuropathies has met with a number of problems. Patients with purely sensory symptoms may have unrevealing electrodiagnostic evaluations. Elbow position markedly influences ulnar conduction velocity, and there has been great difficulty reaching agreement on the best elbow position for performing conduction studies (36). The optimal segment length for across elbow conduction studies remains debatable (16). UNE in some patients affects amplitude and area parameters more than conduction velocity parameters, the "pure axon loss" lesion (3). The relative importance of conduction block v. conduction slowing is disputed. UNE may cause axon loss or focal demyelination, or any combination of the two. Pure axon loss lesions are exceedingly difficult to localize by conduction studies alone.

A recent, literature based practice parameter, similar to the study of CTS, has reviewed the electrodiagnosis of UNE (36). The literature through 1996 was reviewed using six predetermined quality criteria, including a requirement that the diagnosis be based on clinical criteria independent of electrodiagnosis. Only 19 articles met 5 or 6 literature classification criteria, and 13 of these were used to construct tables summarizing the demographics, technical electrophysiologic details, findings in controls and patients, and the sensitivity of various techniques. The conclusions and recommendations of this review are summarized as practice standards or guidelines in Table 17.3.

Ulnar conduction velocity varies markedly with elbow position (36). In extension, the nerve lies lax and coiled in the groove, its redundancy in reserve to play out during flexion. Significant discrepancy thus exists between skin surface length and the greater length of underlying nerve, creating a falsely short distance and a falsely slow CV. Numerous authors have reported slowing across the extended elbow in normal controls (up to 20 m/sec). With full flexion the nerve may slide distally, and in almost 20% of normals it may sublux completely out of the groove and lie anterior to the tip of the ME. This may again produce discrepancies between skin surface distance and nerve length. With subluxation the skin distance is falsely long as the nerve "cuts the corner" across the ME, creating a falsely fast CV. Moderate flexion provides the least variability in motor conduction studies. The most logical position for conduction studies is moderate flexion from the horizontal, with the forearm at an angle of 70–90° from full extension. Reports should specify the position used and the reference values employed. The clinical study should always be done using the same position employed to obtain the reference values, and the same position should be used for both stimulation

TABLE 17.3

Synopsis of the Recommendations of the AAEM Practice Parameter on Ulnar Neuropathy at the Elbow (36)

1. When using moderate-elbow flexion (70–90° from horizontal), a 10 cm across elbow distance, and surface stimulation and recording, the following abnormalities suggest a focal lesion involving the ulnar nerve at the elbow. The most important criterion is the presence of multiple internally consistent abnormalities. Multiple abnormalities are more convincing than isolated abnormalities, which raise the possibility of artifact or technical mishap.
   a. Absolute motor NCV from AE to BE of less than 50 m/sec.
   b. An AE to BE segment greater than 10 m/sec slower than the BE to W segment.
   c. A decrease in compound muscle action potential (M wave) negative peak amplitude from BE to AE greater than 20%.
   d. A significant change in M wave configuration at the AE site compared to the BE site.
2. If routine motor studies are inconclusive, the following procedures may be of benefit:
   a. NCS recorded from the first dorsal interosseous (FDI) muscle.
   b. An inching or short segment study.
3. Needle examination should include the FDI, the most frequently abnormal muscle, and ulnar innervated forearm flexors. Neither changes limited to the FDI, nor sparing of the forearm muscles, exclude an elbow lesion. If ulnar innervated muscles are abnormal, the examination should be extended to include nonulnar C8/medial cord/lower trunk muscles to exclude brachial plexopathy and the cervical paraspinals to exclude radiculopathy.

and measurement to avoid discrepancies produced by altering position in the middle of the examination. There is no consensus regarding the sensitivity of flexion vs. extension in detecting clinically apparent UNEs. There is unanimity that consistency of elbow position and technique is paramount.

Soon after passing beneath the HUA the nerve dives deeply into the substance of the FCU. Surface stimulation much more than 3–4 cm beyond the elbow, especially in large arms, runs a substantial risk of being submaximal.

Debate continues regarding the best distance for across elbow conduction determination (16). A distance of 10 cm correlates best with published norms. But the greater the length of normal nerve included in a CV determination containing a short diseased segment, the less the likelihood of detecting the focal abnormality. A distance of 10 cm may fail to detect significant pathology, or result in an impression of a pure axon loss lesion, when studies of shorter segments are capable of localizing the lesion. The worst possible technique is to establish an above elbow stimulation point just above the ME, then slavishly measure 10 cm distally to a below elbow (BE) point in the mid to upper forearm. This invites gross inaccuracy due to submaximal BE stimulation, coupled with a low likelihood of detecting a lesion.

The M wave negative peak amplitude should not decrease more than 20% from the BE site to the above elbow (AE) site, a conservative criterion. Loss of amplitude greater than 20%, or a significant change in M wave configuration, suggests a focal lesion at the elbow. In the presence of a loss of amplitude or change in configuration on AE stimulation, it is quite simple to perform an inching study by carefully moving the stimulator in sequential steps to detect the point of change. This has a high correlation with the site of the lesion. In the absence of an amplitude or configuration change, "inching" studies require careful measurement of latency changes between successive 1–2 cm segments. Such short segment incremental studies are technically more demanding but potentially rewarding (14,16). A Martin-Gruber forearm anastomosis can cause loss of M wave amplitude on above elbow stimulation. If the BE stimulation site is in the upper forearm, confusion with a pathological conduction block could occur.

Abnormalities of the sensory or compound nerve action potential (NAP) at the wrist can occur with an ulnar neuropathy at any level; loss of amplitude and mild prolongation of latency reflect the loss of axons with random, or perhaps preferential, involvement of the largest fibers. As with CTS, distal NAP abnormalities are nonspecific and nonlocalizing. Across the elbow NAP studies may be occasionally useful for localization of a lesion to the ulnar groove, but are fraught with technical difficulties (36).

Needle electrode examination (NEE) is frequently problematic in UNE. There is often considerable variability in the degree of involvement of different ulnar innervated hand and forearm muscles (9,10,36). The FDI is involved most commonly, and not infrequently is the only muscle to display abnormalities. The ADM is second most commonly involved. The forearm muscles, FCU and FDP are frequently spared, so the lack of abnormality in these muscles in no way excludes a lesion at the elbow. The sparing of the forearm muscles appears related to 1) the severity of the neuropathy—the more severe the slowing and distal M wave amplitude loss, the more likely changes will be found in the forearm muscles; 2) the level of compression—lesions in the ulnar groove are more likely to involve the forearm muscles than compression at the HUA; 3) the redundant innervation via several branchlets—

both FCU and FDP usually receive several small branches from the main ulnar trunk; and 4) the differential susceptibility of fascicles to injury—the location of fascicles within the nerve determines the degree of damage, and the fibers to the forearm flexors run in a deeper and less vulnerable position than the fibers to the small hand muscles. EMG textbooks often provide the specious but incorrect explanation that sparing of the forearm muscles is due to the branch innervating the FCU arising proximal to the elbow (9).

The two surgical procedures most commonly done for UNE at the present time are decompression, by simple release of the HUA, and anterior subcutaneous transposition. Investigators have been hard pressed to demonstrate the superiority of one procedure over the other in any series of unselected patients (43). Payan editorialized the concerns of many in discussing surgery and its complications: "the electromyographer is bound to ruminate on the subject of operative technique because the failures eventually arrive at his door . . . anterior transposition gives rise to a far from negligible morbidity . . ." (46)

There are several regularly recurrent problem scenarios in dealing with suspected ulnar neuropathy at the elbow.

1. The "pure axon loss" lesion at the elbow. In some patients with UNE, it is very difficult to demonstrate focal slowing across the elbow. When the forearm flexors are involved, probable localization to the elbow is still possible by NEE, although it is impossible to exclude a more proximal lesion in the axilla or upper arm. Helpful ancillary techniques in this situation include: 1) recording from the FDI, which may demonstrate focal slowing or CB even though fibers to the ADM do not, and/or 2) a short (1–2 cm) segment incremental study, which can often demonstrate focal slowing missed when studying longer segments. Abnormality of the DUC can at least place the lesion proximal to its takeoff, but the DUC can occasionally be spared in elbow lesions.

2. The patient with purely sensory symptoms and normal routine motor studies. Such patients usually have mild or early UNEs and an adequate evaluation may well be to exclude other pathology, such as brachial plexopathy or cervical radiculopathy, and manage the patient conservatively. To localize the lesion more confidently, FDI recording or SSIS may be useful. NAP recording across the elbow is technically difficult and the results should be interpreted cautiously (Table 17.3).

3. The patient with forearm sparing. When conduction studies place the lesion at the elbow, sparing

of the forearm muscles should be no deterrent to localization. With equivocal conduction studies, the comments in paragraph 1 apply.

4. Wallerian degeneration with confusing distal abnormalities. When severe UNE causes major axon loss distal to the lesion, there may be secondary slowing of the entire distal ulnar nerve and prolongation of the distal motor latency, usually with an absent sensory potential and abundant denervation. In lesions of this severity, NEE abnormalities are usually present in the forearm muscles and FDI recording or SSIS will often place the lesion at the elbow, even if routine studies are equivocal. An occasional error is to diagnose a second lesion at the wrist.

5. Failed ulnar nerve surgery. It is not rare for patients to present with persistent or recurrent symptoms after an unsuccessful operation on the ulnar nerve. Sometimes there are no preoperative studies for comparison, in which case the EMGer is reduced to guesswork. The first order of business should be to establish with certainty that no other process, such as plexopathy or radiculopathy, was responsible for the symptoms initially. Then one should map out the course of the nerve to determine whether or not transposition was done. This procedure alone may sometimes establish, by showing abrupt changes in nerve course, that kinking has occurred due to inadequate distal (more rarely proximal) release. After mapping the course of the nerve, a SSIS study can establish whether there is persistent focal compression or fibrosis, potentially amenable to reoperation, or whether there has been devascularization of a long nerve segment, an essentially endstage condition.

The most convincing localization of a UNE results from multiple internally consistent abnormalities. For example, slowing across the elbow detected during routine conduction studies in the face of no complaints, a normal sensory potential and an absence of changes on NEE is most likely artifactual. Some have argued this represents "subclinical" ulnar neuropathy, an unlikely conclusion. Conversely, there could be no argument regarding localization in the face of a partial conduction block and focal slowing in the across elbow segment, a normal below elbow to wrist segment, an absent sensory potential and fibrillation potentials in ulnar hand muscles and forearm flexors.

RADIAL NEUROPATHY

The radial nerve arises as a direct continuation of the posterior cord of the brachial plexus (see Figure 3.6). Just after passing the teres major muscle, it enters the triceps and sends off innervating branches, then arcs laterally and distally along the spiral groove of the humerus. It pierces the lateral intermuscular septum, then runs between the brachialis and brachioradialis muscles just anterior to the lateral epicondyle. The main trunk innervates the brachioradialis and extensor carpi radialis longus muscles, after which it ends by dividing into superficial and deep branches. The superficial branch travels down the radial aspect of the forearm to supply sensation to the radial aspect of the dorsum of the hand and the radial three and one-half digits. The deep branch passes over the fibrous edge of the extensor carpi radialis brevis and through a slit in the supinator muscle (the arcade of Frohse), then continues as the posterior interosseous nerve, which innervates the extensor carpi ulnaris, finger and thumb extensors, and the abductor pollicis longus.

Acute compression of the radial nerve in the retrohumeral spiral groove, frequently referred to as "Saturday night" or "bridegroom's" palsy, results from sustained compression over a period of several hours during sleep or a drug or alcohol induced stupor (47). Weakness involves all muscles distal to the triceps, which receives its innervation from a branch arising proximal to the spiral groove. The most prominent complaint and finding is wrist drop. Sensory loss is usually present in the superficial radial nerve distribution. Confusion commonly arises on two points: 1) because of mechanical factors, the interossei cannot exert normal power in the face of finger drop and may seem weak; 2) weakness of thumb abduction occurs due to dysfunction of the radial innervated abductor pollicis longus. The apparent weakness of the interossei and of thumb abduction may befuddle the unwary and cause mislocalization. Lesions of the motor cortex can rarely cause a pattern of weakness simulating radial neuropathy (47). The primary differential diagnostic considerations include C7 radiculopathy, posterior interosseous nerve palsy, and lesions involving the middle trunk or posterior cord of the brachial plexus. The radial nerve seems particularly prone to involvement in systemic vasculitis.

Conduction studies are usually performed by recording from a radial innervated forearm muscle, such as the extensor indicis, stimulating at the elbow, and below and above the spiral groove. Surface tape measurement around the curve of the upper arm leads to a surface distance longer than the true nerve course, and radial CVs are typically faster than for other nerves—usually in the 70–80 m/sec range. The primary electrodiagnostic abnormality in most cases is conduction block and slowing involving the spiral groove segment. When axon loss occurs, the M wave amplitude is reduced on distal stimulation, the superficial radial SNAP is reduced in amplitude and fibrillations appear in radial innervated muscles distal to the lesion. Rarely, selective involvement of the posterior interosseous fascicles in a retrohumeral radial neuropathy may lead to confusion with a posterior interosseous nerve palsy.

COMMON PERONEAL NEUROPATHY AT THE FIBULAR HEAD (CPNFH)

The primary root origin of the peroneal nerve is L5, with lesser contributions from L4 (primarily to the tibialis anterior) and from S1 (primarily to the small foot muscles). After traversing the lumbosacral plexus, the peroneal joins the posterior tibial nerve in a common sheath to form the sciatic nerve (see Fig. 3.9). The sciatic exits the pelvis through the sciatic foramen just beneath the piriformis muscle and descends through the posterior thigh. In midthigh, the peroneal division sends a twig to the short head of the biceps femoris, the only peroneal innervated muscle proximal to the knee. At the level of the popliteal fossa, the sciatic divides into the common peroneal and posterior tibial nerves. The common peroneal gives off a sural communicating branch, which joins with a similar branch from the tibial to form the sural nerve. The lateral cutaneous nerve of the calf sends sensory innervation to the lateral lower leg. The peroneal nerve then winds around the head of the fibula, pierces the peroneus longus muscle (the "fibular tunnel") and divides into superficial and deep branches. The superficial branch innervates the peroneus longus and brevis, and terminates as the superficial sensory branch, which provides sensation to the dorsum of the foot. The deep peroneal branch innervates the tibialis anterior, peroneus tertius and long and short toe extensors, and provides sensation to the web space between the first and second toes. Some of the innervation to the extensor digitorum brevis (EDB) may travel via an accessory peroneal branch, a common anomaly. The accessory peroneal arises at the knee and descends on the lateral aspect of the leg, passes posterior to the lateral malleolus and ends in the lateral portion of the EDB.

The peroneal nerve at the fibular head (FH) is superficial, covered only by skin and subcutaneous tissue, not even afforded by nature the protective bony culvert given the ulnar nerve, making it exceptionally vulnerable to external compression (Fig. 17.4). The nerve is also tethered at its point of passage through the peroneus longus muscle, making it susceptible to stretch as well. Rare patients with CPNFH seem to have a true entrapment at the fibular tunnel, but in most instances CPNFH develops in the setting of external pressure.

Habitual leg crossing is a classical cause of CPNFH, producing repetitive trauma to the nerve between the

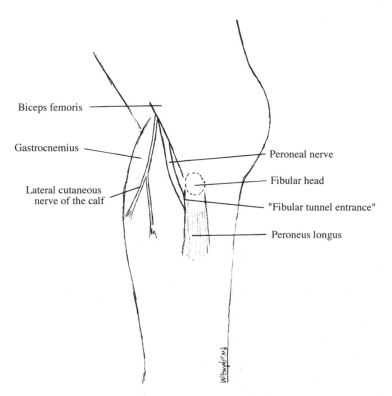

FIGURE 17.4. The peroneal nerve separates from the tibial in the popliteal fossa and angles laterally, emerging beneath the tendon of the biceps femoris. It is covered only by skin and subcutaneous tissue as it curves around the fibular head. It runs through the "fibular tunnel" beneath the superficial head of the peroneus longus, then divides into superficial and deep branches. The lateral cutaneous nerve of the calf does not run through the fibular tunnel.

Biceps femoris

Gastrocnemius

Lateral cutaneous nerve of the calf

Peroneal nerve

Fibular head

"Fibular tunnel entrance"

Peroneus longus

ipsilateral fibular head and the contralateral knee. Occasionally a skin dimple marks the precise site of compression. This type of CPNFH is particularly common in slender or depressed patients, or those who have recently lost weight (slimmer's palsy). Any number of external forces may substitute for the patient's opposite kneecap as the agency of compression, including: plaster casts, knee braces, tight bandages, or even the console of a sports car. In immobile, comatose, paralyzed or anesthetized patients, an ordinary mattress can exert enough force to injure the nerve. Prolonged squatting is another common cause of CPNFH, possibly from a combination of stretch, compression and kinking—a particular hazard for roofers, carpet layers, women who squat in labor (pushing palsy), and farmers (strawberry picker's palsy).

Sudden, forceful plantar flexion or inversion of the ankle may stretch the nerve and cause focal damage at the point where it is tethered in its passage through the peroneus longus. CPNFH is surprisingly common in patients with severe ankle injuries. Transient foot drop is reportedly common in NFL kickers (punter's palsy). Rare causes of CPNFH include true entrapment in the fibular tunnel, Baker's cyst, nerve tumor, ganglion and lipoma.

Physical examination should include detailed assessment of strength in all major lower extremity muscle groups. The status of the ankle invertors is critical information; weakness there excludes CPNFH. The examination of reflexes should include the medial and lateral hamstring jerks. The status of sensation over the lateral calf should be noted, since the lateral cutaneous nerve of the calf does not traverse the fibular tunnel (Fig. 17.4). Tenderness, spasm and range of motion of the lumbosacral spine, and the presence or absence of root stretch signs are highly relevant. Inspection for a skin dimple, discoloration or callus over the fibular head, percussion to elicit Tinel's sign, and careful palpation of the popliteal fossa and fibular head are likewise important.

The most common differential diagnostic exercise is between CPNFH and L5 radiculopathy in the patient with foot drop. The presence of back and leg pain, weakness of foot inversion, positive root stretch signs and depression of the medial hamstring reflex favor radiculopathy. The absence of pain, weakness limited to ankle eversion and foot/toe dorsiflexion, and preservation of the medial hamstring reflex favor CPNFH. The pattern of sensory changes is rarely helpful. In most patients with CPNFH a meticulous history will uncover an explanatory mechanism through external pressure or stretch.

In rare patients, sciatic neuropathy, deep peroneal neuropathy or lumbosacral plexopathy may simulate CPNFH. The development of CPNFH after seemingly trivial compression or stretch suggests an underlying vulnerable nerve syndrome. Peroneal neuropathy may rarely be the presenting feature of vasculitis. A number of generalized conditions may require consideration, especially if foot drop is bilateral, including generalized neuropathies, motor neuron disease and several types of primary muscle disease (e.g., distal myopathy, inclusion body myositis, myotonic dystrophy and scapuloperoneal syndromes).

The standard electrodiagnostic technique is to record from the EDB or tibialis anterior (TA) muscle while stimulating the peroneal nerve above and below the fibular head searching for focal slowing, temporal dispersion or conduction block. With severe neuropathies, often no M wave can be recorded from the EDB, necessitating recording from the TA. Even when an M wave can still be obtained from the EDB, it is often worth recording from the TA, as selective fascicular vulnerability can result in conduction block in fibers innervating the TA but not the EDB (8,17,48).

When stimulating in the popliteal fossa, there is a significant chance of inadvertent spread of the stimulus current to the tibial nerve, which produces spurious and confusing M wave amplitude variations. Because of the dictates of the "10 cm rule" (see above under ulnar neuropathy), many EMGers stimulate below the FH, then measure at least 10 cm into the popliteal fossa. Again, there is a trade off of experimental error against lesion detection, and the proximal stimulation in this instance can become frankly problematic because of stimulus spread. To detect spread, in addition to noting changes in M wave amplitude and waveform, it is useful to observe the motion of the foot. Peroneal stimulation will produce an extension/eversion movement. Tibial stimulation will produce plantar flexion. If both nerves are being stimulated, the foot will simply "quiver" and move neither up nor down.

Because the recording electrode over the EDB detects volume conducted depolarization in tibial innervated muscles, inadvertent spread to the tibial usually results in higher M wave amplitude on proximal than distal stimulation. The increase in amplitude is usually accompanied by a detectable change in waveform. In the presence of an accessory peroneal anomaly (about 20% of the population), the M wave is also higher with proximal stimulation, since the proximal stimulation activates more fibers innervating the EDB than does the distal stimulation, where a portion of the fibers have deviated from the main trunk and are running behind the lateral malleolus (32). Inadvertent spread to the tibial and the presence of an accessory peroneal can thus produce similar M wave amplitude changes. Features favoring an accessory peroneal are lack of change of M wave configuration, elicitation of a small amplitude M wave with stimulation posterior to the lateral malleolus and a pure dorsiflexion foot movement with proximal stimulation.

CPNFH can produce almost any combination of demyelination and axon loss, which may involve any of the target muscles to different degrees (8,17,48). The M wave amplitude with stimulation below the FH, compared with laboratory reference values or the contralateral leg, provides an index of the degree of axon loss. The difference in M wave amplitude with below FH vs. above FH stimulation reflects the degree of demyelinating neurapraxia. Slowing across the FH indicates the CV in demyelinated but not blocked fibers. Which of these features is paramount is a matter of debate. Wilbourn found that M wave amplitude changes, especially when recording from the EDB, were much more helpful than CV changes (17).

The superficial peroneal (SP) NAP is very useful in evaluating CPNFH. Although some mild, demyelinating lesions may spare the SP NAP, with lesions causing any significant axon loss this potential will be reduced in amplitude or absent. In contrast, the most common process mimicking CPNFH, L5 radiculopathy, should leave a robustly normal SP NAP.

Needle electromyography should focus not only on peroneal innervated muscles but non-peroneal L5 muscles, such as the tibialis posterior and flexor digitorum longus, and should always include the short head of the biceps femoris. Since the short head of the biceps is the only peroneal innervated muscle lying proximal to the FH; any abnormality there suggests a lesion above the midthigh. Since a lesion severe enough to cause neurapraxia or significant conduction slowing is usually severe enough to damage at least a few axons, some, occasionally many, fibrillation potentials can be seen in peroneal innervated muscles even with a primarily demyelinating CPNFH. The M wave amplitude and SP NAP amplitude are better indicators of the extent of axon loss. Wilbourn has divided CPNFH syndromes into four types, which are summarized in Table 17.4.

FACIAL NEUROPATHY

The facial nerve provides motor function to the muscles of facial expression and to certain muscles of the scalp, ear and neck, carries special sensory fibers for taste, and conveys parasympathetic fibers to the pterygopalatine and otic ganglia. After exiting the pons and traversing the cerebellopontine angle, the nerve enters the facial canal. The geniculate ganglion is located at the genu of the canal where it makes an abrupt turn posteriorly. Petrosal branches come off in the region of the ganglion to supply lacrimal and salivary glands. More distally, a branch arises to supply the stapedius muscle. Slightly more distally the chorda tympani joins the main trunk. The nerve then exits through the stylomastoid foramen, quickly gives off a branch to the posterior auricular muscle, then elaborates branches to the stylohyoid and posterior belly of the

TABLE 17.4
Patterns of Common Peroneal Neuropathy at the Fibular Head (CPNFH)

	M Wave* Amplitude Stimulating AFH	M Wave Amplitude Stimulating BFH	Amplitude of SP Sensory Potential	Needle Examination
Type 1—Common peroneal, axon loss	Decreased or absent—same potential as BFH	Decreased or absent—same potential as AFH	Decreased or absent	Denervation in common peroneal innervated muscles
Type 2—Common peroneal, conduction block	Decreased or absent	Normal	Normal	"Normal" (see text)
Type 3—Common peroneal, mixed axon loss and conduction block	Decreased or absent	Decreased, but less so than AFH	Decreased or absent	Denervation in common peroneal innervated muscles
Type 4—L5 root/deep peroneal branch axon loss lesion	Same as Type 1	Same as Type 1	Normal	Denervation either (a) involving nonperoneal L5 muscles or b) restricted to deep peroneal distribution

* Either TA or EDB. AFH, above fibular head; BFH, below fibular head; SP superficial peroneal. Modified from Wilbourn A. AAEE Case Report #12: Common peroneal mononeuropathy at the fibular head. Muscle Nerve 1986;9:825–836.

digastric. The nerve then traverses the parotid gland and ends as the superior, temporofacial and inferior cervicofacial divisions.

Acute facial neuropathy produces paralysis in a peripheral facial distribution, i.e., weakness involving both upper and lower face, frequently accompanied by retroauricular pain. Facial weakness of central origin spares the upper facial muscles. Loss of taste on the anterior two thirds of the ipsilateral tongue, hyperacusis and loss of tearing of the ipsilateral eye vary, depending on the level of the lesion in relation to the geniculate ganglion and major intracanalicular branches. The vast majority of patients with acute facial nerve paralysis have Bell's palsy, an idiopathic disorder frequently related to a preceding viral infection. Bell's palsy has almost come to serve as a generic term for any peripheral facial paralysis, and one sees occasional reference to Bell's palsy in diabetes, sarcoidosis and other conditions. The primary differential diagnostic considerations are diabetes, sarcoidosis, HIV infection, H. zoster and Lyme disease. A common problem in neonates is to distinguish obstetrical trauma to the facial nerve from Möebius syndrome.

The electrodiagnostic procedures useful for evaluating facial neuropathy include facial nerve conduction studies, blink reflexes and NEE. Facial conduction studies are done by recording from a facial muscle, usually the orbicularis oculi or nasalis, and stimulating the facial nerve either just anterior to the tragus or just below and anterior to the mastoid, noting the onset latency and M wave amplitude. Care must be taken, especially when the facial paralysis is severe, not to stimulate the masseter muscles and mistake the volume conducted masseter response for a facial response. Blink reflexes use the same recording sites, but the muscle is activated reflexly by stimulating the ophthalmic division of the trigeminal nerve at the supraorbital foramen. The afferent impulse travels along trigeminal pathways to the brainstem to activate the facial nucleus in the pons. The efferent impulse travels along the facial nerve. The early, or R_1 component of the blink reflex, follows a simple oligosynaptic route, but the late, or R_2 component, labors through a complex, polysynaptic pathway before reaching the facial nucleus. Changes in R_1 and R_2 after bilateral stimulation and recording often permit localization of the pathologic process. NEE primarily provides information about the extent of axonal disruption. It can rarely help localize the lesion, e.g., fibrillations in the posterior auricular muscle proves the lesion is not due to obstetrical trauma.

Electrodiagnostic studies in facial neuropathy occasionally serve to localize the lesion along the course of the nerve, but their primary function is prognostic (49). The M wave amplitude and the extent of changes on NEE reflect the degree of axon loss; latency determination is less useful. Since the distal stump of even a severed nerve can continue to conduct for several days, very early studies in facial neuropathy can do little more than determine, from the presence or absence of MUAPs and the status of the blink reflex, whether or not the lesion is complete. After this interval, the M wave amplitude will accurately reflect the extent of axonopathy. Fibrillation potentials will of course not appear in full flower until about three weeks. No presently available technique can accurately prognosticate in the first 24–48 hours; M wave amplitude to direct facial nerve stimulation after 5–7 days is the most reliable predictor of final outcome (49).

Key Points

- Pathological changes involving the myelin sheath are the earliest abnormality in compression or entrapment syndromes. Low force levels selectively damage the paranodal region, crucial for normal impulse conduction. Greater force levels cause segmental demyelination. Depending on the length of the segment involved, conduction velocity may simply slow or conduction may fail entirely, producing conduction block (CB). The electrodiagnostic picture is frequently a complex mixture of CB, varying degrees of focal slowing, and axon loss.

- Experimentally, acute compression neuropathies cause distortion of internodes with intussusception of one internode into the adjacent internode. In chronic compression, there is displacement of myelin from the center of the internode toward the ends. With more severe compression axonal damage occurs.

- Large nerve fibers are more susceptible to pressure than small, and peripheral fibers more vulnerable than central ones; different fascicles may exhibit different susceptibility to injury.

- Recovery after a purely demyelinating injury is generally complete within 12 weeks, although conduction abnormalities may persist. With axonal damage, recovery is more protracted. Collateral sprouts form in the periphery. Growth cones develop in the intact nerve stump and axons then regenerate at about 1–3 mm/day from the injury site to the target. Muscle fibers which have not been reinnervated within one year undergo irreversible changes.

- Seddon's system classifies traumatic nerve injuries into neurapraxia, axonotmesis and neurotmesis. Sunderland's system adds two subclasses of axonotmesis.

- Patients with generalized polyneuropathies are at increased risk of developing a superimposed compression neuropathy—the "vulnerable nerve syndrome."

- Nerve conduction studies and needle electromyography aid in the diagnosis and the management of focal neuropathies. The ideal situation for electrodiagnostic evaluation of focal neuropathy exists when one can stimulate or record proximal and distal to the lesion.

- Abnormalities of the nerve action potential (NAP) often precede abnormalities of motor conduction studies. While sensitive, however, changes in the NAP are often nonlocalizing. Motor conduction studies, while less sensitive, are usually more localizing.

- Several types of abnormalities occur. The most convincing localizing abnormalities in focal neuropathies are CB, partial or complete, or asynchronous focal slowing. In the absence of these, the probability of detecting the lesion depends on the length of nerve segment examined. Studying longer nerve segments produces lower experimental error, but may mask focal slowing. Any process producing axon loss can cause secondary slowing of CV.

- After acute nerve trauma, preserved conduction in the segment distal to the injury in the first 3–10 days may cause a misleading pattern, and pronouncements should be cautious during this interval. The greatest information would accrue from a single electrodiagnostic evaluation if done approximately 3 weeks post injury, but early studies can still provide helpful information.

- CTS, ulnar neuropathy at the elbow, peroneal neuropathy at the knee, retrohumeral radial neuropathy and facial neuropathy comprise the majority of focal neuropathies.

- CTS is often brought on or exacerbated by excessive hand/wrist/finger movements and causes a characteristic clinical picture of hand pain, numbness, and paresthesias (all usually more severe at night), along with varying degrees of weakness. The earliest electrodiagnostic change is prolongation of the median NAP latency. With more severe involvement, there is loss of NAP amplitude, prolongation of the motor distal latency, and the development of denervation in thenar muscles.

- Ulnar neuropathy at the elbow is the most tricky and problematic of all focal neuropathies. Anatomical factors account for much of the susceptibility of the ulnar nerve to injury at the elbow, with at least three potential sites of compression. The terms tardy ulnar palsy and cubital tunnel syndrome invite confusion and should be avoided. Ulnar conduction velocity varies markedly with elbow position. The most logical position for conduction studies is moderate flexion from the horizontal, with the forearm at an angle of 70–90° from full extension. The most convincing localization results from multiple internally consistent abnormalities.

- Compression of the radial nerve in the retrohumeral spiral groove causes weakness of all muscles distal to the triceps and sensory loss in the superficial radial nerve distribution. Apparent weakness of the interossei and of thumb abduction may cause mislocalization. The primary electrodiagnostic abnormality in most cases is conduction block and slowing involving the spiral groove segment.

- The peroneal nerve at the fibular head (FH) is prone to injury because of the lack of protective covering and tethering in its passage through the peroneus longus muscle. Habitual leg crossing and prolonged squatting are the classic causes of compression. The most common differential diagnostic exercise is between peroneal neuropathy and L5 radiculopathy in the patient with foot drop. Almost any combination of demyelination and axon loss can involve any of the target muscles to different degrees. The superficial peroneal NAP is critical for adequate evaluation.

- The vast majority of patients with acute facial nerve paralysis have Bell's palsy, an idiopathic disorder frequently related to a preceding viral infection. Electrodiagnostic studies in facial neuropathy occasionally serve to localize the lesion along the course of the nerve, but their primary function is prognostic. CMAP amplitude to direct facial nerve stimulation after 5–7 days is the most reliable predictor of final outcome.

References

1. Campbell WW. Diagnosis and management of common compression and entrapment neuropathies. Neurol Clin North Am 1997;15:549–567.
   Compression and entrapment neuropathies are common conditions whose diagnosis and management is usually straightforward, but atypical presentations and unusual features require constant vigilance and circumspection. The experimental pathology of acute and chronic compression differ. The clinical pathophysiology includes demyelination, remyelination, axon loss and regeneration. The electrodiagnostic features can be a complex combination of focal slowing, conduction block and axon loss. Selective fascicular involvement and the vulnerable nerve syndrome may further complicate the clinical picture. Anatomical details are important. Careful clinical evaluation can help greatly in narrowing the differential diagnosis and focusing electrodiagnostic and imaging studies. Conservative therapy often suffices, but surgery plays a major role in management of entrapment neuropathies. The most common focal neuropathies are carpal tunnel syndrome, ulnar neuropathy at the elbow and peroneal neuropathy at the fibular head, but many other focal neuropathies due to external compression or entrapment may occur. Rational management depends on accurate localization. The differential diagnosis includes musculoskeletal conditions, plexopathies, radiculopathies and occasionally central nervous system dysfunction.

2. Dawson DM. Entrapment neuropathies of the upper extremities. N Engl J Med 1993;329:2013–2018.
   The three syndromes described in this article were chosen from about a dozen nerve-compression disorders that affect the arm from scapula to digits. They illustrate the range of problems encountered. Some syndromes of nerve compression have important implications for musicians, athletes, and those who place stress on the upper limbs through heavy or repeated use. Well-designed prospective trials are clearly needed to expand our knowledge of the prevention and treatment of the entrapment neuropathies. Much more needs to be known about the long-term natural history of these disorders, since prevention is usually possible.

3. Levin KH. Common focal mononeuropathies and their electrodiagnosis. J Clin Neurophysiol 1993;10:181–189.
   Common focal mononeuropathies can be produced by compression, entrapment, crush, stretch, and transection. Injuries resulting from acute or chronic repetitive external pressure produce compressive neuropathy, whereas chronic distortion or angulation of the nerve from an internal source produces entrapment neuropathy. Electrodiagnostic techniques used in the electromyographic laboratory include nerve conduction studies and the needle electrode examination. Measurement of distal latency, amplitude, conduction velocity, and identification of focal conduction block may help in the localization of focal mononeuropathies. The needle electrode examination gives further information about the distribution of nerve damage, the activity and chronicity of axon loss, and can sometimes date the onset of injury. Basic clinical features and electrodiagnostic patterns are discussed for median, ulnar, radial, and peroneal neuropathies. Differential diagnosis is provided, and illustrative cases are presented.

4. Brown WF, Dellon AL, Campbell WW. Electrodiagnosis in the management of focal neuropathies: the "WOG" syndrome. Muscle Nerve 1994;17:1336–1342.
   The role of electrodiagnosis in managing patients with focal neuropathies is discussed from the differing perspectives of a peripheral nerve surgeon and a practitioner of electrodiagnostic medicine. Both clinical evaluation and electrodiagnosis are useful methodologies, each having limitations. Dr. Dellon labels the overreliance on electrodiagnosis as the "WOG" (Word of God) syndrome, and describes its signs, symptoms, and treatment. Dr. Brown contends Dr. Dellon's crusade is misdirected. The exchange is an eloquent polemic on the virtues and foibles of these different approaches to evaluating peripheral nerve function and the imperative to practice them in a complementary rather than a contentious manner.

5. Dawson DM, Hallett M, Millender LH. Entrapment Neuropathies. 2nd ed. Boston: Little Brown, 1990.

6. Parry GJ. Pathophysiological mechanisms in peripheral nerve injury. In: 1996 AAEM plenary session: physical trauma to peripheral nerves. Rochester: Am Assoc Electrodiag Med, 1996.
   A discussion of the mechanisms of acute and chronic nerve compression, their similarities and differences. Acute compression includes acute physiological block and acute demyelinative block. Chronic compression may produce demyelination or axon loss. The mechanisms whereby compression produces transient symptoms and pathological changes involves a combination of mechanical distortion of the nerve, producing demyelination, and obliteration of the vasa nervorum, causing ischemic axonal degeneration. Which of these mechanisms predominates in a given nerve injury depends on multiple factors including the nature of the compression, the compressing force, the duration of compression, and probably other factors. The role of ischemia in chronic compression is controversial; Dr. Parry makes a convincing case for a greater role than is usually accepted. See also Miller RG. AAEE minimonograph #28: injury to peripheral motor nerves. Muscle Nerve 1987;10:698–710.

7. Wertsch JJ, Oswald TA, Roberts MM. Role of intraneural topography in diagnosis and localization in electrodiagnostic medicine. PMR Clin North Am 1994;5(3):465–475.
   See Chapter 16 for abstract.

8. Brown WF, Watson BV. Quantitation of axon loss and conduction block in peroneal nerve palsies. Muscle Nerve 1991;14:237–244.
   A comparison of conduction in motor fibers supplying the extensor digitorum brevis (EDB) and anterior lateral compartment (AL) muscles to determine whether there were any differences in the relative proportions of degenerated and blocked nerve fibers between the longer EDB and shorter AL fibers. In almost every case the percentage of motor fibers undergoing axonal degeneration was greatest in EDB fibers. Conversely, the percentage of conduction block was greatest in the AL motor fibers. As clinical recovery is dependent on AL muscles rather than EDB, electrophysiological study of the relative proportions of degenerated and blocked fibers in the former should provide a more reliable measure of outcome than similar studies of EDB. Conduction velocity distal to the fibular head was not slowed despite the large loss of EDB motor fibers. Evidence for selective involvement of the larger myelinated fibers is, therefore, lacking. The location of the major conduction abnormalities was in almost every case between the mid-fibular head and popliteal fossa.

9. Campbell WW, Pridgeon RM, Riaz G, et al. Sparing of the flexor carpi ulnaris in ulnar neuropathy at the elbow. Muscle Nerve 1989;12:965–967.
   A common misconception attributes sparing of the flexor carpi ulnaris (FCU) in ulnar neuropathy at the elbow (UNE) to its innervating branch arising "at or above the elbow." We examined the relationship of FCU branches to the medial epicondyle (ME) and humeroulnar aponeurotic arcade (HUA) in 30 cadaver elbows. In only three did the first FCU branch arise at or proximal to the ME. In 36 UNE cases with fibrillations in the first dorsal interosseous, the FCU was normal in 10, mildly abnormal in 11, and severely abnormal in 15. FCU involvement correlated with the severity of the neuropathy and with whether compression was retroepicondylar or at the HUA. We conclude that sparing of the FCU in UNE is unrelated to the level of origin of its innervating branch, but rather is related to the internal neural topography and to the severity and level of compression.

10. Stewart JD. The variable clinical manifestations of ulnar neuropathies at the elbow. J Neurol Neurosurg Psychiatry 1987;50:252–258.
    In twenty-five cases of ulnar neuropathy at the elbow, the involvement of the fibers from three sensory and to four motor branches were examined clinically and, where possible, electrophysiologically. Of the sensory fibers, those from the terminal digital nerves were most commonly involved. The fibers to the hand muscles were much more frequently involved than those to the forearm muscles. These findings suggest that in ulnar neuropathies at the elbow there is variable damage to the fascicles within the nerve.

11. Campbell WW, Sahni SK, Pridgeon RM, et al. Intraoperative electroneurography: management of ulnar neuropathy at the elbow. Muscle Nerve 1988;11:75–81.
    At the elbow, the ulnar nerve may be compressed either in the retrocondylar groove or at the cubital tunnel. Optimal surgical therapy should be directed at the specific site of involvement. Intraoperative electroneurography performed in conjunction with 19 ulnar nerve explorations helped localize the precise site of compression. Of the primary procedures, abnormality was at the retrocondylar groove in 9, cubital tunnel in 4, both locations in 3, and at an unusual distal point in 1; 12 anterior subcutaneous transpositions, 4 cubital tunnel releases, and 1 distal decompression resulted. Intraoperative studies helped

identify residual compression in two patients undergoing re-exploration. Although routine electrodiagnosis may localize an ulnar neuropathy to the elbow, reliably separating retrocondylar from cubital tunnel compression is more difficult. Preoperatively, percutaneous serial short increment studies were more accurate than simple "inching" in predicting the site of compression.

12. Brown WF, Ferguson GG, Jones MW, et al. The location of conduction abnormalities in human entrapment neuropathies. Can J Neurol Sci 1976;3:111–122.
Direct stimulation of 23 median, 13 ulnar, and 2 peroneal nerves at the time of surgical exploration was used to locate and characterize the conduction abnormalities in the nerves. The most frequent location of the major conduction abnormalities in the median nerve was in the first 1–2 cm distal to the origin of the carpal tunnel. In the ulnar nerve the important conduction abnormalities were located most frequently in the segments 1 cm proximal and distal to the medial epicondyle. In the peroneal nerve the major conduction abnormalities occurred proximal or distal to the entry point of the common peroneal nerve into the peroneus longus muscle.

13. Kimura J. The carpal tunnel syndrome: localization of conduction abnormalities within the distal segment of the median nerve. Brain 1979;102:619–635.
Palmar stimulation, including serial stimulation in 1 cm increments, was used to assess median nerve conduction across the carpal tunnel. In 52% of affected nerves, there was a sharply localized latency increase across a 1 cm segment, most commonly 2–4 cm distally to the origin of the transverse carpal ligament. Using these techniques, sensory or motor conduction abnormalities were found in all but 8% of hands. Without palmar stimulation, however, and additional 19% of hands would have been regarded as normal.

14. Campbell WW, Pridgeon RM, Sahni KS. Short segment incremental studies in the evaluation of ulnar neuropathy at the elbow. Muscle Nerve 1992;15:1050–1054.
Conventional electrodiagnosis may localize an ulnar neuropathy to the general region of the elbow. Separating retroepicondylar compression from compression by the humeroulnar aponeurotic arcade from compression by the deep flexorpronator aponeurosis is more difficult. In 35 patients, we compared localization by conventional inching (stimulating stepwise around the elbow searching for focal conduction block or differential slowing) to localization by a more quantitative short segment incremental stimulation (SSIS) technique assessing latency change over consecutive 1 cm segments. Results of percutaneous studies were compared with findings of intraoperative electroneurography. SSIS identifies compression levels more accurately than standard inching. SSIS and intraoperative electroneurography correlate highly, but not perfectly. Studies confined to a search for conduction block or differential slowing are limited by the low incidence of conduction block in chronic compression neuropathies.

15. Stewart JD. Focal peripheral neuropathies. 2nd ed. New York: Raven Press, 1993.
See also Wilbourn AJ, Gilliatt RW. Double crush syndrome: a critical analysis. Neurology 1997;49:21–29.

16. Campbell WW, Geiringer SR. The value of inching techniques in the diagnosis of focal nerve lesions. Muscle Nerve 1997;in press:
A debate on the utility of short segment studies in the evaluation and management of focal neuropathies. See Chapter 9 for summary.

17. Wilbourn AJ. AAEE case report #12: common peroneal mononeuropathy at the fibular head. Muscle Nerve 1986;9:825–836.
Common peroneal mononeuropathies, usually located at the fibular head, are one of the many causes of foot-drop, a condition often evaluated in the electromyography laboratory. If appropriate nerve conduction studies are performed and particular muscles studied on needle myography, a satisfactory diagnosis can almost always be provided for what may be a perplexing problem clinically. With all peroneal mononeuropathies, the compound muscle action potential amplitude of the peroneal motor tibialis anterior nerve conduction studies, stimulating distal to the fibular head, is a semi-quantitative measure of the number of viable fibers supplying the tibialis anterior and allows for accurate prognostication regarding the foot-drop.

18. Kopell HP, Thompson WAL. Peripheral entrapment neuropathies. 2nd ed. Huntington: Robert E. Krieger, 1976.

19. Olney RK, Hanson M. AAEE case report :15: ulnar neuropathy at or distal to the wrist. Muscle Nerve 1988; 11:828–832.
A 56-year-old woman developed insidiously progressive, painless weakness of her left hand. Clinical and electrodiagnostic abnormalities were limited to the motor function of the hand, with the hypothenar less affected than more distal ulnar muscles. Compression of the distal ulnar nerve by a ganglionic cyst was surgically relieved and there was postoperative improvement. The electrodiagnosis of ulnar neuropathy at or distal to the wrist is reviewed together with relevant anatomic and clinical aspects of these uncommon lesions.

20. Campbell WW. AAEE case report #18: ulnar neuropathy in the distal forearm. Muscle Nerve 1989;12:347–352.
A 66 year old professional golf instructor developed pain, numbness and weakness in an ulnar distribution, but the lesion could not be localized to either elbow or wrist by routine nerve conduction techniques. Stimulation along serial 1-cm increments in the distal forearm disclosed a point of focal conduction block approximately 7 cm proximal to the ulnar styloid. At surgery, the flexor carpi ulnaris was enlarged, with muscle fibers extending all along the normally tendinous distal portion. A dense fibrovascular band coursed from the ulnar artery to the abnormal muscle, compressing the adjacent ulnar nerve. Intraoperative electroneurography precisely localized the area of conduction abnormality and helped identify the band as the compressing structure. Within 2 months following surgical decompression there was complete resolution of conduction block with excellent clinical recovery.

21. Lagueny A, Deliac MM, Deliac P, et al. Diagnostic and prognostic value of electrophysiologic tests in meralgia paresthetica. Muscle Nerve 1991;14:51–56.
Electrophysiologic diagnosis of unilateral meralgia paresthetica is usually assessed by side-to-side comparison of SNAP amplitudes, SNCVs, and SEP latencies following stimulation of lateral femoral cutaneous nerves. To determine the relevance for diagnosis of these tests and side-to-side comparison, the results were compared in patients with unilateral meralgia paresthetica and normal subjects. The long-term outcome was also considered, in order to determine whether electrophysiologic findings contribute to the prognosis. In this study, SNAP amplitude comparison was more useful than SNCV and SEP latency comparisons. However the value of the SNAP amplitude on the affected side, just as the results of the other tests,

was not found to be predictive of the outcome. Also the results of the tests depend on the methods used and on the nerve's route.

22. Fardin P, Negrin P, Sparta S, et al. Posterior interosseous nerve neuropathy. Clinical and electromyographical aspects. Electromyogr Clin Neurophysiol 1992;32:229–234.
A clinical and EMG examination of 37 patients with posterior interosseous nerve neuropathy: 5 cases had a traumatic origin, 4 iatrogenic, and 28 non-traumatic. One of the non-traumatic cases had a lipoma, and another had chondroma. In the other cases, nerve entrapment at the level of the arcade of Frohse could be presumed. Acute or chronic onset of the deficit was probably due to repeated pronation-supination hand movements. A motor deficit in finger extension together with a radial deviation of the wrist, was typical. Surprisingly about 50% of the non-traumatic cases showed some sensory disturbance at the forearm, wrist or hand. EMG examination was useful to establish the entity and topography of the deficit.

23. DeLisa JA, Saeed MA. AAEE case report #8: The tarsal tunnel syndrome. Muscle Nerve 1983;6:664–670.
The diagnosis of TTS may be difficult. The symptoms are often vague and the physical findings and signs are not as definite as those noted in the analogous carpal tunnel syndrome. Electrodiagnostic testing may be essential in making the diagnosis. The addition of the averaged sensory latency with the medial and lateral plantar compound nerve action potentials should greatly increase the specificity of diagnosing this condition. The etiologies for the syndrome are multiple, even though this is a relatively rare condition. The results of surgical decompression are variable, but are usually satisfactory enough to justify this mode of therapy if the patient has not responded to conservative treatment.

24. Wertsch JJ. AAEM case report #25: anterior interosseous nerve syndrome. Muscle Nerve 1992;15:977–983.
A case study of a patient with thumb weakness noted while gardening, with difficulty pulling weeds because of an inability to get a firm grip when using the thumb. Physical examination showed weakness of the flexor pollicis longus and flexor digitorum profundus to the index finger. There was no other weakness and no clinical sensory deficit. Electrodiagnostic studies revealed normal median motor and sensory nerve conduction studies with needle examination abnormalities noted only in the flexor pollicis longus, flexor digitorum profundus, and pronator quadratus. The literature on anterior interosseous nerve syndrome (AINS) is reviewed. It is important to differentiate those with idiopathic AINS as part of a neuralgic amyotrophy picture from those with an anatomic cause such as a fibrous band or anomalous muscle. Electrodiagnostic examination can be useful to help make this distinction.

25. David WS, Doyle JJ. Segmental near nerve sensory conduction studies of the medial and lateral plantar nerves. Electromyogr Clin Neurophysiol 1996;36:411–417.
A tarsal tunnel syndrome can be difficult to diagnose: electrophysiologic corroboration is important and has therapeutic implications. Conventional electrodiagnostic techniques are insensitive: motor latency abnormalities exist in only 52%; sensory responses are frequently absent (a nonlocalizing finding). Additionally, previously described near nerve techniques do not isolate CV measurement to the short segment across the flexor retinaculum, which would theoretically improve sensitivity. This study describes a technique which allows for the determination of segmental sensory CVs of the medial and lateral plantar nerves, both below and across the flexor retinaculum.

26. Rosenbaum RB, Ochoa JL. Carpal tunnel syndrome and other disorders of the median nerve. Boston: Butterworth-Heinemann, 1993.

27. Leifer D, Cros D, Halperin JJ, et al. Familial bilateral carpal tunnel syndrome: report of two families. Arch Phys Med Rehabil 1992;73:393–397.
A report of two families in which multiple members had bilateral carpal tunnel syndromes. The pattern was consistent with autosomal dominant inheritance. Electrophysiologic studies on nine of the 15 patients demonstrated bilateral pathology of the median nerves at the wrist in all but one patient, without evidence for subclinical, generalized peripheral neuropathy. Quantitative sensory testing in two cases corroborated the absence of peripheral neuropathy. 5 of 6 patients who underwent carpal tunnel release improved.

28. Ross MA, Kimura J. AAEM case report #2: the carpal tunnel syndrome. Muscle Nerve 1995;18:567–573.
CTS results from entrapment or compression of the median nerve within the carpal tunnel. Electrodiagnostic studies may objectively document the presence of median neuropathy within the carpal tunnel and help distinguish CTS from other disorders such as cervical radiculopathy, neurogenic thoracic outlet syndrome, proximal median nerve compression syndromes, and polyneuropathy which may either mimic or occasionally coexist with CTS. Recording median nerve responses with wrist and palm stimulation allows determination of the wrist segment conduction velocity which is a more sensitive nerve conduction parameter than wrist latency measurements. Electrodiagnostic testing permits estimation of severity and relative contribution of axonal versus demyelinative nerve injury. This information can provide prognostic information and help guide therapeutic decisions.

29. Stevens JC. AAEE minimonograph #26: The electrodiagnosis of carpal tunnel syndrome. Muscle Nerve 1987;10:99–113.
The electrodiagnosis of carpal tunnel syndrome is reviewed, including discussions of old and new techniques of motor and sensory nerve conduction, anomalous innervation, needle electrode examination, and one method of examining a patient with suspected carpal tunnel syndrome. The results of electromyographic testing of 505 patients with carpal tunnel syndrome in Rochester, Minnesota, from 1961 to 1980 are compared with results from previous studies. In the appendixes, a method of performing median motor and sensory nerve conduction studies and Mayo Clinic normal values are provided.

30. Healton EB, Savage DG, Brust JC, et al. Neurologic aspects of cobalamin deficiency. Medicine (Baltimore) 1991;70:229–245.
A review of 153 episodes of cobalamin deficiency involving the nervous system seen in 143 patients over a 17-year period. Pernicious anemia was the most common underlying cause of the deficiency. Neurologic complaints, most commonly paresthesias or ataxia, were the first symptoms of Cbl deficiency in most episodes. The median duration of symptoms before diagnosis and treatment with vitamin B12 was 4 months, although long delays in diagnosis occurred in some patients. Diminished vibratory sensation and proprioception in the lower extremities were the most common objective findings. A wide variety of neurologic symptoms and signs were encountered, however, including ataxia, loss of cutaneous sensation, muscle weakness, diminished or hyperactive reflexes, spas-

ticity, urinary or fecal incontinence, orthostatic hypotension, loss of vision, dementia, psychoses, and disturbances of mood. Multiple neurologic syndromes were often seen in a single patient. In 42 (27.4%) of the 153 episodes, the hematocrit was normal, and in 31 (23.0%), the mean corpuscular volume was normal. In nonanemic patients in whom diagnosis was delayed, neurologic progression frequently occurred although the hematocrit remained normal. In 27 episodes, the serum cobalamin concentration was only moderately decreased (in the range of 100–200 pg/ml) and in 2 the serum level was normal. The extent of neurologic involvement after treatment was strongly related to that before therapy as well as to the duration of symptoms.

31. Jablecki CK, Andary MT, So YT, et al. Literature review of the usefulness of nerve conduction studies and electromyography for the evaluation of patients with carpal tunnel syndrome. AAEM Quality Assurance Committee. Muscle Nerve 1993;16:1392–1414.
   The sensitivity and specificity of nerve conduction studies (NCS's) and electromyography for the diagnosis of carpal tunnel syndrome (CTS) were evaluated by a critical review of the literature. With a search of the medical literature in English through May 1991, 165 articles were identified and reviewed on the basis of six criteria of scientific methodology. The findings of 11 articles that met all six criteria and the results of 48 additional studies that met four or five criteria are presented. The study concludes that median sensory and motor NCS's are valid and reproducible clinical laboratory studies that confirm a clinical diagnosis of CTS with a high degree of sensitivity and specificity. Clinical practice recommendations are made based on a comparison of the sensitivities of the several different median nerve conduction study (NCS) techniques.

32. Gutmann L. AAEM minimonograph #2: important anomalous innervations of the extremities. Muscle Nerve 1993;16:339–347.
   See Chapter 10 for summary.

33. Redmond MD, Rivner MH. False positive electrodiagnostic tests in carpal tunnel syndrome. Muscle Nerve 1988;11:511–518.
   Of 50 normal subjects, 23 (46%) had at least one false positive electrodiagnostic test for carpal tunnel syndrome (CTS). 30% of the subjects had an abnormal median to ulnar sensory amplitude ratio of less than 1.1. In 7 subjects 8 extremities (14%) revealed prolonged residual latencies, and 4 extremities in 4 subjects (8%) had a difference of 0.4 msec between the median and ulnar palmar sensory latencies. The results of this study indicate that certain reported criteria for CTS are abnormal in a high percentage of normal subjects, thereby making them of limited value in the diagnosis of CTS. Of all the criteria studied, it appears that the comparison of the median to ulnar sensory latency across the carpal tunnel is of greatest potential value. However, even here a more conservative difference of 0.5 msec between median and ulnar nerves must be used to avoid false positive tests for CTS.

34. Rivner MH. Statistical errors and their effect on electrodiagnostic medicine. Muscle Nerve 1994;17:811–814.
   See Chapter 5 for abstract.

35. Miller RG. AAEM case report #1: ulnar neuropathy at the elbow. Muscle Nerve 1991;14:97–101.
   A patient with bilateral UNE complicated by anomalous innervation is presented. The electrodiagnostic approach to patients with this neuropathy is reviewed emphasizing new devel-opments. The interpretation of the findings in this patient centers around issues of pathophysiology and methodology.

36. Campbell WW, Greenberg MK, Krendel DA, et al. Literature review of the usefulness of nerve conduction studies and electromyography in the evaluation of patients with ulnar neuropathy at the elbow. Muscle Nerve, in press.
   The sensitivity and specificity of nerve conduction studies and needle electromyography for the diagnosis of ulnar neuropathy at the elbow were evaluated by a critical review of the literature. With a search of the medical literature in English through January 1996, 101 articles were identified and reviewed on the basis of six criteria of scientific methodology. The findings of 6 articles that met all 6 criteria and the results of 22 additional studies that met 4 or 5 criteria are presented. We concluded that ulnar sensory and motor nerve conduction studies and needle electromyography are valid and reproducible clinical laboratory studies that confirm a clinical diagnosis of ulnar neuropathy at the elbow with a high degree of sensitivity and specificity. Clinical practice recommendations are made based on the literature review of several different ulnar nerve conduction study techniques.

37. Folberg CR, Weiss AP, Akelman E. Cubital tunnel syndrome. Part I: Presentation and diagnosis. Orthop Rev 1994;23:136–144.
   Cubital tunnel syndrome (used in the generic sense, WWC) is the second most common entrapment neuropathy after carpal tunnel syndrome. This condition may arise without an obvious compression injury or may be secondary to nerve enlargement or narrowing of the cubital tunnel. Clinical symptoms, radiographic and electrophysiologic findings, and the differential diagnosis of cubital tunnel syndrome are reviewed. See also Orthop Rev 1994;23:233–241.

38. Kincaid JC. AAEE Minimonograph #31: The electrodiagnosis of ulnar neuropathy at the elbow. Muscle Nerve 1988;11:1005–1015.
   Electrodiagnostic testing is useful in evaluating ulnar nerve elbow lesions. A flexed elbow seems preferable for conduction studies, since it eliminates the elbow segment slowing found in normals done in the extended position. Slowing of the motor velocity in the elbow segment was the most frequent abnormality in this study. Sensory conduction studies and needle examination each provided additional helpful data. Latency to ulnar forearm muscles and "inching" stimulations around the elbow are techniques that also deserve to be included in our standard armamentarium.

39. Campbell WW, Pridgeon RM, Riaz G, et al. Variations in anatomy of the ulnar nerve at the cubital tunnel: pitfalls in the diagnosis of ulnar neuropathy at the elbow. Muscle Nerve 1991;14:733–738.
   Two processes account for most instances of ulnar neuropathy at the elbow: compression in the retroepicondylar groove, and compression by the humeroulnar aponeurotic arcade joining the two heads of the flexor carpi ulnaris. While conventional electrodiagnostic criteria may localize an ulnar neuropathy to the elbow, separating retroepicondylar compression from humeroulnar arcade compression is more difficult. In 130 cadaver elbows, we examined the relationships between the medial epicondyle, flexor carpi ulnaris, and ulnar nerve. The humeroulnar arcade lay from 3 to 20 mm distal to the medial epicondyle, the intramuscular course of the nerve through the flexor carpi ulnaris ranged from 18 to 70 mm, and the nerve exited the flexor carpi ulnaris 28 to 69 mm distal to the medial

epicondyle. In 6 specimens, dense fibrous bands bridged directly between the medial epicondyle and the olecranon proximal to the cubital tunnel proper; accessory epitrochleoanconeus muscles were present in 14 specimens: both may cause ulnar neuropathy at the elbow. Anatomical variations may contribute to the difficulty in separating causes of ulnar neuropathy at the elbow.

40. Apfelberg DB, Larson SJ. Dynamic anatomy of the ulnar nerve at the elbow. Plast Reconstr Surg 1973;51:76–81.
The topical and intraneural anatomy of the ulnar nerve at the elbow is reviewed. Dissection of 15 cadaver elbows indicated that the nerve is compressed, stretched, and impacted against unyielding structures during elbow flexion. Measurements of the changing anatomy of the elbow during flexion has allowed a descriptive model of the dynamic stresses on the ulnar nerve.

41. Campbell WW, Pridgeon RM, Sahni SK. Entrapment neuropathy of the ulnar nerve at its point of exit from the flexor carpi ulnaris muscle. Muscle Nerve 1988;11:467–470.
The ulnar nerve normally enters the flexor carpi ulnaris (FCU) proximally and anteriorly between the humeral and ulnar heads of the muscle. After an intramuscular course of several centimeters, the nerve exits the FCU distally to lie in a tissue plane between the FCU and the flexor digitorum profundus (FDP). A patient with ulnar neuropathy studied by intraoperative electroneurography demonstrated major focal conduction block at the point where the nerve exited the FCU. A fivefold increase in amplitude and reversal of a dispersed, irregular compound muscle action potential to a more normal configuration occurred with stimulation just distal to the point of exit. There was no evidence by inspection, probing, or electroneurography of compression in the retrocondylar groove or at the cubital tunnel. In a series of 100 cadaver dissections, the intermuscular septum between FCU and FDP was thick and tough in several specimens. This septum may represent a site of ulnar nerve entrapment.

42. Miller RG. The cubital tunnel syndrome: diagnosis and precise localization. Ann Neurol 1979;6:56–59.
The cubital tunnel syndrome is a subgroup of ulnar neuropathies arising at the elbow, with nerve entrapment under the aponeurosis connecting the two heads of the flexor carpi ulnaris muscle. To separate this condition more clearly from tardy ulnar palsy, the clinical and electrophysiological features of 9 patients are presented, 6 of whom had the syndrome bilaterally. There was no history of trauma and no clinical or roentgenographic evidence of joint deformity in any of the patients. In 9 of the 15 ulnar nerves, abnormal conduction was localized to the level of the cubital tunnel (1.5 to 3.5 cm distal to the medial epicondyle). The findings were confirmed intraoperatively in 7 patients and corresponded to a tight band compressing the ulnar nerve and causing narrowing at the cubital tunnel with swelling proximally. This syndrome represents a common and distinct subgroup of ulnar neuropathies at the elbow.

43. Mackinnon SE, Dellon AL. Surgery of the peripheral nerve. New York: Thieme, 1988;235–247.

44. Feindel W, Stratford J. The role of the cubital tunnel in tardy ulnar palsy. Can J Surg 1958;1:287–300.
In 3 patients, "tardy ulnar palsy" was relieved by simply incising the aponeurotic arch between the two heads of the flexor carpi ulnaris muscle. The term cubital tunnel is proposed for this opening through which the nerve passes. . .the roof is formed by the aponeurosis of the flexor carpi ulnaris and the floor by the medial ligament of the elbow joint. The clinical picture may be termed the cubital tunnel syndrome. . .(to be) distinguished from those cases of tardy ulnar palsy. . .related to gross distortion of the elbow joint.

45. Campbell WW, Buschbacher R, Pridgeon RM, et al. Selective finger drop in cervical radiculopathy: the pseudoulnar claw hand. Muscle Nerve 1995;18:108–110.
A review of the mechanism of the claw or griffe deformity and the syndrome of pseudoulnar claw hand due to posterior interosseous neuropathy. 4 patients with cervical spine disease had a finger drop primarily involving the ring and small fingers which resembled an ulnar or pseudoulnar claw hand.

46. Payan J. An electromyographer's view of the ulnar nerve. J Bone Joint Surg Br 1986;68:13–15.
An editorial reviewing the electromyographer's contribution to management of ulnar neuropathy at the elbow. Reviews diagnostic problems, electrophysiological techniques, indications for operation and surgery and its complications. Replete with pithy observations, a classic.

47. Brown WF, Watson BV. AAEM case report #27: acute retrohumeral radial neuropathies. Muscle Nerve 1993;16:706–711.
Acute radial neuropathies localized to the retrohumeral course of the radial nerve are common. Most individuals fully recover within a matter of days or, at the most, a few weeks. In a few, recovery may take longer and occasionally remains incomplete. In almost all instances the site of injury to the radial nerve can be accurately localized to the region of the spiral groove and the relative contributions of conduction block and axonal degeneration assessed using electrophysiologic techniques.

48. Sourkes M, Stewart JD. Common peroneal neuropathy: A study of selective motor and sensory involvement. Neurology 1991;41:1029–1033.
A prospective clinical and electrophysiologic study of common peroneal (CP) neuropathy to evaluate the extent of involvement of the muscles and cutaneous areas. In 22 patients, seven had more weakness clinically in muscles innervated by the deep peroneal nerve than in those innervated by the superficial peroneal nerve; the reverse never occurred. Statistical paired comparisons confirmed the tendency in the entire group of patients for weakness to be greater in muscles supplied by the deep peroneal nerve. On EMG, denervation was more often present and of more marked degree in muscles supplied by the deep peroneal nerve. Motor nerve conduction studies indicated axonal damage and focal demyelination with similar frequency. Sensory deficits varied in the three areas supplied by the cutaneous branches of the CP nerve: five patients had involvement of all three areas, 11 of two areas, two of one area, and four had no sensory deficit. The most likely explanation for these findings is differing degrees of damage to individual fascicles within the CP nerve.

49. Gilchrist JM. AAEM case report #26: seventh cranial neuropathy. Muscle Nerve 1993;16:447–452.
A patient with acute, bilateral facial palsies had a lymphocytic meningitis, history of tick bites, and lived in an area endemic for Lyme disease, which was ultimately confirmed by serology. Electrodiagnostic investigation, including facial motor nerve study, blink reflex and electromyography of facial muscles indicated a neurapraxic lesion on the right and an axonopathic lesion on the left. The clinical course was consistent with these findings as the right side fully recovered and the left remained plegic. The clinical features of Lyme associated facial neuritis

are reviewed, as is the electrodiagnostic evaluation of facial palsy. The best prognostic indicator is the amplitude of the direct motor response after 5–7 days of illness. When the M wave amplitude is < 10% of that on the healthy side, maximum recovery will be delayed 6–12 months and function will be moderately or severely limited. If the amplitude is 10–30% of the healthy side, recovery may take 2–8 months with mild to moderate residua. If the amplitude is > 30% of normal, full complete recovery can be expected at 2 months after onset.

18

Neuromuscular Transmission Disorders

In the nervous system presynaptic electrical events are converted to chemical events at the synapse, and converted again into electrical events postsynaptically. The neuromuscular junction (NMJ) is a specialized synapse through which electrical events in the peripheral nerve are transduced into chemical events, which then induce depolarization of the postsynaptic muscle membrane, which in turn induces muscle contraction. Disturbed neuromuscular transmission (NMT) results in several different clinical disorders, which are characterized primarily by weakness and fatigability. Electrodiagnostically, NMT disorders produce characteristic changes that allow them to be distinguished from diseases of nerve and from diseases of muscle. This chapter will review the anatomy, physiology, pharmacology and pathology of the NMJ, review the electrodiagnostic techniques that are most useful in evaluating suspected NMT disorders, and conclude with a discussion of the more common and interesting clinical syndromes.

Anatomy and Physiology of the NMJ

As the motor nerve approaches its termination point it divides into fine terminal arborizations. Each twig ends by forming a bulbous swelling, the terminal bouton. The primary synaptic cleft separates the terminal bouton from the postsynaptic muscle membrane, which is in turn divided into a number of secondary synaptic clefts, or junctional folds. The postsynaptic muscle membrane is blanketed by a dense array of nicotinic acetylcholine receptor (AChR) molecules, which extend down into the secondary synaptic clefts. In addition, acetylcholine esterase (AChE) molecules lurk on both presynaptic and postsynaptic membranes (Fig. 18.1A).

The terminal bouton is a beehive of metabolic activity. It is packed with cytoskeletal proteins, mitochondria, and numerous chemicals. Most importantly, it contains vesicles that are membrane-bound collections of acetylcholine (ACh). In the cytoplasm of the terminal bouton, ACh is packaged into these vesicles, which then migrate to and collect at primary release sites, or active zones. The active zones of the presynaptic membrane tend to line up opposite the secondary synaptic clefts of the postsynaptic membrane. The active zones are the sites of both exocytosis of ACh vesicles and ingress of calcium (1).

The presynaptic membrane contains voltage-gated calcium channels (VGCC). In response to nerve depolarization, these channels permit the influx of calcium into the presynaptic terminal, which greatly facilitates the release of neurotransmitter with the next nerve impulse. Magnesium has the opposite effect and inhibits the release of transmitter. After a nerve impulse, calcium diffuses out of the nerve terminal and is largely gone within 100–200 msec. The precise timing of the calcium fluxes is extremely important in determining the response to different rates of repetitive nerve stimulation (RNS). After depolarization, the calcium influx rate exceeds the efflux rate, leading to an accumulation following a series of nerve action potentials. Repetitive nerve impulses also increase the mobilization of ACh vesicles toward the active zones. As a result sustained voluntary muscle contraction has a transient facilatory effect on transmitter release. This effect also comes into play in determining the responses to repetitive stimulation and the phenomena of facilitation and post-activation exhaustion.

Vesicles of ACh are released sporadically and irregularly while the membrane is at rest and are released in flurries when the terminal bouton undergoes depolarization. Each vesicle contains about 5,000–10,000 molecules of ACh. Upon activation the vesicles fuse with the presynaptic membrane and pour their ACh contents out into the primary synaptic cleft. The molecules of ACh diffuse rapidly across the primary synaptic cleft and into the secondary synaptic clefts. Anywhere two molecules of ACh encounter an AChR, a chemical interaction takes place which causes opening of sodium channels in the postsynaptic membrane, producing a brief non-propagated localized depolarization. The depolarization produced by the contents of one vesicle is referred to as a miniature end-plate potential (MEPP).

ACh molecules in the cytoplasm of the terminal bouton are divided into different compartments, pools or "stores." Some ACh is free in the cytoplasm and some is packaged into vesicles, not all of which have migrated to the active zones. Those vesicles at the active zones constitute the readily releasable, or immediately available, store. The mobilization store consists of those vesicles near but not at the active zones. The main store, the largest pool, consists of vesicles randomly in the cytoplasm. At any time there are approximately 200,000–300,000 vesicles in the terminal bouton: about 1,000 vesicles in the readily releasable store, 10,000 in the mobilization pool, and the rest in reserve in the main store. Following a nerve impulse, several seconds are required to completely replenish

Normal Neuromuscular Junction

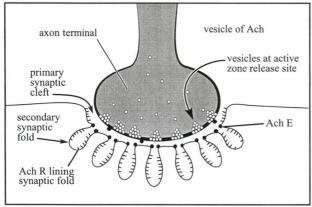

Neuromuscular Junction in Myasthenia Gravis

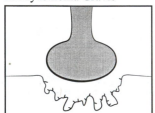

Neuromuscular Junction in Lambert-Eaton Syndrome

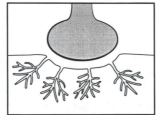

FIGURE 18.1   A. A normal neuromuscular junction. B. A neuromuscular junction in myasthenia, degraded by immunologic attack, simplified and depopulated of AChR. C. A neuromuscular junction in Lambert-Eaton syndrome, highly complex and convoluted with increased surface area.

the immediately available store. This can lead to a temporary decrease in quantal release following serial stimulation.

Freeze fracture techniques show the AChR as large particles concentrated on the tips of junctional folds, extending about halfway down the stalk of the junctional folds. The AChR is a complex structure, consisting of two alpha subunits and beta, gamma and delta subunits, plus an ion channel. The main immunogenic region (MIR) of the AChR is the site that is attacked by autoantibodies in the majority of cases of MG (2).

The 5,000–10,000 molecules of ACh contained within a single vesicle are also referred to as a quantum. The release of one quantum of ACh results in the opening of approximately 1,500 channels in the postsynaptic membrane and produces a MEPP of about 0.5–1.0 millivolt. The summation of many MEPPs produces a localized, nonpropagated depolarization in the region of the end plate, referred to as an end plate potential (EPP). The EPPs in turn summate, and if above threshold spawn a propagated, all or none muscle fiber action potential. The summated electrical activity of hundreds to thousands of muscle fiber action potentials produces the motor unit action potential (MUAP), which can be recorded by needle electromyography.

About 15–20 millivolts is required to produce an EPP. Approximately 60 quanta are released when a nerve impulse invades the terminal bouton. This vast oversupply of quanta and of AChR beyond the minimum required for depolarization is referred to as the safety factor for NMT (3). One of the hallmarks of NMT disorders is diminution in this safety factor. Presynaptic and postsynaptic NMT disorders alter the safety factor through different mechanisms. The events of normal neuromuscular transmission are summarized in Figure 18.2. Defects in neuromuscular transmission may develop at a number of points in the process.

Pathology

Myasthenia gravis (MG) and the Lambert-Eaton myasthenic syndrome (LEMS), the two most common disorders of the NMJ, are both due to autoantibodies. In MG, antibodies to the AChR, in concert with complement, attack and destroy the postsynaptic membrane. The membrane is depopulated of receptors, the primary synaptic cleft is widened, and the secondary synaptic folds disappear. The membrane is simplified and undergoes a drastic reduction in its total surface area, and in the number of AChR (Fig. 18.1B) Following a nerve impulse, the ACh molecules released from the synaptic terminal may diffuse away without ever encountering an AChR to interact with. There is loss of the luxuriant overabundance of ACh-AChR interactions that characterize normal NMT. Safety factor is reduced and transmission may fail. Transmission fails initially under conditions of stress, i.e., after exercise or with increased temperature, producing the characteristic fatigability and fluctuating deficits of NMT disorders. Light microscopy of muscle shows few abnormalities in MG, although occasional round cell collections (lymphorrhages) may be visible. Electron microscopy, however, reveals the devastated postsynaptic membrane.

In LEMS, autoantibodies directed against the VGCC attack the ACh release sites at the active zones on the presynaptic membrane, resulting in a failure of ACh release. The rate of normal spontaneous release decreases, and there is impaired release following a nerve impulse. Deprived of ACh molecules, the postsynaptic membrane begins to increase its surface area in an attempt to increase the likelihood of ligand-receptor interactions. The secondary synaptic clefts become deeper and tertiary clefts develop. The result is a highly complex, convoluted postsynaptic membrane of greatly increased surface area, quite the opposite pathology of MG (Fig. 18.1C). In both MG and LEMS, safety factor declines because there is a decreased number of ACh-AChR interactions; because of a lack of AChR in MG and because of a paucity of ACh molecules in LEMS.

MG and LEMS produce characteristic changes in MEPPs. In MG, only a few ACh-AChR interactions occur after release of the 5,000–10,000 molecules of ACh which comprise a quantum. The result is a decrease in the amplitude of the MEPP, but since ACh release mechanisms are unaffected there is no change in frequency. In LEMS, MEPP amplitude is normal because there is abundant opportunity for ACh-AChR interactions with release of a quantum, but the quanta are released sporadically and at a decreased rate. As a result, the MEPP in LEMS is of normal amplitude but is greatly reduced in frequency (Table 18.1). The gold standard for studying and characterizing NMT disorders is microelectrode analysis of MEPPs in intercostal muscle.

Neuromuscular Junction Pharmacology

The effects of ACh are normally terminated by the hydrolytic action of AChE. Up to half the released ACh

FIGURE 18.2 Schematic of the events of normal neuromuscular transmission.

Events of Normal Neuromuscular Transmission
(events outside box occur in the synaptic cleft)

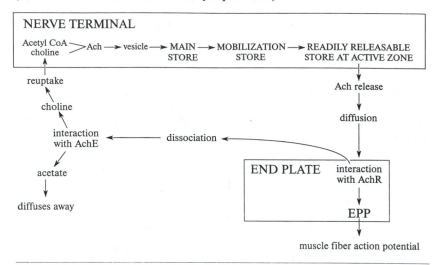

Ach, acetylcholine; AchR, acetylcholine receptor, AchE, acetylcholinesterase; EPP, end plate potential

TABLE 18.1
Electrophysiologic Features of Selected Neuromuscular Transmission Disorders

	Normal	*Myasthenia Gravis*	*Lambert-Eaton Myasthenic Syndrome*	*Mild Botulism*	*Severe Botulism*	*Infantile Botulism*	*Hypermagnesemia*
MEPP frequency	Normal	Normal	Decreased	Decreased	Decreased	Decreased	Decreased
MEPP amplitude	Normal	Decreased	Normal	Normal	Normal	Normal	Normal
CMAP amplitude to single stimulus	Normal	Normal	Low	Normal	Low	Low	Low
Decrement @ 2–3 Hz	No	Yes	Yes	Minimal or absent	Yes	Inconsistent	Yes
Response to 2 Hz RNS after brief isometric exercise or rapid RNS	No change or pseudo-facilitation	Repair of decrement	Marked facilitation	Marked facilitation which may persist	Insignificant facilitation	Marked facilitation, may require 3–10 sec tetanization	Facilitation
Post activation exhaustion	No	Yes	Yes	No	No	No	No

may be hydrolyzed in the primary synaptic cleft before ever reaching the postsynaptic membrane. The surviving ACh molecules react with AChR. After receptor-ligand binding and interaction, there is dissociation, which frees the ACh molecule to interact with another receptor. Without the action of AChE a given molecule of ACh could interact with multiple receptors. AChE cleaves the ACh molecule into choline and acetyl moieties. The choline is taken back up into the presynaptic terminal for resynthesis into ACh, and the acetyl moiety diffuses away. Anti-acetylcholinesterase (anti-AChE) agents are used in the treatment of NMT disorders to increase the likelihood of receptor-ligand interactions by inhibiting the hydrolysis of ACh. A rapidly acting agent (edrophonium) is used in diagnostic testing for MG, and slower acting agents, e.g., pyridostigmine or prostigmine, are used orally or parenterally for treatment.

An excess of ACh can be deleterious to NMT by over stimulating the postsynaptic membrane and keeping it in a perpetually depolarized state. The resting membrane potential cannot be re-established and action potentials cannot be generated, producing weakness, usually accompanied by other evidence of excess ACh activity at muscarinic junctions (e.g., lacrimation, miosis, diarrhea). Chemical warfare nerve agents and organophosphate insecticides are anti-AChE compounds which paralyze by this action. Myasthenic patients sometimes develop increased weakness. It can be difficult to tell whether the weakness is due to an exacerbation of the underlying disease (myasthenic crisis) or to excess effects of anticholinesterase medications (cholinergic crisis).

Neuromuscular blocking agents (NMBAs) are frequently used to paralyze patients in the operating room or ICU (4). There are two varieties of NMBAs. Competitive, or non-depolarizing, agents produce neuromuscular blockade by inhibiting the interaction between ACh and AChR. These agents bind to the AChR molecule and prevent access of the ligand. The prototypic competitive NMBA is curare. Depolarizing NMBAs produce blockade by simulating the action of ACh, producing sustained depolarization of the postsynaptic membrane, causing the same effects as that of overdose with anti-AChE agents. The prototypic depolarizing NMBA is succinylcholine. Many newer agents are available (5).

Overview of the Clinical Manifestations of NMT Disorders

The cardinal manifestation of NMT disorders is weakness. The character and distribution of the weakness and associated manifestations vary among the different conditions. Fatiguable weakness varies and fluctuates with the level of activity and often with the time of day. Patients with MG may have near normal strength with a single muscle contraction, but rapidly become weak with successive contractions. Patients with LEMS may have weakness on the initial contraction, then show increasing strength with successive contractions, followed by relapse of the weakness. These fluctuations in power reflect the physiological changes in the NMJ with rest and with muscle contraction.

In the typical case of MG, weakness prominently involves the eyelids and extraocular muscles, resulting in fluctuating ptosis and diplopia, which varies with the time of day and with activity of the muscles. The ptosis and diplopia are frequently less severe in the morning and grow worse as the day wears on. Ptosis not present at rest can often be elicited by sustained up-gaze, which fatigues the eyelid levators. Where involvement is limited to the extraocular muscles, eyelids and orbicularis oculi the condition is termed *ocular* or *purely ocular* myasthenia (6,7). With some patients the disease may never progress beyond this point. In most, generalized myasthenia eventually develops, with eye symptoms remaining prominent. However, generalized myasthenia with prominent ocular involvement is a vastly different entity therapeutically and prognostically than purely ocular myasthenia with no generalized involvement. The reason for the predilection of MG to involve the extraocular muscles has been a subject of long-standing conjecture (6).

LEMS, in contrast, does not have a predilection for extraocular muscles and tends to involve primarily the hip and shoulder girdles. In most patients, the weakness first appears in the hip and thigh musculature. When the disease is more advanced the shoulder girdle is also weak and generalized weakness may develop, but the eye muscles are relatively spared. Because LEMS is a presynaptic disorder, the patient may become stronger with a series of successive muscle contractions. After five or six quick contractions, a weak muscle may briefly return to nearly normal power. In contrast, myasthenics get weaker with successive contractions. Reflexes in MG are usually normal. In LEMS, the reflexes in the affected areas are usually depressed or absent. However, a 10-second contraction of an affected muscle, e.g., quadriceps, may briefly restore the reflex. Botulism, another presynaptic disorder with impaired ACh release, has a predilection for the eyes and respiratory muscles. Patients usually present with eye muscle involvement, then rapidly develop generalized weakness with respiratory insufficiency. Occasional patients may develop eye muscle weakness, then go into respiratory failure without a great deal of extremity weakness.

Electrodiagnosis of Neuromuscular Transmission Disorders

The primary electrodiagnostic studies used for evaluation of NMT disorders are repetitive nerve stimulation and single-fiber EMG (SFEMG) (8,9). These studies can help define the presence, type, and severity of a neuromuscular junction disorder, provide helpful information regarding therapy, and objectively monitor the response to treatment. Single fiber studies, the most sensitive procedure, are also the most technically demanding. Repetitive stimulation studies are simpler and easier to perform, and more specific for localizing a disorder to the postsynaptic or presynaptic membrane.

REPETITIVE NERVE STIMULATION (RNS) STUDIES

The abnormal response to RNS in MG was first described in 1895 by Jolly, and the procedure is sometimes referred to as the Jolly test or Jolly reaction. RNS studies are performed by stimulating a motor nerve repetitively at different frequencies while recording a serial train of M waves from its target muscle. A train of stimuli is delivered at a rate of anywhere from 2 to 50 Hz, and the amplitudes of the series of evoked M waves are noted. RNS may be carried out in the rested muscle or at various intervals after exercise to further characterize transmission.

The most useful information is usually obtained with a relatively low stimulation frequency, 2–3 Hz (Fig. 18.3). Stimulation at faster frequencies may not detect faulty transmission because transmitter release will be enhanced due to residual calcium in the presynaptic terminal. Frequencies slower than this may mask a transmission disorder because the very low frequency of stimulation, less than 2 Hz, permits mobilization of ACh into the immediately available store with enhancement of transmission. The safety factor for NMT is at its nadir at relatively slow stimulation frequencies. The ideal frequencies lie in between the low frequencies (< 2 Hz), which permit mobilization of transmitter into the readily available store, a slowly developing but long lasting process, and the fast frequencies (> 5 Hz), which permit a stimulus to arrive while the calcium concentration in the presynaptic terminal is still high from the preceding stimulus, a rapidly developing but rapidly dissipating process. The ideal frequency which exploits the low safety factor and brings out abnormalities to best advantage is in the range of 2 to 3 Hz. Stimulation at higher frequencies can sometimes yield additional useful information, especially in presynaptic disorders, but is quite painful. The information obtained with more rapid repetitive stimulation can often be obtained just as readily, and much less painfully, with brief isometric exercise (10).

Presynaptic and postsynaptic NMT disorders produce RNS abnormalities that have some features in common and some features that are different (Table 18.1). Both types produce a decremental response at 2 to 5 Hz stimulation. The decrement tends to stabilize after the 4th or 5th response and then return toward baseline. The abnormal decrement in both types repairs after brief isometric contraction. This repair eliminates the abnormal decremental response in postsynaptic disorders. In presynaptic disorders, there is not only repair but a marked facilitation of

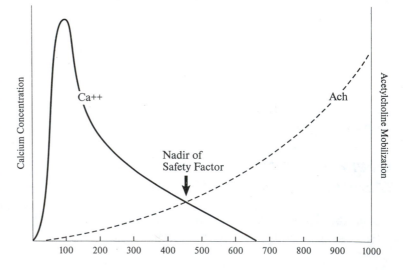

FIGURE 18.3 Curves showing why 2–3 Hz is the optimal stimulation frequency for demonstrating a decremental response in neuromuscular transmission disorders. The calcium concentration in the nerve terminal rises quickly following a nerve impulse, briefly facilitating transmitter release, then decays very rapidly. Transmitter mobilization begins and rises slowly. With very slow stimulation, transmitter mobilization is active and no decrement occurs. With rapid stimulation, calcium facilitates transmitter release and no decrement occurs. The falling curve of calcium concentration crosses the rising curve of transmitter mobilization at about 300–500 msec, which equates to a stimulation frequency of 2–3 Hz, where safety factor is lowest and neuromuscular transmission most vulnerable to failure.

the response, so that the immediate (3–10 sec) post-exercise M wave may be 2 to 5 times larger than the baseline M wave. After the period of activation, whether done by isometric exercise or by rapid repetitive stimulation, the decrement returns, then becomes even more pronounced about 2 to 3 minutes after activation. This phenomenon is referred to as post-activation, post-exercise or post-tetanic exhaustion, occurs for reasons which are not entirely clear, and probably corresponds closest to the fatigable weakness of MG (1). It is most prominent following voluntary or electrical tetanization for 15–30 sec. After about 10 minutes, the M wave amplitude and degree of decrement are about the same as they were in the rested muscle.

Postsynaptic disorders have a fairly normal M wave amplitude to a single shock. There may be a mild diminution in amplitude as compared to normal for a particular patient, but this is subtle and seldom falls outside the normal range. In contrast, the baseline M wave amplitude to a single shock in presynaptic disorders is markedly reduced; one of the hallmarks of presynaptic disorders, and sometimes the first diagnostic clue, is a low baseline M wave. The low amplitude baseline M wave in a presynaptic disorder demonstrates further decrement to low frequency RNS. In a postsynaptic disorder, more rapid stimulation, above 5 Hz, will tend to eliminate any obvious decrement and maintain a fairly normal appearing response. In contrast, in a presynaptic disorder the M wave amplitude shows marked facilitation at faster frequencies, with a tremendous increase in amplitude with successive stimuli. This increase in M wave amplitude may reach 5 or 10 fold.

Rarely other conditions can cause abnormal NMT, but they tend to follow either a pre- or a post-synaptic pattern, as above. Botulism and hyper-magnesemia are presynaptic disorders. Secondary disturbances of NMT may sometimes accompany other neuromuscular disorders, such as ALS and polymyositis, primarily because of the erratic performance of immature, regenerating NMJs. The pattern under these conditions generally resembles that of a postsynaptic disorder.

The decrement is calculated as the difference between the amplitude or area of the first response and that of the lowest ensuing response, generally the fourth or fifth, divided by the amplitude or area of the first response:

$$\text{decrement} = \frac{\text{As} - \text{Ai}}{\text{Ai}} \times 100\%$$

where As = amplitude or area of the smallest M wave and Ai = amplitude or area of the mital M wave.

Decrements up to 8–10% may occur in controls, even more in some muscles (11). The degree of normal decrement varies from muscle to muscle (1,11). Reproducible decrements in excess of 10% are generally indicative of a NMT disorder. Abnormal decremental responses are more likely to be found in warm muscles, proximal muscles, and clinically involved muscles. The pattern of: 1) decrement to 2–3 Hz stimulation in the rested muscle; 2) repair of the decrement (facilitation) after brief isometric exercise; 3) increase in the decrement at 2–5 minutes (postactivation exhaustion); and 4) return to baseline after 10 minutes, is highly suggestive of MG. Elimination of the decrement by intravenous edrophonium is further confirmation. Other disorders only rarely will produce this specific sequence of changes. In presynaptic disorders such as LEMS, the decremental response is more widespread, often detectable in distal as well as proximal muscles.

RNS studies must be done with careful attention to technical detail (3). Technical errors can either produce false positive or false negative studies. Whenever a study appears to show an increment or decrement, it is a wise first assumption that the abnormality is due to artifact. Only when that possibility has been eliminated, and when the abnormal appearing response is reproducible, can one feel confident that a NMT disorder is present. Useful criteria for excluding artifactual changes include: reproducible response; envelope shape of the response and a cycle of changes which conforms to a pattern seen in disease; absence of sudden, erratic, random variations between responses; concordant amplitude and area changes; and response to edrophonium (3).

One of the most common sources of false positive studies is electrode movement. Rapid successive contraction of the muscle due to the repetitive stimulation, or voluntary movement by the patient, can produce changes in electrode position which alter the M wave amplitude. Electrode movement induced M wave amplitude changes are erratic and do not follow any pattern. Although there may appear to be a decrement when the sweeps are superimposed, when the tracings are examined as a series of responses, the variation in amplitude is random and follows no particular pattern. Electrode movement can be minimized by using the least possible amount of electrode gel to increase friction between the electrode and the muscle, by securing the recording and stimulating electrodes well with tape, and by immobilizing the tested part. Intramuscular needle electrodes should never be used for RNS studies, but subcutaneous EEG needle electrodes may be feasible (1).

Submaximal stimulation may produce a low amplitude M wave, and an inconsistent response to RNS, so supramaximal stimulation is an absolute requirement. Muscles innervated by diseased nerves may demonstrate abnormal neuromuscular transmission, particularly in the presence of significant denervation atrophy. Screening nerve conduction studies should establish normality of the nerve-muscle axis to be studied to exclude pre-existent and unrelated disease, such as carpal tunnel syndrome or ulnar neuropathy, before RNS is performed.

Another common technical error is low temperature, often unrecognized, in the tested muscle. The safety factor for transmission increases as the temperature decreases, and low temperature may mask a transmission disorder. Temperature effects at the NMJ are complex; a simplistic but effective way to recall the phenomenon is to imagine decreasing activity of the AChE enzyme with decreasing temperature. Any muscle studied, but particularly hand or foot muscles, should be thoroughly warm at the time of study. In MG, proximal muscles, such as biceps, deltoid, trapezius or facial muscles, have a higher yield in demonstrating abnormal decremental responses. Whether this is due to higher resting temperature, greater tonic resting activity, more involvement in the disease process or some other factor is not clear (1).

Stimulation rates above approximately 10 Hz may produce a phenomenon know as pseudo-facilitation: an increase in the amplitude of the M wave accompanied by a decrease in the duration, without any change in the total area under the curve. Pseudo-facilitation is due to synchronization of the action potentials in muscle fibers, not to any increase in the number of muscle fibers activated. It can produce an increase in M wave amplitude of 50%, which should not be mistaken for abnormal pathological facilitation (3).

NEEDLE ELECTRODE EXAMINATION (NEE) AND SINGLE FIBER EMG (SFEMG)

NEE in most patients with a NMT disorder is normal. In some patients who have significant blocking and transmission failures (see below), a detectable beat to beat variability in the amplitude or configuration of a MUAP can be appreciated at low levels of contraction. Small amplitude, short duration or polyphasic, so-called "pseudomyopathic" units are occasionally seen. Fibrillations can occur in a rare patient with MG, but they are sparse and infrequent and concentrated in bulbar and paraspinal muscles. In botulism, more abundant but frequently tiny fibrillation potentials can occur (1).

The spontaneous, beat to beat variability in the amplitude of a MUAP in NMT disorders is due to the differing number of muscle fiber action potentials that comprise the summated MUAP. When NMT fails at a particular NMJ, no muscle fiber action potential occurs, and that fiber makes no contribution to the MUAP. In a severe NMT disorder, the MUAP may be made up of a different population of muscle fibers with each firing, as random fibers suffer erratic transmission failures and recoveries. In SFEMG, these transmission failures are referred to as blocks. It is the degree of blocking on SFEMG studies that correlates best with MUAP variability on NEE, a decremental response on RNS and with clinical weakness and fatiguability (12).

The details of SFEMG are beyond the scope of this discussion; the following will touch the highlights. See Sanders and Stålberg for a succinct review and Oh for a definitive discussion (1,13). SFEMG studies are done with a special needle electrode that has a side port recording surface 25 μm in diameter, and using a 500 Hz low frequency filter. These features help to focus the recording so that the action potentials of only a handful of muscle fibers are picked up. Muscle fibers belonging to the same motor unit fire in near synchrony. Minor variations in the time the action potentials reach the recording electrode occur because of small differences in the distance to the electrode, as well as differences in the diameter or length of terminal nerve twigs, in the conduction velocity of the muscle fibers and the rise time of the EPP. These variables combine to interfere with the synchrony of firing between fibers. If one fiber of a pair is used to trigger the sweep (the triggering potential), the variations in the arrival time of the second fiber of the pair (the slave or jittering potential) causes a slight instability referred to as jitter. In normal muscle, the jitter is in the range of 10–55 μsec.

NMT disorders cause two types of abnormality detectable by SFEMG: increased jitter and blocking. The paucity and variability of ACh-AChR interactions produces an erratic EPP, which may rise more slowly than normal with one firing, lackadaisically evoking a muscle fiber action potential when interactions are sparse, then rise more rapidly with the next contraction when interactions are more abundant, bringing the muscle fiber to threshold more quickly. The variability in EPP rise time causes increased jitter. On those occasions when ACh-AChR interactions are too few to bring the muscle fiber to threshold, the second potential fails to fire at all, termed an impulse block. Jitter is expressed as a value termed the mean consecutive difference (MCD), the mean difference between consecutive interpotential intervals.

The normal jitter value varies with age and from muscle to muscle; reference data are available for most commonly studied muscles (14). An SFEMG study assesses 20 fiber pairs. A pair is considered abnormal if the jitter exceeds the reference value for the muscle under study, or if there is blocking. Up to 10%

of pairs may be abnormal, including blocking, even in normal muscle. A study is considered abnormal if more than 10% of the pairs are abnormal, or if the mean jitter of all 20 pairs exceeds the reference value for the mean MCD of the studied muscle. A muscle could be declared abnormal because of a high mean MCD even though all individual jitter values fell within the normal range, although in practice this rarely occurs. Obtaining 20 good pairs is often very challenging because of the patient's inability to maintain steady, low level contraction, fatigue (patient's or examiner's), frequent blocking, incidental tremor, or other variables (1). Fatiguing and warming the muscle before examination can make the study less of an ordeal.

Increased jitter and blocking can occur whether the disturbance in NMT is the primary process, as in MG or LEMS, or is secondary to some other neuromuscular disorder. Degenerating or immature, regenerating NMJs may display variable, sometimes unreliable, transmission. Unstable NMJs occur in neurogenic disorders and in some myopathies. Ephaptic transmission may also play a role. Because of the minor, secondary abnormalities of NMT that commonly occur as part of both neurogenic disorders and myopathies, abnormal jitter and blocking is not specific for a NMT disorder. An abnormality of the routine, screening NEE (that should precede the SFEMG), or an abnormal fiber density (see below), may signal the presence of such an underlying disorder. The examiner must always bear in mind that SFEMG is sensitive for detecting NMT disorders, but is not specific.

Another parameter determined by SFEMG is fiber density—the mean number of potentials picked up by the recording electrode at each insertion. Normally, a given insertion detects only a single potential from a motor unit. With careful technique and a cooperative patient, some insertions will achieve needle orientations that pick up two fiber potentials—a pair. Rarely, an insertion will detect three potentials—a triplet. When the muscle under study has undergone reinnervation and the architecture of the motor unit has been altered, the SF electrode may pick up pairs, triplets or multiplets with many insertions. An increase in fiber density can occur in neurogenic disorders, especially motor neuron disease, or in myopathies, especially muscular dystrophy. In neurogenic disorders, the motor unit architecture has been altered because of sprouting and reinnervation; in myopathies, because of fiber splitting, segmental necrosis and the other factors that cause fibrillation potentials and occasional long duration, polyphasic units in myopathy (see Chapters 8 and 19 for further details). An increase in fiber density correlates with fiber type grouping on muscle biopsy, and is a clue that any abnormal jitter

or blocking detected could be secondary to some other disease process and not a NMT disorder. Neurogenic blocking, or group blocking, refers to the simultaneous disappearance of two or more of the jittering potentials from a multiplet, and implies conduction failure at a bifurcation in a reinnervating sprout supplying the blocking potentials.

DISORDERS OF NEUROMUSCULAR TRANSMISSION

Numerous conditions can disturb NMT. The most common conditions encountered clinically are myasthenia gravis and the Lambert-Eaton myasthenic syndrome. The latter has proved an unfortunate choice of words, as the unsophisticated often refer to the patient with vague complaints and findings as possibly having a myasthenic syndrome, when they mean equivocal or minimal myasthenia gravis. In fact, the term myasthenic syndrome refers to a very specific set of clinical, electrophysiological and immunological findings. Other rare disorders that can cause clinically significant NMT disorders include botulism, hypermagnesemia, and exposure to some toxins. Secondary, usually mild, abnormalities of NMT can occur in a variety of neuromuscular disorders.

MYASTHENIA GRAVIS (MG)

Three types of MG are generally recognized: an acquired, autoimmune form, which is most common; a transient neonatal form; and the various syndromes of congenital MG (15). The acquired, autoimmune form, hereinafter referred to simply as MG, results from a complement mediated, autoantibody attack on the postsynaptic membrane (16,17). The transient neonatal variety results from passive, transplacental transfer of autoantibody from an affected mother to an otherwise normal infant, and is usually mild and of brief duration (18). The congenital myasthenic syndromes are a complex group of disorders with several different types of NMT defects (19). MG affects both sexes and all age groups, but with a predominance of younger females and older males. Young females often carry the HLA-B8-DR3 haplotype. There is a significant association with pathology in the thymus gland.(20) Thymic hyperplasia occurs in most young patients. Thymoma occurs in approximately 10% of MG patients, primarily in older males. MG occasionally makes its appearance after removal of a thymoma. There is an increased incidence of thyroid disease, connective tissue disorders and other autoimmune conditions in both patients and their families.

Classical manifestations include weakness which varies with the time of day, increasing with fatigue and decreasing with rest, accompanied by fluctuating ptosis, diplopia, dysarthria and dysphagia. Physical signs may include variable and fatigable ptosis—present at rest or brought out or worsened by sustained upgaze or the application of a warm compress to the eyelid; relieved by rest or the application of a cold pack. Diplopia or extraocular movement limitations may be present in primary gaze or brought out by sustained eccentric gaze. MG can mimic almost any eye movement limitation, including third or sixth nerve palsy or internuclear ophthalmoplegia (myasthenic pseudoINO). Eye closure is usually weak. Speech may be indistinct and nasal, growing worse with prolonged talking or counting. The original patient with MG (described in 1685) became "mute as a fish" with prolonged talking. Weakness tends to involve proximal more than distal extremity muscles, and both flexors and extensors of the neck. With mild disease, weakness may be subtle and best brought out by repetitive contractions or sustained outstretch or arms or legs. In a small minority of patients, the oculobulbar muscles are spared (21). The differential diagnosis of MG includes a horde of neuromuscular and nonneuromuscular conditions. A minimal list includes thyroid eye disease, brainstem disease, mitochondrial myopathy, inflammatory myopathy, oculopharyngeal dystrophy, motor neuron disease, and cranial nerve compressive lesions (22–24).

The diagnosis of MG rests on several lines of evidence: the clinical demonstration of weakness made worse with activity and relieved by rest, pharmacologic testing, AChR antibody assays, and electrodiagnostic testing (25). Seybold recently reviewed the sensitivity, specificity and cost of the various elements of a workup for suspected MG (Table 18.2) (15). The conundrum in MG involves a tradeoff of sensitivity and specificity of the various tests. A typical pattern of abnormality on RNS and positive AChR antibodies are very specific, but of a lower sensitivity, especially in ocular MG. SFEMG is highly sensitive, and may be the only abnormal test in ocular MG, but lacks specificity. Pharmacologic testing and SFEMG run the risk of false positives; RNS and serologic testing run the risk of false negatives, especially in ocular MG. A related issue is technical difficulty and availability. RNS tests are not technically demanding as long as good, basic procedure is followed; they are readily available. SF studies are very demanding, and are not widely available. In the final analysis, the diagnosis rests on the aggregate clinical picture, with the results of all procedures and analyses placed in proper clinical context (26). For example, failure to detect a decrement when recording from a cool, distal muscle in a

TABLE 18.2
Approximate Sensitivity and Specificity of Tests for Myasthenia Gravis

Disorder/test	Sensitivity	Specificity
Generalized myasthenia gravis		
Tensilon test	0.96	0.93
Repetitive nerve stimulation	0.84	0.91
Single fiber EMG	0.96	*
AchR antibody	0.88	0.97
Ocular myasthenia gravis		
Tensilon test	0.83	0.85
Repetitive nerve stimulation	0.44	0.94
Single fiber EMG	0.88	*
AchR antibody	0.63	0.98

* Not determined, but least specific of all.
Modified from Seybold ME. Myasthenia gravis: Diagnostic and therapeutic perspectives in the 1990s. Neurologist 1995;1:345–360.

patient with ocular MG is of little significance in ruling out the diagnosis.

RNS studies are the mainstay of the electrodiagnostic evaluation of suspected MG; studies are positive in approximately 60–70% of patients with generalized disease (1,15). The yield drops in patients with purely ocular MG to <50% (27). Careful attention to technical details is critical, as discussed above. Cool, strong and distal muscles are least likely to demonstrate a decrement, so muscle selection and warming are pivotal. If at least two clinically weak muscles, at least one of which is proximal, are studied with proper warming, the sensitivity is 80+% in generalized MG (15). The diagnostic sensitivity of RNS is directly related to disease severity. The likelihood of an abnormal response increases progressively, from least in ocular MG to maximal in severe, generalized disease (1). The yield of the test also varies with the compulsiveness with which it is conducted and analyzed (1). Efforts to increase the yield of RNS studies, such as with double step or ischemic RNS, or the regional curare test, as well as ancillary tests such as stapedial fatigue, have been largely supplanted by SFEMG.

RNS studies are reasonably specific (90+%). Other neuromuscular disorders can produce a decremental response, but only rarely does it precisely simulate the pattern of MG. To review, the characteristic RNS picture in moderate, generalized MG is: decrement of 10% or greater in the rested muscle, repair of the decrement with brief (10–30 sec) isometric exercise, postactivation exhaustion 2–3 min after exercise, and a return to baseline after 10 minutes. Elimination of the decrement with edrophonium lends further confirmation. Occasional patients have atypical responses to RNS, such as marked facilitation after exercise or a low baseline M wave amplitude. With assessment of the responses to both low and high rate RNS, several patterns of abnormality have been described as consistent with MG; an atypical pattern of response to RNS does not exclude the diagnosis (1). The pattern of abnormality may vary somewhat with disease severity. In patients with severe disease, the decrement may fail to repair with brief exercise, a decremental response may occur to high as well as low rates of stimulation, and postactivation exhaustion may be more difficult to elicit. More prolonged exercise (30–60 sec) may bring out postactivation exhaustion when the disease is mild and the decrement in the rested muscle equivocal.

The NEE in most myasthenics is normal, or shows only beat to beat variability in the amplitude or configuration of a given MUAP at low levels of contraction, as discussed above. However, confusion can arise due to unusual EMG features in occasional patients. Patients with severe disease may have short duration, polyphasic potentials mimicking myopathy. The lymphorrhages and random fiber necrosis seen on biopsy suggest that some secondary minimal myopathic element may occur in some patients. Some patients with long-standing disease may develop a degree of muscle atrophy and have minimal neurogenic abnormalities on NEE. Most authorities believe fibrillations do not occur in MG, but scattered, low grade fibrillations have been reported, especially in bulbar and paraspinal muscles in older patients, or in atrophic muscles of patients with very long-standing, severe disease (1). As a general rule, fibrillations should be considered as consistent with MG only with great reluctance.

SFEMG is very sensitive for the diagnosis of MG; abnormality is detected in 85–90% of patients with ocular MG and in 90–95% of patients with generalized disease. SFEMG is particularly useful for excluding MG: if the jitter is normal in a muscle with definite weakness, MG is effectively excluded. Abnormalities are not specific, however, as discussed, and increased jitter in a weak muscle does not prove the weakness is due to MG. Although SFEMG can be carried out on virtually any muscle (including the anal sphincter!), the muscles most commonly studied are the extensor digitorum communis (EDC) and the frontalis (13). The EDC is usually tested first if generalized disease is suspected. If the EDC is normal, the frontalis is usually examined next. The frontalis is often examined first in ocular MG. Abnormalities in the EDC can be detected in the majority of patients who clinically

suffer from purely ocular disease. The incidence of abnormality is related to disease severity—it is greatest in generalized MG, less in ocular MG and least when the disease is in remission. SFEMG abnormalities correlate imprecisely with severity in a given patient, although decreasing jitter values do roughly parallel clinical improvement. Clinical weakness, and the decrement on RNS, correlate best with the number of pairs which demonstrate blocking.

Jitter and blocking in MG become worse with prolonged activation of a pair, or as the firing rate increases—the effects of neuromuscular fatigue. The classic SFEMG pattern in MG is thus: increased jitter with or without blocking, increasing jitter with a higher discharge rate, and normal fiber density (1).

AntiAChE drugs can become problematic in evaluating suspected MG. They may mask the decrement on RNS studies, and can rarely normalize the SFEMG in patients with mild generalized or purely ocular disease (3). Therapeutic AChE blockade commonly produces fasciculations, which could prove confusing in some patients.

LAMBERT-EATON MYASTHENIC SYNDROME (LEMS)

The clinical and electrophysiological differences between MG and LEMS are summarized in Table 18.3. The autoantibody attack against the VGCC in LEMS produces not only weakness and fatigability, but involvement of muscarinic synapses leads to characteristic signs and symptoms of dysautonomia. Patients frequently have dry mouth, as well as impotence, gastroparesis, constipation, and orthostasis. In males, most cases of LEMS are due to an underlying small cell lung carcinoma (SCLC). In females, about 50% of cases are due to underlying neoplasm, while the remainder appear to represent a primary autoimmune disease. A classic example of LEMS would be: older male; underlying, sometimes not yet diagnosed SCLC; weakness primarily in the hips and thighs which improves with successive contractions; depressed or absent knee jerks which may transiently reappear after brief, isometric quadriceps contraction or repeated taps; minimal ptosis and ophthalmoparesis; and accompanying dysautonomia, especially dry mouth and impotence. Complaints of weakness and fatigue often overshadow demonstrable weakness, probably because of the recruitment phenomenon. The Tensilon test is positive in most patients, although the response is usually not as dramatic as in MG. Serologic testing for VGCC antibodies is available on a limited basis. The differential diagnosis includes MG, inflammatory myopathy, peripheral neuropathy, and primary autonomic failure, among others.

TABLE 18.3
Clinical, Electrophysiologic, and Pharmacologic Comparison Between Myasthenia Gravis and Lambert-Eaton Syndrome

	Myasthenia Gravis	*Lambert-Eaton Syndrome*
Clinical features		
Onset	⅔ of women before 40 yr	After 40 yr
Sex	Women:men, 4:3	Men:women, 5:1
Symptoms	Diplopia; ptosis; dysphagia; limb weakness and fatigability	Weakness and fatigability in legs; difficulty raising arms; dry mouth
Signs	Oculobulbar abnormality common; proximal limb weakness	Weakness of proximal leg; oculobulbar abnormality rare
Reflexes	Normal	Hypoactive or absent, obtainable after brief exercise or repeated taps
Brief exercise	Strength fatigable	Strength initially improves and later declines
Neoplasm	Thymoma in 15%	Small cell carcinoma of lung in 75%
Electrophysiologic features		
CMAP baseline amplitude	Normal	Low
CMAP after exercise	No increase	Increased
RNS		
2–3 Hz	Decremental response	Decremental response
20–50 Hz	Normal or decremental response	Incremental response
Post exercise facilitation	Present	Present
Post activation exhaustion	Present	Present
SFEMG		
Jitter	Abnormal	Abnormal
Rapid discharge rate	Jitter worse	Jitter improved
Needle EMG	Varying MUP amplitude	Varying MUP amplitude
Pharmacologic features		
Tensilon test	Definitely positive	Negative or mildly positive in some

RNS, repetitive nerve stimulation; SFEMG, single fiber electromyography.
Modified from Oh SJ. Electromyography: neuromuscular transmission studies. Baltimore: Williams & Wilkins, 1988.

The typical pattern of abnormality on RNS in LEMS is a low amplitude M wave after a single shock, a decrement to low frequency repetitive stimulation, repair of the decrement and a marked increase in M wave amplitude after brief, isometric exercise, and an incrementing response on high frequency repetitive stimulation (20–50 Hz). The increase in amplitude following exercise or rapid stimulation may be up to 1900%, and tripling or quadrupling is common. Variations from this classical pattern can occur (28). In early LEMS, the M wave amplitude may be relatively preserved, in the low normal range, and the postexercise facilitation less impressive. As the M wave amplitude falls over time, the incrementing response becomes more typical. Some patients may require 2–10 sec of 50 Hz stimulation to bring out the incrementing response (1). The transmission defect is more widespread than in MG, and abnormalities are usually demonstrable in distal and in clinically uninvolved as well as in proximal and clinically weak muscles. Electrophysiologic improvement after Tensilon is minimal or absent.

Routine NEE in LEMS may detect the same beat to beat variation in MUAP amplitude as in any NMT disorder. Short duration, low amplitude MUAPs are common, especially at the start of a muscle contraction. A characteristic finding is a progressive increase in MUAP amplitude as a contraction is sustained, the corollary of the incremental response to rapid RNS or exercise; the opposite pattern may be seen in MG. Fibrillations do not occur. SFEMG in LEMS demonstrates increased jitter and blocking; improvement with sustained contraction or increasing firing rate is characteristic.

OVERLAP SYNDROME

An intermediate state between MG and LEMS, the so-called overlap syndrome, has been observed both clinically and electrophysiologically (29,30). Many examples of the overlap syndrome were reported before the widespread availability of AChR antibody determinations. Some reported cases of typical MG have demonstrated an incremental response of up to 200%; perhaps because the baseline M wave amplitude, while still statistically normal, is relatively depressed. Some patients with the overlap syndrome have had MG clinically, but have had electrophysiologic features typical of LEMS; others have had a mixed picture with some muscles displaying a postsynaptic and others a presynaptic pattern, or with the same muscle having different features at different times. In mild LEMS, a low normal M wave without a dramatic incremental response may resemble MG. Some patients with severe MG may have a low amplitude M wave.

OTHER DISORDERS OF NEUROMUSCULAR TRANSMISSION

Many other conditions can cause neuromuscular transmission. Some of these, such as side effects of many drugs, are subclinical. Most other defects involve presynaptic transmitter release. A number of drugs and toxins can interfere with NMT through a variety of mechanisms (31,32).

There are three types of botulism: foodborne, wound, and infantile, all similar from an electrodiagnostic standpoint. In foodborne botulism, cranial nerve dysfunction appears first. Dilated fixed pupils are classic, but frequently absent. As weakness evolves, respiratory muscles and finally limb muscles are affected. Respiratory failure may occur before any significant limb weakness is evident. Sensation remains normal, the sensorium is clear and reflexes are preserved except in severely weak muscles. The CDC lists five cardinal features of botulism: no fever, normal mental status, normal or slow pulse, no numbness, paresthesias or sensory deficits, and symmetric weakness. Diseases most often confused with botulism include MG, brain stem stroke, Guillain-Barre syndrome, strep throat (because of dry and painful oropharyngeal membranes), bacterial food poisoning, acute surgical conditions of the abdomen, and hysteria (33). In infant botulism, the toxin is produced by C. botulinum colonizing the gut and produces a more indolent picture of generalized weakness, poor suck and cry, hyporeflexia, and constipation.

Most patients with botulism show a defect on RNS that resembles that of LEMS, with a low amplitude M wave, decremental response to slow RNS, and facilitation after brief exercise or on rapid RNS (34,35). The baseline M wave amplitude correlates roughly with the severity of infection. Postexercise and posttetanic facilitation are not as dramatic as in LEMS, and in some patients, especially those with severe intoxication, they may be lacking. When no facilitation occurs after the usual 1–2 sec rapid RNS, more prolonged, 3–10 sec stimulation, may bring it out. A relatively specific finding in botulism is persistence of facilitation for a prolonged period, up to four minutes, after exercise or tetanization. Postactivation exhaustion is frequently lacking (1). The patterns of response in mild vs. severe botulism are slightly different (Table 18.1). The electrodiagnostic aspects of infantile botulism have been recently reviewed (36).

Routine NEE commonly shows fibrillations in botulism. Experience with botulinum injection for movement disorders has shown the toxin readily induces fibrillations, along with a mixture of small, short "myopathic" appearing MUAPs along with complex, polyphasic, rapidly firing units indicative of reinnervation. SFEMG acutely shows normal fiber density, and increased jitter and blocking, which lessen with increasing discharge frequency. Increased jitter may persist after recovery, and abnormal jitter has been found in muscles remote from the site of botulinum injection, indicating that even minute amounts of the toxin may cause a widespread, subclinical disturbance of NMT.

Generalized weakness may follow the administration of magnesium (usually for eclampsia), some antibiotics, and some antiarrhythmics. High magnesium interferes with transmitter release by competing with calcium and blocking its entry into the nerve terminal. Antibiotics, especially aminoglycosides, block transmitter release. Unusual susceptibility to the neuromuscular blocking effects of such agents may signal underlying MG (37). The pattern of the NMT disturbance is that of a presynaptic disorder. Postactivation exhaustion is often absent (Table 18.1). Tick paralysis causes ascending paralysis mimicking Guillain-Barre syndrome. Though often classified as a NMT disorder, the findings are more consistent with an axonopathy affecting terminal nerve twigs. Sensory as well as motor conduction studies are usually abnormal, and there is no abnormal response to RNS (1).

Abnormal responses to RNS have been reported in a number of conditions, including motor neuron disease, myotonic syndromes, periodic paralysis, phosphorylase or phosphofructokinase deficiency, and polymyositis. Most of these have features which differ from those of NMT disorders, but occasionally the pattern can be indistinguishable. In some ALS patients, a pattern similar to that in MG can occur (38). Rare patients have concurrent polymyositis and MG.

Key Points

- The neuromuscular junction is a specialized synapse through which electrical events in the peripheral nerve induce muscle contraction. Disturbed neuromuscular transmission (NMT) results in several different clinical disorders, characterized primarily by weakness and fatigability. NMT disorders produce characteristic electrodiagnostic changes which distinguish them from diseases of nerve and from diseases of muscle.

- The primary synaptic cleft separates the terminal bouton from the postsynaptic muscle membrane, which is in turn divided into a number of secondary synaptic clefts, or junctional folds. The postsynaptic muscle membrane is covered by acetylcholine receptor (AChR) molecules.

- The terminal bouton contains vesicles of acetylcholine (ACh), which line up opposite the primary release sites, or active zones. In response to a nerve impulse, molecules of ACh diffuse across the primary synaptic cleft and interact with AChR to produce a muscle fiber action potential.

- ACh molecules in the cytoplasm of the terminal bouton are divided into different compartments or "stores."

- Safety factor refers to the vast oversupply of ACh and AChR beyond the minimum required for action potential generation. One of the hallmarks of NMT disorders is diminution in this safety factor. Presynaptic and postsynaptic NMT disorders alter the safety factor through different mechanisms.

- Myasthenia gravis (MG) and the Lambert-Eaton myasthenic syndrome (LEMS), the two most common disorders of the NMJ, are both due to autoantibodies. In MG, antibodies to the AChR attack and destroy the postsynaptic membrane. In LEMS, autoantibodies directed against the calcium channel attack the ACh release sites at the active zones on the presynaptic membrane, resulting in failure of ACh release.

- In both MG and LEMS, safety factor declines because there is a decreased number of ACh-AChR interactions; because of a lack of AChR in MG and because of a paucity of ACh molecules in LEMS.

- Rarely, other conditions cause abnormal NMT. Botulism and hyper-magnesemia are presynaptic disorders. Secondary disturbances of NMT may sometimes accompany other neuromuscular disorders, such as ALS and polymyositis.

- The cardinal manifestation of NMT disorders is weakness. The distribution of the weakness and associated manifestations vary among the different conditions.

- The diagnosis of MG rests on several lines of evidence: the clinical demonstration of weakness made worse with activity and relieved by rest, pharmacological testing, AChR antibody assays, and electrodiagnostic testing.

- The primary electrodiagnostic studies used for evaluation of NMT disorders are repetitive nerve stimulation (RNS) and single fiber EMG (SFEMG). SFEMG, the most sensitive procedure, is also the most technically demanding. RNS studies are simpler and easier to perform, and more specific for localizing a disorder to the postsynaptic or presynaptic membrane. The most useful information is usually obtained with a relatively low stimulation frequency, 2–3 Hz, corresponding to the point where the falling curve of calcium concentration crosses the rising curve of transmitter mobilization, at about 300–500 msec following a nerve impulse.

- Presynaptic and postsynaptic NMT disorders produce RNS abnormalities which have some features in common and some features which are different.

- RNS studies must be done with careful attention to technical detail.

- Routine needle examination in most patients with a NMT disorder is normal, or shows beat to beat variability in the amplitude or configuration of a MUAP. NMT disorders cause two types of abnormality detectable by SFEMG: increased jitter and blocking; it is the degree of blocking on SF studies which correlates best with MUAP variability on NEE, a decremental response on RNS, and with clinical weakness and fatiguability.

- The conundrum in MG involves a tradeoff of sensitivity and specificity of the various tests. RNS studies are positive in approximately 60–70% of patients with generalized MG. The diagnostic sensitivity of RNS is directly related to disease severity.

- RNS studies are reasonably specific. The characteristic RNS picture in moderate, generalized MG is: decrement of 10% or greater in the rested muscle, repair of the decrement with brief (10–30 sec) isometric exercise, an increased decrement 2–3 min after exercise, (postactivation exhaustion) and a return to baseline after 10 minutes. An atypical pattern of response to RNS does not exclude the diagnosis.

- SFEMG is very sensitive for the diagnosis of MG; abnormality is detected in 85–90% of patients with ocular MG and in 90–95% of patients with generalized disease, but abnormalities are not specific.

- The typical pattern of abnormality on RNS in LEMS is a low amplitude M wave after a single shock, a decrement to low frequency repetitive stimulation, repair of the decrement and a marked increase in M wave amplitude after brief, isometric exercise, and an incrementing response on high frequency repetitive stimulation (20–50 Hz).

- Most patients with botulism show a defect on RNS which resembles that of LEMS, with a low amplitude M wave, decremental response to slow RNS, and facilitation following brief exercise or on rapid RNS.

References

1. Oh SJ. Electromyography: neuromuscular transmission studies. Baltimore: Williams & Wilkins, 1988.
   An excellent monograph covering all aspects of the electrophysiology of neuromuscular transmission disorders. Detailed discussion of the general concepts, techniques and interpretation of repetitive stimulation and single fiber studies in various diseases.

2. Tzartos SJ, Cung MT, Demange P, et al. The main immunogenic region (MIR) of the nicotinic acetylcholine receptor and the anti-MIR antibodies. Mol Neurobiol 1991;5:1–29.
   MG is caused by autoantibodies against the nicotinic acetylcholine receptor (AChR) of the neuromuscular junction. The anti-AChR antibodies are heterogeneous. However, a small region on the extracellular part of the AChR alpha subunit, called the main immunogenic region (MIR), seems to be the major target of the anti-AChR antibodies. Anti-MIR antibodies are functionally and structurally quite heterogeneous. Anti-MIR MAbs do not affect channel gating, but they are very potent in mediating acceleration of AChR degradation (antigenic modulation) in cell cultures and in transferring experimental MG in animals.

3. Sanders DB. Clinical neurophysiology of disorders of the neuromuscular junction. J Clin Neurophysiol 1993;10:167–180.
   A review of the neurophysiological techniques used clinically to demonstrate abnormalities of neuromuscular transmission. The use of these tests in myasthenia gravis, Lambert-Eaton myasthenic syndrome, congenital myasthenic syndromes, and other conditions with disturbed neuromuscular transmission is presented.

4. Prielipp RC, Coursin DB. Applied pharmacology of common neuromuscular blocking agents in critical care. New Horiz 1994;2:34–47.
   NMBAs are structurally related to acetylcholine and their main site of action is the postjunctional nicotinic acetylcholine receptor. These drugs act to either sustain a depolarization at the postjunctional membrane (succinylcholine), or they inhibit neuromuscular transmission by a competitive (non-depolarizing) blocking mechanism. The metabolism and excretion of NMBAs may be altered in ICU patients with end-organ dysfunction, concurrent medications, electrolyte, acid-base, and nutritional abnormalities, along with underlying nervous system and muscle pathology. Prolonged weakness after discontinuation of NMBAs is increasingly recognized after these agents are used for extended periods. This phenomenon may be related to alterations in the pharmacokinetics and pharmacodynamics, along with altered physiology of the neuromuscular junction, nervous system, or muscle, or other undefined toxic effects.

5. Hunter JM. New neuromuscular blocking drugs. N Engl J Med 1995;332:1691–1699.
   The new nondepolarizing neuromuscular blocking drugs have specific advantages over succinylcholine. Rocuronium has an onset of action that is almost as rapid as that of succinylcholine. This drug may replace vecuronium, since the two agents are otherwise similar. The onset of action of mivacurium is similar to that of atracurium, but recovery from the blockade is more rapid. Although pipecuronium and doxacurium have minimal effects on the cardiovascular system, their long and variable onset and duration of action limit their usefulness. The need for either drug is questionable. There is still a need, however, for a nondepolarizing drug that has an onset of action as rapid as that of succinylcholine but a duration of action similar to that of mivacurium, with no adverse cardiovascular effects and clearance from the body that is independent of organ function.

6. Sommer N, Melms A, Weller M, et al. Ocular myasthenia gravis. A critical review of clinical and pathophysiological aspects. Doc Ophthalmol 1993;84:309–333.
   MG is probably the best studied autoimmune disease caused by autoantibodies against the acetylcholine receptor (AChR) at the neuromuscular junction, subsequently leading to abnormal fatigability and weakness of skeletal muscle. Extraocular muscle weakness with droopy eyelids and double vision is present in about 90% of MG patients, being the initial complaint in about 50%. In approximately 20% of the patients the disease will always be confined to the extraocular muscles. The single most important diagnostic test is the detection of serum antibodies against AChR which is positive in 90% of patients with generalized MG, but only in 65% with purely ocular MG. Electromyographic studies and the Tensilon test are of diagnostic value in clear-cut cases, but may be equivocal in purely ocular myasthenia. Pathogenetically relevant steps of the underlying autoimmune process have been elucidated during the last few years; nevertheless a number of questions remain, especially what starts off the autoimmune process, and why are eye muscles so frequently involved in MG?

7. Weinberg DA, Lesser RL, Vollmer TL. Ocular myasthenia: a protean disorder. Surv Ophthalmol 1994;39:169–210.
   Ocular myasthenia is a localized form of myasthenia clinically involving only the extraocular, levator palpebrae superioris, and/or orbicularis oculi muscles. Ocular manifestations can masquerade as a variety of ocular motility disorders, including cranial nerve and gaze palsies. A history of variable and fatiguable muscle weakness suggests this diagnosis, which may be confirmed by the edrophonium test and acetylcholine receptor antibody titer. This review provides historical background, pathophysiology, immuno-genetics, diagnostic testing, and treatment options for ocular myasthenia, as well as a discussion of drug-induced myasthenic syndromes.

8. Howard JF, Jr., Sanders DB, Massey JM. The electrodiagnosis of myasthenia gravis and the Lambert-Eaton myasthenic syndrome. Neurol Clin 1994;12:305–330.
   Electrodiagnostic studies are valuable in confirming the diagnosis of a disorder of neuromuscular transmission. They are used to distinguish presynaptic and postsynaptic abnormalities. These studies provide an objective measure of the severity of the illness and may be useful in assessing the response to therapy. This article reviews the electrodiagnostic techniques that are commonly used today and highlights their specificity, sensitivity, and pitfalls.

9. Keesey JC. AAEE Minimonograph #33: electrodiagnostic approach to defects of neuromuscular transmission. Muscle Nerve 1989;12:613–626.
   Clinical testing for neuromuscular dysfunction is supported by an extensive amount of excellent basic information about normal and abnormal subcellular physiology and ultrastructure. This information provides an essential frame of reference

for describing the rationale of single-fiber electromyography (SFEMG). SFEMG in turn helps to explain the more conventional clinical testing of neuromuscular function by repetitive nerve stimulation (RNS). Electrical findings in MG, LEMS, and botulinum intoxication are discussed from the subcellular level via the cellular level (SFEMG) to the integrated responses of whole muscle (RNS) as a rational means of understanding the technique of clinical repetitive nerve stimulation.

10. Tim RW, Sanders DB. Repetitive nerve stimulation studies in the Lambert-Eaton myasthenic syndrome. Muscle Nerve 1994;17:995–1001.
    A comparison of the changes in amplitude and area of surface recorded CMAPs during 20-Hz repetitive nerve stimulation and after maximum voluntary contraction in patients with LEMS, MG, and normal controls. There was greater potentiation of CMAP amplitude after voluntary contraction than during 20-Hz stimulation in 10 of 14 LEMS patients; CMAP area increased more after exercise than during 20-Hz stimulation in all LEMS patients. Although abnormal potentiation of CMAP area and amplitude was seen in equal numbers of LEMS patients, more LEMS patients demonstrated a greater than 100% potentiation of CMAP area than of CMAP amplitude. Maximum voluntary contraction is preferable to brief 20-Hz RNS to demonstrate potentiation in LEMS because it is at least as sensitive and is less painful. Measurement of CMAP area in LEMS patients is not better than measuring the change in CMAP amplitude in demonstrating abnormal potentiation. Testing of a single hand muscle for potentiation in LEMS does not demonstrate abnormal potentiation in all LEMS patients.

11. Oh SJ, Head T, Fesenmeier J, et al. Peroneal nerve repetitive nerve stimulation test: its value in diagnosis of myasthenia gravis and Lambert-Eaton myasthenic syndrome. Muscle Nerve 1995;18:867–873.
    Description of an RNS technique for the peroneal nerve. Normal limits for the decremental responses for the anterior tibialis and extensor digitorum brevis muscles are 6–21% at the low rate of stimulation and 44–70% at the high rate of stimulation. These values exceed the normal limits for other commonly tested muscles. This may be due to the lower safety factor for neuromuscular transmission for the anterior tibialis and extensor digitorum brevis muscles. In 4 cases, the peroneal nerve RNS test was crucial for the diagnosis of the limb-girdle form of MG or LEMS. In a small number of patients with neuromuscular transmission disorders, the peroneal nerve RNS test is needed for confirmation of disease.

12. Gilchrist JM, Massey JM, Sanders DB. Single fiber EMG and repetitive stimulation of the same muscle in myasthenia gravis. Muscle Nerve 1994;17:171–175.
    RNS and SFEMG studies were done of the same muscle in 46 patients with MG. Maximum decrement to 3–5-Hz stimulation before and after maximum voluntary exercise, percentage of action potential pairs with increased jitter and blocking, and mean MCD in each study were compared. A significant decrement ($>$ 10% decrease in CMAP area or amplitude between the first and fourth response) was never found without increased jitter and impulse blocking on SFEMG. Increased jitter, blocking, and mean MCD were each correlated with maximum decrement ($r > 0.61$, $P < 0.0001$). Decrement to RNS and impulse blocking on SFEMG likely result from the same physiologic phenomenon, and SFEMG is more sensitive at detecting disordered neuromuscular transmission given its ability to detect impulse blocking at levels below the resolution of RNS and increased neuromuscular jitter when there is not blocking.

13. Sanders DB, Stalberg EV. AAEM minimonograph #25: single-fiber electromyography. Muscle Nerve 1996;19:1069–1083.
    SFEMG is a selective recording technique in which a needle electrode with a small recording surface in the side is used to identify action potentials from individual muscle fibers. The SFEMG parameters of greatest clinical use are fiber density (FD) and neuromuscular jitter. FD reflects the local organization of muscle fibers within the motor unit; jitter reflects the safety factor of neuromuscular transmission at individual neuromuscular junctions. SFEMG can be of great value in demonstrating or excluding abnormalities in mild or questionable disease of nerve, muscle, or the neuromuscular junction. The neuromuscular jitter may be measured during nerve stimulation, which is particularly useful in uncooperative patients or when it is desirable to control the firing rate precisely, or during voluntary muscle activation, which is less subject to technical artifact. The SFEMG findings may not be specific to a particular disease, but they frequently increase understanding of the disease process by demonstrating abnormal neuromuscular transmission or rearrangement of muscle fibers within the motor unit, which complements information from more conventional EMG examinations.

14. Gilchrist JM, et al. Single fiber EMG reference values: a collaborative effort. Ad Hoc Committee of the AAEM Special Interest Group on Single Fiber EMG. Muscle Nerve 1992;15:151–161.
    Presentation of a retrospective and prospective multicenter collection of SFEMG jitter and fiber density data from control subjects obtained for the purpose of defining reference values for many muscles and different ages. The data and calculated upper limits for fiber density, individual pair jitter, and mean jitter are presented for each muscle in tabular and graphical format, for different age groups. See also Bromberg MB, Scott DM, et al. Single fiber EMG reference values: reformatted in tabular form. Muscle Nerve 1994;17:820–821.

15. Seybold ME. Myasthenia gravis: diagnostic and therapeutic perspectives in the 1990's. Neurologist 1995;1:345–360.
    Clinical presentation, response to AChE inhibitors, anti-AChR antibody titer, RNS and SFEMG are used to diagnose MG. All are useful tests in the appropriate setting but not all are necessary in the individual patient. A sequence of utilization that takes clinical presentation and cost into account is recommended by the author.

16. Drachman DB. Myasthenia gravis. N Engl J Med 1994;330:1797–1810.
    Comprehensive, current review with 164 references.

17. Berrih-Aknin S. Myasthenia gravis, a model of organ-specific autoimmune disease. J Autoimmun 1995;8:139–143.
    MG is a neuromuscular disorder of autoimmune origin. Most patients have antibodies directed against the AChR that interfere with neuromuscular transmission. MG is a model of organ-specific autoimmune disease in which the autoantigen, AChR, is well characterized. However, several questions remain unanswered. Why is AChR, which is present in the thymus, not tolerized? Why does the anti-AChR antibody titer not correlate with clinical manifestations, and why do some patients not have such antibodies? What genetic elements are involved in disease susceptibility? How is the expression of AChR regu-

lated after its attack by autoantibodies? Could MG patients benefit from new immunomodulatory treatments?

18. Papazian O. Transient neonatal myasthenia gravis. J Child Neurol 1992;7:135–141.
   Transient neonatal MG is a postsynaptic neuromuscular transmission defect occurring in 21% of infants born to women with active (and, less commonly, in remission) acquired myasthenia gravis. Although passive-transfer AChR antibodies are found in the majority of these newborns, their pathogenic role is questionable because only some infants are symptomatic. Pathogenesis in infants without AChR antibodies is unknown. There is still no biologic marker for prenatal identification of this subpopulation of newborns, although HLA typing may be a promising tool. Sucking, swallowing, and respiratory difficulties are the most common presenting signs in the first day of life. Final diagnosis is done when administration of acetylcholinesterase agents transiently corrects the neuromuscular transmission defect. Serum AChR antibody titers follow the same pattern of those of their mothers. Supportive management and anticholinesterase agents prior to feedings are necessary in about 80% of patients. In the majority of infants the condition resolves spontaneously.

19. Shillito P, Vincent A, Newsom-Davis J. Congenital myasthenic syndromes. Neuromuscul Disord 1993;3:183–190.
   The Congenital Myasthenic Syndromes (CMS) constitute a group of rare genetic disorders affecting neuromuscular transmission. They differ from myasthenia gravis and the Lambert-Eaton myasthenic syndrome, which are autoimmune antibody-mediated conditions. CMS can present at any time from birth to adulthood, though usually within the first 2 yr of life, and result in a spectrum of diseases ranging from mild weakness to severe disability with life-threatening episodes. Several of these syndromes have been well documented, and in recent years fully investigated using a variety of electrophysiological, histochemical, and morphological techniques. This review describes the main results of these investigations, and attempts to classify the disorders into groups that can be recognized by the clinician. They include defects in acetylcholine release, absence of the endplate-specific form of acetylcholinesterase, and alterations in the number or function of postsynaptic acetylcholine receptors. Clinical features are described in detail, and treatment reviewed. These disorders involve a potentially large number of candidate genes.

20. Eymard B, Berrih-Aknin S. Role of the thymus in the physiopathology of myasthenia. Rev Neurol (Paris) 1995;151:6–15.
   In MG, the frequency of histologic abnormalities (hyperplasia in young patients, thymoma in older cases) and clinical improvement after thymectomy indicate involvement of the thymus in the pathophysiology of the disease. MG patient thymuses are characterized by the following features: increased amount of B cells (in hyperplasia) and functional abnormalities, mainly activation of B, T and epithelial cells. Moreover, thymic lymphocytes are sensitized to AChR: first, AChR specific T and B lines can be grown from MG thymus cultures, second, cultured thymic lymphocytes proliferate in the presence of AChR and produce anti-AChR antibodies. AChR molecules are expressed in thymic myoid cells and AChR-like molecules could be displayed at the surface of other cell types. Thus, autosensitization conditions are combined in MG thymus. See also Hohlfeld R, Wekerle H. The role of the thymus in myasthenia gravis. Adv Neuroimmunol 1994;4:373–386.

21. Oh SJ, Kuruoglu R. Chronic limb-girdle myasthenia gravis. Neurology 1992;42:1153–1156.
   The existence of chronic "limb-girdle" form of MG has been questioned. The authors report 12 such patients who constituted 3.8% of 314 MG patients in their study. The duration of disease ranged from 4 months to 7 years before the diagnosis. In almost all cases, the initial diagnosis was other than MG. None of the patients had any oculobulbar weakness. Acetylcholine receptor antibody was positive in five cases, although not all in the first assay. RNS was positive in all cases, although not necessarily the first time. SFEMG was positive in 11 cases. All patients responded to acetylcholinesterase inhibitors, and two thirds underwent immunotherapy. Diagnosis of limb-girdle MG requires a strong index of suspicion.

22. Hopkins LC. Clinical features of myasthenia gravis. Neurol Clin 1994;12:243–261.
   MG can affect any skeletal muscle, and may produce numerous symptoms and signs. To doctors and patients, it may seem like lung disease, stroke, heart disease, or the effects of emotional stress. This article explores the "territory" between MG and diseases of the heart and lungs as well as the other neuromuscular diseases.

23. Emeryk B, Rowinska-Marcinska K, Nowak-Michalska T, et al. Muscular fatigability in mitochondrial myopathies. An electrophysiological study. Electromyogr Clin Neurophysiol 1992;32:235–245.
   The frequent occurrence of ophthalmoplegia and muscle fatigability in mitochondrial myopathy can make its differential diagnosis from myasthenia rather difficult. Neuromuscular transmission was investigated in 9 patients with mitochondrial myopathy and fatigability. There was normal neuromuscular transmission in 5 cases, slight abnormalities in 3 patients, and in 1 case neuromuscular transmission disturbances seemed to be of neurogenic origin. The authors suggest that the causes of muscle fatigability are of a much more complex nature than it has been anticipated. They might depend not only on the metabolic disorders within the muscle fiber itself but also on the impaired function of the peripheral nerve or of the neuromuscular junction. All the mechanisms combined may also play a role, though in individual patients the contribution of particular factors responsible may vary.

24. Krendel DA, Sanders DB, Massey JM. Single fiber electromyography in chronic progressive external ophthalmoplegia. Muscle Nerve 1987;10:299–302.
   A review of the EMG studies of 17 patients with chronic progressive external ophthalmoplegia (CPEO). In 13 of 17 patients, conventional concentric needle EMG demonstrated a "myopathic" pattern, usually predominating in the shoulder muscles. Single-fiber EMG showed increased jitter and/or blocking in at least one muscle in 13 of 16 patients. Jitter was increased in the frontalis muscle in 10 of 13 patients and in an arm muscle in 5 of 12. When both muscles were tested, jitter was greater in the frontalis muscle in 5 patients and in the arm muscle in 2. These observations demonstrate that it may be difficult to distinguish myasthenia gravis from CPEO by EMG. The frequency with which abnormal jitter is found in CPEO suggests that, in addition to a mild generalized myopathy, a primary defect in neuromuscular transmission may be present.

25. Oh SJ, Kim DE, Kuruoglu R, et al. Diagnostic sensitivity of the laboratory tests in myasthenia gravis. Muscle Nerve 1992;15:720–724.
   The diagnostic sensitivity of three laboratory tests, AchR antibody assay, the RNS test, and SFEMG, for MG was compared

in 120 patients. In all cases, at least one of the tests was abnormal. SFEMG was the most sensitive test, being abnormal in 92% of cases, followed by the RNS test (77%) and the AChR-ab assay (73%). SFEMG was abnormal in all cases with negative AChR-ab and RNS tests, in 97% of cases with negative AChR-ab assay, in 89% of cases with negative RNS test, and in 89% of cases with mild MG. Conclusion: one of these three tests is abnormal in all cases of MG, and SFEMG is most sensitive in the diagnosis of MG.

26. Jablecki CK. AAEM case report #3: myasthenia gravis. Muscle Nerve 1991;14:391–397.
A report of the electrodiagnostic findings in a patient with MG who had dysarthria, dysphagia, and dyspnea. The use of RNS and SFEMG studies for the evaluation of patients suspected of MG is reviewed.

27. Oey PL, Wieneke GH, Hoogenraad TU, et al. Ocular myasthenia gravis: the diagnostic yield of repetitive nerve stimulation and stimulated single fiber EMG of orbicularis oculi muscle and infrared reflection oculography. Muscle Nerve 1993;16:142–149.
For the diagnosis of ocular MG, testing of the muscles close to the affected ones may be important. The relative importance of several methods: stimulated SFEMG, RNS of orbicularis oculi muscle, and infrared reflection oculography (IROG) was investigated. Thirty-two patients in whom a diagnosis of ocular MG was considered on clinical grounds were admitted to the study. Based on the results of the three neurophysiological tests, the patients could be divided in three groups: a first group with an abnormal stimulated SFEMG, and an abnormal RNS and/or abnormal IROG; a second group with only a slightly abnormal stimulated SFEMG; and a third group with normal tests in all three tests. The clinical diagnosis of ocular MG was made in all 11 patients of the first group; in 86% (6 of 7) of the patients of the second group; and in 7% (1 of 14) of patients of the third group. This study demonstrates that the orbicularis oculi muscle is a suitable muscle for stimulated SFEMG in patients with ocular MG, and that the results obtained with this technique showed a better relation with the clinical diagnosis than those of the two other techniques. There was no additional value in studying the jitter with different stimulation rates in patients with suspected ocular MG.

28. Oh SJ. Diverse electrophysiological spectrum of the Lambert-Eaton myasthenic syndrome. Muscle Nerve 1989;12:464–469.
Among 13 patients with LEMS, 3 different patterns on the RNS test were observed at the time of initial testing. Type 1 pattern, seen in one patient, had low normal CMAP amplitude, decremental response at the low rate of stimulation (LRS), and relatively normal response at the high rate of stimulation (HRS). Type 2, seen in nine patients, had the classical triad: low CMAP amplitude, decremental response at LRS, and incremental response at HRS. Type 3, seen in three patients, showed low CMAP amplitude, decremental response at LRS, and initial decremental response at HRS. These three patterns probably represent different degrees of blocking in LEMS, from the mildest in type 1 to the most severe in type 3. Since types 1 and 3 can be misinterpreted as myasthenia gravis patterns, they must be recognized in LEMS and an incremental response documented by prolonged stimulation at HRS. See also LoMonaco M, Milone M, Padua L, et al. Combined low-rate nerve stimulation and maximal voluntary contraction in the detection of compound muscle action potential facilitation in Lambert-Eaton myasthenic syndrome. Muscle Nerve 1997;20:1207–1208.

29. Tabbaa MA, Leshner RT, Campbell WW. Malignant thymoma with dysautonomia and disordered neuromuscular transmission. Arch Neurol 1986;43:955–957.
A 42-year-old man had prominent dysautonomia accompanied by clinical and electrophysiological features of both MG and LEMS. AchR antibodies were present in high titer. Invasive thymoma was found at thymectomy; later, a solitary metastasis to the spleen required a splenectomy. Complete remission followed surgery. There was evidence of antibody activity directed against postsynaptic acetylcholine receptors, presynaptic somatic motor terminals, and autonomic effector junctions.

30. Oh SJ, Dwyer DS, Bradley RJ. Overlap myasthenic syndrome: combined myasthenia gravis and Eaton-Lambert syndrome. Neurology 1987;37:1411–1414.
A patient with a known history of pernicious anemia had the combined features of autoimmune MG and the LEMS. Initially, this patient had all the features typical of MG, and after thymectomy developed all the typical features of LEMS. In view of the coexistence of two autoimmune neuromuscular transmission disorders in one patient, the authors term this disorder "overlap myasthenic syndrome."

31. Senanayake N, Roman GC. Disorders of neuromuscular transmission due to natural environmental toxins. J Neurol Sci 1992;107:1–13.
A variety of natural toxins of animal, plant, and bacterial origin are capable of causing disorders of neuromuscular transmission. Animal toxins include venomous snakes and arthropods, venoms of certain marine creatures, skin secretions of dart-poison frogs, and poisonous fish, shellfish, and crabs. There are plant poisons such as curare, and bacterial poisons such as botulinum toxin. These act at single or multiple sites of the neuromuscular apparatus interfering with voltage-gated ion channels, acetylcholine release, depolarization of the postsynaptic membrane, or generation and spread of the muscle action potential. The specific actions of these toxins are being widely exploited in the study of neuromuscular physiology and pathology. Some toxins have proved to be valuable pharmaceutical agents. Poisoning by natural neurotoxins is an important public health hazard in many parts of the world, particularly in the tropics. Poisoning may occur by a bite or a sting of a venomous animal, or by the ingestion of poisonous fish, shellfish or other marine delicacies. Contaminated food is a vehicle for poisons such as botulinum toxin. Clinically, a cardinal feature in the symptomatology is muscle paralysis with a distribution characteristic of myasthenia gravis, affecting muscles innervated by cranial nerves, neck flexors, proximal limb muscles, and respiratory muscles. Respiratory paralysis may end fatally. This paper reviews from the clinical and pathophysiologic viewpoints, naturally occurring environmental neurotoxins acting at the neuromuscular junction.

32. Wittbrodt ET. Drugs and myasthenia gravis. An update. Arch Intern Med 1997;157:399–408.
MG is a disease of the neuromuscular junction in which normal transmission of the neuron-to-muscle impulse is impaired or prevented by AchR antibodies. Several classes of drugs have been associated with clinical worsening of existing MG, and a small subset of drugs, most notably the antirheumatic agent penicillamine, have been implicated in the pathogenesis of a variant of the disease. Recent case reports and other documented evidence link a number of specific agents with clinical worsening of MG.

33. Campbell WW, Swift TR. Differential diagnosis of acute weakness. South Med J 1981;74:1371–1375.

    A discussion of the differential diagnosis of muscle weakness evolving rapidly over hours to days, which demands prompt diagnosis and proper treatment to prevent life-threatening respiratory insufficiency. Such weakness usually results from diseases affecting some portion of the motor unit, such as poliomyelitis, Guillain-Barre syndrome, botulism, and dyskalemic myopathy.

34. Pickett JB, III. AAEE case report #16: Botulism. Muscle Nerve 1988;11:1201–1205.

    Botulinal toxin causes a marked reduction in the number of quanta released by autonomic and motor nerve terminals. As a result it causes blurred vision, inability to move the eyes, weakness of other cranial nerve-innervated muscles, dyspnea progressing to apnea, and generalized weakness. Electrodiagnostic findings in severe botulism can be relatively nonspecific, with low amplitude and short duration motor unit action potentials and small M wave amplitudes. A modest increment in M wave amplitude with rapid repetitive nerve stimulation may help to localize the disorder to the neuromuscular junction. Identification of the toxin in the patient's serum is diagnostic. The treatment of botulism is mainly supportive.

35. Cherington M. Clinical spectrum of botulism. Muscle Nerve 1998;21:701–710.

    The toxin of *Clostridium botulinum* causes skeletal muscle paralysis by producing a presynaptic blockade to the release of acetylcholine. The site of action of the neurotoxin is at the nerve terminal. Five clinical forms of botulism have been described: 1) classic or food-borne botulism; 2) wound botulism; 3) infant botulism; 4) hidden botulism; 5) inadvertent botulism. A clinical pattern of descending weakness is characteristic of all five forms. Almost all human cases of botulism are caused by one of three serotypes (A, B, or E). There are increasing numbers of cases of wound botulism in injecting drug users. Infant botulism, is now the most frequently reported form. In infant botulism spores of *Clostridium botulinum* are ingested and germinate in the intestinal tract. Hidden botulism, the adult variant of infant botulism, occurs in adult patients who usually have an abnormality of the intestinal tract that allows colonization by *Clostridium botulinum*. Inadvertent botulism occurs in patients who have been treated with injections of botulinum toxin for dystonic and other movement disorders. Electrophysiologic studies can provide the presumption of botulism and can be especially helpful when bioassay studies are negative. The most consistent electrophysiologic abnormality is a small evoked muscle action potential in response to a single supramaximal nerve stimulus in a clinically affected muscle. Posttetanic facilitation can be found in some affected muscles. Single-fiber EMG studies typically reveal increased jitter and blocking, which becomes less marked following activation.

36. Gutierrez AR, Bodensteiner J, Gutmann L. Electrodiagnosis of infantile botulism. J Child Neurol 1994;9: 362–365.

    An analysis of the literature on the electrophysiologic features of infantile botulism. Small CMAP amplitude is a very sensitive feature but lacks specificity. The decremental response to 2- to 3-Hz RNS is inconsistent and not a reliable sign. Tetanic and posttetanic facilitation are highly sensitive and highly specific. Absence of posttetanic exhaustion is also highly specific for infant botulism and shared only by hypermagnesemia. The findings of low CMAP amplitude in combination with tetanic facilitation or posttetanic facilitation and absence of posttetanic exhaustion constitute the triad on which the electrodiagnosis of infantile botulism can be supported.

37. Bashuk RG, Krendel DA. Myasthenia gravis presenting as weakness after magnesium administration. Muscle Nerve 1990;13:708–712.

    A report of a patient with no prior history of neuromuscular disease who became virtually quadriplegic after parenteral magnesium administration for preeclampsia. The serum magnesium concentration was 3.0 mEq/L, which is usually well tolerated. The magnesium was stopped and the patient recovered over a few days. While she was weak, 2-Hz repetitive stimulation revealed a decrement without significant facilitation at rapid rates or after exercise, suggesting postsynaptic neuromuscular blockade. After her strength returned, repetitive stimulation was normal, but SFEMG revealed increased jitter and blocking. Her AchR antibody level was markedly elevated. Although paralysis after magnesium administration has been described in patients with known MG, it had not previously been reported to be the initial or only manifestation of the disease. Patients who are unusually sensitive to the neuromuscular effects of magnesium should be suspected of having an underlying disorder of neuromuscular transmission.

38. Bernstein LP, Antel JP. Motor neuron disease: decremental responses to repetitive nerve stimulation. Neurology 1981;31:202–204.

    To 2 Hz repetitive stimulation, six patients with rapidly progressive ALS had a decrement of 7.6 +/− 1.3% at baseline which repaired immediately after exercise and increased to 13.6 +/− 1.2% two minutes after exercise. Only one of eight patients with slowly progressive disease had any decrement. The decrement correlated better with disease progression than with CMAP amplitude. Decrements up to 10% are generally considered normal.

19

Myopathies

Myopathies are those conditions in which there is a primary dysfunction of skeletal muscle. The causes of myopathy are legion, and include, as a partial list: inflammatory myopathies, muscular dystrophies, congenital myopathies, metabolic and mitochondrial myopathies and myopathies arising as a complication of many different systemic disorders. As a broad approximation, myopathies may be divided into those which produce muscle fiber necrosis, which causes characteristic electrodiagnostic abnormalities, and those which do not. The myonecrotic myopathies include the inflammatory myopathies, some dystrophies, some forms of congenital myopathy and other conditions. The bland, nonmyonecrotic myopathies usually occur with metabolic and endocrine disorders. The following sections review the anatomy, physiology, pathology and electrodiagnostic features of myopathies. The concluding sections summarize the findings expected in some of the more common conditions. Related material regarding muscle fiber types and the size principle can be found in Chapter 8 and Table 8.3; and a brief overview of the electrodiagnosis of myopathies is provided in Chapter 11.

Anatomy and Physiology of Muscle

A muscle is composed of hundreds to thousands of individual muscle fibers (Fig. 19.1). Each fiber is a

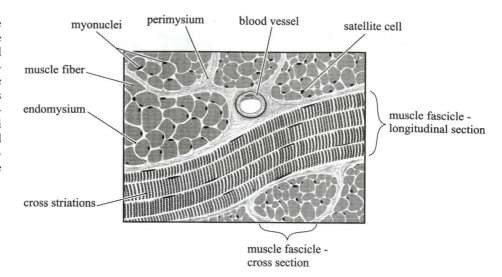

FIGURE 19.1. Cross section of muscle showing several fascicles, with muscle fibers, connective tissue septa and blood vessels. The endomysium surrounds individual muscle fibers, the perimysium surrounds and separates fascicles, and the epimysium surrounds the entire muscle. Myonuclei and satellite cells lie peripherally and cannot be distinguished histologically. Longitudinal fibers demonstrate cross striations.

multinucleated syncytium, roughly cylindrical in shape and encased in a connective tissue covering of endomysium, which extends over a long distance within a muscle fascicle. Fibers are polygonal in cross section; the diameter may vary depending on a number of factors but is relatively constant within a given muscle. A muscle fascicle is a group of fibers lying together within a sheath of perimysium. Intramuscular nerve twigs, capillaries and muscle spindles also occupy the perimysium.

Epimysium separates groups of fascicles and also provides a covering for the entire muscle. The surface epimysium, which encases the muscle proper, is continuous with the fascia which covers the muscle and in turn with the tendons which anchor it at the origin and insertion. The nuclei supporting a fiber lie peripherally just under the sarcolemmal membrane. Just external to the sarcolemma is the dense basement membrane. Satellite cells lie between the basement membrane and the sarcolemma. These dormant, omnipotential stem cells, whose nuclei resemble the sarcolemmal nuclei, can serve as the source of regeneration of muscle fibers following injury (1).

Each muscle fiber is composed of thousands of myofibrils, which are in turn made up of myriad myofilaments, the contractile elements (Fig. 19.2). The myofibril is composed of repeating identical segments called sarcomeres. A sarcomere is anchored at each end by a condensation of protein referred to as a Z disk. From each Z disk arise thin filaments of actin which project toward the center of the sarcomere. From a condensation in the center of the sarcomere, the M line, thick filaments of myosin project outward toward the Z lines. Where the myosin and actin fila-

ments overlap the sarcomere appears denser and transmits less light—the anisotropic or A band. At the sarcomere's ends, where thin actin filaments exist alone, the appearance is lighter—the isotropic or I band. In the paramedian zone, where myosin filaments exist alone, the appearance is intermediate—the H zone. There are twice as many actin filaments as myosin filaments. During muscle contraction, the filaments slide past each other as side arms on the myosin molecule ratchet the actin molecule and draw it past. At maximal shortening, the Z disks are drawn together and the I bands are obliterated as the overall length of the sarcomere decreases (Fig. 19.2).

Myosin is composed of two fragments: heavy meromyosin, which has ATPase activity, and light meromyosin, which does not. Actin is composed of three fragments: actin, troponin and tropomyosin. Troponin can reversibly bind with calcium. A troponin-tropomyosin complex inhibits the interaction of myosin and actin while the muscle is at rest. The binding of calcium to troponin disinhibits the interaction and allows reactions to occur between the cross bridges on the myosin molecule and active sites on the actin molecule.

At the junction of the A and I bands, the transverse (T) tubular systems arise as invaginations of the plasmalemma and ramify as an intricate network within the sarcomere. The T tubules allow communication between the muscle interior and the extracellular space, and are the conduits along which the action potential is transmitted to the depths of the sarcomere. The sarcoplasmic reticulum (SR) is a closed internal labyrinth of vesicles that surrounds the myofibrils. The SR ends as focal dilatations, the terminal cisterns,

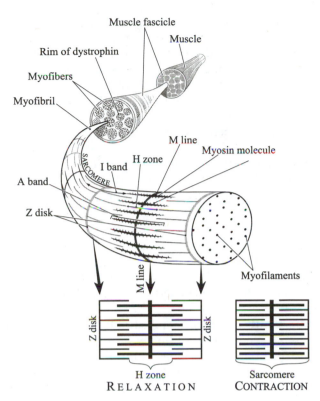

FIGURE 19.2. Myofibrils are composed of repeating sarcomeres. The sarcomere extends from Z line to Z line and consists of the I band (actin filaments only), the A band (actin and myosin filaments overlapping), the H zone (myosin filaments only) and the M line (a central condensation of the myosin filaments). The myosin molecules have cross bridges which interact with the actin molecules. When the muscle shortens the overlapping of the myosin and actin molecules increases as the filaments slide, drawing the Z lines together and obliterating the I band. Dystrophin lies beneath the sarcolemma and helps reinforce it against the stretching and buckling.

which contain calcium. A pair of terminal cisterns abuts a T tubule to form a triad. The action potential conducted into the fiber along the T tubule causes calcium release from the terminal cisterns which in turn activates myosin ATPase and initiates sliding of the filaments. This sequence is referred to as excitation contraction coupling. Following contraction, calcium ions are sequestered back into the terminal cisterns of the SR.

In addition to the contractile elements, skeletal muscle contains important cytoskeletal proteins which help provide it structure. Elastic elements are vital to allow for contraction and relaxation. One of the key cytoskeletal proteins is dystrophin, a large molecule which forms a reinforcing meshwork just beneath the sarcolemma, and links the sarcomere to

the sarcolemma and the extracellular matrix. Dystrophin is not directly connected to the membrane, but anchored to it at each end by a glycoprotein complex (dystrophin associated glycoprotein, or DAG) which spans the membrane and binds externally to laminin in the extracellular matrix. Dystrophin appears to lend mechanical support to the sarcolemma to help stabilize and brace it against the forces of muscle contraction. Genetic derangements of these cytoskeletal proteins underlie many of the muscular dystrophies.

Cellular organelles, glycogen granules, and lipids lie interspersed between the myofibrils and near the sarcolemmal nuclei. The relative abundance of different components varies with the function of a particular muscle. Muscles were broadly divided into red muscle and white muscle, dark meat and light meat, long before the basis for the difference was understood. The red or dark color is now known to result from the presence of the instruments for oxidative metabolism: myoglobin, mitochondria and a vascular network for delivery of oxygen to the metabolizing muscle cells.

The myosin ATPase stain identifies two distinct populations of muscle fibers, referred to as type 1 and type 2; the differences are summarized in Table 19.1. Cross sections reveal a random admixture of the two fiber types creating a checkerboard pattern (see Figs. 3.1 and 3.2). An average muscle contains about 40% type 1 fibers and 60% type 2 fibers, but this ratio varies with the anatomical location and function of the muscle, and similar muscles may vary between individu-

TABLE 19.1
Attributes and Characteristics of Type 1 and Type 2 Muscle Fibers

Attribute	Type 1	Type 2
ATPase stain at pH 4.3	Dark	Light
ATPase stain at pH 9.4	Light	Dark
Oxidative enzymes	High	Low
Lipid	High	Low
Mitochondria	High	Low
Glycogen	Low	High
Glycolytic enzymes	Low	High
Function	Sustained contraction	Brief contraction
Twitch speed	Slow	Fast
Metabolism	Aerobic	Anaerobic
Fatigue	Resistant	Sensitive

als. The fiber type mix in the leg muscles of runners may have some rough correlation with their athletic talents for sprinting as opposed to distance running. All fibers in a particular motor unit are of the same type, and the fiber type mix of a muscle is determined by its innervation and ultimately by its function.

The type 2 fibers stain darkly and the type 1 fibers lightly at pH 9.4; the staining characteristics reverse at pH 4.3. Type 1 fibers are rich in oxidative enzymes and mitochondria but sparse in glycogen, and are designed for sustained, long duration contraction under aerobic conditions. Red meat is high in type 1 fibers, e.g., the leg meat of a bird that mostly walks but the wing meat of a bird that flies long distances. Type 2 fibers are rich in glycogen and glycolytic enzymes, sparse in oxidative enzymes, mitochondria and lipid, and are designed for brief, intense, bursts of activity under anaerobic conditions. The mnemonic *one, slow, red ox* helps recall the essentials: type 1 fibers, slow muscle, red meat, oxidative metabolism. Preincubation at pH 4.6 identifies two kinds of type 2 fibers, type 2A and type 2B. The 2B fibers are the classic fast twitch, fatigue sensitive glycolytic fibers, while 2A fibers have characteristics intermediate between type 1 and type 2B, with some oxidative capability, slower twitch and more fatigue resistance than the 2B fibers. Pathologic processes may cause characteristic abnormalities of fiber type distribution or proportion, or produce changes primarily in one particular fiber type.

Pathology of Muscle

Muscle has a limited repertoire of reactions to injury. Some of the major categories of pathologic change include changes in fiber size and shape, variations in fiber type distribution, internalization of nuclei, fiber necrosis and regeneration, the presence of vacuoles, inclusions or other bodies, morphologic changes in individual fibers and changes in the interstitial compartment. Most pathologic changes are nonspecific but a few are characteristic of particular disease entities. The details of muscle pathology are far beyond the scope of this limited discussion; the following paragraphs can serve at best to highlight a few essentials. The basics of muscle pathology are succinctly reviewed in reference 1. Pathologic and electrodiagnostic features of some disorders affecting muscle are summarized in Figures 19.3 and 19.4.

One of the commonest changes in sick muscle is variation in fiber size and shape. Normal muscle fibers are polygonal in cross section and of more or less the same size. Denervation atrophy tends to produce small, angular fibers with sharp outlines. Primary muscle disease tends to cause random variation in fiber size and rounding up of involved fibers. Atrophy selectively affecting type 2 fibers is a nonspecific change typically seen in disuse atrophy and in steroid myopathy. Selective atrophy of type 1 fibers occurs in myotonic dystrophy, and selective hypertrophy of type 1 fibers is characteristic of Werdnig-Hoffman disease (SMA-I).

Normal muscle is a random mosaic of fiber types, the checkerboard pattern. Fibers of the same type congregating in groups most often occur with denervation and reinnervation, or in congenital fiber type disproportion. Small groups of atrophic fibers suggest denervation. Large group atrophy with vast expanses of atrophic fibers of the same type suggests Werdnig-Hoffman disease. Atrophy concentrated around the periphery of fascicles is characteristic of dermatomyositis.

Muscle fiber nuclei lie subsarcolemmal in 97% of fibers (1). A collection of nuclei in the center of more than 10% of fibers is abnormal but nonspecific. Many internal nuclei in many fibers suggests congenital centronuclear (myotubular) myopathy or myotonic dystrophy. Morphologic changes which deform and disfigure the sarcoplasm include moth eaten, target, split and ring fibers. Target fibers are characteristic of denervation; the other morphologic aberrations occur most often in primary muscle disease. Various abnormal forms may be present inside a muscle fiber, such as rods in nemaline myopathy, vacuoles in inclusion body myositis, and various "bodies" (fingerprint, zebra, cytoplasmic and others). A lack of oxidative enzyme staining in the center of fibers is characteristic of central core disease. Muscle fiber necrosis occurs most commonly in the dystrophies and inflammatory myopathies. Necrotic fibers are phagocytosed by macrophages. Regeneration of fibers occurs from satellite cell metamorphosis into myoblasts, or by budding from surviving sarcoplasm. Pathologic changes also take place in the interstitial connective tissue and blood vessels of muscle. Inflammatory cell infiltrates are typical of the inflammatory myopathies. Replacement of necrotic, degenerated muscle by fat and fibrous tissue is characteristic of the dystrophies.

Electrodiagnosis of Myopathies

Electrodiagnosis is one of the major tools for evaluating patients with suspected muscle disease and can provide a great deal of valuable information, but it has limitations (2). The typical changes associated with myopathy can occur in other conditions, and the

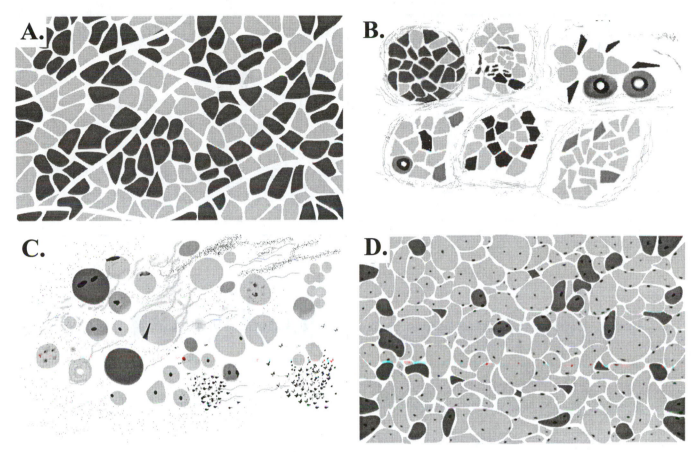

FIGURE 19.3. A. Normal muscle. B. Denervation atrophy—note scattered small angular fibers, small groups of atrophic fibers (small group atrophy), large fields of atrophic fibers (large group atrophy), type grouping due to reinnervation, and target fibers. C. Myonecrotic myopathy—note random variation in fiber size, large and small round fibers, many internal nuclei, inflammatory infiltrates, fiber necrosis, moth eaten and ring fibers, fibrosis and fatty infiltration. D. Nonmyonecrotic myopathy—note mild variation in fiber size and many internal nuclei.

range of possible findings in myopathy is very wide, from no detectable abnormality to widespread and severe alterations. Widely different categories of muscle disease, such as inflammatory myopathies and muscular dystrophies, can produce an identical pattern on needle electrode examination. The abnormalities found are never diagnostic of any specific disease process, although in certain instances they are highly suggestive. For all these reasons, the final diagnosis in myopathy is more likely to be found under the pathologist's microscope than on the EMGer's oscilloscope. See Chapter 8 for a discussion of remodeling of the motor unit in myopathy and resultant changes in the motor unit action potentials (MUAPs).

Some of the patterns of abnormality that can be seen on the needle electrode examination in myopathies are summarized in Table 8.6. The essential pathophysiologic abnormality in all myopathies is a decrease in the contractile power of muscle fibers.

This is reflected on needle electromyography as an overabundance of active MUAPs in proportion to the force of contraction (Fig. 19.5). Since individual muscle fibers can muster less contractile power, more fibers must be recruited in order to deliver a given level of strength. A minimal level of contraction which might cause the activation of only a few MUAPs in a normal individual, may produce a profuse shower of MUAPs as the muscle futilely attempts to marshal enough fibers to generate normal strength. Several descriptive terms have been used to describe this excess of active MUAPs for the force of contraction, such as early, increased, rapid or myopathic recruitment.

In addition to increased numbers, the MUAPs may be of decreased amplitude, shortened duration and demonstrate increased complexity (Fig. 19.5). The amplitude is attenuated since the individual muscle fibers contributing to the MUAP are usually atrophic and generate less than a normal change in electrical

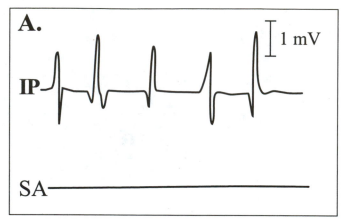

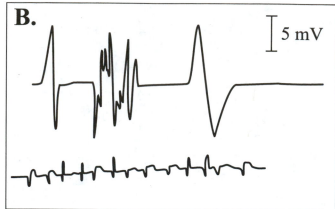

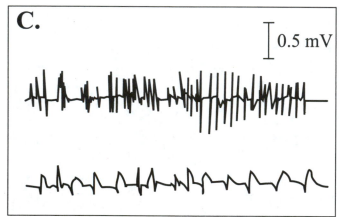

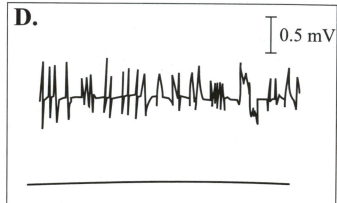

FIGURE 19.4. Needle electrode examination findings at slight contraction which correspond to the histology shown in Figure 19.3. A. Normal size, configuration and number of MUAPs; no spontaneous activity. B. A decreased number of large, complex MUAPs which fire rapidly; spontaneous spike fibrillations and positive waves. C. An increased number of MUAPs for the force of contraction, small MUAPs and many polyphasic potentials; spontaneous spike fibrillations and positive waves. D. An increased number of MUAPs for the force of contraction, small MUAPs and many polyphasic potentials; no abnormal spontaneous activity.

potential with contraction. The duration is short because the needle electrode picks up fewer of these low ionic flux distant fibers. The complexity may be increased because of the variability of fiber size, fiber splitting and similar pathologic changes which increase the disparity in conduction velocity along the muscle fibers, creating desynchronization and more discrete, identifiable components in the MUAP. Satellite potentials are small, trailing late components which may arise from atrophic fibers with extremely slow conduction velocity (3).

Rapid and early recruitment of small, short duration, polyphasic potentials recruited in numbers out of proportion to the strength of muscle contraction, producing an abnormal abundance of MUAPs with even minimal exertion, is the electrodiagnostic hallmark of all primary muscle disorders. The acronym "BSAP" serves as a mnemonic for this pattern: *brief,*

small, abundant, potentials. Rather than use this term descriptively, or the term "myopathic", it is preferable to state the approximate size of the MUAPs numerically and give as quantitative a description as possible of the recruitment characteristics (4). Other processes can sometimes cause confusion. Newly reinnervated motor units are frequently small and highly polyphasic. The MUAPs in neuromuscular transmission disorders and very early denervation may be low amplitude and short duration. Rarely, neuropathies selectively affecting terminal nerve twigs can produce a pattern simulating myopathy.

Some muscle disorders are associated with necrosis and degeneration of individual fibers. Segmental necrosis may incidentally involve intramuscular nerve twigs or isolate part of the fiber from its nerve supply. Some fibers may split, which can also isolate part of a fiber from its nerve supply. Because of this "myogenic

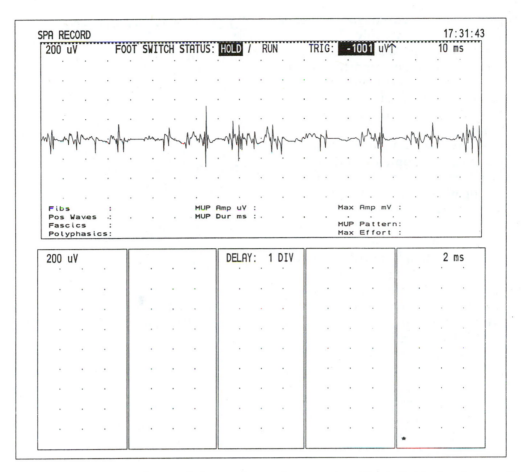

FIGURE 19.5. Motor unit action potentials recorded at minimal contraction with a concentric needle electrode from the deltoid muscle of a 73-year-old man with polymyositis. There are an excessive number of units present for the force of contraction. The individual units are of short duration, low amplitude or polyphasic. Some display all these features.

denervation" and likely for other reasons as well, some primary muscle disorders produce EMG changes which are more commonly and classically associated with neurogenic processes (see Chapter 8). Myopathies producing a great deal of necrosis, such as inflammatory myopathies and dystrophies, are particularly likely to be associated with spontaneous and increased insertional activity: fibrillation potentials, positive sharp waves, and occasionally CRDs. A stronger association exists between fibrillations and the presence of necrosis and regeneration than between fibrillations and "inflammation"(2). Fibrillation potentials in myopathy are often of very low amplitude, because the muscle fibers which generate the spontaneous discharges are atrophic, and may discharge slowly. Searches for spontaneous activity made at high gain (50 µV per division) and in a methodical manner are more likely to be productive.

Myopathies may therefore be broadly classified into those which produce myonecrosis, which is associated with fibrillation potentials, and those which do not cause myonecrosis and do not display either spontaneous or increased insertional activity (Table 8.6). Very long-standing, chronic myopathies sometimes produce large amplitude, fast firing MUAPs: the "neurogenic" pattern of very chronic myopathy (5). Inclusion body myositis and alcoholic myopathy are particularly prone to display a mixed picture of concomitant neuropathy and myopathy. Distinctive and characteristic electrical discharges occur in the myotonic disorders.

In some myopathies, the electrodiagnostic abnormalities are very subtle, with the only abnormality consisting of a slight change in MUAP amplitude or duration, or a mild increase in the proportion of complex units. Occasionally, the abnormalities can be detected only by quantitative MUAP studies. The distribution of electrical changes may vary. Examination of clinically weak muscles is usually the most informative. Abnormalities are generally most obvious in proximal and axial muscles. Some conditions, such as inclusion body myositis, myotonic dystrophy, or hereditary distal myopathies, have a predilection for distal muscles. Occasionally, especially in the inflammatory myopathies, the most striking abnormalities are seen in the paraspinal muscles.

Except for loss of M wave amplitude recorded from an atrophic muscle, nerve conduction studies are normal in most myopathies. As in other situations, there may be abnormalities on repetitive nerve stimulation in some patients with a primary myopathy. This ostensibly reflects incidental damage to terminal nerve twigs or to neuromuscular junctions. The abnormality is characteristically mild and does not follow the typical pattern of a primary neuromuscular transmission disorder. The propensity of needle electromyography to cause CK elevation and artifactual changes on muscle biopsy must be constantly borne in mind when evaluating patients with suspected myopathy.

Common Myopathies

The conditions which can cause myopathy are numerous. (Table 19.2 and Table 8.6). For purposes of this discussion we will divide myopathies into those which are inherited and those which occur sporadically, as this is often the initial step in clinical differential diagnostic thinking. This scheme is not absolute; inclusion body myositis is usually sporadic but can occur as an inherited disorder, most channelopathies are inherited but some are sporadic, and so forth.

Inherited Myopathies

MUSCULAR DYSTROPHY

The muscular dystrophies (MD) are inherited disorders that usually become symptomatic in childhood or early adulthood with subsequent steadily progressive weakness leading to major disability or death. Rare cases occur sporadically. The most common forms of MD are myotonic dystrophy and those disorders associated with an abnormality of dystrophin. The spectrum of clinical expression of dystrophinopathies is much broader than previously recognized (6).

Duchenne muscular dystrophy (DMD) is a severe disorder with onset before age 5, producing unremit-

---

TABLE 19.2
Common Primary Muscle Diseases

I. Inherited diseases
  A. Dystrophies
    1. Dystrophinopathies (Duchenne muscular dystrophy, Becker muscular dystrophy, others)
    2. Myotonic dystrophy
    3. Facioscapulohumeral dystrophy
    4. Limb-girdle dystrophy
    5. Congenital dystrophies (Fukayama, etc.)
  B. Metabolic
    1. Mitochondropathies (ragged red fiber diseases)—Kearnes-Sayre syndrome, MELAS, MERRF, etc
    2. Glycogenoses (McArdle's disease, phosphofructokinase deficiency)
    3. Lipid myopathies (carnitine deficiency, carnitine palmityl transferase deficiency)
  C. Congenital myopathies
    1. Nemaline myopathy
    2. Central core disease
    3. Myotubular myopathy
    4. Congenital fiber type disproportion

  D. Channelopathies
    1. Myotonia congenita
    2. Periodic paralysis
    3. Malignant hyperthermia
II. Acquired diseases
  A. Inflammatory myopathies
    1. Polymyositis, dermatomyositis
    2. Inclusion body myositis
    3. Myopathies related to infection (HIV, HTLV-1, parasites)
  B. Myopathies complicating systemic illness
    1. Endocrine myopathies
    2. Sarcoidosis
    3. Critical illness myopathy
  C. Toxic myopathies
  D. Rhabdomyolysis

ting, predominantly proximal weakness, calf hypertrophy, contractures and frequently scoliosis. The CK is invariably elevated, often spectacularly. Pathologically there is marked fiber necrosis and regeneration, followed eventually by fibrosis and fatty infiltration. Most patients succumb in their teens to cardiac and pulmonary complications. The disease is X-linked and due to a deletion (65%) or a mutation (35%) in the DMD gene, located on the short arm of the X chromosome at the Xp21 locus. Becker muscular dystrophy (BMD) is a milder dystrophinopathy than DMD in which the dystrophin is functionally abnormal or decreased quantitatively, but not severely reduced or absent as in DMD. The dystrophin abnormalities in most BMD patients are due to DNA deletions that do not alter the translational reading frame. The onset of BMD is later, the weakness milder and the progression slower.

The EMG in DMD/BMD displays a myonecrotic pattern with many brief, low amplitude, early recruited units plus fibrillations and complex repetitive discharges. Short duration potentials in the 3–7 msec range occur most often in proximal muscles, whereas polyphasic potentials are more prominent in distal muscles (7). Long duration polyphasic potentials with late components can appear; their inclusion in mean duration calculations may obscure the contribution of short duration potentials (5). On delay line analysis, these late components, or satellite potentials, can follow the main spike by 25 msec or more and likely contribute to the appearance of an excess number of MUAPs by routine needle exam. Both the EMG abnormalities and the pathologic changes in BMD are qualitatively similar to but less severe than those in DMD.

Myotonic dystrophy (MyoD) is an autosomal dominant disorder linked to chromosome 19, where a mutation causes repeats of the cytosine-thymidine-guanine sequence in the gene which codes for myotonin protein kinase. Up to 40 CTG repeats occur in normals, while MyoD patients may have 50–200 (1). The clinical manifestations of the disease are extremely variable and severity seems related to the number of CTG repeats. Presentation is usually in adolescence or early adulthood, but the disease may become apparent anywhere from the neonatal period to old age. Weakness is most severe in distal muscles. The cardinal manifestation is myotonia, an inability of muscle to relax after contraction or on percussion. The face is typically thin and myopathic with bilateral ptosis and prominent atrophy of the temporalis and sternomastoid muscles. Numerous nonneuromuscular manifestations attest to the systemic nature of the disease process, including cardiac conduction defects, insulin resistant diabetes mellitus, testicular atrophy, baldness, and cataracts. Typical pathologic findings include selective atrophy of type 1 fibers, many internal nuclei, ring fibers, sarcoplasmic masses, necrosis, regeneration and fibrosis (1). Proximal myotonic myopathy (PROMM) is a recently described dominant disorder which resembles MyoD, with myotonia, weakness of proximal but not distal muscles, strange myalgias and cataracts, but is not associated with abnormal CTG repeats of the myotonic dystrophy gene (8).

The EMG in MyoD reveals the expected short duration, low amplitude, polyphasic MUAPs, most prominent in affected muscles and distal muscles, and accompanied by fibrillation potentials. Some MUAPs in some patients may be long duration and increased amplitude, and rarely a bimodal pattern of MUAP changes is present with a short duration, low amplitude subpopulation and a long duration, high amplitude subpopulation. The myotonia induced by muscle contraction and needle movement often obscures the MUAPs and makes analysis of the interference pattern and appreciation of the characteristics of individual MUAPs difficult. Nerve conduction studies are usually normal, but a mild generalized axonopathy has been reported. M wave amplitudes recorded from atrophic distal muscles may be reduced. A decremental response sometimes occurs with rapid repetitive stimulation in the rested muscle which repairs with exercise and can superficially resemble a defect in neuromuscular transmission (9).

The myotonia in myotonic dystrophy is due to abnormal function of the sodium channel, and the presence of myotonic discharges identifies the disorder electrically. Occasionally local cooling and sampling of multiple muscles may be required to bring these out. Myotonic discharges originate from a single muscle fiber and most commonly occur as a train of positive sharp waves (2). The discharges vary spontaneously and erratically in both amplitude and frequency, producing a waxing and waning pattern (see Chapter 8). Myotonic discharges may be induced by muscle contraction or percussion, nerve stimulation or needle movement.

Myotonic discharges are not specific for MyoD and can occur in other conditions as well, including myotonia congenita, paramyotonia congenita, the myotonic subtype of potassium sensitive periodic paralysis, acid maltase deficiency, myotubular myopathy and possibly hypothyroidism (see Table 8.6).(2) Some of the other myotonic disorders are discussed in the subsequent section on channelopathies.

There are numerous other forms of muscular dystrophy, most of which have the same electrodiagnostic pattern of myonecrotic myopathy as the dystrophino-pathies (10). The clinical, pathological and electrodiagnostic medical aspects of some of these are summarized in Table 19.3.

CONGENITAL MYOPATHY

The congenital myopathies (CMs) are conditions which usually present in infancy and are major considerations in the differential diagnosis of infantile hypotonia (11). Most are nonprogressive and hereditary. Some can result in severe disability. The original handful of CMs has now expanded to about forty different conditions. The classical CMs include such conditions as central core disease, centronuclear/myotubular myopathy, nemaline or rod body myopathy, and congenital fiber type disproportion. Juvenile and adult subtypes occur in several of the syndromes. CMs are generally designated by some disease-specific mor-

phological feature, such as rods, cores or various inclusions. Some have associated abnormalities such as kyphosis, scoliosis, high arched palate, facial dysmorphism, extraocular muscle palsies, short stature and joint contractures. Some CMs carry an increased risk for malignant hyperthermia.

Most CMs show only an increased proportion of brief duration, small amplitude, polyphasic units with an early recruitment pattern. In some, the needle examination is completely normal. Fibrillations may occur with the nemaline and centronuclear/myotubular myopathies. Myotubular myopathy may also display CRDs and myotonic discharges.

METABOLIC MYOPATHY

The metabolic myopathies are inborn errors of metabolism which may produce a wide variety of neuromuscular signs and symptoms, including exercise intoler-

TABLE 19.3
Other Forms of Muscular Dystrophy

Condition	Clinical Features	Pathology	Electrodiagnostic Picture
Facioscapulohumeral (FSH) dystrophy	Autosomal dominant, chromosome 4, onset 5–20, extremely variable expression from minimal facial weakness to severe disability, deltoids and forearm spared; Popeye arm appearance	Myopathic changes; moth eaten fibers, occasional inflammatory infiltrates	Nonmyonecrotic myopathy, i.e., MUAP changes without fibrillation potentials; with early or mild disease may be normal
Limb-girdle dystrophy	Usually recessive, sometimes dominant; slowly progressive pelvic and shoulder girdle weakness, deltoids involved; variable expression, heterogeneous disorder; CK elevated 5–10x normal	Fiber atrophy, marked fiber hypertrophy, fiber splitting, necrosis and regeneration, dysmorphic fibers, fibrosis	Myonecrotic myopathy
Emery Dreifuss dystrophy	X-linked; humeroperoneal wasting and weakness; early prominent contractures–especially elbow flexion and neck extension; striking cardiac abnormalities	Varies from selective type 1 atrophy to typical dystrophy, may have features of neurogenic atrophy	Features of both myopathy and neuropathy
Oculopharyngeal dystrophy	Autosomal dominant; adult onset of ptosis, dysphagia and mild limb girdle weakness; variable, mild EOM weakness	Fiber size variability subsarcolemmal rimmed vacuoles, 8.5 mm tubular filaments in myonuclei	Nonmyonecrotic myopathy, i.e., MUAP changes without fibrillation potentials; may have neurogenic feature; abnormalities most obvious in shoulder girdle musculature
Congenital muscular dystrophy	Heterogeneous; usually autosomal recessive; infantile onset of progressive hypotonia and weakness; prominent contractures; EOM's full; variable CNS involvement (severe in Fukuyama type)	Nonspecific myopathy with necrosis and regeneration	Myonecrotic myopathy

ance, cramps, rhabdomyolysis, progressive weakness and others (12). Some are part of a more widespread disorder with other neurologic or systemic manifestations. This discussion will cover the metabolic myopathies affecting glycogen and lipid metabolism. Mitochondrial myopathies and channelopathies will be considered in separate sections.

The ATP required to drive muscle contraction may come from four different sources. For immediate use, energy stored as phosphocreatine can convert ADP to ATP through the action of creatine kinase. Phosphocreatine stores are limited, and the expended energy requires quick replacement. Metabolic processes can convert glucose, lipid, nucleotides or protein into ATP. For muscle, the most important energy sources are glucose and lipid. Brief, intense muscle contraction is primarily fueled by glucose in type 2 muscle fibers. More sustained contraction is primarily fueled by lipid in type 1 fibers. Metabolic errors involving these two systems have quite different clinical profiles.

The muscle's energy factories are its mitochondria. Essential enzymes are located on the inner and outer mitochondrial membranes. The sequential steps of glycolysis result in the ultimate formation of pyruvate, which enters the mitochondria, undergoes oxidative decarboxylation and is converted into acetyl-CoA which enters the tricarboxylic acid (TCA) cycle to produce NADH and FADH. Under the control of carnitine palmityl transferase (CPT), long chain fatty acids (LCFAs) combine in the cytosol complex with carnitine for transport across the mitochondrial membranes. In the mitochondrial interior, these LCFAs undergo beta oxidation with the ultimate formation of acetyl-CoA for the TCA cycle, as well as the formation of NADH and FADH directly. The dinucleotides derived from beta oxidation and the TCA cycle enter the electron transport (respiratory) chain, a series of oxidation-reduction reactions mediated by 5 different "complexes" of multienzymes located on the inner mitochondrial membrane. Oxidative processing through the respiratory chain produces ATP which exits the mitochondria and returns to the cytosol where, under the influence of myosin ATPase, it powers the cross bridges that slide the actin filaments and result in muscle contraction.

These complex metabolic processes can go awry in a number of ways, resulting in a metabolic myopathy. Defective glycolysis may fail to supply enough glucose for brief, high intensity activity, resulting in cramps (more accurately painful contractures), exercise intolerance and rhabdomyolysis: McArdle's disease and related conditions (13). Carnitine deficiency results in an inability to transport LCFAs into the mitochondria, resulting in accumulation of lipid in muscle cells and impaired energy metabolism. In CPT deficiency, LCFAs are not available as an energy source, leading to rhabdomyolysis after sustained exertion. There are many variations on this essential theme related to specific, rare enzyme deficiencies. In most the EMG is normal or shows only minimal myopathic changes. In the syndromes involving abnormal glycogen metabolism, the electrodiagnostic features can provide important clues to the diagnosis. The clinical, pathological and electrodiagnostic medical aspects of some of the more common disorders are summarized in Table 19.4. The diagnosis of some of the metabolic myopathies may be possible through recent additions to the diagnostic armamentarium, sparing patients the rigors of the traditional workup (14,15).

MITOCHONDRIAL MYOPATHY

The mitochondrial myopathies (MMs) are disorders which are akin to the metabolic myopathies, characterized by some abnormality of mitochondrial metabolism and sometimes accompanied by abnormalities of mitochondrial structure or number (16). Clinical abnormalities are rarely limited to the neuromuscular system, and in fact some mitochondropathies have no obvious neuromuscular involvement, e.g., Leber's optic atrophy or Leigh's syndrome.

The MMs share a distinguishing but not invariably present feature, the ragged red fiber (RRF). The RRF, usually a type 1 fiber, appears reddish against the green background of the modified Gomori trichrome stain, with subsarcolemmal and intermyofibrillar collections of irregular red material reflecting the presence of abnormal mitochondria. RRFs are not specific for mitochondropathies and can occasionally appear in other conditions. Electron microscopy discloses a variety of abnormalities: an increased number of normal mitochondria, abnormally large or morphologically deformed mitochondria, or mitochondria with paracrystalline inclusions. Mitochondrial DNA is inherited solely from the mother, so these disorders may display maternal inheritance. The metabolic aberration most often involves one of the respiratory chain enzyme complexes. While these diseases usually begin in childhood or young adulthood, late life onset can occur (17). The frequency of ophthalmoplegia and fatiguability may cause confusion with myasthenia gravis (18).

Electrodiagnostically, the MMs are by and large bland, with either no abnormalities or changes limited to the MUAPs, without fibrillations, CRDs or myotonia. A mild peripheral neuropathy is not uncommon (19). The clinical, pathological and electrodiagnostic

TABLE 19.4
Summary of Selected Metabolic Myopathies

Condition	Clinical Features	Pathology	Electrodiagnostic Picture
McArdle's disease (myophosphorylase deficiency)	Exercise intolerance; cramps and stiffness precipitated by brief, high intensity exercise; onset 2nd–3rd decade; autosomal recessive, chromosome 11; male predominance; second wind phenomenon; no rise in venous lactate; occasional rhabdomyolysis; fixed proximal weakness with advancing age in 1/3; variants: late life progressive proximal weakness; fatal infantile form	PAS positive, subsarcolemmal vacuoles, negative phosphorylase stain, fiber size variability, occasional degenerating and regenerating fibers	Early recruitment of short duration, low amplitude MUAPs and polyphasics, especially with increasing age; fibrillation potentials; electrically silent painful contractures induced by exercise; decremental response to 20 Hz repetitive nerve stimulation
Tarui's disease (phosphofructokinase deficiency)	Rare; same as McArdle's disease, but no fixed weakness; +/− hemolytic anemia; no second wind	Same as McArdle's but negative PFK stain and positive phosphorylase stain	Same as McArdle's
Pompe's disease	Floppy baby; onset by 3 months; progressive weakness; cardiomyopathy; respiratory insufficiency; death by age 2; autosomal recessive	Severe vacuolar myopathy, glycogen storage	MUAP changes as above, profuse fibrillation potentials, positive sharp waves, CRDs, and myotonic discharges, especially in paraspinal muscles, in the absence of clinical myotonia
Adult acid maltase deficiency	Progressive proximal weakness plus respiratory insufficiency in adolescence or early adulthood; mimics polymyositis or limb-girdle dystrophy; may present with respiratory failure	Vacuolar myopathy with glycogen storage	Same as infantile form
Carnitine deficiency	Childhood or early adult onset of progressive proximal weakness; +/− hypertrophic cardiomyopathy	Lipid storage, primarily in Type I fibers	Normal or minimal MUAP changes, occasional fibrillation potentials in some cases
CPT deficiency	Recurrent attacks of rhabdomyolysis beginning in adolescence, precipitated by prolonged exercise, fasting; myalgia and stiffness common but no true cramp, no second wind; normal exam between attacks	Normal, or changes secondary to rhabdomyolysis, minimal lipid accumulation in 1/3 of cases	Normal, or MUAP changes only interictally; myonecrotic myopathy pattern during attacks
Myoadenylate deaminase deficiency	Exercise intolerance, exertional myalgias, adult onset, failure of ammonia to rise after forearm exercise; a controversial entity	Normal except for absence of staining for the enzyme	Normal

medical aspects of some of the more common disorders are summarized in Table 19.5.

CHANNELOPATHY

The term channelopathy refers to a condition affecting one of the voltage-gated ion channels in skeletal muscle or peripheral nerve (see Chapter 4). Molecular genetics has shown that abnormalities, usually inherited, of the sodium, potassium, chloride or calcium channel underlie many clinically diverse conditions, including: the congenital myotonias, the periodic paralyses, neuromyotonia, episodic ataxia, and malignant hyperthermia (20).

The electrodiagnostic picture in the channelopathies is varied and often complex. Myotonia occurs in myotonic dystrophy and in the sodium channelopathies (hyperkalemic periodic paralysis and paramyotonia congenita). The different forms of myotonia congenita are associated with mutations in the chloride channel gene (21). Potassium channel abnormalities are important in the syndromes of continuous muscle fiber activity (22). Mutations in the calcium channel gene are pivotal in the predisposition to develop malignant hyperthermia.

Most channelopathies are clinically heterogeneous. Since most dominantly inherited diseases result from a change-of-function alteration in a mutant gene's protein product, heterozygotes have both mutant and normal proteins. One possible mechanism for clinical variability could be the difference in relative levels of mutant vs. normal mRNA in different patients with the same mutation. The clinical variability and severity may ultimately relate to the ratio of mutant and normal channels. For instance, the dominantly inherited form of myotonia congenita, Thomsen's disease, is usually a mild disorder with considerable clinical heterogeneity. The EMG picture correlates most closely with mutation data, still some mutation-positive patients may fail to demonstrate myotonia on at least one occasion, and rare patients may never have electrical myotonia. Only about half of the mutation-positive patients have obvious percussion myotonia.

Myotonia is a kind of sustained contraction of a muscle, an inability to relax, which is usually nonpainful. It should not be confused with cramp, spasticity, rigidity, dystonia or myoedema. It may be brought on by contraction of the muscle (e.g.,grip myotonia), percussion (APB and EDC work well), or during EMG by needle movement. The distribution may vary in the different myotonic syndromes. In myotonic dystrophy, myotonia is most obvious in affected muscles and distal muscles; it may disappear as muscle atrophy sets in with disease progression. Mild myotonia may only be visible in the facial muscles or eyelids. Clinical myotonia improves with repeated contractions, the warm up phenomenon, and may worsen in the cold or after prolonged rest. Paradoxical myotonia is that which worsens after repetitive contraction. Myotonia can occur in other circumstances, for instance: Isaac's syndrome, chondrodystrophy, Schwartz-Jampel syndrome, periodic paralysis, acid maltase and debrancher deficiency, myotubular myopathy and due to the effects of certain drugs.

The clinical and electrodiagnostic features of some of the nondystrophic myotonic syndromes are summarized in Table 19.6. Myotonic discharges on percussion or needle movement are common to all, although those in paramyotonia congenita are sparser and somewhat atypical with less waxing and waning. Myotonic discharges generally become slightly more prominent with cooling, but in paramyotonia congenita marked cooling may cause not only disappearance of the myotonia but paralysis of the muscle. MUAPs and recruitment are normal in Thomsen's disease but small polyphasics are present in distal muscles in some patients with recessive myotonia congenita; analysis of MUAPs and recruitment is often difficult due to the interference of the myotonia. A decremental response may occur on rapid (>30 Hz)

TABLE 19.5
Summary of Mitochondrial Myopathies

Condition	Clinical Features	Pathology	Electrodiagnostic Picture
Kearns-Sayre syndrome	Progressive external ophthalmoplegia; retinitis pigmentosa; short stature; heart block; variable weakness; peripheral neuropathy	Myopathy with ragged red fibers	"Myopathic" MUAP changes; no fibrillation potentials; may have mild generalized axonopathy; may have abnormal SFEMG simulating a neuromuscular transmission disorder; normal study in most cases
Myoclonic epilepsy and ragged red fibers (MERRF)	Heterogeneous picture; proximal weakness (no PEO); ataxia; cognitive impairment	Myopathy with ragged red fibers	Usually normal
Mitochondrial myopathy, lactic acidosis and stroke like episodes (MELAS)	Heterogeneous picture; short stature; recurrent focal neurological deficits; seizures; vomiting; migraine; increased lactate	Myopathy with ragged red fibers	Usually normal, sometimes with mild MUAP abnormalities

TABLE **19.6**
Myotonic Syndromes Other Than Myotonic Dystrophy

Condition	Clinical Features	Pathophysiologic Features	Electrodiagnostic Features
Myotonia congenita, dominant form (Thomsen's disease)	Onset in infancy; non-progressive, generalized stiffness and myotonia worse in the cold; no weakness; muscle hypertrophy common, especially masseters (characteristic facies); stiffness and myotonia decrease after exercise	Absence of type 2B fibers, decreased chloride conductance, probable abnormality of chloride channel	Widespread, profuse myotonic discharges; decremental response on rapid repetitive nerve stimulation or after brief isometric exercise
Myotonia congenita, recessive form (Becker's disease)	Later onset; progressive generalized stiffness and myotonia that decrease after exercise; legs > arms; transient weakness that resolves with exercise; fixed weakness in some; can simulate myotonic dystrophy	Absence of type 2B fibers, decreased chloride conductance; probable abnormality of chloride channel	Same as dominant form except more marked decremental response; small polyphasic MUAPs in distal muscles in some
Paramyotonia congenita	Autosomal dominant; onset in infancy; mild to moderate stiffness and myotonia, primarily in hands and face; nonprogressive; attacks of weakness precipitated by cold or exercise; stiffness and myotonia increase with exercise (paradoxical)	Abnormal Na+ channel function	Mild to moderate myotonia with less waxing and waning; myotonia decreases with cooling; with extreme cold myotonia disappears and the muscle becomes paralyzed; no decrement on rapid repetitive nerve stimulation or after brief, isometric exercise
Proximal myotonic myopathy (PROMM)	Onset in early adulthood, peculiar muscle pain, proximal weakness without atrophy, cataracts, intermittent clinical myotonia, absence of chromosome 19 CTG repeats	Mild myopathic changes on muscle biopsy, no DNA linkage to muscle chloride or sodium channel genes	Myotonic discharges, no decrease in M wave amplitude following 1 minute of isometric exercise

repetitive stimulation, causing loss of M wave amplitude of up to 50% in dominant and 80% in recessive myotonia congenita. This decremental response is not present in paramyotonia congenita.

The periodic paralysis (PP) syndromes are a group of diseases characterized by episodic weakness. PP can secondarily complicate a number of systemic diseases which produce aberrations of K^+ concentration. The primary PP syndromes are divided into hypokalemic and K^+ sensitive forms. In the K^+ sensitive forms, the administration of K^+ induces weakness. Most of these are due to abnormalities of the Na^+ channel. The familial hypokalemic form is due to an abnormality of the dihydropyridine receptor. Thyrotoxicosis can cause a sporadic syndrome closely resembling familial hypokalemic PP. Paramyotonia congenita is also due to an abnormality of the Na^+ channel and is closely related to PP (21).

All the forms of PP have features in common: attacks of weakness with hyporeflexia, sparing bulbar and respiratory function, which are provoked by rest following exercise; eyelid myotonia; normal interictal strength during the early course; and the development of permanent weakness in some patients. In the hypokalemic form, onset is usually in adolescence, attacks last for many hours, the weakness is severe, and attacks may be precipitated by carbohydrate ingestion. In the hyperkalemic, or K^+ sensitive, form, onset is usually in childhood, attacks last less than 2 hours, the weakness is mild, and attacks may be precipitated by fasting. The episodic weakness in paramyotonia congenita closely resemble those in hyperkalemic PP except the attacks are also provoked by cold; the underlying defect involves the same gene and both conditions are due to dysfunction of the Na^+ channel. Hyperkalemic PP has been further divided into a form in which there is clinical and electrical myotonia and a form without this feature.

The electrodiagnostic picture in PP is markedly different during attacks vs. between attacks. As an attack evolves, the M wave amplitude progressively falls and the muscle may eventually become inexcitable if paralysis is severe. Brief exercise or brief rapid repetitive stimulation may temporarily return the M wave amplitude toward normal (7). Needle examination shows a progression toward low amplitude, short duration MUAPs and decreased insertional activity as weakness progresses; with severe weakness the patient may lose the ability to recruit units and the muscle may become electrical silent. Occasionally, fibrillation potentials appear as weakness develops. Recovery follows the reverse sequence, MUAPs reappear and regain their amplitude and the M wave returns to normal. Patients with the myotonic subtype of hyperkalemic PP may display myotonic discharges at the onset of the attack, which disappear as weakness develops and resurface with recovery.

The interictal electrodiagnostic features depend on whether the patient has developed fixed weakness. If not, routine studies are normal. If so, the needle examination may show early recruitment and small, polyphasic units. Patients with the myotonic subtype of K$^+$ sensitive PP display the characteristic discharges.

The diagnosis can sometimes be made by the exercise test, which is positive in 70% of patients (23). After establishing a consistent baseline M wave amplitude in a well immobilized hypothenar muscle, the patient exercises vigorously for 3–5 minutes, pausing only as necessary. The M wave is then recorded every minute during exercise and for 30–45 minutes afterward. In controls, only minimal changes in M wave amplitude occur during this procedure. In PP, an abnormal increase in M wave amplitude occurs immediately postexercise (> ±30%), followed by a greater than normal decrement postexercise (> ±30%). The maximal decrement generally occurs in the first 20 minutes after exercise.

Malignant hyperthermia (MH) is a rare and dramatic disorder usually triggered by anesthetic agents, such as halothane, or muscle relaxants, such as succinylcholine (24). The temperature typically begins to soar during the induction of anesthesia, sometimes accompanied by muscular rigidity, especially masseter spasm, accompanied by other manifestations of intense hypermetabolism. The temperature can reach levels of 105–110° F. Patients surviving the acute phase often develop rhabdomyolysis with marked weakness and extreme elevations of CK. The mortality currently is about 30%, usually due to cardiac arrest presumably mediated by K$^+$ release, acute renal failure or DIC (1). MH is associated with a variety of neuromuscular disorders, especially central core disease. Patients with dystrophinopathies are at increased risk. In some patients, the only clue to MH

susceptibility is unexplained CK elevation, and many patients are totally asymptomatic before the event. About 1/3 have a positive family history of MH episodes, but there is genetic heterogeneity.

Susceptibility to MH in many instances results from a mutation of the gene for the ryanodine receptor, which makes up the calcium release channel of the sarcoplasmic reticulum. Dysfunction of the channel in response to a triggering agent or event causes an outpouring of calcium from the terminal cisterns resulting in generalized muscular overactivity and hypermetabolism. The normal relaxation mechanisms for resequestering calcium after shortening fail and muscle contraction continues, leading to rhabdomyolysis and the cascade of complications. The proximity of the abnormal gene causing central core disease to the ryanodine receptor gene on chromosome 19 may explain the increased risk.

There are several diseases associated with excess motor unit activity (25). These include the stiff man syndrome, tetanus, Isaac's syndrome (neuromyotonia, continuous muscle fiber activity) and others. Though most channelopathies are inherited disorders, Isaac's syndrome (IS) is sporadic and usually due to autoantibody attack against the voltage gated K$^+$ channel (VGKC) (26). The pathophysiology in the other conditions is varied (22).

The stiff man syndrome presents with chronic, progressive, fluctuating muscle stiffness and frequent painful spasms. Autoantibodies to glutamic acid decarboxylase are present in about half the patients. These presumably interfere with GABA activity and cause a generalized central disinhibition. EMG needle examination shows continuous firing of normal MUAPs, which the patient is unable to suppress. The excess activity subsides with sleep, anesthesia and nerve block, indicating central origin. Facial muscles are usually spared. Tetanus resembles stiff man syndrome in many respects, but presents as a fulminant disease with severe, generalized spasms which involve the face and jaw.

Typical symptoms of IS include muscle stiffness, cramps, impaired relaxation, myokymia, and hyperhidrosis. IS is associated with other autoimmune diseases, and can complicate thymoma. It responds to immunosuppressive treatments. An autoantibody directed against the VGKC probably suppresses the outward K+ current, destabilizes the membrane and causes nerve hyperexcitability. IS is usually a sporadic condition but may occur in hereditary peripheral nerve disorders and in other settings (25).

The characteristic electrodiagnostic features of IS are continuous MUAP activity not under voluntary control; spontaneous firing of MUAPs as doublets, triplets or multiplets; myokymia; fasciculations;

TABLE 19.7
Common Inflammatory Myopathies

Condition	Clinical Features	Pathology	Electrodiagnostic Features
Polymyositis	Symmetrical, progressive, predominantly proximal weakness; dysphagia, ↑ CK, (5–10×); myalgias uncommon; no skin lesions; increased risk of malignancy likely	Necrosis, inflammatory infiltration with CD8+ T lymphocytes and macrophages, most intense infiltrate around muscle fibers	Normal NCS; needle EMG abnormalities vary from fibrillation potentials only (early disease) to full blown myonecrotic myopathy to MUAP abnormalities only in remission; occasional long duration polyphasic unit with late components in chronic disease
Dermatomyositis	Symmetric, progressive, predominately proximal weakness; dysphagia; ↑ CK; myalgias common in children; contractures; skin rash (periorbital edema, heliotrope cyanosis, Gottron's nodules, scaly erythema over MP and IP joints, knees and elbows; disease is a vasculitis in childhood dermatomyositis; increased risk of malignancy in adult dermatomyositis; rash is usually the first symptom; scarring and calcinosis common in children	Necrosis, inflammation, infiltration with B and CD4+ T lymphocytes, perifascicular atrophy, perivascular infiltrates, most intense infiltrate around blood vessels	Same as polymyositis
Inclusion body myositis	Older patients; male predominance; slowly progressive/indolent, painless, often asymmetric weakness of proximal and distal muscles of arms and legs; weakness of wrist and finger flexors > deltoid and quadriceps > hip flexors; CK < 12× normal; relatively resistant to immunosuppressant treatment; ESR usually normal; not associated with malignancy	Same as polymyositis plus rimmed vacuoles, 15–18 nm tubofilaments, amyloid deposition, angular fibers and small group atrophy common	Same as polymyositis; questionable increased frequency long duration polyphasic units ("neurogenic features")

cramp discharges and very high frequency (150–300 Hz) bursts of MUAPs referred to as neuromyotonia. These findings persist after proximal nerve block and likely arise from distal nerve terminals which lie beyond the protection of the blood nerve barrier and are susceptible to circulating autoantibodies.

Patients with the cramp fasciculation syndrome typically present with cramps. Fasciculations are particularly obvious in the small foot muscles. The needle examination is normal except for fasciculations; there are no fibrillations, CRDs or myokymia. Repetitive nerve stimulation produces a shower of afterdischarges (27).

Acquired Myopathies

The common acquired myopathies include the inflammatory myopathies (polymyositis, dermatomyo-sitis and inclusion body myositis), critical illness myopathy, toxic myopathies and rhabdomyolysis. Less common syndromes are summarized in the tables.

INFLAMMATORY MYOPATHY

The inflammatory myopathies (IM) of primary clinical concern are polymyositis (PM), dermatomyositis (DM) and inclusion body myositis (IBM) (28–30). PM is a cell mediated autoimmune attack directly on muscle fibers. In DM, a humorally mediated autoimmune attack primarily against intramuscular blood vessels leads to an ischemic-inflammatory myopathy. IM can complicate connective tissue disorders and other systemic diseases, as well as infections, most notably HIV. The clinical, pathologic and electrodiagnostic features of IM are summarized in Table 19.7. The differential diagnosis of the IM syndromes is extensive, and basically includes any condition which can cause the picture of myonecrotic myopathy.

The electrodiagnostic picture of an active IM syndrome is that of a myonecrotic myopathy. The findings vary with the stage and activity of the disease (Fig. 19.6). In early disease, fibrillations are more prominent than MUAP changes; in remission MUAP changes are more prominent than fibrillations. In active disease, the classic triad of increased insertional activity with CRDs, fibrillations and positive waves and small, polyphasic, short duration, rapidly recruited MUAPs is typical (28). The yield of the EMG examination increases with the number of muscles examined. The incidence of fibrillation potentials is highest in the paraspinal muscles, and in some patients they are limited to the paraspinal muscles. Fibrillations may be of small amplitude. The paraspinal fibrillations are not limited to the multifidus muscles as often occurs in radiculopathy, and examination of the superficial paraspinals may be more rewarding. Long duration, complex polyphasics can occur in IM, as in any chronic myopathy, but seem more frequent in IBM, perhaps reflecting the indolence of that condition. Greater intensity of fibrillations in wrist and finger flexors compared to shoulder muscles and quadriceps and anterior tibialis compared to hip flexors would suggest IBM.

Muscle disease can complicate a host of systemic illnesses. Table 19.8 summarizes the clinical, pathological and electrodiagnostic features of some of these. Thyrotoxicosis can cause a myopathy, but may also be associated with myasthenia gravis or produce a periodic paralysis syndrome (31). Thyrotoxic PP oc-

curs primarily in Oriental males, and has been reported with factitious hyperthyroidism; the clinical features closely resemble familial hypokalemic PP. Hypothyroidism typically causes a bland myopathy. True myotonic discharges have been reported but must be extremely rare. The often striking elevation of CK seems inconsistent with the paucity of electrical or pathological evidence of myonecrosis. Some patients develop muscle enlargement: the Kocher-Debré-Sémélaigne (infant Hercules) syndrome in children or the Hoffman syndrome in adults. Steroid myopathy is classically a chronic, low grade, bland myopathy that arises as a complication of steroid treatment of a systemic illness. Recently a more acute form has been recognized (32). Sarcoidosis commonly involves muscle pathologically but does not often cause clinical symptoms (33).

CRITICAL ILLNESS MYOPATHY

Critical illness myopathy, also referred to as acute quadriplegic myopathy, thick filament myopathy, post paralysis and acute necrotizing myopathy of intensive care, is an entity still being clarified. Affected patients usually develop a flaccid quadriplegia, the "floppy person syndrome," with variable preservation of reflexes and a muscle biopsy demonstrating marked fiber atrophy with disorganized myofibrils and selective loss of thick (myosin) filaments with relative preservation of thin (actin) filaments and Z-discs, especially in type 2 fibers. Most cases follow prolonged use of neuromuscular blocking agents (NMBAs), especially pancuronium and vecuronium, and concomitant high dose corticosteroids. The majority of the patients have received NMBAs plus corticosteroids, a few have received NMBAs alone and the rest received corticosteroids alone (34). However, pancuronium and vecuronium are members of a series of synthetic *bis*-quaternary-ammonium steroids, and the ring structure of these compounds bears a striking resemblance to the structure of corticosteroids. In effect, all patients with critical illness myopathy have thus received steroids.

The pathology resembles that seen experimentally with high dose corticosteroids following denervation, and the NMBAs could be causing functional denervation. The syndrome has occurred in a patient whose neuromuscular blockade was due to myasthenic crisis. Risk factors include hepatic dysfunction, acidosis, renal failure and female sex. Critical illness myopathy does not seem to share critical illness polyneuropathy's association with sepsis. CK elevation is variable; it may be low as in typical chronic steroid myopathy or extremely elevated if the patient has suffered rhabdomyolysis. The NMBAs, especially vecuronium, may

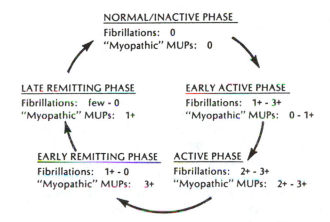

FIGURE 19.6. The cycle of changes on needle electrode examination that can be seen during the various stages of a reversible necrotizing myopathy, such as polymyositis. Reprinted with permission from Wilbourn AJ. The electrodiagnostic examination with myopathies. J Clin Neurophys 1993;10: 132–148.

TABLE 19.8
Myopathy Complicating Systemic Illness

Condition	Clinical Features	Pathology	Electrodiagnostic Picture
Hyperthyroidism	Proximal weakness and atrophy; brisk reflexes; eye signs; fasciculations; weight loss; low CK; may co-exist with myasthenia gravis	Usually normal; mild, nonspecific changes in some	Myopathic EMG with occasional fibrillations; fasciculation potentials; myokymia
Hypothyroidism	Weakness; stiffness; cramps; myalgias; associated carpal tunnel syndrome; myoedema; muscle enlargement in some; marked elevation of CK; hung up reflexes	Usually normal	Normal to mild MUAP changes; occurrence of true myotonia debatable
Steroid myopathy	Proximal weakness; mild atrophy; normal reflexes; normal or low CK; greatest risk is with high dose, daily halogenated steroids in women	Selective type 2 fiber atrophy	Usually normal; minimal MUAP changes in some patients
Sarcoidosis	Young adults; muscle involvement common but rarely symptomatic; progressive weakness and wasting; myopathy may be "atrophic" or "nodular"	Inflammatory myopathy with noncaseating granulomas	Myonecrotic myopathy; can have myotonic discharges
Critical illness myopathy	Prolonged paralysis in association with critical illness, usually after prolonged neuromuscular blockade, with or without concomitant steroids; variable CK elevation; ± rhabdomyolysis	Severe atrophy, selective lysis of thick filaments especially in type 2 fibers, ± fiber necrosis, ± vacuoles	↓ M wave amplitudes; normal sensory potentials; normal NCVs; ± fibrillations; MUAPs normal or short duration polyphasic

be more prone to produce CK elevation and rhabdomyolysis. In some patients, the post paralysis syndrome is due to the prolonged effect of NMBAs; such patients demonstrate a decremental response on 2 Hz repetitive stimulation long after the time when the NMBA effect should have faded (35). Critical illness myopathy is much less common than critical illness polyneuropathy. In the weak ICU patient, it may be clinically difficult to sort out prolonged neuromuscular blockade from critical illness myopathy from critical illness polyneuropathy, and electrodiagnostic studies can help greatly in the differential diagnosis.

TOXIC MYOPATHY

Many different chemicals and drugs are toxic to skeletal muscle. Some cause acute rhabdomyolysis, but most cause an indolent, low grade syndrome of progressive weakness or an asymptomatic elevation of CK. Any number of drugs can cause weakness or muscle dysfunction through the induction of electrolyte imbalance, changes in calcium or magnesium metabolism, or the induction of an autoimmune process. A few agents, such as cimetidine or penicillamine can induce an inflammatory myopathy. Some agents are toxic to both nerve and muscle and affected patients can have evidence of both processes. A more myopathic EMG picture in proximal muscles evolving into a more neuropathic picture in distal muscles, especially when associated with sensory symptoms or minor slowing of NCVs, suggests the possibility of a combined toxic effect, most often due to alcohol, occasionally due an agent such as colchicine or vincristine. Needle EMG in most chronic toxic myopathies shows early recruitment of short duration, low amplitude polyphasics with low grade spontaneous activity. Some toxins can produce myotonic discharges, usually without concomitant clinical myotonia. Cholesterol lowering agent myopathy (CLAM) can complicate therapy with any of the antilipid agents. The clinical picture may vary from asymptomatic CK elevation to cramps and myalgias with variable weakness to rhabdomyolysis.

The pathology is frequently helpful. Zidovudine causes a mitochondrial myopathy with ragged red fibers which is distinctly different from the inflammatory myopathy of AIDS. The presence of autophagic vacuoles and myelin figures suggests colchicine or chloroquine.

Alcohol is of course the archetypal myotoxin. It can lead to rhabdomyolysis by causing prolonged coma, electrolyte imbalance or seizures, or possibly by a direct toxic effect. Alcoholics may also develop an acute myopathy with cramps and myalgias and tubular aggregates on biopsy. Whether chronic myopathy can be attributed to alcohol alone remains debatable.

RHABDOMYOLYSIS

Rhabdomyolysis (RM) refers to acute, fulminant muscle necrosis which leads to weakness, myalgias, myoglobinuria, and often to acute renal failure and a host of complications (36). RM can occur in anyone under proper circumstances, but patients who have recurrent episodes often have an underlying metabolic myopathy, most commonly CPT deficiency.

RM was originally described in patients who had suffered crush injuries from prolonged external pressure while trapped in bombed out buildings during World War II (37). The pressure from prolonged immobility, as in coma or a drug stupor, can produce RM through the same mechanism. RM has been reported many times in apparently normal individuals under conditions of intense physical exertion. Conditions of high ambient temperature and dehydration, especially with hypokalemia, predispose. Seemingly ordinary activities, such as weight lifting, mountaineering, Marine boot camp, or pick-up basketball, can induce acute muscle necrosis. Patients in status epilepticus suffer RM frequently. Numerous toxins can cause RM, most notably drugs of abuse, such as alcohol, heroin and cocaine, which can cause prolonged immobility, possibly confounded by a direct myotoxic effect. Many drugs and chemicals can cause RM, including cholesterol lowering agents, antifibrinolytics, cyclosporine, zidovudine, NMBAs, amphetamines, finasteride, licorice and others. Malignant hyperthermia and the neuroleptic malignant syndrome are special instances of RM related to specific drugs. Other etiologies include compartment syndromes and muscle ischemia. The electrodiagnostic picture in acute RM is that of a myonecrotic myopathy. Rarely does the EMG provide any clues to a specific etiology in the acute setting.

Key Points

- Myopathies are those conditions in which there is a primary dysfunction of skeletal muscle. There are numerous etiologies, including inflammatory myopathies, dystrophies, congenital myopathies, metabolic myopathies and

myopathies due to underlying systemic disorders. Most myopathies produce some changes in recruitment patterns and alterations in the individual MUAP, with a tendency toward low amplitude, short duration and polyphasic potentials. The myonecrotic myopathies are those which also induce abnormal insertional and spontaneous activity: fibrillation potentials, positive waves, and CRDs. Typically myonecrotic myopathies include the inflammatory myopathies, some dystrophies, some forms of congenital myopathy and other conditions. Nonmyonecrotic myopathies usually occur with metabolic and endocrine disorders.

- A muscle fascicle is a group of fibers lying together within a sheath of perimysium. The myonuclei lie peripherally just beneath the sarcolemma. Muscle fibers are made up of myofibrils, which are in turn made up of myofilaments, the contractile elements. The myofibril is composed of repeating identical segments called sarcomeres. During contraction, the myofilaments slide past each other to generate contractile power. Calcium is an important mediator of excitation contraction coupling. In addition to the contractile elements, skeletal muscle contains important cytoskeletal proteins which help provide it structure. One of the key cytoskeletal proteins is dystrophin, which reinforces the sarcolemma against the forces of muscle contraction. The ATPase stain separates muscle fibers into primarily oxidative type 1 and primarily glycolytic type 2 fibers.

- Muscle has a limited repertoire of reactions to injury. Some of the major categories of pathologic change include changes in fiber size and shape, variations in fiber type distribution, internalization of nuclei, fiber necrosis and regeneration, the presence of vacuoles, inclusions or other bodies, morphologic changes in individual fibers and changes in the interstitial compartment. Most pathologic changes are nonspecific but a few are characteristic of particular disease entities.

- Electrodiagnosis can provide valuable information in evaluating myopathies, but has limitations. Abnormalities found are seldom diagnostic of any specific disease process. Rapid and early recruitment of small, short duration, polyphasic potentials recruited in numbers out of proportion to the strength of muscle contraction, producing an abnormal abundance of MUAPs with even minimal exertion, is the electrodiagnostic hallmark of myopathies. Disorders associated with myonecrosis often produce spontaneous and increased insertional activity as well. Fibrillation potentials in myopathy are often of very low amplitude, and may discharge slowly.

- The muscular dystrophies are inherited disorders. The most common forms are myotonic dystrophy and the dystrophinopathies. The congenital myopathies are conditions which typically present in infancy and are nonprogressive, such as central core disease, centronuclear/myotubular myopathy, nemaline myopathy, and congenital fiber type disproportion. The metabolic myopathies are inborn errors of metabolism which may cause exercise intolerance, cramps, rhabdomyolysis, and weakness. The mitochondrial myopathies are characterized by an abnormality of mitochondrial metabolism and produce the distinctive ragged red fiber. The metabolic aberration most often involves one of the respiratory chain enzyme complexes. Channelopathies affect one of the voltage-gated ion channels in skeletal muscle or peripheral nerve, and include the congenital myotonias, the periodic paralyses, and malignant hyperthermia.

- The common acquired myopathies include the inflammatory myopathies (polymyositis, dermatomyositis and inclusion body myositis), myopathies which complicate systemic disease, critical illness myopathy, toxic myopathies and rhabdomyolysis.

References

1. Heffner RR, Schochet SS. Skeletal Muscle. In: Damjanov ILinder J, eds. Anderson's pathology. 10th ed. St. Louis: Mosby, 1996;2653–2690.
   An excellent short review of both clinical and pathological aspects of myopathies. Covers normal anatomy and physiology, procedures and techniques for muscle biopsy, general reactions of muscle to injury, and the pathological findings in common myopathies.

2. Wilbourn AJ. The electrodiagnostic examination with myopathies. J Clin Neurophysiol 1993;10:132–148.
   The values and limitations of the electrodiagnostic examination in assessing patients with possible myopathies are discussed. Limitations include: (1) no findings are specific for muscle disease; (2) the particular changes may be quite diverse; (3) myopathies of different etiologies may have the same presentation, whereas the same myopathy may have different presentations at different times; (4) a specific myopathy cannot be diagnosed; and (5) the ability to diagnose myopathy may be seriously compromised by the presence of certain disorders. Benefits include: (1) widespread muscle sampling; (2) help in determining most appropriate muscle for biopsy; (3) ascertaining, to some extent, the type of myopathy present, depending on the particular findings; (4) distinguishing entities often confused clinically with myopathies; (5) recognizing abnormalities (e.g., myotonic discharges) otherwise undetectable. Both the clinical and electrodiagnostic presentations of myopathies are discussed. Regarding the latter, the potential or actual changes seen with each component of the electrodiagnostic assessment (nerve conduction studies, late responses, repetitive stimulation studies, needle electrode examination, quantitative electromyographic studies) is reviewed.

3. Cruz Martinez A, Lopez Terradas JM. Conduction velocity along muscle fibers in situ in Duchenne muscular dystrophy. Arch Phys Med Rehabil 1990;71:558–561.
   The muscle fibers of the biceps brachii muscle were stimulated distally with two monopolar needles while recording proximally with a SFEMG electrode in 14 boys with DMD. The mean CV of 508 muscle fibers in situ (MFCV) calculated with this method shows that MFCV in DMD patients ($2.38 \pm .94$ m/sec) is significantly slower than in 20 control children of the same age ($3.24 \pm .53$ m/sec). The distribution frequency of MFCV in all fibers tested in healthy children shows a Gaussian distribution (mode = 3.2 m/sec). In DMD patients the distribution frequency is bimodal with spikes at 1.2 and 2.4 m/sec. Significant decrease in minimum propagation velocity and increased SD values were other striking results in patients with DD. Slowing and large variation in MFCV were significantly correlated with some findings in a coaxial needle EMG such as long polyphasics and MUAPs followed by satellites. Satellites might arise from atrophic muscle fibers with slow conduction velocity.

4. Daube JR. The description of motor unit potentials in electromyography. Neurology 1978;28:623–625.
   A plea for quantitative description of MUAPs rather than use of terms such as myopathic. Reviews the origin of the MUAP and the technical and biologic factors that can produce alterations in it. An accurate description of EMG data includes statistical description of the characteristics of a population of MUAPs, and these can be assessed at least subjectively even for routine EMGs, including recruitment patterns, duration and variability.

5. Uncini A, Lange DJ, Lovelace RE, et al. Long-duration polyphasic motor unit potentials in myopathies: a quantitative study with pathological correlation. Muscle Nerve 1990;13:263–267.
   In most myopathies, the duration of MUAPs is shorter than normal. However, polyphasic MUAPs of duration longer than 20% of the control mean, (long-duration polyphasic potentials, or LDPPs) may be seen. The authors analyzed the incidence and meaning of LDPPs using quantitative MUAP analysis in 41 patients with different myopathies. The mean duration of all potentials was reduced in only 64% of patients because LDPPs increased the mean. When only simple potentials were considered, however, the mean duration was decreased in 95% of patients. This observation confirms the need to exclude LDPPs when calculating the mean duration of MUAPs for diagnosis. LDPPs occurred most often in chronic polymyositis and in one patient with BMD. LDPPs are attributed to desynchronization of single-fiber potentials within the MUAP and may be due to slow conduction in regenerating muscle fibers.

6. Samaha FJ, Quinlan JG. Dystrophinopathies: clarification and complication. J Child Neurol 1996;11:13–20.
   A review of the clinical applications of advances made in molecular genetics, primarily with regard to Becker muscular dystrophy. A new classification is required to clarify such syndromes as DMD and BMD. Dystrophinopathies can be seen in patients with early onset and a severe course (DMD), patients with later onset and milder weakness (BMD), patients with myalgia and cramp syndrome, and patients with dilated cardiomyopathies. Dystrophin testing in muscle is the most sensitive test for identification of dystrophinopathy patients, although gene deletion studies can make the diagnosis in most cases.

7. Griggs RC, Mendell JR, Miller RG. Evaluation and treatment of myopathies. Philadelphia: F.A. Davis Company, 1995.

8. Moxley R T 3rd. Proximal myotonic myopathy: mini-review of a recently delineated clinical disorder. Neuromuscul Disord 1996;6:87–93.
   A mini-review describing proximal myotonic myopathy (PROMM), a recently delineated, dominantly inherited disorder similar to but distinct from myotonic dystrophy. PROMM is not linked to the gene locus for myotonic dystrophy or to the loci of the genes of the muscle sodium and chloride channels associated with other myotonic disorders. Patients often present with myotonia and peculiar muscle pain in early adulthood and develop weakness of the thigh muscles later in life.

Cataracts that are indistinguishable from those in myotonic dystrophy also occur commonly. The gene defect responsible for PROMM awaits discovery. Because of the clinical similarities between PROMM and myotonic dystrophy, clarification of the genetic differences will not only shed light on the pathomechanism of proximal myotonic myopathy, but may also increase our understanding of myotonic dystrophy. See also Sander HW, Tavoulareas GP, Quinto CM, et al. Exercise test distinguishes proximal myotonic myopathy from myotonic dystrophy. Muscle Nerve 1997;20:235–237.

9. Jablecki CK. Myopathies. In: Brown WF, Bolton CF, eds. Clinical electromyography. 2nd ed. Boston: Butterworth-Heinemann, 1993;653–689.

10. Nonaka I, Kobayashi O, Osari S. Nondystrophinopathic muscular dystrophies including myotonic dystrophy. Semin Pediatr Neurol 1996;3:110–121.
The spectacular progress concerning dystrophin and its pathology, the dystrophinopathies, has led to a somewhat arbitrarily separated heterogeneous group of nondystrophinopathic muscular dystrophies that currently comprise the Emery-Dreifuss type, the nosologically heterogeneous autosomal-recessive limb-girdle muscular dystrophy, the severe childhood autosomal-recessive muscular dystrophy, the merosin-positive and -negative congenital muscular dystrophies, the autosomal-recessive distal muscular dystrophy of Miyoshi, the facio-scapulo-humeral muscular dystrophy, and myotonic dystrophy, both the adult and neonatal variants. Deficiencies of adhalin in a particular form of limb-girdle muscular dystrophy, and of merosin in a particular form of congenital muscular dystrophy as well as the newly discovered principle of abnormal tri-nucleotide repeats in myotonic dystrophy are evidence of progress that has also amplified the notion of the dystrophinopathies that the protein-deficient muscular dystrophies can now be considered examples of contributions of the dystrophin-glycoprotein complex across the muscle fiber plasma membrane.

11. Goebel HH. Congenital myopathies. Semin Pediatr Neurol 1996;3:152–161.
The congenital myopathies (CM) are a group of nonprogressive neuromuscular conditions, often hereditary, delineated by morphological techniques, i.e., enzyme histochemistry and electron microscopy. The catalogue of CM entailing well known "classic" conditions as central core disease, nemaline myopathy, and centronuclear myopathy has continuously been expanded, now comprising some 40 conditions. Nosologic advances have occurred with immunohistochemical techniques that show generalized or focal protein abnormalities within muscle fibers of certain CM, but at much slower pace as to localization of CM genes. So far, only those for central core disease, nemaline myopathy, and myotubular myopathy have been reported. Epidemiological rarity and nosographic controversy of CM have contributed to this lack of molecular genetic progress in CM. See also Bodensteiner JB. Congenital myopathies. Muscle Nerve 1994;17:131–144.

12. Wortmann RL. Metabolic myopathies. Curr Opin Rheumatol 1991;3:925–933.
The term metabolic myopathy refers to a heterogeneous group of conditions that have in common abnormalities of muscle energy metabolism that result in skeletal muscle dysfunction. Most recognized metabolic myopathies are considered primary, represent inborn errors of metabolism, and are associated with known or postulated defects that affect the ability of muscle fibers to maintain adequate ATP concentrations.

Traditionally, these diseases are grouped into abnormalities of glycogen, lipid, purine, and mitochondrial biochemistry. This discussion reviews the basic metabolic pathways that regulate normal muscle function; recent observations involving glycogen storage diseases, carnitine deficiency states, and myoadenylate deaminase deficiencies; and lastly, newer techniques available to assess patients with myopathic disorders.

13. Servidei S, DiMauro S. Disorders of glycogen metabolism of muscle. Neurol Clin 1989;7:159–178.
Glycogen is a crucial source of energy in the initial stages of muscle activity and during exercise of high intensity. There are 10 well-defined biochemical defects of glycogen metabolism expressed in muscle and affecting the following enzymes: alpha 1,4 glucosidase (glycogenesis type II), debrancher enzyme (III), brancher enzyme (IV), phosphorylase (V), phosphofructokinase (VII), phosphorylase b kinase (VIII), phosphoglycerate kinase (IX), phosphoglycerate mutase (X), lactate dehydrogenase (XI). These disorders cause two main syndromes: one characterized by exercise intolerance with cramps and myoglobinuria, the other by fixed weakness. However, there are examples of clinical and biochemical heterogeneity for each disease, and molecular genetic analysis is already showing evidence of genetic heterogeneity.

14. el-Schahawi M, Tsujino S, Shanske S, et al. Diagnosis of McArdle's disease by molecular genetic analysis of blood. Neurology 1996;47:579–580.
An analysis of leukocyte DNA from 32 patients with suspected McArdle's disease, 24 of whom had biochemically or histochemically proven myophosphorylase deficiency. 19 were homozygous for the most common mutation, 2 were compound heterozygotes, and 1 was a manifesting heterozygote. Findings indicate that the diagnosis of McArdle's disease can be established in approximately 90% of patients using DNA isolated from leukocytes, thereby avoiding muscle biopsy.

15. Bank W, Chance B. An oxidative defect in metabolic myopathies: diagnosis by noninvasive tissue oximetry. Ann Neurol 1994;36:830–837.
This study used a noninvasive optical technique to measure oxygen consumption in the exercising limb in normal subjects and patients with metabolic myopathies. Noninvasive tissue oximetry during exercise demonstrates specific abnormalities in a variety of metabolic myopathies, indicating abnormal oxygen utilization, and will be a useful addition to the clinical investigation of exercise intolerance.

16. Lombes A, Bonilla E, DiMauro S. Mitochondrial encephalomyopathies. Rev Neurol (Paris) 1989;145:671–689.
This review deals with the morphological, clinical, biochemical and genetic aspects of mitochondrial encephalomyopathies. The various morphological abnormalities of mitochondria are described. These are not specific of any particular disease. They may be present in some non-mitochondrial diseases and may be lacking in diseases due to specific defects of mitochondrial enzymes (e.g. carnitine palmityl-transferase or pyruvate dehydrogenase). The clinical classification of mitochondrial encephalomyopathies is discussed. There are two main schools of thought: the "lumpers" do not recognize specific syndromes within the spectrum of mitochondrial "cytopathies"; the "splitters" try to identify specific syndromes while recognizing the existence of borderline cases. The following syndromes are described: chronic progressive external ophthalmoplegia (CPEO), Kearns-Sayre syndrome (KSS), MERRF syndrome (myoclonic epilepsy with ragged-red fibers), MELAS syndrome

(mitochondrial myopathy, encephalopathy, lactic acidosis, stroke-like episodes) and Leigh and Alpers syndromes. The biochemical classification comprises five types of abnormalities: defects of transport through the mitochondrial membrane, of substrate utilization, of Krebs' cycle, of oxidative phosphorylation and of various complexes of the respiratory chain. The clinical pictures corresponding to these defects are briefly described. The genetic aspects of these diseases are especially interesting because mitochondria have their own genome coding for thirteen proteins, all of them belonging to the respiratory chain. Genetic mitochondrial diseases may result from alterations of the nuclear genome, which are transmitted by Mendelian inheritance, but they may also be due to alterations of the mitochondrial genome and transmitted by non-Mendelian "maternal" heredity. A few examples are discussed, including Leber's optic atrophy and MERRF syndrome.

17. Johnston W, Karpati G, Carpenter S, et al. Late-onset mitochondrial myopathy. Ann Neurol 1995;37:16–23.
In the majority of patients with mitochondrial encephalomyopathies, signs and symptoms appear in the first three decades of life. This report describes a group of 9 older patients (>69 years old) with late-onset skeletal myopathy characterized by focal accumulations of deleted mitochondrial DNAs (mtDNAs) and altered muscle energy status, suggestive of a primary mitochondrial disease. The clinical phenotype was somewhat variable. However, all patients shared a common feature of insidious moderate proximal muscle weakness; some also showed fatigability and axial muscle weakness. In situ hybridization analysis demonstrated accumulations of messenger RNAs transcribed from deleted mtDNAs in a relatively large number of muscle fibers in the patient group. These fiber segments appeared as ragged red with the modified Gomori trichrome stain and hyperreactive with a modified succinate dehydrogenase stain. The myopathy in this group of patients appears to result from mitochondrial dysfunction related to the clonal expansion of different mtDNA deletions in individual fiber segments. While the origin of the mtDNA mutations is not clear, the phenotype seems to represent an exaggerated form of what is observed in the normal aging process.

18. Emeryk B, Rowinska-Marcinska K, Nowak-Michalska T, et al. Muscular fatigability in mitochondrial myopathies. An electrophysiological study. Electromyogr Clin Neurophysiol 1992;32:235–245.
The frequent occurrence of ophthalmoplegia and muscle fatigability in mitochondrial myopathy can make its distinction from myasthenia difficult. Neuromuscular transmission was investigated in 9 patients with mitochondrial myopathy. Normal neuromuscular transmission was present in 5 cases, in 3 there were slight abnormalities of neuromuscular transmission, and in 1 case neuromuscular transmission disturbances seemed to be of neurogenic origin.

19. Yiannikas C, McLeod JG, Pollard JD, et al. Peripheral neuropathy associated with mitochondrial myopathy. Ann Neurol 1986;20:249–257.
20 patients with mitochondrial myopathy were investigated for the presence of peripheral neuropathy. There were clinical features of a mild sensorimotor neuropathy in 5 patients (25%) and nerve conduction studies were abnormal in 10 patients (50%). Electrophysiological studies of the whole group showed significant impairment of motor and sensory conduction, compared with controls. Sural nerve biopsy and morphometric studies were performed on 4 patients with clinical neuropathy. There was a reduction in density of myelinated fibers and electron microscope features of axonal degeneration affecting myelinated and unmyelinated fibers. Abnormal mitochondria containing paracrystalline inclusions were seen in the Schwann cell cytoplasm of two nerves.

20. Hoffman EP. Voltage-gated ion channelopathies: inherited disorders caused by abnormal sodium, chloride, and calcium regulation in skeletal muscle. Annu Rev Med 1995;46:431–441.
The pathological genetic defects in the inherited myotonias and periodic paralyses were recently elucidated using molecular genetic studies. These disorders are usually transmitted as a dominant trait from an affected parent to a child. The many clinical symptoms include cold-induced uncontrollable contraction of muscle, potassium-induced contraction and paralysis, myotonia with dramatic muscular hypertrophy, muscle stiffness, and insulin-induced paralysis (in males). Horses afflicted with the disorder can suddenly collapse, despite an impressive physique. These disorders share a common etiology: subtle defects of ion channels in the muscle-fiber membrane. Although the specific ion channel involved varies depending on the disease, most patients have single amino acid changes in the channel proteins, with both normal and mutant channels present in each muscle fiber.

21. Ptacek LJ, Johnson KJ, Griggs RC. Genetics and physiology of the myotonic muscle disorders. N Engl J Med 1993;328:482–489.
A review of the heterogeneous but clinically similar diseases which share the feature of myotonia. Genetic studies have pinpointed the lesions to chromosomal loci encoding specific ion channels and a protein kinase. In the new classification scheme there are sodium channel diseases (hyperkalemic periodic paralysis with or without myotonia, and paramyotonia congenita—chromosome 17q), chloride channel diseases (Thomsen's dominant and Becker's recessive types of myotonia congenita—chromosome 7q), protein kinase-related disease (myotonic dystrophy—chromosome 19q), and still uncharacterized disorders (chondrodystrophic myotonia and Andersen's syndrome).

22. Gutmann L. Axonal channelopathies: an evolving concept in the pathogenesis of peripheral nerve disorders. Neurology 1996;47:18–21.
Abnormalities of peripheral nerve Na+ and K+ channels result in clinical manifestations unrelated to axonal degeneration or demyelination. Na+ channel blockade causes weakness and sensory loss associated with slowed conduction and decreased motor and sensory action potential amplitudes. K+ channel abnormalities result in high frequency repetitive action potentials (e.g., myokymia). Ion channel abnormalities may also play an important role in electrophysiologic changes seen in demyelinating disorders.

23. McManis PG, Lambert EH, Daube JR. The exercise test in periodic paralysis. Muscle Nerve 1986;9:704–710.
Of 21 patients with clinically definite hypokalemic, hyperkalemic, or normokalemic periodic paralysis, 15 (71%) had a greater than normal increase in compound muscle action potential amplitude during 2–5 minutes of intermittent strong voluntary contraction of the muscle. This increase was followed by a progressive decline in amplitude, which was greater than in a control population and which was most rapid during the first 20 minutes after exercise. The amplitude often decreased to a level below the preexercise level. A similar response was seen in six of nine patients with periodic paralysis second-

ary to disorders such as thyrotoxicosis. This test may have value in the identification of patients with periodic paralysis.

24. Allen GC. Malignant hyperthermia and associated disorders. Curr Opin Rheumatol 1993;5:719–724.

Malignant hyperthermia is a pharmacogenetic disorder of skeletal muscle that may cause a life-threatening reaction during administration of general anesthesia. It is inherited in an autosomal dominant pattern and, at least in some families, is caused by a mutation in the ryanodine receptor-calcium-release channel gene on chromosome 19. Malignant hyperthermia displays heterogeneity, making the development of a simple screening test difficult. Malignant hyperthermia may be caused by other biochemical defects affecting intramyoplasmic calcium. Some myopathies, such as central core disease, are frequently associated with malignant hyperthermia susceptibility. In other myopathies, like Duchenne muscular dystrophy, unusual compensatory mechanisms may produce a hypermetabolic state identical to that of malignant hyperthermia.

25. Auger RG. AAEM minimonograph #44: diseases associated with excess motor unit activity. Muscle Nerve 1994;17:1250–1263.

Stiff-man syndrome is due to hyperexcitability of anterior horn cells, possibly related to interference with the synthesis or action of gamma-aminobutyric acid. Unexpected acoustic and exteroceptive stimuli produce exaggerated muscle responses. Needle electrode examination of involved muscles yields nonspecific findings and demonstrates involuntary motor unit activity. The appearance and firing pattern of motor units are normal except that agonist and antagonist muscles may contract concurrently. Continuous muscle fiber activity (Isaacs' syndrome) comprises a heterogeneous group of hereditary and acquired disorders that cause hyperexcitability of peripheral nerves. Some are associated with electrophysiologic evidence of peripheral neuropathy and some are not. Repetitive afterdischarges often follow the M-, H-, and F-waves. Needle electrode examination reveals an abnormal pattern of motor unit firing, consisting of myokymic discharges, doublets and multiplets, neuromyotonic discharges, and fasciculations. These abnormalities may occur alone or in combination.

26. Arimura K, Watanabe O, Kitajima I, et al. Antibodies to potassium channels of PC12 in serum of Isaacs' syndrome: Western blot and immunohistochemical studies. Muscle Nerve 1997;20:299–305.

An investigation into the pathophysiology of nerve hyperexcitability in Isaacs' syndrome, demonstrating immunological involvement of the voltage dependent potassium channels located along the distal motor nerve or at the nerve terminal.

27. Tahmoush AJ, Alonso RJ, Tahmoush GP, et al. Cramp-fasciculation syndrome: a treatable hyperexcitable peripheral nerve disorder. Neurology 1991;41:1021–1024.

9 patients described with muscle aching, cramps, stiffness, exercise intolerance, and peripheral nerve hyperexcitability with a shower of after discharges following the M wave after repetitive stimulation. These patients did not have continuous muscle fiber activity. Repetitive nerve stimulation in both Isaac's and cramp fasciculation syndrome can produce showers of afterdischarges. Both Isaac's and the cramp fasciculation syndrome are hyperexcitable peripheral nerve disorders and the difference in clinical symptoms is due to differences in degree of hyperexcitability: in Isaac's the terminal axon in very excitable and continuously firing; in CF syndrome patient's have mild hyperexcitability with rare firings, which become

more frequent after voluntary activity (exercise) or nerve stimulation.

28. Robinson LR. AAEM case report #22: polymyositis. Muscle Nerve 1991;14:310–315.

Polymyositis usually presents with progressive proximal muscle weakness, increased serum levels of muscle enzymes, inflammatory changes on muscle biopsy, and characteristic electromyographic (EMG) abnormalities. Motor unit action potential (MUAP) changes of configuration, duration, and amplitude are the most frequently observed EMG abnormality. Fibrillation potentials are commonly seen and tend to reflect active disease, diminishing after successful medical management or disease regression. Other muscle diseases can present with similar electromyographic abnormalities, thereby necessitating muscle biopsy for definitive diagnosis.

29. Amato AA, Gronseth GS, Jackson CE, et al. Inclusion body myositis: clinical and pathological boundaries. Ann Neurol 1996;40:581–586.

Inclusion body myositis (IBM), polymyositis (PM), and dermatomyositis are three distinct categories of inflammatory myopathy. Some have noted selective early weakness of the volar forearm muscles, quadriceps, and ankle dorsiflexors in IBM. The most important feature distinguishing IBM is lack of responsiveness to immunosuppressive treatment. Although most patients with IBM have characteristic muscle biopsy findings, some cannot be distinguished histologically early from PM. Predicting responsiveness to immunosuppressive medications, independent of muscle histology, would be valuable to clinicians. This study retrospectively reviewed the pattern of weakness and other clinical features of 46 patients newly diagnosed with either IBM, PM, or dermatomyositis. Asymmetrical muscle weakness with prominent wrist flexor, finger flexor, and knee extensor involvement was specific for IBM and unresponsive PM. Male sex, lower creatine kinase levels, slower rate of progression, and peripheral neuropathy were also more common in IBM and unresponsive PM than in responsive PM and dermatomyositis patients. Repeat muscle biopsy in 2 patients in the unresponsive PM group demonstrated histological features of IBM. Patients with clinical features of IBM but lacking histological confirmation may nonetheless have IBM. This study supports the recently proposed criteria for definite and possible IBM. See also Griggs RC, Askanas V, DiMauro S, et al. Inclusion body myositis and myopathies. Ann Neurol 1995;38:705–713.

30. Dalakas MC. Polymyositis, dermatomyositis and inclusion-body myositis. N Engl J Med 1991;325:1487–1498.

A review of the pathogenesis, clinical manifestations, diagnostic criteria, pathology, electrodiagnostic picture and treatment of PM, DM and IBM.

31. Kelley DE, Gharib H, Kennedy FP, et al. Thyrotoxic periodic paralysis. Report of 10 cases and review of electromyographic findings. Arch Intern Med 1989;149:2597–2600.

A review of the clinical characteristics of 10 patients with thyrotoxic periodic paralysis. In these patients, a relatively uniform group of young men, the periodic paralysis developed nearly concurrently with the onset of hyperthyroidism. The attacks were precipitated most frequently by rest and by exercise and, occasionally, by ingestion of a large carbohydrate load. In each patient, the paralysis resolved on return of euthyroidism. The approximate incidence rate for thyrotoxic periodic paralysis in this largely white North American patient population (all hyperthyroidism cases) ranged from 0.1% to 0.2%, which is one tenth the rate reported for Oriental populations. In 7 patients, electrodiagnostic testing revealed characteristic changes in compound muscle action potential amplitude in response to exercise of the muscle being tested.

32. al-Lozi MT, Pestronk A, Yee WC, et al. Rapidly evolving myopathy with myosin-deficient muscle fibers. Ann Neurol 1994;35:273–279.

Five patients with rapidly evolving, severe weakness had an unusual myopathy with virtually complete loss of myosin in 5 to 40% of muscle fibers. Three of the 5 patients began to develop weakness 1 to 2 weeks after lung transplantation. The fourth became weak after a febrile illness. The fifth presented with diabetic ketoacidosis and weakness. All patients had received corticosteroid therapy. In all cases the weakness was progressive and led to severe disability, with respiratory failure in 4 patients. Initial diagnostic testing did not localize an underlying cause for the weakness. Creatine kinase was normal or minimally elevated. Electromyography generally showed mildly myopathic or nondiagnostic changes. However, muscle biopsy revealed numerous small angular fibers with no myosin ATPase staining at any pH. Immunocytochemical staining and ultrastructural studies confirmed a severe loss of myosin in many fibers. This rapidly evolving myopathy with myosin-deficient muscle fibers appears to be different clinically and pathologically from previously described syndromes involving rapidly progressive weakness. Slow recovery over a period of months is the most common outcome.

33. Chapelon C, Ziza JM, Piette JC, et al. Neurosarcoidosis: signs, course and treatment in 35 confirmed cases. Medicine (Baltimore) 1990;69:261–276.

Thirty-five cases of biopsy-proven sarcoidosis with neurologic manifestations are reported. Neurosarcoidosis was the presenting symptom in 31% of cases and the only clinical manifestation in 17%. Mean follow-up time was 48 months. Central nervous system involvement was observed in 37% and meningitis in 40% of patients. Other manifestations were cranial nerve palsies (37%), peripheral neuropathy (40%), and myopathy (26%). Multiple neurologic manifestations were present in 51% of cases. All but 4 were treated with corticosteroids. Another immunosuppressive agent or cerebral irradiation was added in 6 and 2 patients, respectively. Complete recovery was observed in 46%, improvement in 46%, 4% remained stable, and 4% worsened. There were no deaths. The authors advocate treating neurosarcoidosis with corticosteroids as early as possible. If the patient's condition worsens, additional immunosuppressive agents or cerebral irradiation is warranted.

34. Zochodne DW, Ramsay DA, Saly V, et al. Acute necrotizing myopathy of intensive care: electrophysiological studies. Muscle Nerve 1994;17:285–292.

A series of recent reports have identified cases of a quadriplegic myopathy characterized by myofiber necrosis and loss of myosin filaments associated with the use of nondepolarizing muscle blocking agents and glucocorticoids. This study reports electrophysiological findings in 7 intensive care unit patients who developed evidence of an acute myopathy in association with the use of nondepolarizing muscle blocking agents. Several important features were identified: (I) a neuromuscular transmission deficit was observed in 3 patients up to 7 days following withdrawal of vecuronium; (ii) motor M potentials were of low amplitude, there was mild abnormal spontaneous activity on needle electromyography, and sensory conduction was relatively preserved; (iii) not all patients received glucocorticoids or were asthmatic; (iv) 2 patients given vecuronium had very high creatine kinase levels and developed acute renal failure associated with myoglobinuria; and (v) rises in motor M potentials accompanied clinical recovery. This complication of intensive care may be severe, but is reversible and possibly avoidable. The findings implicate nondepolarizing muscle blocking agents in the development of the myopathy. Electrophysiological studies provide important prognostic guidance.

35. Gooch JL. AAEM case report #29: Prolonged paralysis after neuromuscular blockade. Muscle Nerve 1995;18:937–942.

Nondepolarizing neuromuscular blocking agents (NMBA) are being used with increasing frequency in critically ill patients. Recently, many centers have described patients with prolonged muscle weakness after long-term use of these agents, either alone or in combination with other agents or disorders. Brief weakness lasting several hours to several days is probably the result of prolonged neuromuscular blockade, while more prolonged weakness lasting several weeks to months is, in all likelihood, caused by a myopathy. Patients with this myopathic disorder have flaccid paralysis with intact cognition and sensation. Electrodiagnostic findings include decreased M-wave amplitudes, positive waves and fibrillations, and rapid recruitment of small amplitude short duration, polyphasic motor unit potentials. Muscle biopsy findings include atrophy of type I and type II fibers, myofiber necrosis, and selective loss of thick myofilaments. The myopathy is believed to be related to the prolonged use of NMBA either alone or in combination with other disorders or medications, particularly corticosteroids. The weakness experienced by these patients leads to additional respiratory compromise, difficulty weaning from the ventilator, and prolonged hospitalization.

36. Knochel JP. Mechanisms of rhabdomyolysis. Curr Opin Rheumatol 1993;5:725–731.

Rhabdomyolysis is a common disorder that occurs as a primary disease or as a complication of a broad spectrum of other diseases. Although some cases are caused by hereditary metabolic or structural abnormalities of the skeletal muscle cell, the majority of cases occur in healthy persons as a result of exhaustive exercise, infections, intoxications, deficiency states, or trauma. Although the causes of rhabdomyolysis are diverse, current evidence suggests that there may be a common final pathway that mediates cellular injury. Thus some noxious factor, perhaps a drug that injures the plasma membrane of the cell, a toxin that activates a cytolytic enzyme, a factor that interferes with metabolism and disrupts the integrity of the skeletal muscle cell, a cytokine such as tumor necrosis factor, or simple hypoxia that reduces energy production by the cell, serves to increase cellular permeability to sodium ions. When sodium ions accumulate in the cytoplasm of the cell, an increase of cytosolic or mitochondrial calcium follows. Calcium activates a variety of proteolytic enzymes that injure the cell membrane, allowing efflux of cellular components into the circulation. The ability to identify some of these components, such as myoglobin or creatine kinase, facilitates clinical recognition of rhabdomyolysis. The cytosolic components released into the circulation, under appropriate conditions, may be life threatening, eg, release of potassium causes hyperkalemic cardiotoxicity. This review attempts to describe a variety of factors that are known to be injurious to skeletal muscle cells and, when possible, describes the apparent mechanism whereby these factors result in injury and disruption of the muscle cell.

37. Better OS. The crush syndrome revisited (1940–1990). Nephron 1990;55:97–103.

A review of the local and systemic effects of crush injury.

Within minutes to hours after extrication of survivors trapped under fallen masonry (and immediately following decompression of limbs), a massive volume of extracellular fluid is lost into the injured muscles, leading to circulatory failure. Solutes leaking out of damaged muscles cause a spectrum of metabolic disturbances. Chief among them are hyperkalemia and hypocalcemia which, synergistically, have a lethal cardiotoxic potential, particularly in hypotensive patients. Early volume replacement, preferably already started at the rescue site, may combat shock and correct the hyperkalemia. If urine flow is established, this regimen should be followed by a forced solute-alkaline diuresis for the prevention of myoglobinuric and uricosuric acute renal failure, which is a common and ominous late complication of crush injury.

Modeling of Waveforms With the Electromyograph

By adjusting the filters, stimulus duration and other parameters, the EMG machine itself can be used to illustrate some of the waveforms seen on the needle examination in patients. Try the following exercises.

The spike fibrillation potential is a high frequency positive-negative wave that typically fires at 2–10 Hz. The normal settings for motor CV studies are approximately LFF 2 Hz and HFF 20 Hz. For a Nicolet Viking IV, the LFF range for motor conduction studies is from 0.2–5.0 kHz, and the HFF range from 30–20 kHz. The shock artifact can be used to simulate the shape and sound of various potentials, using the settings in Table 1. A spike fibrillation potential is a high frequency waveform, therefore the LFF is increased to the maximal (5 kHz) to exclude low frequency components, while the HFF is increased to the maximal to include all high frequency components. This shifts the bandwidth to permit maximum detection of high frequencies and maximum rejection of low frequencies. The bandwidth is shifted to the opposite end of the scale to simulate the predominately low frequency PSW.

To simulate a spike fibrillation, hold the prongs of the stimulator close to the input jacks of the preamplifier with the anode of the stimulator closest to the cathode of the preamp (Fig. 1). With some minor positioning adjustments, a waveform should appear on the screen which has an initial positive component followed by a sharp negative spike, firing with metronomic regularity at the frequency selected. To see and hear a simulated positive wave, change the filters as in Table 1 and use the same anode to cathode position. To see a train of PSWs, use these filter set-

tings with the machine in repetitive stimulation mode. Trigger the sweep and a series of potentials closely simulating the sight and sound of a train of PSWs will appear (Fig. 2). Make the train die out by smoothly and quickly turning down the stimulus intensity or moving the stimulator away from the preamp; depending on the length of the train, this can simulate anything from prolonged insertional activity, to unsustained PSWs to a long train slowly dying away which would qualify as spontaneous activity. For an even more impressive simulation, soak a 4 × 4 sponge with normal saline and wad it into a ball, insert a CNE into one side and stimulate on the opposite side. This can also be done by inserting stimulating and recording needle electrodes into a piece of citrus fruit. By adjusting the CNE position, the filters and other parameters, a convincing replication of different waveforms can be created and recorded with an ordinary needle electrode.

As discussed in detail in Chapter 8, there has been a long-standing controversy over the relationship, similarities and differences, between spike fibrillation and positive sharp wave fibrillation potentials. One possibility for the difference between these two waveforms that does not appear to have been previously considered in the literature is that tissue filtering and the spatial relationships between the various fibrillating fibers and the recording electrode can alter the shape of the fibrillation potential. Tissue has filtering effects, particularly on the high frequency components of a waveform. By simply changing the filter settings to shift the bandpass to filter out either high or low frequencies and making minor adjustments in the orien-

TABLE 1
Simulation of EMG Needle Examination Waveforms with the Electromyograph Apparatus

Simulated Waveform	Stimulus	Recording	LFF	HFF	Stimulus Duration	Frequency	Comment
Spike fibrillation	Anode of stimulus prongs	Cathode of preamp, or CNE	5 kHz	20 kHz	0.1 msec	2 Hz	Amplitude varies with stimulus intensity, use NCV mode, recurrent stimulation. Position stimulator to get an initial positive deflection
Sustained positive sharp wave	Anode of stimulus prongs	Cathode of preamp, or CNE	150 Hz	1 kHz	0.1–1.0 ms	2 Hz	Amplitude varies with stimulus intensity, use NCV mode, recurrent stimulation. Position stimulator to get an initial positive deflection
Increased insertional activity	Anode of stimulator prongs	Cathode of preamp, or CNE	150 Hz	1 kHz	0.1–1.0 ms	2–5 Hz	Rep stim mode, deliver a train at 3–5 Hz
Unsustained PSWs	Anode of stimulator prongs	Cathode of preamp, or CNE	150 Hz	1 kHz	0.1–1.0 ms	2–5 Hz	Rep stim mode, deliver a train of 5–10 stimuli while smoothly decreasing the stimulus intensity
End plate spikes	Cathode of stimulator prongs	Cathode of preamp, or CNE	5 kHz	20 kHz	0.1 msec	50 Hz	Rep stim mode, deliver maximum length train the system will permit, high intensity to achieve spike amplitude of 100–300 μV. Potentials will lack the sputtering irregularity of real end plate spikes
End plate noise	Cathode of stimulator prongs	Cathode of preamp, or CNE	5 kHz	20 kHz	0.05 msec	50 Hz	Same as for end plate spikes but with stimulus intensity adjusted to give an amplitude of 10–20 μV. A suboptimal simulation because apparatus will not deliver a frequency high enough to obscure the baseline

tations of the stimulator prongs, the shape of the shock artifact can be changed back and forth between that of a spike fibrillation and that of a positive sharp wave. The ability in these modeling schemes to so readily alter the waveform by changing the filter settings raises the possibility that the passive electrical properties of the recording medium may have an important effect on the morphology of the waveforms (Fig. 3).

Even more complex potentials, such as CRDs, and myotonia can be simulated with varying effectiveness

(Fig. 4). Varying the stimulus intensity during a long repetitive train simulates the waxing and waning of a myotonic discharge.

To get a feel for the small, short duration MUAPs typical of myopathy, insert a CNE into the muscle of a control, such as your own anterior tibialis, or a random patient with a normal study. During moderate contraction, increase the LFF to 500 Hz (the setting used for single fiber EMG). This LFF setting eliminates low frequency components, shortening the duration and lowering the amplitude of the MUAPs, mak-

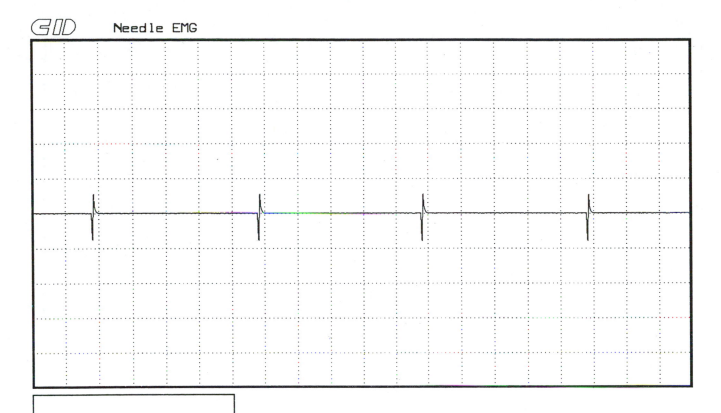

Needle EMG

generic
Mar 12 98 17:15:10
Patient:
  test
  1234

Sweep Speed	=	10 ms/d
Gain	=	2.0 mU/d
High Filter	=	15 kHz
Low Filter	=	500 Hz
Notch Filter	=	Off

FIGURE 1. Simulation of a spike fibrillation and a positive sharp wave using the EMG apparatus.

The stimuli were delivered using a Nicolet Viking IV, set on repetitive stimulation mode to deliver a long train at 20 Hz. The stimulator prongs were held near the preamplifier jacks of a Clark Davis electromyograph, with the anode of the stimulator opposite the cathode of the preamp, and the cathode of the stimulator opposite the anode of the preamp, Filter settings as shown. Stimulus duration 0.1 ms. See text and Table 1 for details. With minor adjustments of the position of the stimulator prongs the stimulus artifact can be made to resemble a spike fibrillation, with an initially positive component followed by a sharp negative spike.

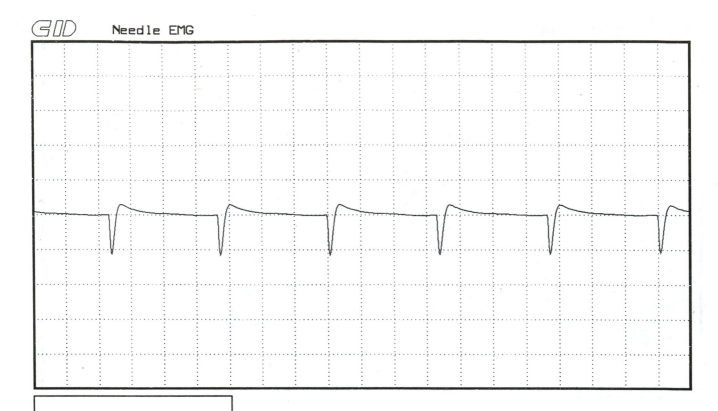

Needle EMG

```
generic
Mar 12 98 17:09:36
Patient:
 test
 1234
```

```
Sweep Speed  =  10 ms/d
Gain         =  1.0 mV/d
High Filter  = 200 Hz
Low Filter   =  20 Hz
Notch Filter = Off
```

FIGURE 2. The exact same set up was used as for Figure 1, except the filter settings were changed as shown and the stimulus rate was increased to 30 Hz. The stimulus artifact now strikingly resembles a train of positive sharp waves.

FIGURE 3. Hypothesis for the difference between spike and positive sharp fibrillation potentials. Consider a recording needle electrode inserted into a group of muscle fibers which are all fibrillating. The fibers labeled "A" lie immediately adjacent to the electrode and deliver a spike fibrillation directly to the recording surface. These same "A" fibers, however, lie between the "B" fibers and the electrode and could filter out the high frequencies from the fibrillations arising from the "B" fibers, converting them from spike fibrillation potentials into positive sharp waves. The admixture of spike and positive sharp fibrillation potentials seen in well established denervation might result from a combination of the effects of tissue filtering and the spatial relationships between the muscle fibers and the recording surface. This theory would not explain all the curiosities about fibrillations and positive sharp waves, such as why the latter typically appear sooner.

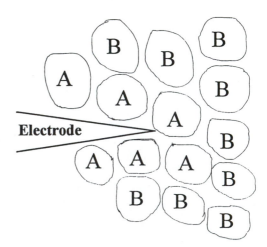

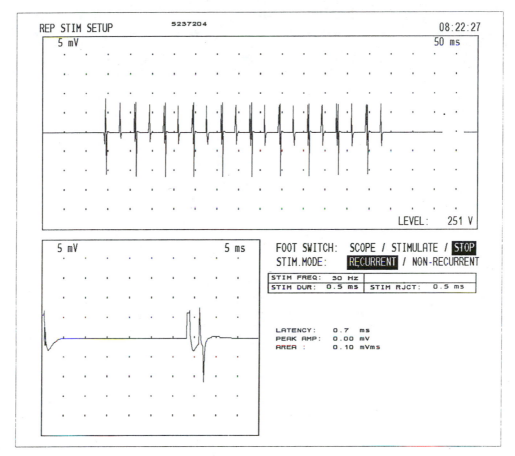

FIGURE 4. Simulation of a complex repetitive discharge (CRD) using two EMG machines. Filters are set as for a spike fibrillation. Recording was done with a CNE inserted into an orange. Stimulation was delivered via two sets of needle electrodes, one inserted into the opposite pole and the other at right angles. Using a long train of repetitive stimulation, with one machine delivering stimuli at a frequency of 30 Hz with the other machine delivering stimuli at 15 Hz. The two stimulus trains are triggered as simultaneously as possible. This simulates two different waveforms firing in time-locked synchrony, with abrupt onset and termination. The sound produced bears a striking relationship to a CRD. This can also easily be done just by holding the stimulator handles from the two machines close to the input jacks. *Obviously, one must take great care not to touch the two stimulator handles together.*

ing them appear "myopathic." Full contraction at this LFF setting recruits a host of small, short potentials which fire at normal rates, and looks and sounds like the increased recruitment often seen in primary muscle disorders. "Neuropathic" recruitment is difficult to simulate because normal MUAPs cannot fire at the high rates necessary. Delivery of a percutaneous, subthreshold high frequency repetitive train, recording with an intramuscular electrode, works but is uncomfortable for the subject.

Index

Page numbers in italics (set in italics) denote figures; those followed by a "t" denote tables.

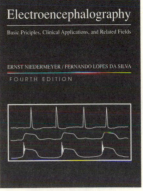
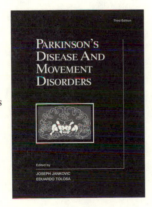
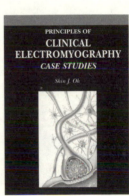